QUALITY CONTROL OF HERBAL DRUGS: STANDARDISATION AND REGULATIONS

QUALITY CONTROL OF HERBAL DRUGS: STANDARDISATION AND REGULATIONS

SI Deore

Associate Professor
Govt. College of Pharmacy,
Kathora naka, Amravati- 444604

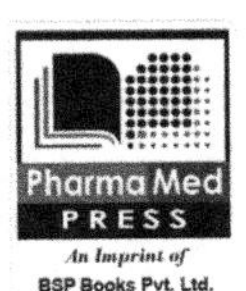

PharmaMed Press

An imprint of BSP Books Pvt. Ltd.
4-4-309/316, Giriraj Lane,
Sultan Bazar, Hyderabad - 500 095.

Quality Control of Herbal Drugs: Standardisation and Regulations
by SI Deore

Published by

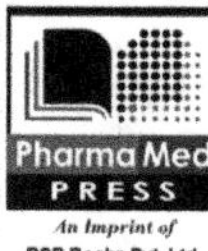

PharmaMed Press
An imprint of BSP Books Pvt. Ltd.
4-4-309/316, Giriraj Lane, Sultan Bazar, Hyderabad - 500 095.
Phone: 040-23445688; Fax: 91+40-23445611
E-mail: info@pharmamedpress.net
www.bspbooks.net/www.pharmamedpress.net

ISBN: 978-93-90211-94-4 (Hardback)

Preface

Market of herbs and derived products has increased globally. Herbal products are not just used for primary health care in developing countries, but now component of national health care system in many parts of world.

A wide variety of herbal medicines in different categories (indigenous herbal medicines, traditional system herbal medicines, modified herbal medicines, herbal supplements, and or pure phytochemicals) are readily available in the market all over the world. Herbal cosmetics and toiletry preparations are second largest share in Herbal Products. Health awareness among world population is increasing market of herbal nutraceutical products.

With the rising utilisation of herbs and derived products, regulations of these products are public health concern. Many countries have published regulatory guidelines covering quality, safety and efficacy while many other countries are in process to publish. However, WHO or ICH guidelines are applicable to herbal products as global documents.

In this book **35** chapters are divided into seven sections: **Section 1.** Herbal Products and Regulations **Section 2.** Herbs and Derived Products, **Section 3**. Traditional Medicines Regulations, **Section 4.** Quality Control Regulations for Herbal Products, **Section 5.** Pre-clinical and Toxicity Regulations for Herbal Products, **Section 6.** Pharmacovigilance and Clinical Trial Regulations for Herbal Products and **Section 7.** Herbal Industry, IPR and Regulatory Affairs. QR codes provided after each chapter can be scanned for relevant supportive knowledge.

This book of "Quality Control of Herbal Drugs: Standardisation and Regulations" systematically compiled all relevant guidelines and extensive data related to quality, safety and efficacy of herbs and derived products starting from scientific cultivation to processing, formulation development, manufacturing, sell and IPR with appropriate regional, national and or international regulations.

This book has complied regulatory frameworks for herbal raw material, traditional medicines, modern herbal medicines, herbal cosmetics and herbal nutraceutical supplements. This book will be comprehensive reference for academic as well industry professionals, students and researchers.

I would first and foremost like to acknowledge the authors and publishers of various guidelines, books, research articles, journals, websites and other sources that have been referred to make this book an unique source of reference.

I am thankful to my guide, mentor and fatherly figure Dr. S. S. Khadabadi, Principal, Govt. College of Pharmacy, Amravati for his teachings and guidance.

I am thankful to my Ph.D and M.Pharm Students- Anjali Kide, Bhavana Shende, Kirti Deshmukh, Vikas Ghait and Jayesh Vighne for valuable inputs in construction of this book content. I would also like to thank all my B.Pharm & M.Pharm students since year 2006, Pharm.D Students since 2011 and who have monumental for publishing this text and their inputs has made this book complete.

I am grateful to Publisher **Mr. Anil Shah** (Director) for giving me this opportunity and moral support throughout the journey of writing this book. I am thankful to **Mr. Naresh Davergave** (Production Manager) for pointing out errors and offering suggestions for improvement.

Finally, I express deep gratitude and love to my wise family- husband Bhushan Baviskar, Sons- Prathaam and Aadeet, for offering tower of support and every back-up to make this book reality.

Few errors and deficiencies crept in despite best efforts are mine responsibility. I will be grateful to the readers if they point them out and offer their constructive comments. Lastly I am wishing readers "An Informative Reading Experience" through this book.

Sharada L. Deore

Contents

Annexures

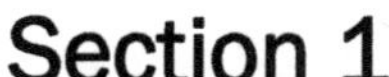

Section 1

Herbal Products and Regulations

CHAPTER 1

Overview on Herbal Product Regulations: Challenges and Solution

Introduction

There is rapid growing demand of medicinal and aromatic plants in pharmaceutical, cosmetic, agriculture and nutraceutical sector. The sector is currently engaged in a modernisation and standardisation process aiming at an increase of its market share, while trying to meet the demand to deliver better quality herbal products. To ensure both safety and efficacy of herbal medicines, implementation of and adherence to guidelines and regulations specific to step must be followed.

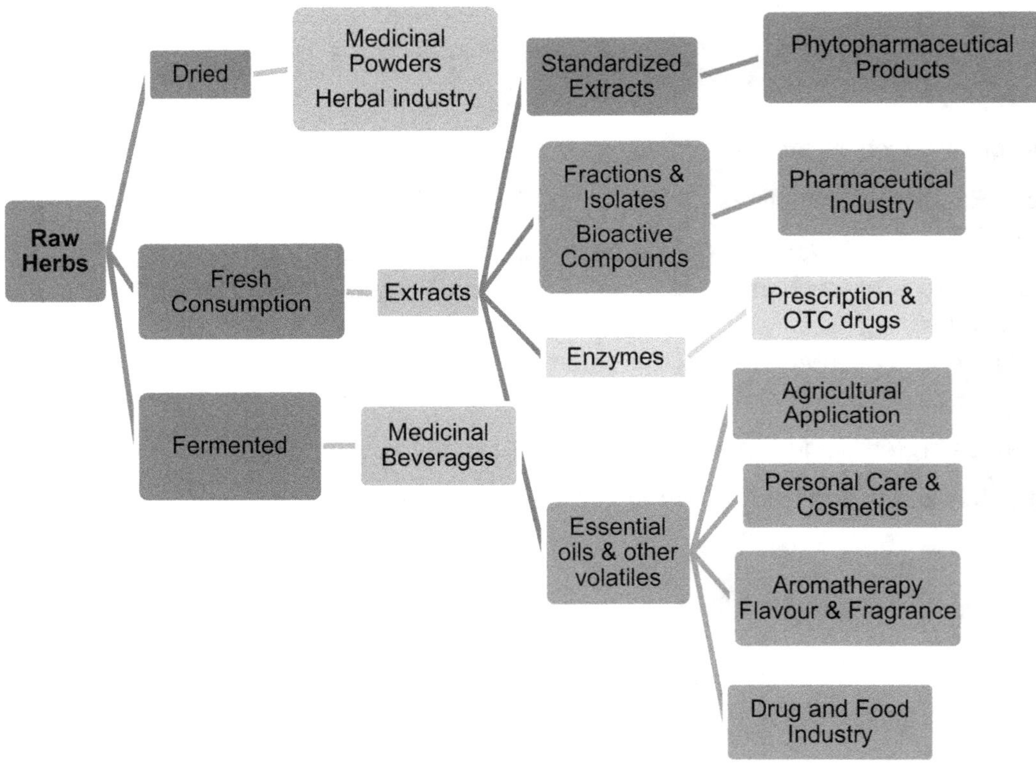

Figure 1.1 Potential Market Herbs derived Products.

Herbal products related terminologies in different parts of World		
Official terminology of Country	**Terminology**	**Definition**
United States	Dietary supplements	In the USA, the term dietary supplements are legally defined for the product "The Federal Food, Drug, and Cosmetic Act defines a dietary ingredient as a vitamin; mineral; herb or other botanical; amino acid; dietary substance for use by man to supplement the diet by increasing the total dietary intake; or a concentrate, metabolite, constituent, extract, or combination of the preceding substances

Contd...

Herbal products related terminologies in different parts of World		
Official terminology of Country	**Terminology**	**Definition**
		Unlike drugs, supplements are not intended to treat, diagnose, prevent, or cure diseases. That means supplements should not make claims, such as "reduces pain" or "treats heart disease." Claims like these can only legitimately be made for drugs, not dietary supplements. Dietary supplements include such ingredients as vitamins, minerals, herbs, amino acids, and enzymes. Dietary supplements are marketed in forms such as tablets, capsules, softgels, gelcaps, powders, and liquids".
	Functional food	There is no defined and legal terminology, however, it is used as an alternative term for the 'nutraceutical,' with the concept that foods can have some health benefits. Functional food can be an extract, powder, or other processed forms originated from normal food such as gapes and peanuts that contain resveratrol with antioxidant properties. Health Canada has the definition of 'nutraceutical,' and is considered as the product originated from the food. In the EU legislation, "functional foods" or "nutraceuticals" are not recognized categories.
Japan and China	Health food	Japan and China mainly use the term health food, but with different regulatory processes. The general concept of health food is that the food contains nutrient as well as health benefits. Thus, some permitted health-related claims can be made. In Japan, health and nutrition claims handled separately, processing via different regulatory route while, in China, the claims are restricted to the pre-defined twenty-seven health claims.
Canada	Natural Health Products	Natural Health Products (NHP) is the category created for a variety of products that are naturally sourced products intended for improving human health. This is well defined in Canada and contains a variety of products like vitamins, minerals, herbal and homeopathic medicine and traditional medicines (e.g., Traditional Chinese Medicine).
	Food supplement	These foods are packed with nutrients or other substances with a nutritional or physiological effect, and mainly contained in the concentrated form and available in specific dosage form to supplement the normal diet. Food supplements can bear approved nutritional and health claims, but medical claims are not permitted. Food supplements are defined in EU as food and monitored through centralized legislation.
EU, Canada, Australia	Novel food	Novel food is mainly defined in EU and Canada and Australia, to deal with the category of the food that was not consumed as food historically in that region. Certain alterations to the regular food could be considered as novel food such as using new technologies or production processes (e.g., bioengineering, nanotechnology, or UV treated food, etc.), or upgraded with the addition of nutrients, or used the new sources for known products.
Australia	Complementary medicine	It is mainly used in Australia as a regulatory term. It denotes to all the health care practices that are not conventional part of a country's health care practices. Health care system from those countries is not integrated with these practices.

Contd...

Herbal products related terminologies in different parts of World		
Official terminology of Country	**Terminology**	**Definition**
	Traditional medicine	These are practices that have a long history of usage in particular jurisdiction. The practice could be a combination of beliefs, knowledge, and skills in addition to medicine. It could be used for preventative, diagnosis, or treatment of physical and mental health.
China	Traditional Chinese medicine (TCM)	It is part of ancient Chinese healthcare system. This system includes medicines, practices, acupuncture, massage and have preventative health as well as restoring the health. The medicines can be single herb, complex combination from plant or animal origin. Some of the cases prescribed by the health care practitioner. TCM are still integral part of Chinese healthcare system with hospitals and health care practitioners are there to monitor as well as prescribe the medicine or combination of therapy to the patients.
Japan	Kampo medicine	It is popular in Japan and derived from the ancient version of Traditional Chinese Medicine. Although Kampo medicine and TCM share a similar philosophy, the ingredients are different. Specifically, Kampo medicine has evolved and modified to incorporate materials from Japanese origin.
India	ASU drugs - Ayurveda, Siddha, Unani, Drugs	ASU drugs include all medicines intended for internal or external use for or in the diagnosis, treatment, mitigation, or prevention of disease or disorder in human beings or animals exclusively in accordance with the formulae described in the authoritative books.
UAE	Product derived from plant origin [traditional herbal medicine]	"Product derived from plant origin is a finished labelled medicinal product that contains as active ingredients aerial or underground parts of plants, or other plant materials or combinations thereof, where in the crude state or as plant preparations intended for prophylactic or therapeutic or other human health benefits" "Plant preparations are herbal ingredients present in a form other than the crude medicinal plant material including powdered plant material, balsams, dried and fluid extracts, tinctures, essential oils etc., prepared from plant material, and plant preparations obtained by fractionation, purification or concentration, without chemically defined isolated constituents regardless of whether or not its therapeutically active constituents have been identified"

Various Regulatory Guidelines for Herbs and Derived Products

Regulatory bodies are agencies which look after implementation of the legislation related to safety, efficacy and quality of drugs. They work under the Ministry of Health and Family Welfares. Each country has its own regulatory body. WHO (World Health Organization) and ICH (International Conference on Harmonization) are some important organizations who proposed guidelines for the Quality Standards of Herbal products. Following are various guidelines for herbs and derived products:

Various Regulatory Guidelines for herbs and derived products are as follows:	
WHO Traditional and Modern Herbal Products	• WHO - General Guidelines for Methodologies on Research and Evaluation of Traditional Medicine 2000 • WHO Guidelines for Assessment, Evaluation of Toxicity, Safety and Efficacy of Herbal Medicines 2000 • WHO Good Agricultural and Collection Practices [GAP, GCP, GACP] 2003 • WHO guidelines on safety monitoring of herbal medicines in pharmacovigilance systems 2004 • WHO Guidelines for assessing quality of herbal medicines with reference to contaminants and residues 2007 • WHO Guidelines for Quality control of herbal materials 2011 [Updated edition of Quality control methods for medicinal plant materials, 1998] • WHO Guidelines for Selecting Marker Substances of Herbal Origin for Quality Control of Herbal Medicines 2017 • WHO guidelines on Good Herbal Processing Practice for Herbal Medicine 2018
AYUSH, India (Traditional Medicines)	• NMPB Guidelines and Standards for Good Field Collection Practices for Indian Medicinal Plants 2009 • AYUSH General Guidelines for Safety/Toxicity Evaluation of Ayurvedic Formulations 2018 • AYUSH Guidelines of Good Clinical Practices 2018 • General Guidelines for Drug Development of Ayurvedic Formulations, 2018
CDSCO, India (AYUSH and Modern herbal Products)	• Drug and Cosmetics Act, 1940. • Drug and Magic Remedies Act, 1954. • Narcotic Drugs and Psychotropic Substances Act, 1985. • CDSCO Guidelines of Good Clinical Practices 2013
Other acts, India	• Industries (Development Regulation) Act 1951. • Trade and Merchandise Marks Act 1958. • Indian Patents and Design Act 1970. • Factories Act 1948. • Indian Forest Act 1927 • Wild Life Protection act, 1972 • Geographical Indications of Goods (Registration and Protection) Act, 1999 • Biodiversity Act, 2002
ASEAN	• ASEAN Guidelines on Labeling Requirements for Traditional Medicines, 2015 • ASEAN Guidelines on Stability Study and Shelf-Life of Traditional Medicines, 2013

Contd...

Various Regulatory Guidelines for herbs and derived products are as follows:	
Nutraceuticals	• Food Safety and Standards act, 2006 • Dietary Supplement Health and Education Act of 1994 [DSHEA]
Cosmetics	• Drug and Cosmetics Act, 1940. • BIS/ISI Regulations

Global Overview of Regulations of Herbs and Derived Products

In 2003, a global survey of international health authorities indicated that most responding member 92 countries had regulations covering herbal medicines, whereas 85 countries reported having a registration system for herbal medicines.

Comparison of regulatory requirements when natural products are classified as "SUPPLEMENT"			
Country	**Regulatory Agency**	**Classified as Supplements**	**Regulatory Requirements**
USA	Dietary Supplement Health and Education Act (DSHEA) 1994	**Dietary Supplement - Center for Food Safety and Applied Nutrition (CFASN)/FDA** • Herbs/Botanicals • Vitamin • Minerals • Amino Acids • Dietary substance for use by man to supplement the diet by increasing the total intake • Concentrate, metabolite, constituent, extract or combination of the preceding substances.	➢ **Allowed route of admin- Oral only** ➢ **Pre-market approval - no** ➢ **Therapeutic claims- no** ➢ **Recommended dosing - yes** ➢ **Addition of new compound-Via NDI Notification***
Australia	Food Standards Australia New Zealand (FSANZ)	**Novel Food** • Foods and extracts from plants, animals, etc., • Foods and their extracts resulting from production processes and practices, and new technologies.	➢ **Allowed route of admin- NA** ➢ **Pre-market approval-NA** ➢ **Therapeutic claims- NA** ➢ **Recommended dosing- NA** ➢ **Addition of new compound-NA**
New Zealand	New Zealand Ministry for Primary Industries (MPI)	**Supplemented food** • Foods modified or with added substances so that they perform a physiological role	**Allowed route of admin- Oral only** ➢ **Pre-market approval-No** ➢ **Therapeutic claims-No** ➢ **Recommended dosing- If Supplemented food- no; If Dietary supplements- yes** ➢ **Addition of new compound- Active ingredient must be listed on website**
New Zealand	New Zealand Medicines and Medical Devices Safety Authority (Medsafe)	**Dietary supplements**	

Contd...

Comparison of regulatory requirements when natural products are classified as "SUPPLEMENT"			
New Zealand	Food Standards Australia New Zealand (FSANZ)	**Novel Food** • Foods and extracts from plants, animals, etc., • Foods and their extracts resulting from production processes and practices, and new technologies.	
China	China Food and Drug Administration (CFDA)	Health foods	➢ Allowed route of admin- Oral only ➢ Pre-market approval- yes ➢ Therapeutic claims- Only from one of 27 predefined ➢ Recommended dosing -yes ➢ Addition of new compound-Apply for registration and show toxicity data
Japan	Ministry of Health, Labor and Welfare (MHLW) for Medicines Consumer Affairs Agency (CAA) for Supplements	Health foods	➢ Allowed route of admin- Oral only ➢ Pre-market approval- no ➢ Therapeutic claims- FOHU and FFC can have health claim ➢ Recommended dosing- yes ➢ Addition of new compound- Needs to go through the registration process
EU Member States	**National competent authorities European Food Safety Authority (EFSA) if centralized procedures apply**	**Substances with a nutritional or physiological effect (vitamins, minerals, botanicals, etc.)**	**➢ Allowed route of admin- Oral only ➢ Pre-market approval- Only if considered as "novel foods" safety assessment by EFSA ➢ Therapeutic claims- No ➢ Recommended dosing- yes ➢ Addition of new compound- Apply for registration**
India	**FSSAI**	**Eight categories of Functional foods, namely, Health Supplements, Nutraceuticals, Food for Special Dietary Use, Food for Special Medical Purpose, Specialty food containing plant or botanicals, Foods containing Probiotics, Foods containing Prebiotics and Novel Foods.**	**➢ Allowed route of admin- Oral only ➢ Pre-market approval- Only if considered as "novel foods" safety assessment by EFSA ➢ Therapeutic claims- No ➢ Recommended dosing- yes Addition of new compound- Apply for registration**

Comparison of regulatory requirements when natural products are classified as "MEDICINE"			
Country	**Regulatory Agency**	**Classified as Medicines**	**Regulatory Requirements**
United Kingdom	Food and Drug Administration (FDA)	Botanical Drug Products	➢ Pre-market approval- yes ➢ Clinical trial data- yes ➢ Therapies- Medicine only ➢ Reported adverse reactions/poisonings- yes ➢ Historical usage- yes
	Medicines and Healthcare products Regulatory Agency (MHRA) Committee on Herbal Medicinal Products (HMPC) Traditional Herbal Registration Scheme (THRS).	Complementary and alternative medicine	➢ Well-established use (marketing authorisation) and traditional use (simplified registration)
USA	Food and Drug Administration (FDA)	**Botanical drugs - Center for Drug Evaluation and Research (CDER)/FDA**	➢ Pre-market approval- yes ➢ Clinical trial data- yes ➢ Therapies- Medicine only ➢ Reported adverse reactions/poisonings- yes ➢ Historical usage- yes
Australia	Therapeutic Goods Administration (TGA)	**Complementary Medicines - Complementary and OTC Medicines Branch/TGA** • Herbs • Vitamin • Minerals • Nutritional supplements • Homeopathy • Microorganism (whole extracted) etc.	➢ Pre-market approval- Yes ➢ Clinical trial data- Yes ➢ Therapies- Medicines Homeopathy Aromatherapy ➢ Reported adverse reactions/poisonings- Yes ➢ Historical usage- Yes
New Zealand	Food Standards Australia New Zealand (FSANZ)	**Herbal Remedies**	➢ Pre-market approval- Yes ➢ Clinical trial data- Yes ➢ Therapies- Medicine Only ➢ Reported adverse reactions/poisonings- Yes ➢ Historical usage- Yes
Canada	Health Canada (HC)	**Natural Health Products** • Traditional medicine • Herbal Medicine • Homeopathy	➢ Pre-market approval- Yes ➢ Clinical trial data- Yes ➢ Therapies- ➢ Reported adverse reactions/poisonings- Yes ➢ Historical usage- Yes

Contd...

Comparison of regulatory requirements when natural products are classified as "MEDICINE"			
Country	**Regulatory Agency**	**Classified as Medicines**	➢ **Regulatory Requirements**
China	China Food and Drug Administration (CFDA)	Traditional Chinese Medicine	➢ Pre-market approval- Yes ➢ Clinical trial data- Yes ➢ Therapies- Medicine and Procedure ➢ Reported adverse reactions/poisonings- Yes ➢ Historical usage- Yes
Japan	Ministry of Health, Labor and Welfare (MHLW) for Medicines Consumer Affairs Agency (CAA) for Supplements	**Kampo Medicine**	➢ Pre-market approval- Yes ➢ Clinical trial data- Yes ➢ Therapies- Medicine and Procedure ➢ Reported adverse reactions/poisonings- Yes ➢ Historical usage-
EU	European Medicines Agency (EMA)	**Herbal Medicinal Products** National competent authorities of EU Member States	➢ Pre-market approval- Yes ➢ Clinical trial data- Yes/No ➢ Therapies- Medicine Only ➢ Reported adverse reactions/poisonings- Yes ➢ Historical usage- Yes
India	Drugs and Cosmetics Act, 1940 Drugs and Cosmetics Rules, 1945	**ASU drugs** -Ayurveda, Siddha, Unani, Drugs	➢ Pre-market approval- Yes ➢ Clinical trial data- Yes/No ➢ Therapies- Medicine Only ➢ Reported adverse reactions/poisonings- Yes ➢ Historical usage- Yes

Challenges in Herbs and Derived Product Regulations

Global promotion and acceptance of traditional as well as herbal medicines are facing following various challenges mainly in developed nations despite of promising evidence-based history.

Raw Material Standardization	Selection, identification, reproducibility, inter/intra species variation due to environmental factors, plant part used, time of harvesting, post harvesting factors, contaminants, pesticides, fumigants and toxic metals are the factors responsible for quality raw material. Poor cultivation and collection practices, lack of pre and post-harvest processing techniques, adulteration, misidentification of plant, faulty collection and preparation are major hurdles to get quality raw materials. Major percentage of medicinal plant raw materials from natural sources is creating environmental and social issues and affecting biodiversity. Poor implementation of

Contd...

	Good collection practices as well as *in situ* and *ex situ* conservation strategies is another problem for sustainable, socio-culturally equitable and safe supply of herbal drugs. Biodiversity, scarcity and conservation of raw material issues are causing the hinder in the availability of quality raw material.
Finished products standardization	***"Only quality raw material/s can give quality finished product/s."*** Poor implementation and regulation of the quality control guidelines in small and medium scale industries especially evaluation of pesticide residue, trace metal content, microbial and aflatoxins contamination leading to poor efficacy of herbal products.
Inadequate research and modernization	Decisive gap in traditional *and modern herbal drug research with reference to* pharmacokinetics studies, pharmacovigilance (toxicity, assessment of adverse reactions and drug-food interactions), active constituents-based monographs, clinical trials to endorse safety and efficacy
Skilled personnel and Infrastructure Development	Unethical practice of herbal medicine by non-qualified health workers responsible for exposure of unreliable and misleading information. Unregulated irrational practice of herbal drugs due to lack of trained personnel is major obstacle all around the world. Lack of knowledge of Intellectual Property Rights (IPR) of traditional medicines and modern herbal drugs with reference to biodiversity and biopiracy are creating confusions and demotivation in herbal drug research. Infrastructure facilities for processing, sophisticated modern analysis, manufacturing and research are not sufficient.
Fragmentation of the industry	Traditional medicines, modern herbal products, nutraceuticals and herbal cosmetics have different quality, safety, efficacy, labeling and marketing standard requirements at local, national and international levels lead to poor control and compliance for global commercialization of herbal raw materials.
Regulations	Lack of uniform regulations, stringent control, proper monitoring along with absence of focused marketing and branding creating chaos in herbal industry. There is especially a great confusion between regulations of traditional medicines, modern herbal products, nutraceuticals and herbal cosmetics.

Regions, category of registration of herbal products and their regulatory hurdle		
Region	**Category of registration**	**Major regulatory hurdle**
ASEAN	1. Traditional herbal medicines 2. Indigenous herbal medicine. 3. Modified herbal medicine 4. Imported products with a herbal medicine base	1. Country-wise different National regulation 2. Product category is based on sample dossier. 3. Certain markers closely associated with a plant restricted by Health Sciences Authority, Singapore 4. Many categories of registration
Canada	1. Natural Health Product	1. Herbal products are not allowed as herbal medicine. 2. Single category as Natural Health Product 3. No scope to file as traditional herbal medicine.

Contd...

USA	1. Dietary supplement 2. Botanical drug	1. No therapeutic claims is allowed for dietary supplements 2. Botanical drug are under New drug application (NDA)
Europe	1. Traditional use registration 2. Well-established use marketing authorization 3. Stand-alone or mixed application 4. A simplified registration	1. 30 years Rule (15 +15 years) to qualify for well-established use – Traditional Herbal Medicinal Product (THMP) 2. EU GMP approved manufacturing / Research and development laboratories. 3. Stringent heavy metal / microbial contamination control. 4. Well established identified principle active marker control.
UK	1. Traditional herb registration (THR)	1. Evidence of quality as per the GMP standards 2. Evidence of safety and efficacy based on long traditional use of 30 years overall and 15 years in EU, 3. The label should carry that the THR certification mark and a statement that the product is "exclusively based on long term use". 4. For major health claims, or the products that calls for a medical prescription, 5. Market Authorization is required.
India	1. Traditional herbal medicines 2. Indigenous herbal medicine. 3. Modified herbal medicine	1. Evidence of safety and efficacy based on traditional texts 2. Many categories of registration 3. Must follow Drug Controller General of India (DCGI's) regulations

Solutions in Herbs and Derived Product Regulations

- Uniform herbal drug registration process, dossier submission, pharmacopoeias, related policies and regulations for ensuring uniformity in quality, safety, and efficacy of the one herbal product globally
- Biodiversity and traditional knowledge should be major control factors for herbal product marketing.
- Geographical location-based group farming, strengthening of indigenous techniques of cultivation, buy-back process, promotion of value-added products, industry tie-ups for medicinal plant cultivation should be encouraged to get quality raw material.
- Quality propagation material in consideration to therapeutic efficacy and safety should be get available from certified regional facilitation centers.
- Although medicinal and aromatic plants have been used for thousands of years, basic research programmes and administrative actions need to be focused on the quality raw material supply. To control raw material contamination and maintain uniformity in raw materials of different locations, it is necessary to implement standard operating

procedures (SOPs) for collection, cultivation and processing of medicinal plants and derived value-added products.

- Knowledge of cultivation, collection, pre- and post-harvesting techniques, IPR and marketing strategy and latest developments and policies related trainings of herbal raw material can be shared by participatory learning among cultivars, growers, traditional healers, researchers and manufactures.
- Proper implementation of uniform regulations, development of more elaborate guidelines on quality control and quality assurance aspects, and development of marker-based standards are needed to produce safe and effective herbal medicines.

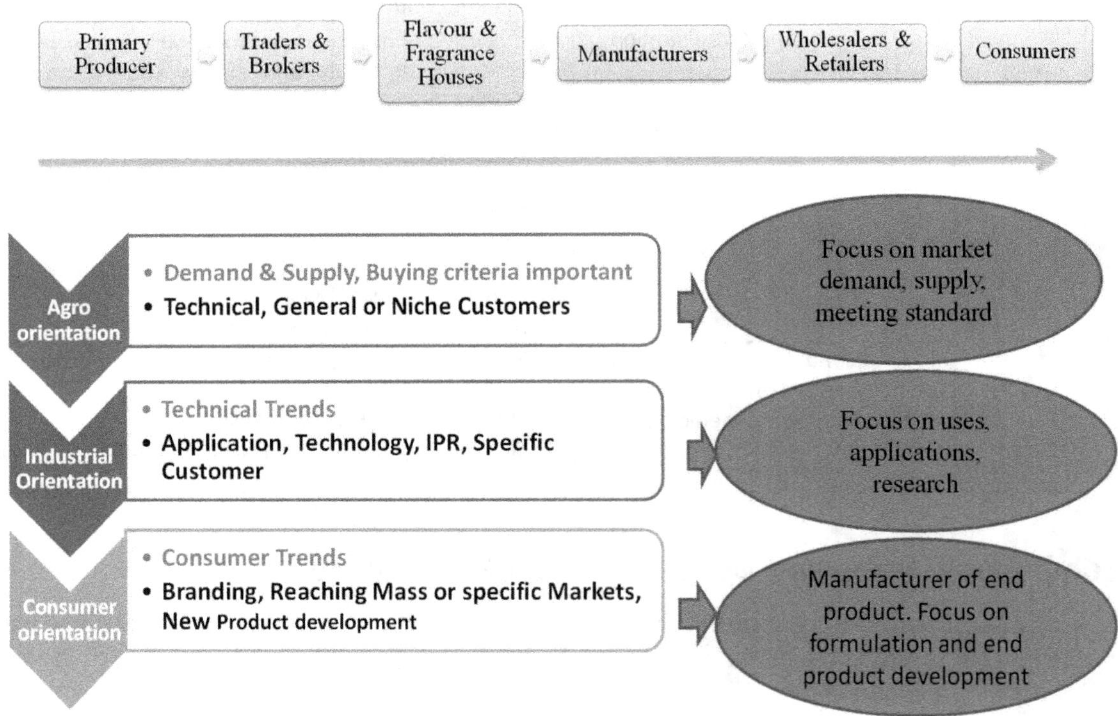

Figure 1.2 Solutions in Herbal Product Regulations.

Further Reading

1. European Medicines Agency 2006a. Guideline on Quality of Herbal Medicinal Products/Traditional Herbal Medicinal Products (CPMP/QWP/2819/00 Rev)
2. European Medicines Agency 2006b. Guideline on Specifications: Test Procedures and Acceptance Criteria for Herbal Substances, Herbal Preparations and Herbal Medicinal Products/Traditional Herbal Medicinal Products (CPMP/QWP/2820/00 Rev)

3. European Medicines Agency 2008. Reflection Paper on Markers used for Quantitative and Qualitative Analysis of Herbal Medicinal Products and Traditional Herbal Medicinal Products (EMEA/HMPC/253629/2007).
4. JuntraKarbwang, Francis P. Crawley, Kesara Na-Bangchang, Cecilia Maramba-Lazarte, "Herbal Medicine Development: Methodologies, Challenges, and Issues", Evidence-Based Complementary and Alternative Medicine, vol. 2019, Article ID 4935786, 2 pages, 2019. https://doi.org/10.1155/2019/4935786
5. Li S, Han Q, Qiao C, et al. . Chemical markers for the quality control of herbal medicines: an overview. Chin Med 2008;3:7.
6. NiharikaSahoo, PadmavatiManchikanti. Herbal Drug Regulation and Commercialization: An Indian Industry Perspective. J Altern Complement Med. 2013 Dec 1; 19(12): 957–963. doi: 10.1089/acm.2012.0275
7. Prakash C. Phondani, Indra D. Bhatt, Vikram S. Negi, Bhagwati P. Kothyari, Arvind Bhatt, Rakesh K. Maikhuri. Promoting medicinal plants cultivation as a tool for biodiversity conservation and livelihood enhancement in Indian Himalaya.Journal of Asia-Pacific Biodiversity. 2016; 9 (1): 39-46.
8. S. Sen, R. Chakraborty. Toward the integration and advancement of herbal medicine: a focus on Traditional Indian medicine. Bot Target Ther, 5 (2015), pp. 33-44
9. S. Sen, R. Chakraborty. Traditional knowledge digital library: a distinctive approach to protect and promote Indian indigenous medicinal treasure. CurrSci, 106 (2014), pp. 1340-1343
10. S. Thillaivanan, K. Samraj. Challenges, constraints and opportunities in herbal medicines – a review Int J Herb Med, 2 (2014), pp. 21-24
11. S.C. Mandal, M. Mandal. Quality, safety, and efficacy of herbal products through regulatory harmonization. Drug Info J, 45 (2011), pp. 45-53
12. Sahoo N, Manchikanti P, DeySH.Herbal drugs standards and regulation. Fitoterapia 2010;81:462–471
13. SaikatSen, Raja Chakraborty. Revival, modernization and integration of Indian traditional herbal medicine in clinical practice: Importance, challenges and future. Journal of Traditional and Complementary Medicine. 2017;7 (2):234-244.
14. Saxena PK, Cole IB, MurchSJ.Approaches to quality plant based medicine: significance of chemical profiling. In: Applications of Plant Metabolic Engineering, Verpoorte R, Alfermann AW, Johnson TS, eds. Dordrecht, the Netherlands: Springer; 2007:311–330
15. World Health Organization Guidelines on good agricultural and collection practices for medicinal plants [homepage on the Internet]. Online document at: http://whqlibdoc.who.int/publications/2003/9241546271.pdf
16. World Health Organization Traditional medicine, fact sheet no. 134 [homepage on the Internet]. Online document at: http://www.who.int/mediacentre/factsheets/fs134/en/
17. MalathiSeshasayeeKonda Ramadoss &KailasamKoumaravelou. (2019). Regulatory compliance of herbal medicines – A review. International Journal of Research in Pharmaceutical Sciences, 10(4), 3127-3135. https://doi.org/10.26452/ijrps.v10i4.1609

Scan QR code to view the website/guidelines

- National policy on traditional medicine and regulation of herbal medicines-

National policy on traditional medicine and regulation of herbal medicines : report of a WHO global survey

- International Regulatory Cooperation for Herbal Medicines (IRCH)-

International Regulatory Cooperation for Herbal Medicines (IRCH) (who.int)

- Herbal medicinal products-

Herbal medicinal products | European Medicines Agency (europa.eu)

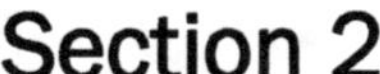

Section 2

Herbs and Derived Products

CHAPTER 2

Extraction, Purification, Preliminary Phytochemical Screening and Structural Elucidation of Natural Products

Introduction

Important Definitions Related to Herbs

Herbs, Medicinal Plants, Sources of Herbs, Herbal Materials, Herbal Medicines, Herbal Medicinal Products, Herbal Preparations, Finished Herbal Products

Factors Responsible for Quality of Herbal Raw Material

Processing of Herbal Raw Materials

Collection, Harvesting, Post Harvest Processing, Drying, Pulverisation, Garbling /Cleaning/Dressing, Packing, Storage

Extraction

Extraction Steps, Types of extracts, Choice of Extraction Method: Key Points

Methods of Extraction

Maceration, Percolation, Hot Continuous Counter-current Extraction, Infusion, Decoction, Distillation (For volatile oil), Expression (For volatile oil), Enfleurage (For volatile oil), Ultrasound Extraction, Extraction by Electrical Energy or Microwave Assisted Extraction, Couther Current Distribution (CCD), Droplet Counter Current Chromatography (DCCC), Accelerated Solvent Extraction (ASE), Supercritical Fluid Extraction (SCF), Solid-Phase Extraction (SPE), Liquid-liquid Extraction (LLE), Phytonics, Turbo Extraction (Vortical Extraction)

Purification Methods

Choice of Purification Method, Removal of Common Interfering Substances, Various Purification Methods

Filtration, Separation, Chromatographic Methods, Electrophoresis, Concentration/ Evaporation, Crystallization

Preliminary Phytochemical Testing (Qualitative Testing)

Quantitative Estimation of Phytochemicals

Structural Elucidation of Natural Products

Introduction, Computation Techniques in Structural Elucidation

Spectroscopic Elucidation of Phytoconstituents

Introduction

- Ultraviolet (UV) and Visible Spectroscopy
- Infrared Spectroscopy
- Mass Spectrometry
- Nuclear Magnetic Resonance Spectroscopy

Role of Spectroscopy in Structural Elucidation

Examples - Atropine, Caffeine

Role of Hyphenated Techniques in Structural Elucidation

Introduction

Preliminary phytochemical screening involves four major steps: Extraction, Purification, Qualitative Chemical evaluation and Quantitative Chemical estimation. Qualitative Chemical evaluation is the step after extraction in order to identify different classes of constituents that can be present in extracts, i.e., carbohydrates, proteins, lipids, flavonoids, tannins, glycosides, alkaloids, and essential oils. Always choose a solvent of extraction whose solubility and/or polarity is same as that of the constituents, i.e., use polar solvents only to obtain polar components. After detecting the particular class, one can perform specific chemical tests for whole crude drug or individual constituents to confirm any known drug or component. The present chapter elaborates maximum available tests that can be performed for preliminary phytochemical screening.

Important Definitions Related to Herbs

- **Herbs** include crude materials which could be derived from lichen, algae, fungi or higher plants, such as leaves, flowers, fruit, fruiting bodies, seeds, stems, wood, bark, roots, rhizomes or other parts, which may be entire, fragmented or powdered.
- **Medicinal Plants** are plants (wild or cultivated) used for medicinal purposes. medicinal plant materials – see herbal materials.
- **Sources of Herbs**: herbs are generally obtained from wild sources or commercial sources depending upon geographical location.
- **Herbal Materials** include, in addition to herbs, fresh juices, gums, fixed oils, essential oils, resins and dry powders of herbs. In some countries, these materials WHO guidelines on good manufacturing practices (GMP) for herbal medicines may be processed by various local procedures, such as steaming, roasting or stir baking with honey, alcoholic beverages or other materials.
- **Herbal Medicines** include herbs, herbal materials, herbal preparations and finished herbal products.
- **Herbal Medicinal Products** are defined as any medicinal product, exclusively containing as active ingredients one or more herbal substances, one or more herbal preparations, or a combination of the two.
- **Herbal Preparations** are the basis for finished herbal products and may include comminuted or cut herbal materials, or extracts, tinctures and fatty oils of herbal materials. They are produced by extraction, fractionation, purification, concentration, or other physical or biological processes. They also include preparations made by steeping or heating herbal materials in alcoholic beverages and/or honey, or in other materials.
- **Finished Herbal Products** consist of herbal preparations made from one or more herbs. If more than one herb is used, the term "mixture herbal product" can also be used. Finished herbal products and mixture herbal products may contain excipients in addition to the active ingredients. However, finished herbal products or mixture herbal products to which chemically defined active substances have been added, including synthetic compounds and/or isolated constituents from herbal materials, are not considered to be herbal

Factors Responsible for Quality of Herbal Raw Material

The increasing demand for herbal medicine both in developing and developed countries has inevitably led to maintaining the quality and quantity of the herbal raw materials and finished products. To control the quality of the starting material, the following aspects need to be considered.

- Selection of appropriate medicinal plant species
- Correct botanical identity &Authenticity and homogeneity of herbal raw materials
- Reproducibility of herbal raw materials
- Inter/intra species variation in plants
- Environmental factors
- Time of harvesting
- Post harvesting factors
- Contaminants of herbal ingredients and decontamination methods
- Plant part adulterations
- Pesticides, fumigants and toxic metals (Lead, cadmium, mercury, thallium and arsenic)

Processing of Herbal Raw Materials

Before using a crude drug for production of herbal formulations, it should be properly processed so that, the active constituents and the appearance of the drug do not deteriorate. For raw materials of botanical identity with scientific and common names, plant parts, the state (Example- fresh, dried), macroscopic and microscopic description, therapeutic and toxic constituents or marker compound(s), if applicable, should be provided. The preparation of a crude drug for the market depends on the following major processes.

Collec-tion	Collection of drugs from cultivated plants instead of wild sources always ensures a true natural source and reliable products. It may require unskilled native labour for few plants and skill worker with highly scientific skills for few plants. The age and season of plant governs not only the quality but total quantity of active constitutes too
Harves-ting	Harvesting is the process of collection of the highest quality crude drug from its original source in the appropriate season and time of the day. ➢ Leaves are collected from plants during the flowering season when the plant is very active. ➢ Barks should be collected in early summer or spring. ➢ Flowers are collected about the time of pollination in dry weather in the forenoon when the dew has disappeared and dried in shade. ➢ Roots and tubers are collected in autumn when the plant is inactive and the vegetative process has ceased and contain the maximum active constituents. ➢ Fruits must be harvested ripe or unripe based on constituent quality and quantity

Contd...

<table>
<tr><th colspan="2">Post Harvest Processing</th></tr>
<tr><td>Drying</td><td>Drying is essential for maintaining the quality of crude drugs after collection to avoid decomposition, microbial growth, enzyme activation and other possible chemical changes. Herbal raw drugs are dried prior to extraction to avoid deterioration on storage and transport as well as to facilitate grinding. In the preparation of crude drugs, drying is usually designed to yield a stable, homogenous product which is easy to manipulate in subsequent operation of storage and packaging.
Drying is defined as the removal of a liquid or moisture contents from a material (herbal drugs) by the application of heat and is accomplished by the transfer of a liquid or moisture content from a surface into an unsaturated vapour phase.
Proper and successful drying depends on control of temperature and regulation of air flow. Drying process is to be done depending upon source of herbal crude drug and its chemical nature.
• If enzymatic action is to be encouraged, slow drying is necessary at moderate temperature. Example- Orris rhizome, Vanilla pods, Cocoa seed, Gentian root.
• If enzymatic action is not desired, drying should take place as soon as possible after collection. Drugs containing volatile oil are liable to lose their aroma if not dried or if the oil is not distilled from them immediately.
Two types of drying are classified as follows:
1. Natural drying (sun drying)
(a) Direct sun drying (outdoor drying): The crude drugs can be dried directly in sunshine if the contents of crude drugs are quite stable to the temperature and sunlight. Example: Gum acacia, seeds, fruit are dried by direct sun drying method.
(b) Shed drying: Shed drying is prepared when the natural colors of the drug (digitalis leaves, clove, senna leaves) and volatile principles of the drug (Example- Peppermint) are to be retained. Drying in the shed at the air temperature is frequently adopted especially for leaves containing oil.
2. Artificial drying
(a) Tray dryer: (truck dryer): This is most commonly used method in the pharmaceutical plant operation. Tray dryers are used for drying heat stable plant material. Example- roots, barks. In this process, hot air of desired temperature is circulated through the dryers and this facilitates the removal of water content of the drugs. This is simplest and inexpensive method. Disadvantage of tray dryersis deterioration of material due to high residence time at high temperature.
(b) Vacuum dryer: In this method, vacuum facilitates drying of plant material at low temperature. It can handle sticky, free flowing, hygroscopic, heat sensitive plant materials. Examples- Tannic acid, Digitalis leaves.
(c) Spray dryer: This is used for non-hygroscopic products. This is continuous, thermally efficient dryer where filtered atmospheric hot air comes in contact with atomized fine mist of the feed and instantly evaporates the water in the feed droplets. The fluidized mixture of air and powder get separated in cyclone separator. This method of drying retains all the original properties of plant material such as color, aroma, efficacy, density</td></tr>
</table>

Contd...

	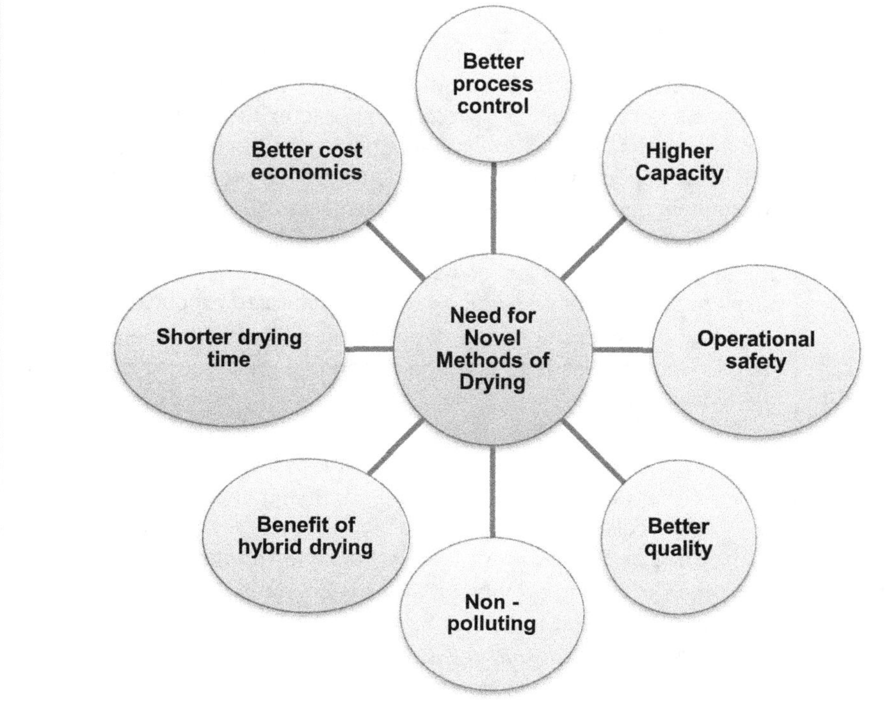 **Figure 2.1** Need for Novel Methods of Drying.
Pulverisation	Pulverisation or comminution is a process of fragmenting a substance into small particles by mechanical forces. It is one of the important process operation and inevitable in very first step of herbal extraction. Size reduction, pulverization, Comminution or grinding is a process of reducing large solid or liquid particles into small, coarse particles or fine particles. Size reduction process by mechanical means is called as Milling. The size reduction of solids is called as grinding or cutting and of liquids called as emulsification or atomization. Uniform powders instead of polydisperse powders are perfect for herbal formulation development. Hence, size reduction along with size separation is always crucial step in herbal product manufacturing. Various factors like size, shape, hardness, stickiness, friability, moisture content, thermal stability, abrasiveness and ratio of feed size to product size, affect the size reduction. Advantages of size reduction of herbal drugs and or crude drugs are content uniformity, uniform mixing, drying and flow, effective extraction of drug, effective drying, improved stability, dissolution rate, rate of absorption, surface area and bioavailability. Disadvantages of size reduction are drug degradation, poor mixing and contamination. **Objectives of Understanding Size Reduction are s**ize reduction is necessary for uniform mixing, to increase surface area, therapeutic effectiveness, rate of absorption and or bioavailability. Herbal capsules, insufflations, suppositories and ointments require particles size to be below 60 mm size. Herbal suspensions of finer particle size reduces rate of sedimentation. Fine size globules of emulsions increase its stability. All the ophthalmic preparations must be free from gritty particles to avoid irritation. The physical appearance of herbal ointments, pastes and creams depends on particle size.

Contd...

Various Size Reduction Equipments are as follows:	
Rotary Cutter Mill	Sharp knife performs successive cutting / Shearing of herbal material like tough - fibrous materials.
Roller Mill	Size is reduced by application of stress and attrition through rotating heavy wheels, Muller or Rollers. It is generally useful for crushing of seeds before extraction of fixed oils
Hammer Mill	Rapidly moving hammers mounted on rotor helps in size reduction of stationary powder material. It is useful to brittle and fibrous material
Disintegrator	Size is reduced by heavy impact and useful to powder all types of drugs including very hard drugs.
Ball Mill	Size is reduced by principle of impact and attrition in closed system hence suitable for size reduction of toxic substances as well.
Fluid Energy Mill	Size is reduced by impact and attrition. It is useful to grind heat sensitive materials.
Spray drying	This is most preferred method to get size reduced uniform dried powder of liquid samples.
Supercritical fluid process	Herbal extracts or phytochemicals are solubilised in super critical fluids and re-crystallized to get size reduced uniform powder.
Sono-crystallization	Herbal extracts or phytochemicals are reduced to fine size crystallization by exposing to ultra sound of frequency 20 – 100 kHz.
Micron technologies	Herbal extracts or phytochemicals are subjected to high pressure air / gas causing particle collision and micronization to give particles smaller than 20 microns
Micro fluidizer	The ultra-high shear developed by the micro fluidizer processor reduces the particle size and high turbulence prevents agglomeration.

Comminution of different parts of the herbal drugs can be explained as followed.

Crude Drug	Details and type of mills useful
Leaf drugs	Leaf drugs are predominant in herbal industry. • Shredding mills - medicinal leaves and herbs with high content • of stem and stalk • Hammer mills- for resinous and friable leaf drugs • Pin mills – leaf drugs with high fat content or ethereal oil.
Roots and barks	Roots and barks are moderately hard or woody but sometimes brittle and friable also. Example- Cinnamon, Quercus, Ipecacuanha • Shredder mills- cutting and shredding • Hammer mills- grinding
Seeds and fruits	The comminution of seeds and fruits offer proves to be particularly difficult because of their content of fats and ethereal oils. Example- coffee and cocoa beans. • Shredder mills – comminution
Other drug plant materials	These include flowers, part of flowers and products such as alginates, agar, and gelatins • Shredder mills – Comminution

Contd...

Garbling / Cleaning/ Dressing	This step is the final step in preparation of crude drugs for market. This involves removal of foreign matter like soil, sand, animal excreta, dirt, or other parts of the same plants (Example- roots from stem, stalks from flower buds etc). Presence of foreign matter affects pharmacopoeial limits of standard values of physicochemical parameters.
Packing	The morphological and chemical nature of the drug, its ultimate use and effect of climatic conditions during transportation and storage should be taken into consideration while packing of herbal raw material. **Examples**: ➢ Colophony and balsam packed in kerosene tins. ➢ Asafoetida is stored in well-closed container to prevent loss of volatile oil. ➢ Cod liver oil is sensitive to sunlight so it should be stored in sunlight proof containers. ➢ Leaf drug like senna, vinca are pressed and baled. ➢ Digitalis, ergot, squills like crude drug are very sensitive to moisture and costly at the same time need special attention to be stored in moisture resistant containers. ➢ Colophony needs to be packed in big masses to control auto oxidation. ➢ Crude drugs like roots, seeds and other part can be packed in gunny bags. ➢ Weight of certain drug in lots need to be kept constant Example: Indian opium. **Packing material and specific storage of Raw Herbs** • Hard Woody parts like stem, root bark etc.: Gunny bags and woven sacks • Soft parts like creepers, leaves etc.: High gauge HMHD bags, woven sacks with LD liner, High gauge polyethylene bags • Fleshy parts like fruits, rhizomes etc.: High gauge HMHD bags, woven sacks with LD liner, wooden boxes. • Flowers, anthers, stigma, petals, seeds etc.: Corrugated box with polypropylene woven sacks, HDPE containers, Fiber board's drums • Volatile contents: Air tight HDPE containers, Air tight HDPE carboys, Card board box with polyethylene liners • Herbal extracts and compounds: Air tight HDPE containers, corrugated box with polyethylene woven sacks and fiber board's drums with polyethylene bags. HDHM (High molecular weight high density polyethylene), LD liner (Low density liner bags), HDPE (High density polyethylene)
Storage	• Proper storage and preservative are important factors in maintaining a high degree of quality of Herbal Raw material. • Warehouse should preferably be of fire proof, steel, concrete or brick construction, and unheated and rodent proof. • Hard packed bales usually reabsorb little moisture. This is also true of barks and resinous drug but leaf, herbs, and roots drugs that are not well packed tend to absorb moisture up to 10%, 15%, or 30% of weight of drug. • Excessive moisture not only increases the weight of the drug. Thus reducing the % of active constituents but also favours enzymatic activity and facilitates fungal growth. Example: Digitalis glycoside is deteriorate when moisture in the drug reaches 8% or higher. • Liquid adversely affects drugs, which are higher colored, rendering them unattractive and possibly causing undesirable changes in constituents. It has been shown that polarized light changes more rapidly the ordinary light.

Contd...

	• The oxygen of the air increase oxidation of the constituent so of the drugs, especially when oxidases (oxidizing enzymes) are present. • Insects also attack on crude herbal drugs so to prevention of their attacks a number of methods have been employed. The simple method of all being to expose the drug to a temperature of 65°C. They also prevent form determination. • The fumigation of large lots of crude drugs such as stored in warehoused and manufacturing plants, the use of methyl bromide. • Small lots of drugs may readily be stored in air-light, moisture proof and lightproof containers. • If drugs in small quantities are stored in air-tight containers, insect attack can be controlled by the addition of a few drops of chloroform or CCl_4. • Certain drugs such as biologics must be stored at a temperature between 2° and 10°C

Extraction

Extraction is the process of separation of desired constituents from the crude drug by efficiently dissolving and separating with appropriate solvents. The properties like polarity, pH and thermal stability of secondary metabolites decides solvent selection for extraction. The extraction of crude drugs involves a separation of solid or liquid chemical constituents from solid components. Initially plant cells are disintegrated in suitable solvent/s with or without application of temperature and or shear for specific time. Swelling mediated increase in the permeability of the cell walls lead to penetration of the solvent into the plant cells, further diffusion and then dissolution of phytochemicals.

Plant and plant derived products are gaining world wide acceptance due to several advantages including easy availability, possible source of lead molecules, synergism with modern drugs, and their significant patent opportunities. World Health Organisation (WHO) and other regulatory bodies have emphasized research, especially in extraction and isolation of phytomedicines from the herbs utilized in complementary and alternative medicines (CAM) which can be useful for affirming scientific evidences along with setting good quality control parameters. Here, we will first discuss the basic concepts of extraction methods which is the very first step in any herbal research.

The extraction solvents should be non-inflammable, inert, non-toxic, easy to remove, and should dissolve the maximum amount of desired phyto-constituents. Polarity is the major criteria in the selection of solvents. A number of extraction techniques are utilized by researchers; drawbacks of traditional extraction systems like poor solubility in solvents, time and energy consumption along with thermal degradation led to the development of various modern alternative extraction methods which are rapid, solvent free, and compatible with thermo labile substances. These modern methods are more promising and found to be fruitful but are very costly. Some of the traditional (e.g. maceration, decoction, percolation, soxhlet extraction) as well as modern (Example- super critical fluid (SCF), accelerated, ultrasound, microwave) extraction methods have been discussed as possible effective methods as per desired phytoconstituents.

Extraction Steps

In order to extract medicinal ingredients from plant material, the following sequential steps are involved:

- **Drying:** Drying of crude drugs after collection and before extraction is necessary to avoid microbial growth, prevent chemical degradation, and determine the final weight of raw material. The time and choice of drying method depend on physical and chemical nature of the crude drug. The delicate parts like leaves and flowers require less time and temperature for drying. Hard materials like bark, roots, and fruits require high temperature and longer time for drying. Even high water containing plant takes a long time to dry, and volatile oil containing drugs should be dried with extreme care.
- **Size reduction or Pulverization [Refer above]**
- **Extraction:** The choice of an extraction method depends on factors like sample size, quantity of extract required, extraction time, choice of solvent, and lastly, the overall cost of selected extraction method. Often the extraction method suitable for laboratory scale process is found to be useless at the industrial level due to high scale.
- **Filtration**: Filtration is a mechanical means of separating solids from a liquid suspension via a porous medium or screen that permits the liquid to pass while retaining the solids. Filtration may be necessary in the early stages of sample preparation to separate materials that are either solids in liquids or the other way round. There are several laboratory filtration techniques depending on the desired outcome namely, hot, cold and vacuum filtration. Two main types of filter media are employed in laboratories:
    - ***Surface filters***: solid sieves which trap the solid particles intact, with or without the aid of filter paper (Example- Buchner funnel, belt filter, rotary vacuum-drum filter, cross-flow filters, and screen filter).
    - ***Depth filters***: a bed of granular material with greater surface area which do not retain the solid particles intact as they pass (Example- sand filter) but are less prone to clogging.
- **Solvent evaporation and Concentration**: Rotatory evaporation is most preferred method for thermo stable phytochemicals. Spray drying is quick system of drying and preferred over other systems of drying particularly in case of heat sensitive product. Spray dryer is also used for entrapping volatile constituents of extract within the particle and this process is called micro encapsulation. After liquid extraction, we may have to go for further purification either by repeated solvent fraction or crystallization in order to isolate active ingredients fluidized bed dryer is generally preferred for drying. Vacuum tray dryer is also used in at a temperature. Not exceeding 60°C in cases where products are prone to oxidation.

The critical problem with herbal extracts is drying after extraction which is a must to stabilize them for storage. The volatile solvents like pet ether or acetone can be easily removed but alcoholic and aqueous extracts are difficult to dry. The moisture containing extracts are sensitive to microbial growth and can activate enzymes like glycosidase associated with glycosides or can deteriorate the whole product. Hence, it is necessary that the final moisture content of the extract powder must be as low as possible. The temperature and heat sensitivity of herbal extracts requires extremely gentle drying and should also be performed at a low temperature and lowest possible pressures. Following are a few of the methods which are commonly used to dry the herbal extracts:

- **Vacuum Drying:** This is the method of drying which uses the combination of low-pressure and low-temperature to ensure a good quality product without oxidation/degradation. Many commercial vacuum dryers are available in the market to fulfill the requirement. This is the most cost effective method of drying.
- **Spray Drying:** Here, the specially designed spray nozzle disperse the purified liquid extract into small drops of uniform size which are quickly dried up using a hot and dry air or gas current. The dry product which is always a free flowing powder is collected in a cyclone. This method is applicable to food materials, colouring, and flavouring phytoconstituents as well as for microencapsulation of phytopharmaceuticals.
- **Freeze Drying:** This is also known as lyophilization and is the most gentle and highly recommended method for thermolabile components where the water from the product is first frozen, then slowly heated under vacuum to allow the sublimation of water. The sublimation should always be carried out at pressure below the triple point of water. Disadvantage of this method is that it is highly complex and costly and is used for high value products only.
- **Rotary evaporation Drying:** It is an efficient, fast, gentle, and the most widely used method for drying of herbal extracts. The removal of solvent by rotary evaporator involves evaporation of the solvent from extract under controlled temperature in applied vacuum. It also involves the rotation of the extract containing flask in a water bath which enables effective heat transfer and prevents local overheating. This is also the method of choice for pre-concentration stage prior to final drying of extracts.

Types of Extracts

- **Standardized (Adjusted) extracts** are adjusted within an acceptable tolerance to a given content of constituents with known therapeutic activity; Standardization is achieved by adjustment of the extract with inert material or by blending batches of extracts.
- **Quantified extracts** are adjusted to a defined range of constituents; adjustments are made by blending batches of extracts.
- **Other extracts** are essentially defined by the production process (state of the herbal drug or animal matter to be extracted, solvent, extraction conditions) and their specifications.
- **Soft extracts** are semi-solid preparations obtained by evaporation or partial evaporation of the solvent used for preparation.
- **Dry extracts** are solid preparations obtained by evaporation of the solvent used for their production. Dry extracts usually have a loss on drying or water content not greater than 5 per cent m/m.
- **Liquid extracts** are liquid preparations of which, in general, 1 part by mass or volume is equivalent to 1 part by mass of the herbal drug or animal matter. These preparations are adjusted, if necessary, so that they satisfy the requirements for the content of the solvent and, where applicable, for the constituents.
- **Tinctures** are liquid preparations which are usually obtained using either 1 part of herbal drug or animal matter and 10 parts of extraction solvent or 1 part of herbal drug or animal matter and 5 parts of extraction solvent.

Contd...

> - Depending on the physical state of an extract the following types can be distinguished: - **Liquid preparation:** liquid extracts (fluid extract, tincture), oily macerates, - Semi-solid preparations: soft extracts.
> - The difference between **fluid extract and tincture** is that tinctures are diluted preparations.

Choice of Extraction Method: Key Points

- After collecting the plant material for research, authenticate its species from a competent botanist to avoid the use of improper or toxic species.
- Dry the raw material using an appropriate method of drying to avoid bad effects of moisture.
- Always use coarse powder of plant material for extraction instead of fine powder because the latter causes coagulation. Coarse powder gives sufficient space for solvent surrounding it, and thus, helps proper penetration.
- Successive extraction is suitable to extract the constituents of different polarity. It involves extraction of the same plant material with solvents of different polarity ranging from non-polar to polar. Polarity preference can be given as: Petroleum ether < Chloroform < Methanol < Ethyl acetate < Water
- Petroleum ether extract will give lipids, fatty acids, sterol, steroids or aglycone moieties of glycosides. Chloroform extract will give sugars or mainly alkaloids. Methanol extract will give glycosides, saponins or a few phenolic constituents. Ethyl acetate extract will give flavonoid or tannins. Water will solublize all polar constituents like few glycosides, alkaloids, sugars or tannins.
- Soxhlet or decoction method of extraction should be preferred for hard plant materials like bark, stem etc. To extract soft materials, hot or cold maceration methods of extraction should be used.
- For extraction of thermolabile constituents, ultrasound or SCF extraction method should be used. In case, if Soxhlet extraction method is unavoidable, then maintain the temperature below 55° C.
- To obtain water or hydroalcoholic extracts, do not use soxhlet extraction method as boiling point of water is very high and extraction takes a long time.
- Select the solvents according to the polarity of the desired constituents (e.g. glycosides, being polar in nature, are soluble in polar solvents only). Avoid the use of toxic solvents like benzene or chloroform.
- Use double or triple distilled solvents for extraction because presence of water molecules changes the polarity of solvent and thereby, extraction efficiency.
- To extract enzyme associated plant materials, use alcohol soaked powder to deactivate enzymes.
- For the complete extraction of alkaloids, add ammonia in small quantities to chloroform. Alkaloids are always associated with acids; the alkali liberates the free alkaloid bases.
- To remove impurities like chlorophyll pigments, lipids, and other fatty substances from the plant material, especially leaves or seeds, initially extract the powder using petroleum ether which is called defatting.

- Liquid extraction is the best option to separate different chemical classes and to isolate desired constituents from plant extract. For example, water extract can be portioned with n-hexane to separate polar classes from non-polar one. Saponins can be separated from the aqueous solution of methanolic extract by partitioning with n-butanol.
- As phytochemicals are very unstable in nature and undergo derivatization, solvent should be removed immediately after extraction.

Methods of Extraction

In this section, different traditional and modern methods of extraction of desired constituents are explained.

Maceration	As per IP 1966 maceration is : "Place the solid material with the whole of the menstruum in a closed vessel and allow it to stand for 7 days, shaking occasionally, and strain, pressing the marc and mixing the liquids obtained. Clarify by subsidence or filtration". Seven days are considered to be an adequate period of time to bring about equilibrium between solute and solvent. Closed vessel is preferred to avoid undue loss of solvent due to evaporation and contamination.
Percolation	As per IP 1966 percolation is carried out as follows: "Moisten the solid materials with sufficient quantity of the menstruum, allow it to stand for 4 hours in a well closed vessel, packed in a percolator, and add sufficient of menstruum to saturate the material. When the liquid commences to drop from the percolator, close the outlet, add sufficient amount of the menstrum to leave a layer above the drug and allow it to stand for 24 hours. Allow percolation to proceed slowly until the percolate measures about three quarters of the volume required for the finished tincture. Press the marc, mix the expressed liquid with the percolate, and sufficient of menstrum to produce the required volume. Clarify by subsidence or filtration.
Hot Continuous Counter-current Extraction	This is also called as Soxhlet extraction due to specially designed apparatus. It is the process where the same quantity of solvent is made to circulate through the extractor of drug by evaporation and subsequent condensation. With less solvent complete extraction is possible. But this method is not suitable for thermolabile components.
Infusion	This is a very simple method of extraction used for vitamins, volatile ingredients and soft ingredients in which the powdered drug is extracted with hot or cold water.
Decoction	The word decoction means to concentrate by boiling. In this method, the drug powder can be boiled with water for a few minutes to hours and then filtered.
Distillation (For volatile oil)	This method is useful for extraction of essential oils. It involves the heating of plant material with water in a distillation unit. The vapours of the volatile oil component are passed towards the condenser along with the steam vapours. The oil and water layer separate on cooling.
Expression (For volatile oil)	It is a purely mechanical technique which involves sponge, ecuelle and mechanical methods to extract essential oils. Volatile oil absorption on sponge by rupturing the oil glands from citrus peels by squeezing is the best example of sponge method. In Ecuelle method, the sharp projection containing vessel is used to rupture the glands from the citrus peels.

Contd...

Enfleurage (For volatile oil)	This method is useful for extraction of essential oils from delicate plant parts like rose oil from rose petals. Fatty material is spread evenly into the glass plate as a thin layer. The petals or inflorescences are spread on this fatty layer. The material is allowed to extract completely in fat by keeping for 24 hours. Then, again fresh petals are loaded. This process continues till the fatty layer is saturated with volatile oil.
Ultrasound Extraction	It is also called as sonication extraction. In this method, sound wavesof high-frequency pulses of 20 kHz are generated in suitable vessel containing mixture of herb and appropriate solvent. Mechanical stress generated from the sound waves cause easy penetration of solvent to the cell membrane. This further lead to extraction of phytochemicals.
Extraction by Electrical Energy or Microwave Assisted Extraction	Microwaves (frequency 300 MHz to 300 GHz) are non-ionising electromagnetic waves which are useful in the extraction of phytoconstituents. The principles on which microwave works is that the high temperature produced by microwaves evaporates the moisture present in the plant powder which dehydrates cellulose, ruptures the cell walls and thus solubilises phytoconstituents. It gives rapid exhaustive extraction within 5-10 min.Fast heating with less energy, reduced both extraction time as well as volume of solvent are major advantages of microwave assisted extraction compared to conventional extraction methods.
Couther Current Distribution (CCD)	This is a liquid-liquid extraction process and is based on the principle of partition coefficient i.e. the liquid to be isolated is much more soluble in either one of the two immiscible liquids. The apparatus (**Craig Apparatus)**consists of a series of interconnected tubes in order to repeat the same cycle of process for efficient separation. The first tube in the series contains three liquids • Heavy stationary phase liquid • Mixture to be separated • Light mobile phase liquid.
Droplet Counter Current Chromatography (DCCC)	DCCC is based on the combined principle of liquid-liquid extraction and column chromatography. It is a simpler modification of counter current distribution (CCD) principle of Craig apparatus. Here, the mobile phase moves in the form of small droplets or plates. Hence the solute separates by distributing between stationary and droplets according to the partition coefficient differences. Stationary and mobile phase moves in the counter current direction and hence it is called as counter current chromatography.
Accelerated Solvent Extraction (ASE)	It is also known as pressurised solvent extraction (PSE) and is very similar to a Soxhlet extraction. This is a relatively new fully automated technique which operates at high temperatures and pressures (100–200 bars) ,but at the same time, keeps the solvents in liquid form during the extraction process. The solvents used are near their supercritical state where they have high extraction properties. It is very similar to supercritical fluid extraction, the only difference is the pressure is high but below the supercritical point and ACE does not involve the use of carbon dioxide.

Contd...

Supercritical Fluid Extraction (SCF)	This is organic solvent free extraction method. At super critical point (temperature and pressure above critical point) gas converts to fluid. Such super critical fluid solvent mediated extraction is a process, very similar to simple extraction where solvent passes through the coarsely powdered sample and extracts its constituents. The only difference here is that there is a special assembly to control temperature and pressure. It is easy to remove the solvent extract because carbon dioxide escapes as gas as the pressure is released. Gas can be re-cycled and reused.
Solid-Phase Extraction (SPE)	Solid-phase extraction (SPE) is a modern chromatographic separation technique. It separates the individual components from the liquid mixture in accordance with their physical and chemical properties. It is of three types i.e. normal, reversed or ion exchange SPE. Unlike liquid-liquid extraction, it doesn't form emulsion. SPE uses the principal of chromatographic separation.
Liquid-liquid Extraction (LLE)	Liquid-liquid extraction or solvent extraction is the most preferred extraction/ separation method of choice in organic chemistry. This process is based on partition coefficient that allows the separation of components of mixture due to their unequal solubility in two immiscible liquid phases.
Phytonics	"Phytonics process" is patented technology by Advanced Phytonics Limited (Manchester, UK). It is process of extraction of herbal drugs by using fluorocarbon solvents especially 1,1,2,2-tetrafluoroethane, better known ashydrofluorocarbon-134a (HFC-134a) with low residual solvent below levels of detection invariably less than 20 parts per billion hence do not require further critical purification steps. HFC-134a has boiling point -25° C, vapor pressure of 5.6 bar. It is neutral, non-flammable, non- toxic and non-ozone depleting. It is a poor solvent hence not able to extract plant wastes like plant lipids or triglycerides. It requires a minimum amount of electrical energy, ambient temperature and can be completely recycled. This technique is found useful for extraction of high-quality essential oils, natural colors, flavors and other phytochemical extracts.
Turbo Extraction (Vortical Extraction)	Turbo extractors, based on "Hot Break/Cold Break" or Zenith Chrono inactivation technology, are specifically designed for separation of fruit juice from peels, seeds and foreign matters. Hence it is suitable for refining fluid-based products which requires separation of liquid from solids like tomato and other fruit puree and or juices. Recently, the turbo-extraction or turbolysis, performed using a high shear stirrer Ultraturrax found to be useful in extraction of glycosides from stevia using 70-90% ethanol. Stirring and simultaneous high shearing force mediated reduction of particle size results in a rapid exhausted dissolution of the phytochemicals in minimum time.

The conventional extraction methods like **maceration, decoction, percolation**, **reflux and Soxhlet extraction** requireslong time and large quantity solvent/s for extraction. While modern extraction methods likesuper **critical fluid extraction (SFC), pressurized liquid extraction**

(PLE), microwave assisted extraction (MAE) and Phytonics extraction requires lessor no organic solvent/sand minimum time.

Comparative summary of various extraction methods is as follows:

Method	Solvent	Temperature	Pressure	Time	Solvent requirement
Maceration	Water or organic solvents	Room temperature	Atmospheric	24 hr to 7 days	Large
Percolation	Water or organic solvents	Room temperature	Atmospheric	24 hr	Large
Decoction	Water	High temperature based on phytochemical and solvent	Atmospheric	1-2 hr	None
Reflux extraction	Water or organic solvents		Atmospheric	1-3 hr	Moderate
Soxhlet extraction	Organic solvents		Atmospheric	Upto 8 hr	Moderate
Pressurized liquid extraction	Water or organic solvents		High	1-2 hr	Small
Supercritical fluid extraction	Supercritical fluid of gases usually CO_2	Near room temperature	High	1-2 hr	None or small
Ultrasound assisted extraction	Water or organic solvents	Room or High temperature based on phytochemical and solvent	Atmospheric	1-2 hr	Moderate
Microwave assisted extraction	Water or organic solvents	Room or High temperature based on phytochemical and solvent	Atmospheric	Less than 1 hr	None or moderate
Pulsed electric field extraction	Water or organic solvents	Room or High temperature based on phytochemical and solvent	Atmospheric	Less than 1 hr	Moderate
Enzyme assisted extraction	Water or organic solvents	High temperature enzyme treatment	Atmospheric	2-4 hr	Moderate

Purification

Choice of Purification Method

Purification by chromatographic method depends on properties of phytochemical/s to be isolated. Reverse Phase-HPLC is useful to separate polar phytochemicals, affinity chromatography to separate enzymes and antigens, gel-filtration chromatography to separate large size biomolecules. Due to advancement in various processing technologies, phytochemicals can be isolated in less time with minimal contaminations and maximum yield.

Removal of Common Interfering Substances	
Lipids, pigments, and tannins	Lipids, pigments, and tannins are the most common interfering substances in the isolation of secondary metabolites. Defatting with non-polar solvents (e.g., benzene and petroleum ether) prior to isolation can be effective for the removal of these substances.
Lipids	Liquid chromatography–Mass spectrometry (LC-MS) and Gas chromatography–Mass spectrometry (GC-MS) analysis can be useful in identification of lipids while Vacuum liquid chromatography (VLC) is useful in separation.
Plant pigments	Plant pigments can be removed by either of the following methods: • Liquid–liquid extraction using two different immiscible solvents (Example n-hexane or petroleum ether and 90% methanol) separates phytochemicals based on their relative solubilities or partition coefficient. It can be performed by separating funnels or countercurrent distribution equipment. • Vacuum Liquid chromatography (VLC) with adsorbent Diaion LH-20 resin as stationary phase and 50 % aqueous methanol as mobile phase • Open column chromatography using mobile phase consisting of methanol and acetone in 1:1 ratio.
Tannins are polyphenolic compounds	Tannins are polyphenolic compounds present in high concentration mostly in water or alcoholic plant extracts. Tannins can be separated by partitioning with 1% NaOH solution or precipitation by 5% w/v NaCl and 0.5% w/v gelatin.

After the removal of these substances, the methods usually adapted for purification of phytoconstituents are as follows:

Various Purification Methods	
Filtration	➢ Filter press (Filtration by high pressure), Membrane/Ultra/Nano filtration (use of pressure to filter material through a semi permeable material)
Separation	➢ Liquid-Liquid Extraction (separation by using immiscible solvents) ➢ Separation, based on size, mass, charge, lipophilicity, solubility, thermostability
Chromato-graphic Method	➢ **Chromatographic separation and Purification: Following are** chromatographic techniques useful for separation and isolation of phytochemicals from extracts:

Contd...

	Liquid Chromatographic (LC)Techniques - **A. Column Chromatography** • Open Column Chromatography (CC) • High performance Liquid Chromatography (HPLC) • Gas Chromatography (GC) • Affinity chromatography (AC) • Ion exchange chromatography (IEC) • Gel filtration chromatography **B. Planar Chromatography** • Planar Chromatography (PC) • Thin layer chromatography (TLC) • High performance Thin layer chromatography (HPTLC) • Reversed Phase Thin layer chromatography (RPC) • Optimum performance laminar chromatography or Over Pressured Layer Chromatography (OPLC)
Electrophoresis	Electrophoresis is an easy and comparatively inexpensive and powerful molecular separation technique for DNA, proteins and or enzymes. Electrophoresis is based on the principle that charged particles in a liquid media under the influence of an electric field will migrate to the electrode of the opposite charge. Positive ions (cations) will migrate to the cathode (negative electrode) and negative ions (anions) will migrate to the anode (positive electrode).
Concentration/ Evaporation	Concentration is to get more solid matter by evaporating liquid matter.
Crystallization	Crystallization is the (natural or artificial) process of solid-liquid separation by formation of solid crystals precipitating from a solution. Crystallization is also a chemical technique, in which mass transfer of a solute from the liquid solution to a pure solid crystalline phase occurs. Nucleation (gathering of solute into clusters) and crystal growth (growth to critical cluster size) are two major events of crystallization process. Recrystallization can be Single-solvent (through addition of mallest amount of hot solvent to mixture) or Multi-solvent (two or more solvents use).

Preliminary Phytochemical Testing (Qualitative Testing)

Class of Drugs	Procedure	Inference
Carbohydrates		
Molisch's test [Dissolve 3.75 g of 1-naphthol in 25 ml of Ethanol 99%.]	Mix 1 ml reagent in 2 ml of test solution. Add 1 ml of concentrated sulfuric acid.	Red to violet ring depending on the amount of sugar appears at the junction of the two liquids.
Iodine test for starch	Mix 0.5 ml of iodine solution with 1 ml of the test solution.	Starch gives deep blue color.
Fehling's test [Fehling's "A" is 7 g copper(II) sulfate pentahydrate dissolved in distilled water containing 2 drops of dilute sulfuric acid.	Mix 1 ml of Fehling's solution 'A' with 1 ml of Fehling's solution 'B' and 1 ml of test solution. Then, boil it.	Yellow to red precipitate indicates presence of reducing sugars

Contd...

<table>
<tr><th>Class of Drugs</th><th>Procedure</th><th>Inference</th></tr>
<tr><td>Fehling's "B" is 35g of potassium tartrate and 12g of NaOH in 100 ml of distilled water. These two solutions should be stoppered and stored until needed.]</td><td></td><td></td></tr>
<tr><td>Benedict's test
[Benedict's reagent is prepared by mixing 17.3 grams of copper sulfate pentahydrate, 100 grams of sodium carbonate, and 173 grams of sodium citrate in distilled water (required quantity).]</td><td>Mix 2 ml of Benedict's reagent with 2 ml test solution. Boil it in a water bath.</td><td>Formation of red, yellow or green colored precipitate depending on the sugar concentration indicates presence of reducing sugars<table><tr><th>Colour of the Precipitate</th><th>Approximate percentage of Reducing Sugar</th></tr><tr><td>Green</td><td>0.5%</td></tr><tr><td>Yellow</td><td>1%</td></tr><tr><td>Orange</td><td>1.5%</td></tr><tr><td>Red</td><td>2%</td></tr></table></td></tr>
<tr><td>Barfoed's test
[Barfoed's reagent is 0.33 molar solution of copper (II) acetate in 1% acetic acid solution.]</td><td>Mix 2 ml of Barfoed's reagent with 1 ml of the test solution. Boil it and wait.</td><td>Brick-red precipitate of monosaccharides.</td></tr>
<tr><td>Seliwanoff's test for ketohexoses
[Seliwanoff's Reagent is 110 mg of Resorcinol in 220 ml of 3N HCl.]</td><td>Mix 2 ml of Seliwanoff's reagent with 1 ml of test solution. Boil.</td><td>Deep red color due to ketohexoses.</td></tr>
<tr><td>Bial's test for pentoses
[Bial's reagent is 0.4 g orcinol, 200 ml of concentrated hydrochloric acid and 0.5 ml of a 10% solution of ferric chloride.]</td><td>Mix 5 ml of Bial's reagent with 1 ml of test solution. Warm slowly.</td><td>Green color precipitate due to pentoses.</td></tr>
<tr><td>Gum</td><td></td><td></td></tr>
<tr><td>Fehling's or Benedict's test.</td><td>Take the powder of gum sample and add HCl to hydrolyze the polysaccharides. Now, perform Fehling's or Benedict's test.</td><td>Positive test.</td></tr>
<tr><td>Mucilage</td><td></td><td></td></tr>
<tr><td>Ruthenium red test</td><td>Treat the powder with ruthenium red.</td><td>Red color</td></tr>
<tr><td>Swelling test</td><td>Dissolve the powder in water.</td><td>Powder swells</td></tr>
<tr><td>Fatty Oil</td><td></td><td></td></tr>
<tr><td>Filter paper test</td><td>Press the powder between filter paper.</td><td>Permanent oily spot.</td></tr>
<tr><td>Solubility test</td><td>Mix oil in alcohol.</td><td>Insoluble</td></tr>
</table>

Contd...

Proteins		
Biuret test [Biuret reagent is prepared by mixing 1.5 gram of pentavalent copper sulphate ($CuSO_4$), 6 gram of Sodium potassium tartarate (chelating agent) in 500 ml of distilled water and 375 ml of 2 molar Sodium hydroxide Mix and make final volume to 1000 ml by adding distilled water.	Mix 2 ml test solution with 2 ml Biuret reagent.	Violet to pink color
Millon's test [Millon's reagent is Mercuric Nitrate-160 g, Mercurous Nitrate-160 g, Conc. Nitric acid-400 ml and Distilled water-600 ml	Mix 2 ml test solution with 2 ml Millon's reagent. Boil it.	Red color
Lead acetate test	Mix 2 ml test solution with 2 ml of 40% NaOH and 0.5 ml lead acetate solution. Boil it.	Black to brown color
Amino Acids		
Ninhydrin test [Ninhydrin reagent is 0.2 grams of ninhydrin in 10ml of either ethanol or acetone]	Mix 2 ml test solution with 1 ml of 5% ninhydrin solution. Boil for 5 minutes in water bath.	Blue or purple color.
Tyrosine test	Mix 2 ml test solution with 1 ml Millon's reagent and boil the solution.	Dark red color.
Alkaloids		
Dragendorff's reagent (Potassium Bismuth iodide)	Mix 2 ml of reagent with 2 ml filtrate of plant drug extract.	Reddish brown precipitate.
Modified Dragendorff's reagent (Kraut's reagent) (Potassium Bismuth iodide + Nitric acid)	Mix 2 ml of reagent with 2 ml filtrate of plant drug extract.	Precipitate
Hager's reagent (Picric acid)	Mix 2 ml of reagent with 2 ml filtrate of plant drug extract.	Yellow color precipitate
Mayer's reagent (Potassium mercuric iodide)	Mix 2 ml of reagent with 2 ml filtrate of plant drug extract.	Cream colored precipitate
Wagner's reagent (Potassium iodide)	Mix 2 ml of reagent with 2 ml filtrate of plant drug extract.	Reddish brown precipitate.

Contd...

Class of Drugs	Procedure	Inference
Glycosides		
General test	**Solution A:** Extract sample powder with alcohol or water, and then, add Fehling Solution. **Solution B:** Add sulfuric acid and then add Fehling Solution to water or alcoholic extract	If solution B has dark color than solution A (if sugar content is high in solution B than solution A), it indicates the presence of glycosides. **Note**: Acid hydrolyzes glycone and aglycone moiety and thus, sugar content is increased in solution B.
Cardiac Glycosides		
Kedde's test [Kedde Reagent A: Dissolve 3,5-dinitrobenzoic acid (2 g) in 90% ethanol). Kedde Reagent B: Dissolve sodium hydroxide (5 g) in distilled water 000 ml)]	Mix 1 ml of test solution with 2 ml reagent.	Blue to purple color
Baljet reagent (Bufadienolides)	Mix 2–3 mg of sample in 2 ml sodium picrate solution.	Yellow and orange to deep red color
Keller-kiliani test for digitoxose sugar	To the alcoholic extract of sample, add 5 ml of water and 0.5 ml of strong solution of lead acetate. Filter and treat the clear filtrate with equal volume of chloroform, and evaporate to yield dry residue. Add glacial acetic acid, 0.5 ml of ferric chloride solution, and 2 ml of concentrated sulfuric acid.	The initial red-brown layer changes to blue green.
Legal's test (Cardenolides)	Mix 1 ml of test solution with 2 ml pyridine and sodium nitroprusside.	Pink or red color
Raymond test (alkaline m-dinitrobenzene)	Mix alcoholic extract of sample in 0.1 ml of Raymond's reagent and add 2-3 drops of 20% NaOH solution.	Violet color changes to blue
Flavonoids		
Shinoda test	Add magnesium powder and a few drops of concentrated HCl or H_2SO_4 to 2 ml of sample solution.	Flavones, flavonols and xanthones: Orange, pink, red, and purple. Flavanones and flavononols: weak pink to magenta colors, or no color at all.
Modified Shinoda test	The procedure is same as above except the use of zinc powder instead of magnesium.	Flavanonols: Deep-red to magenta color

Contd...

Class of Drugs	Procedure	Inference
Sulphuric acid	Add 3 ml of H_2SO_4 in sample.	Flavones and flavonols: Deep yellow color. Chalcones and aurones: Red or red-bluish. Flavanones: Orange to red colors.
Lead acetate	Mix test solution with lead acetate.	Yellow precipitate
Alkali test	Treat test solution with increasing amount of NaOH.	Yellow coloration which decolorizes after addition of acid
Tannins		
Ferric chloride test	Mix 2 ml of test solution with 5% of ferric chloride solution.	Blue, blue-black or blue-green color reaction
Gelatin-salt test	Prepare three test tubes of extract solution. To the first, add 1% solution of NaCl; to the second, add 1% NaCl and 5% gelatin solution; and to the third, add $FeCl_3$ solution.	Formation of a precipitate in the second treatment suggests the presence of tannins and a positive response after addition of $FeCl_3$ to the third portion supports this inference.
Lead acetate test	Mix test solution with lead acetate solution.	White precipitate
Bromine water test	Mix test solution with bromine water.	Discoloration of original solution
Dilute iodine test	Mix test solution with dilute iodine solution.	Red color to solution
Triterpenoids		
Liebermann–Burchard test	Mix 2 ml test extract with 1 ml chloroform, 1 ml acetic anhydride, and add one drop concentrated H_2SO_4.	Blue-green to red-orange color. A bluish-green or blue color indicates presence of steroids, and a pink-violet color indicates terpenoids.
Noller's test	Mix 2 ml test extract with small quantity of tin and thionyl chloride.	Pink coloration indicates the presence of triterpenoids.
Sannie test	Mix 2 ml extract with stannous chloride, acetic acid and carbon tetrachloride (6:50:50). Heat at $100^{o}C$	Brown color
Steroids		
Liebermann test	Mix 2 ml test extract with 2 ml acetic anhydride. Boil and add 0.5 ml of H_2SO_4.	Blue color.
Zimmermann test (% dinitrobenzene)	Mix 2 ml test extract with 1 ml of 2N KOH in alcohol and 1 ml 1% dinitrobenzene in alcohol. After 10 min add this mixture to 8 ml alcohol.	Violet color
Salkowski reaction	Dissolve 1–2 mg of the sample in 1 ml of $CHCl_3$ and add 1 ml concentrated H_2SO_4.	**Chloroform** layer shows red color and acid layer shows green fluorescence

Contd...

Class of Drugs	Procedure	Inference
Saponins		
Foam test	Shake aqueous solution of a saponin containing sample producing foam, which is stable for 15 seconds or more.	Foam lasts for more than 15 seconds
Hemolysis test	Mix red blood sample with sufficient quantity of extract solution. Shake and observe.	Clear red solution
Anthraquinone Glycosides		
Borntrager's test o-glycosides	Take a little quantity of aqueous solution of sample; add H_2SO_4, then add CCl_4 or ether in it. Separate the organic layer and shake with dilute ammonia.	Rose pink color of ammonia layer.
Modified anthraquinone test for C-glycosides	Take little quantity of aqueous solution of sample; add ferric chloride solution, HCl, and then add CCl_4 or ether. Separate the organic layer and shake with dilute ammonia.	Rose pink color of ammonia layer
Cyanogenetic Glycosides		
Sodium picrate test (Guignard picrate test)	Take the aqueous test solution of sample in test tube and add dilute H_2SO_4; suspend sodium picrate treated filter paper.	Hydrogen Cyanide (HCN) turns the paper to brick red color due to formation of sodium iso-perpurate.
Mercurous nitrate test	Mix 2 ml test extract solution with 3% aqueous mercurous nitrate solution.	Formation of metallic mercury
Guaiacum test	Dip strip of paper in guaiacum resin, then, moisten with dilute $CuSO_4$ and exposed to cut surface of crude drug.	Paper turns to blue due to HCN.
Coumarin Glycosides		
Odour test	Take the odour of powder or extract.	Aromatic smell.
Alkali test	Mix the test solution with alkali.	Blue green fluorescence
Fluorescence filer paper test	Take the moist powder of drug in test tube, cover test tube with alkali moist filter paper. Heat the test tube and observe paper under UV light.	Yellow green fluorescence
Essential Oil		
Sudan red III test	Treat the test solution with Sudan red III.	Red color
Tincture alkana test (Alkannatinctoria roots)	Treat the test solution with tincture alkana.	Red color
Solubility test	Dissolve the oil in alcohol.	Completely soluble

Quantitative Estimation of Phytochemicals

Estimation of primary (carbohydrates, proteins, lipids/fats, enzymes) and secondary metabolites (alkaloids, glycosides, saponins, flavonoids, phenolics, tannins, steroids) along with vitamins, minerals helps in screening of nutrional, nutraceutical and pharmaceutical potential of herbal drugs. Gravimetric, colorimetric, spectrophotometric and chromatographic estimation methods and or assay and their modifications are explored by many researchers and authors.

Structural Elucidation of Natural Products

Introduction

Chemical fingerprints obtained by chromatographic and spectroscopic techniques have become the most preferred tools for structural elucidation of phytochemicals. Further, the combination of qualitative fingerprinting and quantitative multi-component analysis is a novel and rational method to address the key issues of structural elucidation of phytochemicals. The progression of analytical techniques serves as a quick and precise tool in the structural elucidation of phytochemicals.

Computation Techniques in Structural Elucidation

Till date, structural elucidation of phytochemicals is a major challenge due to its time-consuming process. Recently, Computer-aided structure elucidation is getting popularity due to generation of matching list of possible chemical structure/s and by ranking these structures in order of probability.

NMR/LC-MS and X-ray spectroscopy based Bruker Complete molecular confidence (CMC) helps in automated verification of molecular formulae and structure through analysis information-rich spectroscopic techniques data.

ACD/Structure Elucidator Suite automatically compares predicted and experimental NMR and or mass spectra by collectively applying all possible analytical data in one place. It suggests match as well as alternatives to a proposed structure.

Spectroscopic Elucidation of Phytoconstituents

Introduction

Spectroscopy is analytical technique use to study interaction between electromagnetic radiation (EMR) and matter. It measures amount of radiation transmitted or absorbed which is specific for each molecule/s. Spectroscopic methods can be classified according to the region of the electromagnetic spectrum involved in the measurement. The regions that have been used include gamma-ray, X-ray, Ultraviolet (UV), Visible, Infrared (IR), Microwave and Radio frequency (RF).

Spectroscopic methods are classified as atomic, molecular or ionic based on their application. Most acceptable classification is based on EMR interactions is as follows:

- ***Absorption spectroscopy***: Infrared, ultraviolet, visible and microwave spectroscopy
- ***Emission spectroscopy***: Fluorescence spectroscopy, flame photometry
- ***Scattering spectroscopy***: Raman spectroscopy.

Ultraviolet (UV) and Visible Spectroscopy is concerned with the study of absorption of UV-visible radiation. Radiation wavelength range from UV-radiation: 200-400nm, visible 400-800nm. When light is absorbed by a material, valence (outer) electrons are promoted from their normal (ground) states to higher energy (excited) states. This is called transition due to characteristic spectrum is obtained according to nature of substances. The absorption is characteristic and depends on the nature of electrons present .The intensity depends on the concentration and path length. This spectroscopy is useful in identification of unsaturation and or aromatic nature of phytochemicals. Isolated double bonds, α, β-unsaturated esters, acids, lactones also have characteristic maxima

Infrared Spectroscopy uses electromagnetic spectrum between the visible and microwave regions which is divided into three regions: the near (12500-4000 cm^{-1}), mid (4000-400 cm^{-1}), and far IR (400-10 cm^{-1}). Mid infrared radiation interaction with organic molecules converts energy of molecular vibration or rotational energy which generates fingerprint spectrum signifying functional groups present in isolated phytochemicals- Example-hydroxyl (-OH) group (~3400cm^{-1}), *oxo*(-O) group (saturated 1750-1700cm-1)

Mass Spectrometry is a powerful analytical technique used to elucidate molecular weight and chemical structure of phytochemicals. A mass spectrometer generates multiple ions by fragmentation, separates them based on mass-to-charge ratio (m/z), and then records the relative abundance of each separated ion. Mass spectrum is a plot of ion abundance versus mass-to-charge ratio.

Nuclear Magnetic Resonance Spectroscopy measures the interaction of nuclei of atoms that possess both "magnetic moments" and "angular momentum" under external magnetic field. NMR is useful to determine quality and quantity of hydrogen, carbon routinely. Simple phytochemical structures are determined by one dimension (1D-NMR) while larger and complex structures are determined by two dimensions- (2D-NMR: COSY, NOESY, HSQC, HMBC, TOCSY) or three dimensions (3D-NMR) NMR techniques.

Thus following important points cane be considered while elucidating molecule's structure:

- Calculate Index of Hydrogen Deficiency (IHD) from molecular formula because once, the molecular formula of an unknown compound is known, structural information can be elucidated by IHD.
- List important structural information of a molecule available from UV-VIS, IR, ^{1}H-NMR, ^{13}C-NMR, and mass spectra.
- Correlate the signals and their intensities, integrate the information in different types of spectra of a molecule to similar structures.
- Predict and verify the spectral information from molecule's structural formula.

Role of Spectroscopy in Structural Elucidation

Different types of molecular spectra of same phytochemical contain important key information and can be efficiently used for the structure elucidation of the organic molecules. This is done by correlating the spectral signals to different structural units present in the molecule, comparing them with available library of similar and or alternative structures and predicting molecule as well as its structure. In this context, use the information available from UV-Vis, IR, ^{1}HNMR, 13CNMR and mass spectrometry. UV spectrum is used to predict whether compound is aromatic or aliphatic and saturated or unsaturated. Fingerprint region of IR spectrum gives details of functional groups present in a molecule. NMR yields information about quality and quantity of hydrogen and carbon atoms in the structure. Mass spectroscopy is useful to determine molecular weight and fragmentation pattern of a molecule. Thus, every spectroscopic data is very useful for detail construction of molecule's architecture.

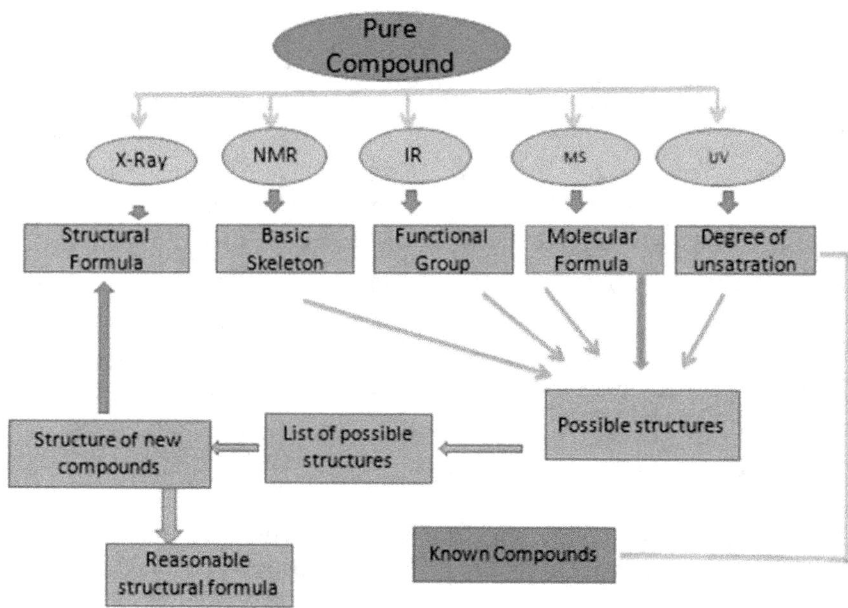

Figure 2.2 Role of Spectroscopy In structural elucidation.

EXAMPLE 1: ATROPINE

Chemical Name: (1R, 5S)-8-methyl-8-azabicyclo [3.2.1] octan-3-yl 3-hydroxy-2-phenolpropanoate

Chemical Formula: $C_{17}H_{23}NO_3$

Exact Mass: 289.17

Molecular Weight: 289.37

Element Analysis: C, 70.56; H, 8.01; N, 4.84; O, 16.59

M.P.: 118°C

Atropine

IR (Kbr cm^{-1}): 750, 1050, 1080, 1180, 1250, 1430, 1710, 2990

MS: 290, 284, 261, 231, 207, 187, 141, 141, 112, 89, 77, 54.

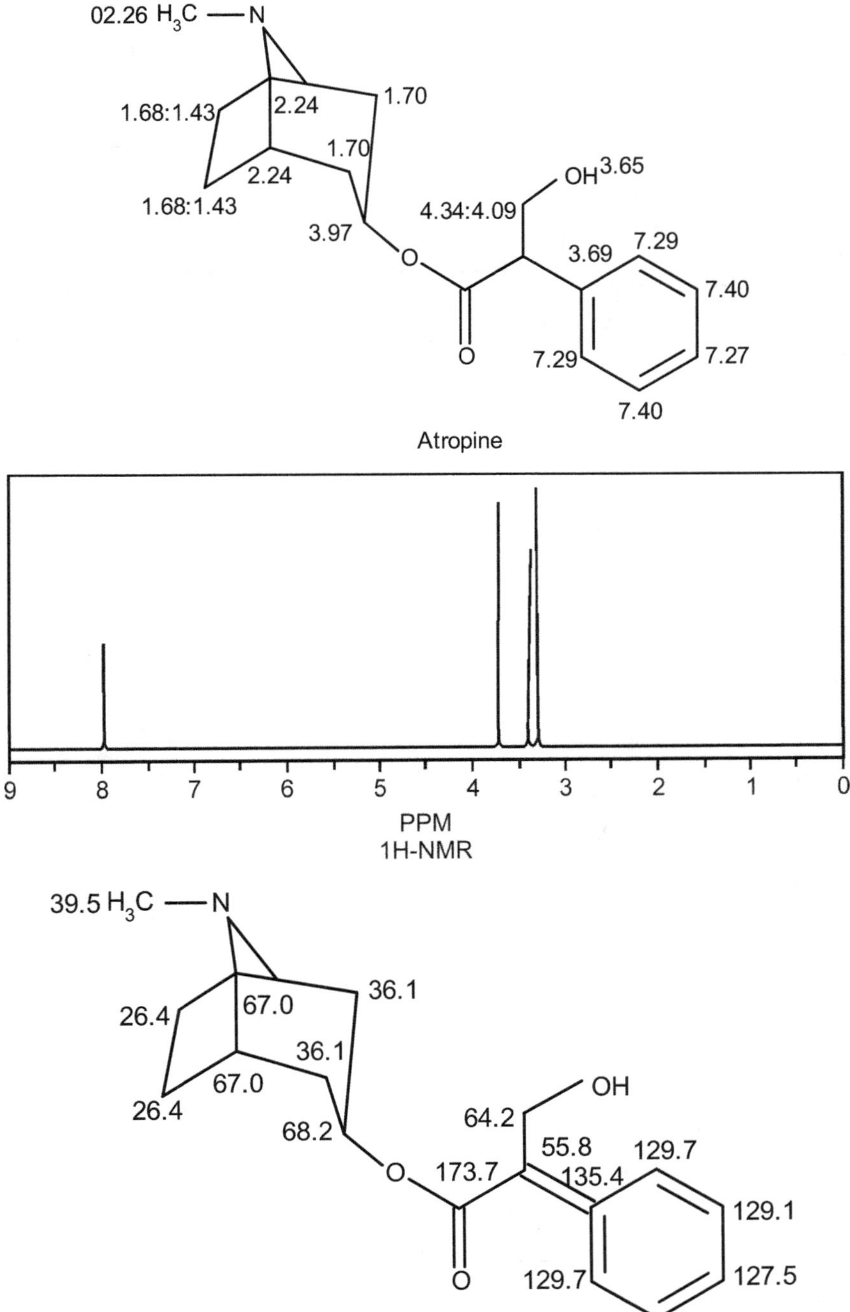
02.26 H_3C — N
1.68:1.43
2.24
1.70
1.70
2.24
1.68:1.43
3.97
4.34:4.09
OH 3.65
3.69
7.29
7.40
7.27
7.29
7.40
O
O
Atropine
9 8 7 6 5 4 3 2 1 0
PPM
1H-NMR
39.5 H_3C — N
26.4
67.0
36.1
36.1
67.0
26.4
68.2
64.2
OH
55.8
173.7
135.4
129.7
129.1
127.5
129.7
129.1
O
O

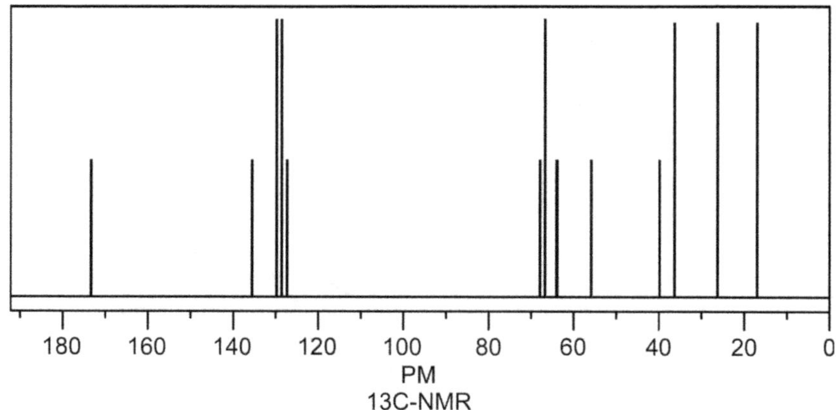

EXAMPLE 2: CAFFIENE

Chemical Name: 1, 3, 7-trimethyl-1H-purine-2, 6(3H, 7H)-dione

Chemical Formula: C8H10N4O2

Exact Mass: 194.08

Molecular Weight: 194.19

Element Analysis: C, 49.48; H, 5.19; N, 28.85; O, 16.48

M.P.: 228 – 235°C

IR (KBr cm–1): 1703 (C=O), 974 (C–CStr), 1361 (C–H bend), 2953 (C–H), 1546 (C–N Str.),1548.89, 3111 (N–H Str.)

MS: 194, 165, 137, 109, 97, 94, 82, 67

Caffiene

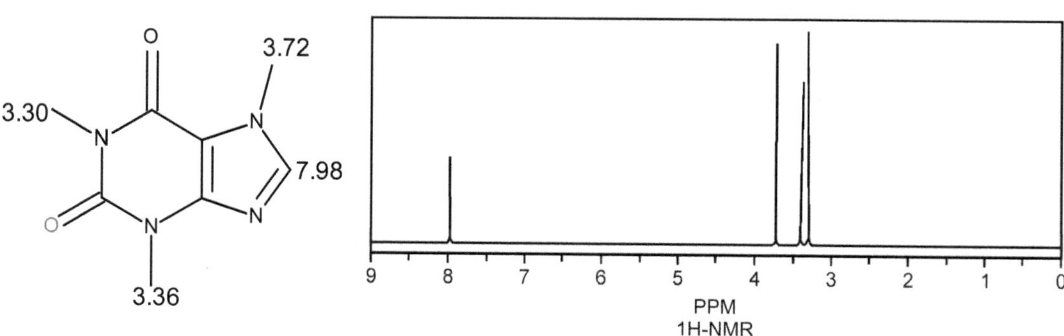

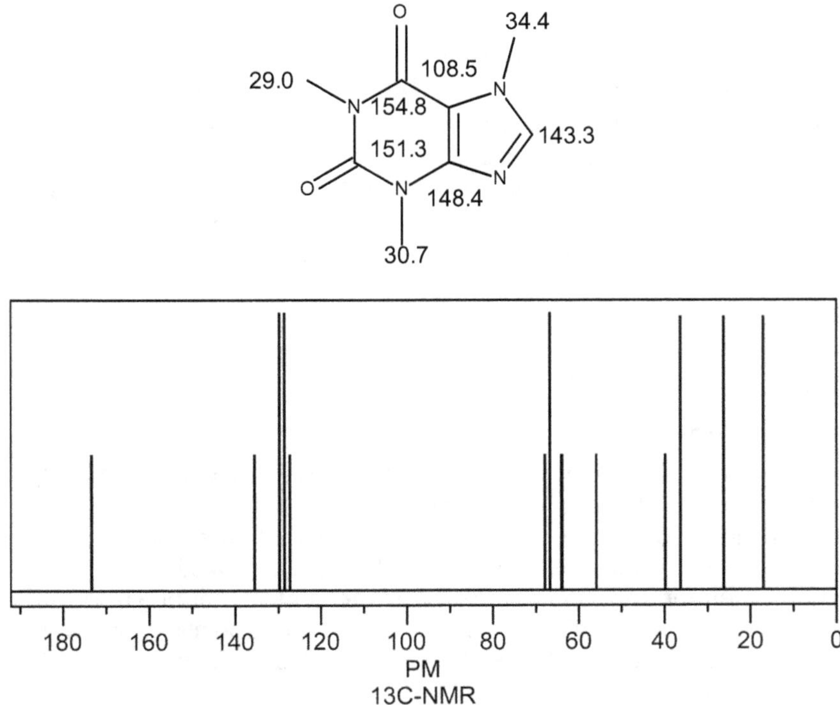

Role of Hyphenated Techniques in Structural Elucidation

Known or new phytochemicals can be identified and characterized rapidly with the help of combined application of modern hyphenated techniques without time-consuming and costly isolation and or purification steps.

Combining chromatography with spectrometry provides the advantage of both chromatography as a separation method and spectrometry as an identification method. Gas chromatography-Mass Spectrometry (GC–MS), first successful hyphenated technique, is widely used in the structural analysis of volatile chemicals from herbal drugs. GC-FTIR found useful in analysis of simple to complex components in herbal extracts.

Liquid chromatography mass spectrometry (LC-MS), highly sensitive and specific hyphenated technique, helps in specific detection and potential identification of individual phytochemicals in the mixture. Raw materials like honey and animal fats can be authenticated by this technique and the spectral fingerprints of them can be generated.

Liquid chromatography- Nuclear magnetic resonance (LC-NMR) and LC-PDA-NMR-MS has been demonstrated to be a valuable analytical tool for the analysis pharmacokinetics, toxicity studies, and thus drug discovery process due to improved speed and sensitivity of detection.

Conclusion

Present chapter has summarized various steps of processing of herbal raw material, extract preparation, qualitative evaluation, and quantitative estimation and chromatography-spectroscopy applications in chemical composition screening of herbs or derived extracts. Herbal extracts are used in medicine, cosmetics, nutraceuticals and agriculture industry. The therapeutic or physiological benefits are due to different chemical constituents present in extracts. Phyto equivalence or bioequivalence for Herbal products is still under development due to multicomponent nature of the herbal extracts and to the natural variability of their constituents.

Further Reading

Processing of Herbal Raw Materials

1. WHO guidelines on good agricultural and collection practices (GACP) for medicinal plants. Geneva: World Health Organization; 2003.
2. WHO guidelines on assessing quality of herbal medicines with reference to contaminants and residues. Geneva: World Health Organization; 2007.
3. WHO guidelines for selecting marker substances of herbal origin for quality control of herbal medicines. In: WHO Expert Committee on Specification for Pharmaceutical Preparations: fifty-first report. Geneva: World Health Organization; 2017: Annex 1 (WHO Technical Report Series, No. 1003).
4. WHO good manufacturing practices (GMP): supplementary guidelines for the manufacture of herbal medicines. In: WHO Expert Committee on Specifications for Pharmaceutical Preparations: fortieth report. Geneva: World Health Organization; 2006: Annex 3 (WHO Technical Report Series, No. 937).
5. WHO guidelines on good manufacturing practices (GMP) for herbal medicines. Geneva: World Health Organization; 2007.
6. WHO good manufacturing practices (GMP): supplementary guidelines for the manufacture of herbal medicines. In: WHO Expert Committee on Specifications for Pharmaceutical Preparations: fifty-second report. Geneva: World Health Organization; 2018: Annex 2 (WHO Technical Report Series, No. 1010).
7. Quality control methods for herbal materials. Geneva: World Health Organization; 2011.
8. Good manufacturing practices for pharmaceutical products: main principles In: WHO Expert Committee on Specifications for Pharmaceutical Preparations: forty-eighth report. Geneva: World Health Organization; 2014: Annex 2 (WHO Technical Report Series, No. 986).
9. Safety issues in the preparation of homeopathic medicines. Geneva: World Health Organization; 2009.
10. The International Pharmacopoeia, seventh edition. Geneva: World Health Organization; 2017.
11. WHO monographs on selected medicinal plants, volume 1. Geneva: World Health Organization; 1999.
12. WHO monographs on selected medicinal plants, volume 2. Geneva: World Health Organization; 2002.
13. WHO monographs on selected medicinal plants, volume 3. Geneva: World Health Organization; 2007.

14. WHO monographs on selected medicinal plants, volume 4. Geneva: World Health Organization; 2009.
15. WHO monographs on selected medicinal plants commonly used in the Newly Independent States (NIS). Geneva: World Health Organization; 2010.
16. General guidelines for methodologies on research and evaluation of traditional medicine Geneva: World Health Organization; 2000 (WHO/EDM/TRM/2000.1)
17. European Medicines Agency 2006a. Guideline on Quality of Herbal Medicinal Products/Traditional Herbal Medicinal Products (CPMP/QWP/2819/00 Rev)
18. European Medicines Agency 2006b. Guideline on Specifications: Test Procedures and Acceptance Criteria for Herbal Substances, Herbal Preparations and Herbal Medicinal Products/Traditional Herbal Medicinal Products (CPMP/QWP/2820/00 Rev)
19. European Medicines Agency 2008. Reflection Paper on Markers used for Quantitative and Qualitative Analysis of Herbal Medicinal Products and Traditional Herbal Medicinal Products (EMEA/HMPC/253629/2007).
20. WHO guidelines on good herbal processing practices for herbal medicines. WHO Technical Report Series, No. 1010, 20

Extraction, Purification and Preliminary Phytochemical Screening

1. Altemimi A, Lakhssassi N, Baharlouei A, Watson DG, Lightfoot DA. Phytochemicals: Extraction, Isolation, and Identification of Bioactive Compounds from Plant Extracts. Plants (Basel). 2017;6(4):42.
2. VenketeshwerRao, Leticia Rao. Phytochemicals: Isolation, Characterisation and Role in Human Health. BoD – Books on Demand, 2015
3. W. David Ollis, Edi.Sir Derek Barton, W. David Ollis. Advances in Medicinal Phytochemistry. J. LibbeyEurotext, 1986.
4. Cannell R J P. Natural Products Isolation. New Jersey: Human Press Inc; 1998. pp. 165–208.
5. Fabricant D S, Farnsworth N R. The value of plants used in traditional medicine for drug discovery. Environ Health Perspect. 2001;109:69–75.
6. Huie C W. A review of modern sample-preparation techniques for the extraction and analysis of medicinal plants. Anal Bioanal Chem. 2002;373:23–30.
7. Heftmann F. Chromatography: Fundamentals and Application of Chromatographic and Electrophoretic Techniques. 5th edn., Elsevier, Amsterdam, The Netherlands. 1992.
8. Weiss J, wesiss T. Handbook of Ion Chromatography. Wiley-VCH, Weinheim, Germany. 2004.
9. Harborne JB. Phytochemical Methods: A guide to modern techniques of plant analysis. 2nd Edition. Chapman and Hall publishers: 3, Springer. Germany. 1998.
10. Sherma J, Zweig G. Paper Chromatography. Academic Press, New York., USA. 1971.
11. Stahl E. Thin Layer Chromatography. Springer-verlag, Berlin. 1965.
12. Hahn-Deinstrop E. Applied Thin Layer Chromatography: Best practice and avoidance of Mistakes. Wiley-VCH, Weinheim, Germany. 2000.
13. Littlewood AB. Gas Chromatography Principle, Techniques and Applications. Academic Press, London, U.K. 1962.
14. Burchfield AP, Storrs EE. Biochemical Applications of Gas chromatography. Academic press, New York., USA. 1962.
15. Hancock WS. High Performance Liquid Chromatography in Biotechnology. Wiley-Interscience, New Jersey, USA. 1990.

16. Katz ED. High Performance Liquid Chromatography: Principle and Methods in Biotechnology (Separation science Series). John wiley& sons, New Jersey, USA. 1995.
17. J. B. Harborne, H. Baxter, and G. P. Moss, Phytochemical Dictionary: Handbook of Bioactive Compounds from Plants, Taylor & Francis, London, UK, 2nd edition, 1999.
18. GS Kumar. KN Jayaveera. A Textbook of Pharmacognosy and Phytochemistry. S CHAND & Company Limited. India. 2014.
19. Simone BadalMccreath. RupikaDelgoda. Pharmacognosy-Fundamentals, Applications and Strategies. Elsevier Science. 2017
20. Biren Shah, Avinash Seth. Textbook of Pharmacognosy and Phytochemistry. Elsevier Health Sciences. 2014
21. AshutoshKar. PharmacognosyAndPharmacobiotechnology. New Age International (P) Limited. 2003
22. Michael Heinrich, Elizabeth M. Williamson, Joanne Barnes, Simon Gibbons, Jose Prieto-Garcia Fundamentals of Pharmacognosy and Phytotherapy E-Book. Elsevier Health Sciences. 2017
23. W.C.Evans, Trease and Evans Pharmacognosy, 16th edition, W.B. Sounders & Co., London, 2009.
24. Jean Bruneton. Pharmacognosy, Phytochemistry, Medicinal Plants. Technique & Documentation. 1999
25. Luqi Huang. Molecular Pharmacognosy. Springer Netherlands. 2012
26. Gunnar Samuelsson. Drugs of Natural Origin-A Textbook of Pharmacognosy. Apotekarsocieteten. 1999
27. A.N.M. Alamgir. Therapeutic Use of Medicinal Plants and Their Extracts: Volume 1
28. Pharmacognosy- Volume 1. Springer International Publishing. 2017
29. Michael Heinrich, Joanne Barnes, Simon Gibbons. Fundamentals of Pharmacognosy and Phytotherapy. Churchill Livingstone/Elsevier. 2012
30. K. Mangathayaru. Pharmacognosy: An Indian perspective. Pearson Education India. 2013
31. Mohammad Ali. Pharmacognosy and Phytochemistry, CBS Publishers & Distribution, New Delhi.2019
32. C.K. Kokate, Purohit, Gokhlae. Text book of Pharmacognosy, 37th Edition, NiraliPrakashan, Pune. 2007
33. Kaliya.A. Text Book of Industrial Pharmacognosy. CBS Publishers & Distributors, Delhi. 2009
34. Rangari VD. Pharmacognosy& Phytochemistry. Career Publication, Nashik. 2008
35. James Bobbers, Marilyn KS, VE Tylor. Pharmacognosy&Pharmacobiotechnology. Williams & Wilkins. 1996.
36. H. Ansari. Essentials of Pharmacognosy. Second edition, Birla publications, New Delhi, 2007
37. S. S. Handa. Pharmacognosy. VallabhPrakashan, New Delhi. 1989
38. N P S Sengar, Ashwini Singh, RiteshAgrawal. A Textbook of Pharmacognosy. PharmaMed Press. 2018
39. Kendall Jefferson. Pharmacognosy and Phytotherapy. Foster Academics.2019
40. C. S. Shah, J. S. Qadry. A Textbook of Pharmacognosy. Messrs B.S. Shah 1971
41. Alice Kurian, M. AshaSankar Medicinal Plants. New India Publishing Agency. 2007
42. T. C. Denston. A Textbook of Pharmacognosy. Read Books. 2012
43. S. S. Agarwal, M. Paridhavi. Herbal Drug Technology. Universities Press. 2012

44. SaikatSen, Raja Chakraborty Herbal Medicine in India-Indigenous Knowledge, Practice, Innovation and Its Value. Springer Singapore. 2019
45. Kokate CK. Practical Pharmacognosy. VallabhPrakashan, Delhi. 2005
46. K. R. Khandelwal. Practical Pharmacognosy. NiraliPrakashan, Pune. 2008
47. Joshi Saroja, VidhuAeri. Practical Pharmacognosy. Frank Brothers. 2009.
48. M AIyengar. Pharmacognosy of Powdered Crude Drugs. PharmaMed Press. 2017
49. M AIyengar, S G K Nayak. Pharmacognosy Lab Manual. PharmaMed Press. 2019
50. M AIyengar. Study of Crude Drugs. PharmaMed Press. 2016
51. Christophe Wiart, Ashok Kumar. Practical Handbook of Pharmacognosy-Preliminary Techniques of Identification of Crude Drugs of Plant Origin. 2000
52. Steven E. Ruzin. Plant Microtechnique and Microscopy.1999
53. VidhuAeri, D.B. AnanthaNarayana, Dharya Singh. Powdered Crude Drug Microscopy of Leaves and Barks. Elsevier Science. 2019
54. Nilambari S. Gurav, Shailendra S. Gurav Indian Herbal Drug Microscopy. Springer New York. 2013
55. AnjooKamboj, MoronkolaDorcasOlufunke Practical Pharmacognosy. Scitus Academics LLC. Thomas Edward Wallis. Practical Pharmacognosy. Churchill. 2018

Structural Elucidation of Natural Products

1. Jeffrey B. Harborne. Phytochemical Methods-A Guide to Modern Techniques of Plant Analysis. Springer Netherlands. 2012
2. Satyajit D. Sarker, LutfunNahar. Computational Phytochemistry. Elsevier. 2018
3. VenketeshwerRao, Leticia G. Rao. Phytochemicals Isolation, Characterisation and Role in Human Health. IntechOpen. 2015
4. Richard J. P. Cannell. Natural Products Isolation. Humana Press. 1998
5. Alexander I. Gray, Satyajit D. Sarker, ZahidLatif. Natural Products Isolation. Humana Press. 2006
6. Juliana M Prado, Mauricio A Rostagno. Natural Product Extraction-Principles and Applications. Royal Society of Chemistry. 2013
7. CorradoTringali. Bioactive Compounds from Natural Sources-Isolation, Characterization and Biological Properties. Taylor & Francis. 2003.
8. Indrayanto G. Validation of Chromatographic Methods of Analysis: Application for Drugs That Derived From Herbs. Profiles Drug SubstExcipRelatMethodol. 2018;43:359-392.
9. Joseph Sherma, Monika Waksmundzka-Hajnos. High Performance Liquid Chromatography in Phytochemical Analysis. CRC Press. 2010
10. Raphael Ikan. Natural Products-A Laboratory Guide. Elsevier Science. 2013
11. T.A. Scott, Sabine Bladt, Eva M. Zgainski. Plant Drug Analysis-A Thin Layer Chromatography Atlas. Springer Berlin Heidelberg. 2013
12. Stefan Berger, Dieter Sicker. Classics in Spectroscopy-Isolation and Structure Elucidation of Natural Products. Wiley. 2009
13. Joseph Sherma, Monika Waksmundzka-Hajnos, Teresa Kowalska. Thin Layer Chromatography in Phytochemistry. CRC Press. 2008
14. N. Raaman. Phytochemical Techniques. New India Publishing Agency. 2006
15. Elke Hahn-Deinstrop. Applied Thin-Layer Chromatography-Best Practice and Avoidance of Mistakes. Wiley. 2007
16. Bernard Fried. Handbook of Thin-Layer Chromatography. Taylor & Francis. 2003
17. M.R.F. Ashworth. Egon Stahl. Thin-Layer Chromatography-A Laboratory Handbook. Springer Berlin Heidelberg. 2013

18. Reiner Westermeier. Electrophoresis in Practice-A Guide to Methods and Applications of DNA and Protein Separations. Wiley. 2016
19. Fraiture MA, Herman P, Taverniers I, De Loose M, Deforce D, Roosens NH. Current and new approaches in GMO detection: challenges and solutions. Biomed Res Int. 2015;2015:392872.
20. T. RabilloudProteome Research: Two-Dimensional Gel Electrophoresis and Identification Methods. Springer.2000

Scan QR code to view the website/guidelines

- Guidelines on minimum requirements for the registration of herbal medicinal products in the Eastern Mediterranean Region-

Microsoft Word - EDBrevisedfinalformat.doc (who.int)

- IMPPAT-

IMPPAT | IMPPAT: Indian Medicinal Plants, Phytochemistry And Therapeutics (imsc.res.in)

CHAPTER 3

Herbal Formulations: Traditional, Conventional and NDDS

Traditional Dosage Forms

Ayurveda, Siddha, Unani, Chinese and Homeopathy based medicine systems have their own different dosage forms which can be categorize as solid, semisolids and liquid dosage forms. Most of these preparations are polyherbal or herbomineral compositions. Detail methods, specific procedures and steps are well explained in traditional manuscripts, authenticate books, pharmacopoeias of respective traditional alternative medicines systems which are unable to get covered in this book.

Ayurvedic Dosage (Kalpana) Form

Ayurvedic name	English name
Vati	Tablet
Gutika	Pill
Churn	Powder
Kwath churn	Coarse powder
Swarasa	Expressed juice
Pravahikwath	Preserved decoction
Asava and arishta	Fermented Alcoholic liquid
Arka	Distilled medicated water
Avleha	Jam like formulation
Pakakhand	Confectionary like formulation
Ghrita	Butter based formulation
Taila	Oil based formulation
Lepa	Paste
Malhara	Ointment
Satva	Water extract
Panaka	Syrup
Aaschayotana	Eye drops
Karnbindu	Ear drop
Nasaya	Nasal drop
Bhasma	Calcinated ash
Lauh and mandora	Iron ash based formulation
Ras yoga	Herbo mineral metallic formulation

Shelf life of Ayurvedic drugs

Sr.No	Dosage form	Shelf life or date of expiry with effect from the date of manufacture
(i)	Anjana	
	(a) Anjana made from Kasthaushadhi	1 year
	(b) Anjana made from Kasthaushadhi along with Rasa/Uprasa/Bhasma	2 years
	(c) Anjana made only from rasa/Uprasa/Bhasma	3 years

Contd...

(ii)	Arka	1 year
(iii)	Asava Arista	10 years
(iv)	Avaleha, Khanda, Paka, Guda	3 years
(v)	Chuma, KwathaChuma, LepaChuma, DantaManjan, (Chuma)	2 years
(vi)	Dhoopan	2 years
(vii)	Dravaka, Lavana, Kshara	5 years
(viii)	Ghrita	2 years
(ix)	Guggulu	5 years
(x)	Gutika/Vati	
	(I) Gutika or Vati containing Kasthaushadhi along with Rasa / Uprasa/ Bhasma/ Guggulu (including LepaGutika and GhanVati)	5 years
	(II) Gutika or Vati containing only Kasthaushadhi (including LepaGutika and GhanVati)	3 years
	(III) Gutika / Vati containing only Ras / Uprasa / Bhasmaexcept Naga, Vanga and TamraBhasma	10 years
(xi)	Kama/ Nasabindu	2 years
(xii)	KupipakvaRasayana	10 years
(xiii)	Malahar	3 years
(xiv)	Mandura-Lauha	10 years
(xv)	Naga Bhasma, Vanga Bhasma and TamraBhasma	5 years
(xvi)	Netrabindu	1 years
(xvii)	Parpati	10 years
(xviii)	Pishti and Bhasma except Naga, Vanga and TamraBhasma	10 years
(xix)	PravahiKwatha	3 years
(xx)	Rasayoga	
	(I) Rasayoga Containing only Rasa / Uprasa / Bhasma except Naga, Vanga and TamraBhasma	10 years
	(II) Rasayoga Containing Rasa / Uprasa/ Bhasma along with Kasthaushadhi/Guggulu	5 years
(xxi)	Sattva (derived from medicinal plant)	2 years
(xxii)	Sharkar / Panak/Sharbat	3 years
(xxiii)	Shvetaparpati	2 years
(xxiv)	Taila	3 years
(xxv)	Varti	2 years

Unani System Dosage Form (Unani Murakkabat)

Unani names	English name
Sufoof	Powder
Zarur	Dusting powder
Kohal	Kajal
Nufookh	Insufflation
Ghaza	Face powder
Ghalia	Perfumed body powder
Noorah	Hair remover
Habb	Pills
Qurs	Tablet
Shiyaf	Suppositories
Firzaja	Pessary
Tila	Liniment
Sanoon or manjan	Tooth powder
Barood	Microfine powder for eye
Joshanda	Decoction
Khesanda	Infusion
Haleeb	Milk
Zulal	Purified water
Mahlool	Solute
Nabeez	Drink
Sharbat	Syrup
Arq	Distillate
Lakhlakha	Inhalation
Bakhoor	Fumigation
Looq	Linctus
Laboob	Pulp
Marham	Ointment
Qaturat	Drops

Siddha System Dosage Forms

Name in siddha system	English Name
Caru	Juice
Karkam	Herbal paste
Churanam	Herbal powder
Vadagam	Lozenges
Manappahu	Syrup
Ennai	Medicated oil

Contd...

Name in siddha system	English Name
Mathirai	Pills
Mezhugu	Medicinal wax
Kuzhampu	Medicinal Semi liquid
Patru	Paste
Pasai	Ointment
Podi	Dusting powder
Gulligai	Tablet
Lehyam	Confections
Bhasmam	Calx prepared by calcination
Kashayam	Extract
Ghrtam	Medicated ghee
Chenduram	Metal complex

Conventional Dosage Forms

Processing of Herbal Dosage Forms

The appropriate and technically sound manufacturing process for herbal dosage forms should be developed indicating raw materials, vehicles if any, critical steps with specific precautions (light, moisture, miscellaneous contamination, and temperatures) to get routine and consistent quality production. Each and every step with sufficient time for operation must be optimized.

Control of critical steps and intermediates involves process and analytical validation and/or evaluation, from initial step to final step should be carried. It is necessary to reference the official Pharmacopoeial manufacturing method if available. Information of characterization of active constituents as well as impurities originating from the raw material(s) and or arising from the manufacturing process should be provided. Impurity degradation products analysis, limits of detection of various analytical parameters - like foreign matters including pesticides should be provided. Quality control tests like chromatographic analysis to confirm composition, loss on drying reference materials or marker analysis. Proper container closure system(s) specifications based on the stock stability studies should be selected for storage of all types of herb derived products. Batch stability data or re-testing (for immediately non-processed material) or post-approval stability protocol required for all types of herb derived products.

Table 3.1 Summary of Processing of Herbal Dosage Forms.

Raw material	Source identification, Process validation from cultivation to collection and its packing
Storage of raw material	Analysis of stores material at the time of use, proper storage conditions
Manufacturing process	Well defined processes, In-process analysis, Temperature effect, residual solvent, organic and inorganic impurities, microbial limits etc
Intermediate materials	Analysis of excipients, proper storage before packaging

Contd...

Finished product	Description of dosage forms and it's State (Solid, liquid, semisolid), Stability, proper container, labels
Quality of herbal drug preparation	Assay, specific tests, aflatoxin, heavy metal and pesticide residue determination
Phytochemical characteristics	Identification by chromatographic methods
Stability of active constituents	Formulation packaging
Specific tests	Oral liquids: uniformity, ph, water content, specific gravity, microbial limits, antimicrobial and antioxidant preservative content, alcohol content, particle size distribution, reconstitution time Tablet, capsule: Dissolution, disintegration, hardness, friability, uniformity of dosage forms, water content, microbial limit,
Safety and efficacy consideration	Clinical and preclinical studies

Herbal Tablets

Tablet are the solid unit dosage forms containing a medicament or mixtures of medicament and excipients compressed or molded into solid cylindrical shape having either flat or convex surface. Monoherbal tablets are having only single herb as an active ingredient, while poly herbal tablets are having more than one active herb within it.

Preparation Methods

Compressed tablets can be prepared by any one of the three basic methods. Each method has its own advantages, disadvantages and limitation.

Wet granulation method

- This is oldest and still most widely used method of tablet preparation. The powdered and mixed tablet constituents are converted to a moist coherent mass by wet screening. The process essentially involves a series of operations such as weighing, mixing, granulation, screening the damp mass, drying, drying screening, lubrication, finally compression. However as all of these operations are time consuming and costly the process does not tend its self to automation.
- ***Procedure:*** The active ingredient, diluent and disintegrant are mixed and blended well. The blended material is then shifted through a screen of suitable mesh to remove or break the lumps. The solution of binding agent is added to the powder with stirring till the mass attains consistency. The damp mass is then forced through 6 and 8 mesh screen. The granular material thus obtained is dried. During drying the particles may agglomerate and form lumps and therefore a dry screening operation is usually required after drying. This followed by the addition of lubricant as a fine powder.

Dry- granulation method

- It is also known as slugging, double compression or recompression method. It can be used when the tablet ingredients are sensitive to moisture or are unable to withstand elevated temperatures during drying. Under these circumstances, dry granulation is the method of choice provided the tablet ingredients have sufficient inherent binding or cohesive properties. Essential steps in this method include weighing, mixing, slugging, dry screening, lubrication and compression. Thus the slugging method requires fever steps than wet granulation and avoids the time handling required for a drying step. A slow production rate is the major disadvantage of this method.

Direct compression:

- The method consists of compressing tablets directly from powdered material without modifying the physical nature of the material itself. This method special interest for a small group of crystalline chemicals having all the physical characteristics necessary for the formation of good tablet. Advantage of the method are simplicity of the process, absence of granulating step, avoidance of moisture and drying steps, minimum material handling, rapidity of the total process and optimum possible bioavailability of the drugs from the resulting tablets. Excepting the limitation that only a few crystalline drugs lend themselves to direct compression, the process has no other major disadvantage.

Evaluation Parameters:

(a) **General appearance:** it includes overall appearance of the tablet like size, shape, odour, taste, colour, surface, consistency, textures physical flaws. Tablet thickness should be controlled with ± 5% variation of standard value.

(b) **Weight variation test:** Twenty tablets are weighed randomly in a batch, and the average weight of the tablet is determined. As per the IP specification, if the tablets weight is

< 80mg- deviation upto 10% is allowed

80-250mg - deviation upto 7.5% is allowed

>250 mg- deviation upto 5% is allowed

(c) If any tablet deviates from the specification, another 10 tablets are selected from the batch and the same procedure is repeated. In case of 30 tablets, not more than one tablet should deviate.

(d) **Hardness test:** It is defined as the force required to break the tablet. This test is performed in order to ensure that the tablet withstands mechanical shocks during manufacture, packaging and shipping of tablet. Various types of hardness testers are used to measure the hardness of the tablet like: Monsanto hardness tester, strong cobb tester, Pfizer tester etc. The tablet hardness should be 2.5-5kg/cm^2 (for conventional tablets), for extended-release tablets hardness should be 5-7.5 kg/cm^2.

(e) **Friability test:** Friability test is performed, in order to ensure the mechanical strength of the tablet during transportation, packing etc. Roche friabilator is the instrument, used to carry out the friability test, in which tablets are weighed before fibrillation, and subjected to fibrillation with a speed of 25 rpm. Thus, the tablets are weighed after fibrillation, and the percentage friability is determined. The deviation should be between **0.5-1%.**

(f) **Disintegration test:** Disintegration is the breakdown of tablet into finely divided particulates or granules in gastrointestinal tract. The time required to disintegrate is called as Disintegration time. Complete disintegration is defined as that state in which any residue of the tablets, except fragments of insoluble coating in the auxiliary tube, is a soft mass having no palpably firm core. The rate of disintegration depends on the type of tablet. The tablets which dissolved by slow solution in mouth or chewed or are to be dissolved in water before administration do not need a disintegration test. The disintegration time is as short as one minute and in other cases it may be as long as 30 min. In general pharmacopeia prescribed limit for 15 min the most of tablet otherwise indicated in monograph.

Assembly of disintegration apparatus contain six cylindrical glass tubes which are transparent with transparent plate having holes. Woven wire gauze made up with stainless steel is attached to the lower plate. This assembly is suspended in 1000 ml beaker and having six discs to protect tablet going out from tubes. Hot plate maintains body temperature and an electrical motor rotates basket as like gastric motion.

For Immediate Release Tablet: Unless otherwise specified, place one tablet to each of the 6 tube of the basket; add the disc to each tube. Maintain apparatus water temperature to35to37-degree Celsius. Operate apparatus for 15 min. Observe the tablets after 30 minutes of operation for uncoated tablets and after 60 minutes for coated tablets, unless otherwise specified. The test is met if all of 6 tablets in the auxiliary tubes have disintegrated completely. If 1 or 2 tablets fail to disintegrate, repeat the test on 12 additional tablets. The test is met if not less than 16 of the total of 18 tablets tested are disintegrated.

For Enteric coated Tablet Unless otherwise specified, perform the following two tests, (a) the test with 1st fluid for disintegration test and (b) the test with the 2nd fluid for disintegration test, separately.

1. Enteric coated tablet and capsule:

(a) *The test with 1st fluid for disintegration test:* Carry out the test for 120 minutes, using 1st fluid for disintegration test according to the procedure described in immediate release preparations. The test is met if none of six dosage units is disintegrated. If 1 or 2 dosage units are disintegrated, repeat the test on additional 12 dosage units. The test is met if not less than 16 of the total of 18 dosage units tested are not disintegrated.

(b) *The test with 2nd fluid for disintegration test*: According to the procedure described in immediate-release preparations, carry out the test with new dosage units for 60 minutes using 2nd fluid for disintegration test and determine if the test is met or not.

Dissolution test: the time required for the given percentage of drug in tablet, to go into solution, under specified set of conditions as in in-vitro test. It can also be considered as solubilisation of drug in dissolution media. Several dissolution apparatuses like paddle over disk, flow through cell, cylindrical apparatus, paddle over disk, etc. used depending on the type of dosage form. For tablets, rotating basket and rotating paddle type is most commonly used. The tablet passes the test if for each of five tablets the amount of active ingredient is in solution is not less than 70% of stated amount.

Herbal Capsules

Capsules are the solid unit dosage form of medicament in which the drug is enclosed in a practically tasteless, hard or softsoluble shell made up of a suitable form of gelatin. Hard capsules are used for filling the solid substances where as soft capsules are used for filling the liquid and semisolids. Monoherbal capsules are having only single herb as an active ingredient, while poly herbal capsules are having more than one active herb encapsulated within it. Capsule shell is made up of gelatin, colorants, opaquing agent, preservatives, water etc.

Preparation Methods(Soft Gelatin Capsule)

Plate process(die press simultaneously seals and cuts out the capsules filled with material) and **Rotary Die process** (large-scale method involves spreading the solution into two rotating drums to form a pair of continuous sheets of gelatin) are commonly used to prepare soft gelatin capsules.

Preparation Methods (Hard Gelatin Capsule)

Automatic process of dipping, spinning, drying, stripping, trimming and joining the capsule is followed to prepare hard gelatin capsules.

Evaluation Parameters

1. **Stability test:** for capsules are performed to know the integrity of gelatin capsule shell (but not to know the stability of therapeutically active agent) and for determining the shelf life of capsules. The tests help in improving the quality of contents of capsule shell and for choosing the appropriate retail package.

   Before actually performing the test following facts:

   (i) the capsule shell is to be stabilized to know atmospheric condition with relative humidity about 20-30 % and temperature about 21-24°c.

2. **Shell integrity test:** This test is performed to find out the integrity of capsule shell. The standard capsule shells kept at the room temperature 40 °c and 80% RH becomes more soft, sticky and swollen. Determination of self-life: Shelf life or the expiry date of packed capsules is determined under normal storage conditions.

3. **Invariability test:** The invariability in the medicaments packed in the capsule shells can be determined by performing the following tests:

   (a) Weight variation test: use 20 hard gelatin capsules are weighted individually average weight per capsule is determined the capsule passes test by if average wt. of capsule is less than 500 mg then % of deviation will be 10 and weight is 500 mg or more than 7.5 % of deviation.

   (b) Content uniformity test: is required all capsule which administered orally the assay done as per monograph of drug in pharmacopeia. Following are some limits to pass test.

Weight of medicament in each capsule	Subtract lower sample	From limit of	The for a	Add For	Upper The	Limit sample
	15	10	5	15	10	5
0.12 gm or less	0.2	0.7	1.5	0.3	0.8	1.8
More than 0.12 gm and less than 0.3	0.2	0.5	1.2	0.3	0.6	1.8
0.3 or more	0.1	0.2	0.8	0.2	0.4	1.0

4. **Disintegration test:** is a method to evaluate the rate of disintegration of solid dosage forms. Disintegration is defined as the breakdown of solid dosage form into small particles after it is ingested.

   Enteric coated granules and capsules containing the enteric coated granules: Shake granules or contents taken out from capsules on a No. 30 (500 pm) sieve as directed in

   1. Granules under Particle Size Distribution Test for Preparations <6.03>, transfer 0.10 g of the residue on the sieve to each of the 6 auxiliary tubes, secure the 6 tubes to the bottom of the basket tightly, and operate the apparatus, using the 1st and 2nd fluids for disintegration test.

      (a) *The test with 1st fluid for disintegration test*: According to the procedure described in immediate-release preparations, carry out the test for 60 minutes, using 1st fluid for disintegration test. The test is met if particles fallen from the openings of the wire gauze number not more than 15.

      (b) *The test with 2nd fluid for disintegration test:* According to the procedure described in immediate-release preparations, carry out the test with new samples for 30 minutes, using 2nd fluid for disintegration test and determine if test is met or not.

5. **Dissolution test**: is an official method to determine the dissolution rate of a solid dosage form. Dissolution rate is defined as the rate at which the drug is released into the systemic circulation from the dosage from.

6. **Moisture permeation test:** This test is to assure the suitability of containers for packaging capsules. The moisture permeating feature of capsules packaged in single unit containers – blister pack or strip pack unit dose containers – glass or plastic bottles are to be determined.

Herbal Semisolid Dosage Forms

Ointments

Ointments are semisolid preparations intended for external application to the skin and mucous membranes. They are composed of fluid hydrocarbons mashed in a matrix of higher melting solid hydrocarbons. Due to high oil content, ointments tend to be greasy and messy to use. This greasiness can be reduced by adding solid components, such as microcrystalline cellulose, which give a dry feel on the skin. Ointment bases may be used for their physical effects or as vehicle for medicated ointments. They are classified into four general groups: Oleaginous base, Absorption base, Water removable base and water soluble base. **Example**- Calendula Ointment

Preparation Methods: Ointments are prepared by two methods, a) incorporation and b) fusion, depending primarily on the nature of the ingredients.

Trituration or Incorporation: The components are mixed until a uniform preparation is attained by mortar and pestle, or rubbing by spatula on an ointment slab in small scale.

Fusion: In this method, allointment base components of formula are mixed and melted together. Other ingredients are added to the congealing mixture in warm condition with stirring. Add heat labile and or volatile ingredients lastly.

Evaluation Parameters

1. **Spredability:** Spredability of the formulation can be determined by an apparatus consists of a wooden block, provided by a pulley at a one end. Fix a rectangular glass plate (ground plate) on this block. Place an excess of ointment (about 3 gm) under study on this ground plate. Sandwich ointment between this plate and another glass plate of same dimension of fixed ground plate and provided with the hook. Place 1 Kg weight on the top of the plates for 5 minutes to expel air and to provide a uniform film of the ointment between the plates. Scrap off excess of the ointment from the edges. Subject the top plate to pull of 80 gms with the help of string attached to the hook and note the time (in seconds) required by top plate to cover a distance of 10 cm. A shorter interval indicates better Spredability. Spredability is given in unit gm.cm/sec Spredability of the formulation may be determined by the following formulation, $S = M \times L/T$ Where, L = length moved by glass slide, T = Time in seconds, M = Weight in pan & S = Spredability
2. **Particle size Consideration:** Particle size can be in the range of 0.2- 20 microns. It can be determined by particle size analyzer instrument.
3. **Penetration:** Rub weighed quantities of the ointments over definite areas of the skin for a given length of time. Collect unabsorbed ointment from the skin and weigh. The difference between the two weights roughly represents the amount absorbed.
4. **Rate of release of drug:** Place small amount of the ointment on the surface of nutrient agar contained in a petri dish or if the medicament is bactericidal, the agar plate is previously seeded with a suitable organism like *S. aureus*. The zone of inhibition is correlated with the rate of release. Another method is filling previously smeared the internal surface of test tubes with thin layers of ointment with saline or serum and after interval of time, estimate the amount of drug present in the serum/saline.
5. **Irritant Effect:** In general, no ointment should possess an irritant effect on the skin or mucous membranes. Irritant effect is determined on skin and eyes of rabbits or the skin in ratsat intervals of 24, 48, 72, and 96 h. Lesions on the cornea, iris, and conjunctiva are eye irritation symptoms while patches on the skin within 2 weeks are indication of skin irritation symptoms.
6. **Viscosity:** capillary tube (Ostwald), coaxial cylinder (Brookfield, Couette) and falling sphere (Hoeppler) type of viscometers are routinely used to measure viscosity at a given temperature.

Consistency type	Approximate viscosity in cps at 25°C	Pharmaceutical example
Soft, spreadable	100,000-300,000	w/o, o/w Cream
Plastic flow, spreadable	300,000-1,000,000	Ointment

7. **Content Uniformity:** Content uniformity is vital in process control parameter and this governs product stability too. Particle size, shear rate, and mixing efficiency are responsible to attain and maintain uniformity of the active drug component.
8. **Tube Extrudability:** Quantity extruded by measuring the force required to extrude the material from tube is extrudability. The semi-solid herbal formulations (cream, ointment etc.) under study should be filled in clean, lacquered aluminum collapsible tube with nozzle of 5mm opening and applies pressure on tube by the help of finger.

Cream

Creams are viscous semisolids for external use. They are usually either o/w emulsions, i.e. aqueous creams or w/o emulsions, i.e. oily creams. Different types of cream available are antiseptic cream, cold cream, anti-acne cream, anti-wrinkle cream etc. e.g. Aloe cold cream

Method of preparation: Emulsified creams are prepared by heating the components of the oily phase (usually including the emulgent) until molten and then cooling to 60°C. The components of the aqueous phase are mixed in a separate vessel and also heated to 60°C. The aqueous phase is then added to the oily phase at the same temperature. This is important and a thermometer should be used. The resulting emulsion should be stirred until cool. Rapid cooling may result in separation of high melting point components. Excessive aeration caused by vigorous stirring may also lead to a granular product. If necessary the product may be homogenized after cooling.

Gels

Gels are semisolid system in which a liquid phase is constrained within a three-dimensional polymeric matrix (consisting of natural or synthetic gums) in which a high degree of physical (or sometimes chemical) cross- linking has been introduced. The polymers used to prepare pharmaceutical gels include the natural gum tragacanth, pectin, carrageen, agar and alginic acid and some synthetic and semi-synthetic materials as methyl-cellulose, hydroxyethylcellulose, car-boxymethylcellulose and the carbopols. **Example**- V-gel by Himalaya

Preparation Methods: It may be prepared by either a fusion process or a special procedure necessitated by the gelling characteristics of the gallant.

Types of Gels	
1.Based on nature of solvent	
Hydro (water based)gels	Gels in which water as continuous liquid phase. Example-Gelatin, cellulose derivatives, poloxamer gel.
Organic (non-aqueous solvent based)Gels	Gels in which non-aqueous solvent as continuous phase. Example-plastibase (polyethylene dissolved in mineral oil), metallic stearate in oils.

Contd...

Xerogels	Solid gels with low solvent concentration produced by evaporation of solvent or freeze drying and can be easily reconstituted by swelling in contact with fresh fluid. Example-Tragacanth ribbons, βcyclodextrin,.
2. Based on rheological properties	
Usually gels exhibit non-Newtonian flow properties. They are classified into,	
Plastic gels	Above yield value of rheogram, elastic gel distorts and begins to flow.Example- flocculated suspensions of Aluminum hydroxide
Pseudo plastic gels	With no rheogramyield value, the viscosity of these gels decreases with increasing rate of shear. Example- Liquid dispersion of tragacanth, sodium alginate
Thixotropic gels.	The bonds between gel particles broken down by shaking and revert back to again gel due to linking together (the reversible isothermal gel-solgel transformation). Example- Kaolin, bentonite and agar.
3. Based on physical nature	
Elastic gels	The fibrous molecules of gels of agar, pectin, guar gum and alginates linked at junction by relatively weak bonds such as hydrogen bonds and free –COOH group forms additional bonding by salt bridge between two adjacent strand networks.
Rigid gels	This rigid gel with network of pores can be formed from macromolecule in which the framework linked by primary valance bond. Example-silica gel

Herbal Liquids

Monoherbal liquids are the liquid dosage forms taken orally and consist of single herbal drugs which is dissolved, dispersed or suspended in a suitable vehicle and polyherbal liquids are those which consist of two or more herbal drugs dissolved, dispersed or suspended in the suitable vehicle in the same dosage form.

Syrups: Syrups are sweet, viscous, concentrated aqueous solutions of sucrose or other sugars. Medicated syrup contains a therapeutic or medicinal agent. Syrups containing flavouring agents but no medicinal substances are called flavouring or flavoured syrups. Syrups offer a pleasant means of administering disagreeable testing (nauseous, saline or bitter) drugs. Sucrose is partly hydrolysed into reducing sugars, levulose and dextrose. This helps in retarding oxidation. Syrups often contain vegetable drug extracts which are liable to decomposition. Strong solutions of sucrose prevents such decomposition by exerting direct osmotic pressure and inhibits the development of bacteria, fungi and molds. Besides, syrups are good demulcents and soothing agents and hence they are of special value in cough syrup. Sucrose is most commonly used in the preparation of syrups but it may be replaced in whole or in part by their sugars such as dextrose and non-sugars such as sorbitol, glycerin and propylene glycol. All these substance are glycogenic (converted to glucose into the body). Non-glycogenic substances like methylcellulose or hydroxymethyl-cellulose can also be used for replacing glycogenic materials in the preparation of syrups and are particularly suitable for diabetic patients. Concentration of sucrose in sugar based syrup is very important. A dilute solution of sucrose supports the growth of micro-organisms whereas a saturated solution may lead to crystallization of a part of sucrose under conditions of varying temperature. If syrups contain 65% by weight or more of sugar, the solution will retard the growth of micro-organism. Syrup I.P. is a 66,7% w/w solution of sucrose whereas syrup USP is 85% w/v (corresponding to 64.74% w/w) solution of sucrose is purified H2O. **Example:** Tolu balsam syrup- mono-herbal syrup and Live-52 Polyherbal syrup.

Preparation Methods

Hot process: This method is used when the active constituent is neither volatile nor heat labile. Desired amount of sucrose is weighed in a tarred dish, purified water is added and heated on a water both till a solution is obtained. The product is strained and enough boiling purified water is added to adjust the desired weight or volume. **Example:** Syrup IP, Acacia syrup NF, Cocoa syrup NF, and Tolu syrup IP are prepared by this method.

Percolation (Cold process): This process is employed in the preparation of syrup USP. Sucrose is placed in suitable percolator and purified H2O or an aqueous solution is allowed to pass slowly through sucrose. The neck of the percolator is packed with loosely compressed cotton. Rate of percolation regulates the rate of dissolution of sucrose.

Addition of a Medicating or Flavouring liquid to syrup: The method is useful when fluid extracts, tinctures or other liquids are to be added to syrup. Alcohol is present in these liquids to dissolve resinous or oleo resinous substances. Addition of these liquids to syrup may cause precipitations of alcohol – soluble materials due to dilution with water. Alcohol also acts as preservative.

Agitation without heat: The method is suitable for preparing syrups containing heat-labile constituents. Sucrose and other ingredients if any are dissolved in purified water by placing the ingredients in a bottle of about twice the volume required for the syrup. This permits thorough agitation. The bottle is stoppered to avoid contamination and loss of H_2O by evaporation. The bottle is allowed to lie upon its side when not being agitated. For large scale preparation of syrups by this method glass lined tanks with mechanical agitators are employed.

Preservation and storage: Syrups should be prepared in such quantities which can be used within a month. Syrup should be stored at a temperature not exceeding 25°C. When the concentration of the sucrose in the syrup is low then, the preservatives like glycerin, methyl paraben, benzoic acid, sodium benzoate. Syrups are stored in well dried, completely filled and carefully stoppered bottles in a cool dark place.

Elixirs

Elixirs are defined as clear, sweetened, aromatic hydro alcoholic liquids intended for oral use. Elixirs frequently contain considerable quantity of alcohol. They provide a palatable means of administering potent or nauseous drugs. Elixirs are less sweet and less viscous than syrups and may contain less or no sucrose. Elixirs are more stable than syrups and hence are preferred over syrups from a manufacturing viewpoint. Preservatives are not needed in elixirs as their alcohol content is sufficient to render them self-preserving. It provides palatable means of administering – potent and nauseous drugs. These are more stable than mixtures and less sweet and less viscous than syrups. **Example:** Digoxin Elixir, USP

Methods of preparations: Elixirs are commonly prepared by simple dissolution with agitation and / or by admixture of two or more liquid components. Ingredients are dissolved in their respective solvents **Example**-alcohol soluble ingredients in alcohol and water-soluble ingredients in H_2O. In order to maintain optimum alcoholic strength and to avoid separation of alcohol – soluble ingredients, as a rule the aqueous solution is always added to alcoholic solution. The mixture is then made up to the volume with the solvent or vehicle specified in the formulation and filtered.

Aromatic Waters

Aromatic waters are clear, saturated aqueous solutions of volatile oils or other aromatic or volatile substances. They are mainly used as flavouring agents. **Example**: Concentrated peppermint water

Preparation Methods

Distillation: In distillation methods, the crude drugs are placed with sufficient purified water in a suitable still. Most of the water is distilled over the steam and condensed distillate contains dissolved aromatic principle. The main disadvantage of this method is that they all are expensive and tedious. **Example** strong rose water N.F. orange flower water N.F.

Solution method: In solution method, the volatile oil is shaken for 15 min with sufficient water (500 times) to make the solution (Repeat shaking is done to distribute the oil uniformly). The solution obtained is set aside for 12 hrs, to allow the freely divided globules of suspended to coalesce, then filtered through wetted filter paper to prevent passage of excess oil. **Example:** Dill water, peppermint water etc.

Emulsion

An emulsion is a biphasic system in which one phase is intimately dispersed in the other phase in the form of minute droplets ranging in diameter from 0.1nm to 100nm. It is a thermodynamically unstable system which can be stabilized by the presence of a emulsifying agent. The dispensed phase is called internal phase or the discontinuous phase while the outer phase is called dispersion medium, external phase or continuous phase. Emulsifying agent is called intermediate phase or inter-phase. Milk is an e.g. of natural emulsion. Micro emulsion, however contain globules that have diameters of less than 0.1nm, Droplets of such dimension cannot refract light and are transparent. The emulsion is which oil is distributed in the form of finely subdivided globules would be called as oil-in-water (O/W) emulsion and when water is dispersed in oil it is called as water in oil (W/O) emulsion. **Example:** Peppermint emulsion B.P.C.

Preparation Methods

- **Continental or dry gum method**: In this method emulsifying agent is mixed with oil before the addition of water. The method is also referred to as 4:2:1 method because primary emulsion preparation uses 4 parts of oil, 2 parts of water and 1 part of gum.
- **English or wet gum method:** In this method emulsifying agent (gum) is mixed with water before the addition of oil. This method uses the same proportion of oil, water or gums as in dry gum method.

- **Bottle method**: In this method, mix emulsifying agent (gum)with 2 parts of oils by thorough shaking in the capped container. Then add volume of water approximately equal to oil. Mix thoroughly by shaking after each addition.

Evaluation Parameters

Cracking	It means separation of two layers.
Creaming	it is formation of layer of dispersed globules at the surface of emulsion
Phase inversion	It is change in one type of emulsion in other. **Example**- O/W to W/O

1. **Phase separation:** Keep measured volume of emulsion in graduated cylinder and measure rate and degree of phase separation by measuring the volume of separated phase with or without centrifugation at low/moderate speeds at valid time intervals. Creaming or coalescence of globules causes phase separation.
2. **Globule Size:** Globule size is an indicator of physical stability and indication of flocculation.
3. **Rheological Properties:** The creaming tendency, consistency in shelf life can be determined by rheological properties of an emulsion based on globule size, emulsifier, and its concentration, phase volume ration, *etc*.
4. **Effect of Thermal Stresses:** Exposure to too high (60 °C for a few hours)and low temperatures (0 to 40 °C) in alternating cycles governs thaw stability.

Suspensions

A pharmaceutical suspension is a biphasic system composed of finely divided insoluble solid material suspended in a liquid medium. The average size of the suspended particles ranges from 0.5 nm to 5 nm in most of the pharmaceutical suspensions. **Example:** Cascara sagrada suspension

Preparation Methods

Small scale preparation of the suspension can be carried out by employing a maximum of equipment. The insoluble material is ground or levigated in the mortar to a smooth paste with the suspending agent previously dispersed in water to form mucilage. Levigation is the most common technique and propylene glycol and glycerin are the most commonly used levigating agents. After a smooth paste is obtained, rest of vehicle is added in divided portions. Soluble drugs if any, flavouring agents and colouring materials etc. are added to this part of the vehicle. Instead of using the mucilage of the suspending agent, it may also be mixed with other powders in this formulation. Prior to the formation of the smooth paste. The suspension is then transferred to a measure and final portions of the vehicle are used to rinse the mortar and pestle and the product made up to the required volume. The degree of dispersion of the final product may further be improved by passing through a hand homogenizer as used in the homogenization of emulsion.

For large scale preparation of the suspensions, mixing tanks fitted with a variable speed stirring device such as propeller or a turbine impeller may be used. The product is then passed through a homogenizer or a colloid mill. Suspension containing 50% or more of solids behaves as dilatant materials and is particularly troublesome. They flow freely into the colloid mill but set up a high shearing rate and produce overheating and stalling of the motor.

Evaluation Parameters

Sedimentation rate	It is ratio of ultimate height to initial height.
Rheological properties	Viscosity and flow properties can be determined
Electro kinetic properties	It involves measurement of zeta potential

Evaluation of suspension

(a) **Sedimentation volume:** Sedimentation volume (F) is a ratio of the final volume of sediment (Vu) to the original volume of sediment (Vo) before settling. Take suspension in 50 ml measuring cylinders and record the volume of sediment formed at every 24 hr for 7 days. Calculate sedimentation volume F (%), using the formula: **F = 100 Vu/ Vo**

(b) **Viscosity measurement:** The viscosity of the samples is determined at 25°C using the Brookfield viscometer. The suspension viscosity increases with increasing solid fraction and it decreases with increasing average particle size.

(c) **Particle size measurement:** The particle size in suspensions is measured by optical microscopy using a trinocular microscope at100x (10×10) magnification. The average particle size of 100 particles should be determined.

(d) **Dissolution study/Drug release:** There are number of methods to determine the drug release from suspensions. The drug release aliquot/s may differ from the therapeutic dose.

Herbal Parenterals

Parenteral preparations are sterile preparations like solutions, suspensions, emulsions, powders for injection or infusion, gels for injection and implants, intended to be administrated directly into the systemic circulation in humans or animals. Parenteral preparations must be sterile, pyrogen-free, clear or free from visible particles, no phase separation in case of emulsions and easy dispersion of particles on shaking in case of suspensions. They are usually supplied in single dose glass or plastic containers or more and more in pre-filled syringes or pens to facilitate the ease of use.

Types of parenteral preparation:

Sr.No.	Route	Injection site
1	Intravenous (IV)	Vein
2	Intramuscular (IM)	Muscle tissue
3	Intradermal (ID)	Dermis of the skin
4	Subcutaneous (SC)	Subcutaneous tissue of the skin
5	Intrathecal	Subarachnoid space of the spinal cord
6	Epidural	Epidural space of the spinal cord
7	Intra- arterial	Artery
8	Intra-articular	Joint space
9	Intracardiac	Heart
10	Intraocular	Eye
11	intraperitoneal	Peritoneal cavity

Advantages as compared to other dosage forms

- An immediate physiological response can be achieved if necessary.
- It provides a direct route for achieving the drug effect within the body.
- Modification of the formulation can however slow down the onset and prolong the action. This may also be achieved by the change in the route of injection.
- When food cannot be taken by mouth, total nutritional requirement can be supplied by the parenteral route.
- Low drug concentration
- Low toxicity as compared to solid dosage form
- Most suitable route for those drugs which are degraded or erratically or unreliably absorbed when administered orally
- Most suitable if the patient is unconscious, difficult to swallow drug etc.

Disadvantages:

- Requirement of aseptic technique in production and handling of product
- Requirement of skilled personnel for administration.
- Painful administration.

Examples of Parenteral Administration of Herbal Drugs

Sr. no	Name of Herbal drug	Biological source	Property of preparation	Use of Herbal drug	Dose quantity	Route of administration
1	Morphine	*Papaverso-mniferum.*	Morphine Sulphate form due to solubility issue	Moderate to severe pain	15 mg/mL	Intravenous, intramuscular and subcutaneous
2	Artem-isinin	Artemisia annua	Rapidly converted in the bloodstream to dihydroartemisinic (DHA), which has 5–10 times greater antimalarial potency than artemisinin.	Treat fever and malaria	1.2 ml	intravenous and intramuscular
3	Vincris-tine (vinca)	Catharan-thusroseus.	Vincristine sulphate li posome injection (VS LI, sphingomyelin and cholesterol nanoparticle vincristin e (VCR), facilitates VCR dose-intensification and densification plus enhances target tissue delivery	To treat acute leukaemia, non–Hodgkin's malignant lymphomas, rhabdomyosar coma,	2 mL	Intravenous

Contd...

Sr. no	Name of Herbal drug	Biological source	Property of preparation	Use of Herbal drug	Dose quantity	Route of administration
4	Digoxin	*Digitalis lanata*	Parenteral administration of digoxin should be used only when the need for rapid digitalization is urgent or when the drug cannot be taken orally	Heart failure and atrial fibrillation	0.125-0.25 mg	Intravenous
5	Atropine	*Atropab-elladona*	The signs of overdose are dilation of the pupils, difficulty in swallowing, hot dry skin, flushing and inability to pass urine. Rapid breathing, increased heart rate and hyperactivity may also occur.	Brady-arrhythmia Anaesthesia, Anticholinesterase Poisoning Rhi norrhea, AV Heart Block, Head Injury, Peptic Ulcer, Organophosphate Poisoning Nerve Agent Poisoning	(0.05 mg/mL; 0.1 mg/mL; 0.4 mg/mL	Intravenous and intramuscular
6	Paclitaxel	Yew tree- *Taxus-baccata., Taxus-brevifolia*	Antineoplastic by promoting intracell-ular tubulin polymeri-zation and stabilizes abnormal microtubule structures against depolymerization	Treatment of lung, ovarian, and breast cancer, it also used in Kaposi sarcoma.	6mg/ml	Intravenous infusion.
7	Podophyl lotoxin	*Podophyllum peltatum*	It is 4'-demethylepip-odophyllotoxin 9-[4,6-0-(R)-ethylidene-β-D-glucopyranoside].a semisynthetic derivative of podoph-yllotoxin	Treatment of certain neoplastic diseases	(20 mg/mL)	Intravenous solution
8	Vinblas-tine	*Catharanthu sroseus.*		To treat acute leukaemia, non–Hodgkin's malignant lymphomas, rhabdomyosar coma,	3.7 mg/m2	intravenous

Novel Dosage Forms

Introduction

Poor water solubility hence frequent dosing, more side effects, poor site-specific action, and poor bioavailability and thus drug release are major drawbacks of conventional formulations. To overcome these issues and to improve patient compliance, recently, novel drug delivery systems (NDDSs) and dosage forms have gained much attention mainly in chronic disease (Cancer, arthritis, immunodeficiency diseases etc.) due to their target specificity, high efficacy and stability. Following are few different NDDSs:

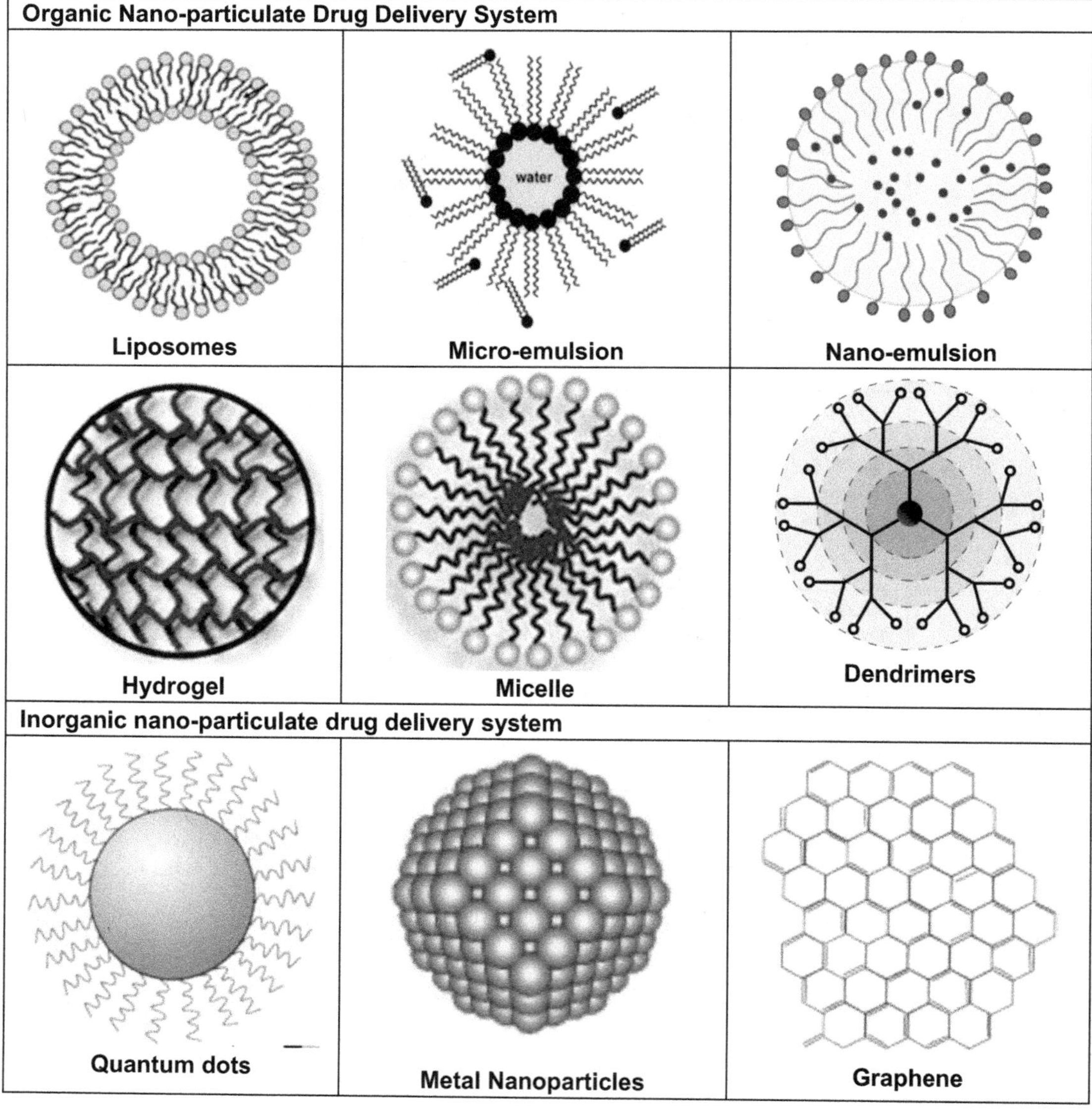

Contd...

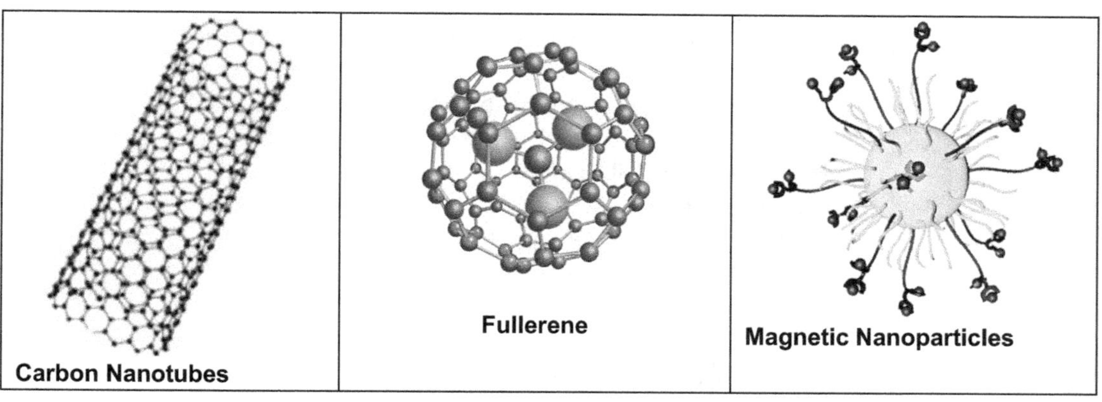

Different types of Novel Drug Delivery Systems (NDDSs)	
Modified release dosage forms	Modified-release dosage unlike immediate-release dosage delivers a drug with a delay after its administration (delayed-release dosage) or for a prolonged period of time (extended-release dosageconsists of either sustained-release (SR) or controlled-release (CR) dosage) or to a specific target in the body (targeted-release dosage). SR maintains drug release over a sustained period but not at a constant rate. CR maintains drug release over a sustained period at a nearly constant rate. Examples: controlled delivery (CD), controlled release (CR), delayed release (DR), extended release (ER, XL, XR, XT), immediate release (IR), long-acting (LA), long-acting release (LAR), modified release (MR), prolonged release (PR), sustained action (SA), sustained release (SR), timed release (TR)
Vesicular Carriers	Liposomes, Phytosomes, Niosomes, BilosomesTransfersomes, Ethosomes, Emulsones, Pharmacocomes, Invasomes, Layerosomes,
Micellar Carriers	Polymeric micelles, Dendrimers. Mixed micelles, Phospholipid based micelles
Particulate Carriers	Solid lipid nanoparticles, Nanostructured lipid carriers, Polymeric nanoparticles
Emulsified Carriers	Microemulsions, Nanoemulsions, Lipid emulsions
Other Novel NDDS	Oral Films, Transdermal patch

Vesicular Carriers	
Liposomes	Liposomes, sphere-shaped vesicles consisting of one or more phospholipid bilayers, were first described in the mid-60s. Very small globule size (0.025 μm to 2.5 μm) and hydrophobic as well as hydrophilic character makes liposomes choice of drug delivery. Liposomes are artificially prepared vesicles made of lipid bilayer which vastly improves drug absorption and bioavailability. Materials commonly used for the preparation of transferosomes are phospholipids (soya phosphatidyl choline, egg phosphatidyl choline), surfactant (tween 80, sodium cholate) for providing flexibility, alcohol (ethanol, methanol) as a solvent, dye for confocal scanning lasermicroscopy

Contd...

	(CSLM) and buffering agent (saline phosphate buffer pH 7.4), as a hydrating medium. **Types:** On the basis of their size and number of bilayers, liposomes are classified as follows: Multilamellar vesicles (MLV) Unilamellar vesicles Large unilamellar vesicles (LUV) Small unilamellar vesicles (SUV) **Preparation Methods** • Following are different methods in preparation of liposomes: • Detergent removal method • Dialysis • Dried reconstituted vesicles • Ethanol injection • Ether injection (solvent vaporization) • Extrusion • Freeze-thawed liposomes • Gel-permeation chromatography • Lipid film hydration • Mechanical dispersion method • Membrane extrusion • Micro-emulsification • Passive loading techniques • Reverse phase evaporation method • Solvent dispersion method • Sonication **Procedure:** liposomes can be prepared by four basic steps: drying lipophilic phase from organic solvent, dispersing the lipophilic phasein aqueous phase, purifying the resultant liposome and analyzing the final product. There is no single universal encapsulation method hence each drug requires a different approach to manage all of its properties. ***Evaluation parameters***: Liposomal drug delivery system involves following evaluation parameters: Rheological properties like Viscosity Electro kinetic properties like zeta potential, surface charge, polydispersity Particle size, lamellarity Drug entrapment efficiency and drug release.
Phytosomes	Phytosome is a patented technology to incorporate standardized plant extracts into phospholipids to produce phytosomes. Liposomes forms without chemical bondswhile phytosomes are formed by chemical bonds.Extract or phytochemicaltophosphatidylcholineratio is usually 1:1 or a 2:1
Niosomes	Niosomes are made up of cholesterol and nonionic surfactantsand small amount ofanionic surfactant such as diacetyl phosphate. Niosomes are chemically more stable and economical than liposomes.

Contd...

Ethosomes	Ethosomes are composed of phospholipids, (phosphatidylcholine, Phosphatidyl serine, phosphatitidic acid), high concentration of ethanol and water. These are more malleable and of better drug distribution capability in skin than liposomes.
Transfersomes	Transfersomes are composed of phospholipids and edge activator (Sodium deoxycholateTween 80, Span 80 and sodium cholate) as membrane-softening agent (such as) to produce self-optimizing deformabilityhavingultraflexible lipidcomplexeswhich can easily cross even the very narrow skin pores.
Bilosomes	Bilosomearenon-lipoidalbiocarriers composed of nonionic surfactants and bile salts and useful for vaccine oral delivery due to its enzymes and bile salts resistance in the gastrointestinal tract as well as drug permeation across biological membranes.
Emulsomes	Emulsome is composed of solid lipid core material (solid at room temperature-25°C)stabilized by cholesterol and soya lecithin. These are prepared by melt expression or emulsion solvent diffusive extraction.
Pharmacosome	**Pharmacosome**are composed of optimum ratio of polyphenol with phospholipids to formcomplex vesicular system.Hydroxyl moiety of the lipid converts freeamino, hydroxyl groups of drug to an ester to formprodrug.
Invasomes	Invasomes are composed of phospholipids, ethanol, and terpeneto improve transdermal penetration to increase the permeability of the drug into the skin and decrease absorption into the systemic circulation.
Layersomes	The layersomes are conventional liposomes coated with one or more layers of biocompatible polyelectrolytes in order to stabilise their structure. The formulation strategy is based on an alternative coating procedure of positive poly(lysine) and negative poly(glutamic acid) (pGA) polypeptides on initially charged small unilamellar liposomes (SUVs). The size distribution and the zeta potential of the final entity depend on the number of layers and the charge of the last coating layer.

Micellar Carriers	
Mixed Micelles	The solubilization of lipid bilayer by surfactant is accompanied by morphological change of bilayer and emergence of mixed micelles. From the phase equilibrium perspective, the lipid, surfactant, water system is in two phase area during the solubilization a phase containing mixed micelles is in equilibrium with bilayer structure of laminar phase. In some cases, three phases are present the single micelles phase is replaced by a concentrated and dilute solution phase in the case of non-ionic surfactant. The lipid bilayer reach saturation when mixed micelles often flexible rod like or thread like start from it aqueous solution at the constant chemical proportion of surfactant.
Polymeric Micelles	They are formed from self-aggregation of amphiphilic block / graft co-polymers with the hydrophobic part of the polymer on the inside (core) and hydrophilic on the outside (shell). In drug delivery, PM are classified under the "Nano carriers". A polymeric micelle usually consists of several

Contd...

	hundred block copolymers and has a diameter of about 20-50 nm. They have Self-assembled supramolecular core-shell structure. Core is a dense region consisting of the hydrophobic part of the amphiphilic polymer. Core serves as a reservoir for drugs with low aqueous solubility. Shell consisting hydrophilic portion of the co-polymer. the morphology of micelles is the hydrophilic– hydrophobic balance of the block copolymer defined by the hydrophilic volume fraction, f (f>45% form PM)
Solid Lipid Nano-particle	Colloidal particles ranging in size between 10 & 1000 nm are known as nanoparticles. Solid lipid nanoparticle (SLNs)are new generation of submicron sized lipid emulsion where the liquid lipid(oil) has been substituted by a solid lipid. Advantages of SLNs over polymeric NPs Polymeric Nanoparticles Solid Lipid Nanoparticles Residual Contamination Avoid residual contamination Possible toxicity problems No toxicity problems Expensive production & a lack of large scale production method Cost effective methods are available Lack of suitable sterilization method Feasible sterilization method available Not stable as compared to SLNs SLNs formulation stable for even three years have been development. General ingredients include solid lipid, emulsifier & water, Lipid contains triglycerides, partial glycerides, fatty acids, steroids, waxes Combination of emulsifier might prevent particle agglomeration, Emulsifier include soybean lecithin, egg lecithin, poloxamer etc.
Phospholipid-based Micelles	The self-assembly of amphiphilic surfactants in solution is an interesting phenomenon that has wide significance in fields ranging from fundamental biology to chemical engineering and biotechnology. Particularly interesting biological surfactant self-assemblies are formed by phospholipids. Besides their essential role in the cell membrane of most organisms, phospholipids are present and form various aggregates and colloidal assemblies in many bioproducts, including all plant oils and their derivatives, and have various industrial applications as surface-active components. A commonly employed phospholipid surfactant is lecithin, which is an amphiphilic substance mostly consisting of glycerol-based phospholipids extracted from food sources such as eggs and soybeans. This makes it biocompatible and nontoxic. Most widely studied and applied self-assembling lecithin systems include ternary mixtures of lecithin, water, and an organic solvent of low polarity (oil), which typically take the form of an emulsion with the hydrophobic tail of the lecithin molecule residing in the nonpolar oil phase and the hydrophilic headgroup being in contact with the water.

Particulate Carriers	
Nanostructured Lipid Carrier	NLC (Nanostructured lipid carrier) which are second generation of SLN. NLC composed of binary mixture of solid lipid and a spatially different liquid lipid as hybrid carrier. Average size between 10-500 nm. NLC consist of a mixture of specially blended solid lipid (long chain) with liquid lipid (short chain), preferably in a ratio of 70:30 to 99.9:01. Objectives of NLCTo overcome disadvantages of SLN such as Tendency for particle growth.

Contd...

	Unpredictable gelation tendency. Poor drug loading capacity. Drug expulsion after polymeric transition during storage. High water content in dispersions have been observed i.e.70-99.9%. The Excipients used in NLC¬ Solid lipids A mixture of several chemical compounds which have high melting point (higher than 40ºC). These solid lipids are well tolerated of GRAS status. Accepted for human use. Also in vivo biodegradable. Liquid lipids (OIL) These solid lipids are well tolerated of GRAS status. Emulsifying agents It is an surfactant, which is adsorbed at interfaces and lowers the interfacial tension. UV blockers Help to protect the skin from the ultraviolet radiation of the sun. Lowering the risk of skin cancer. Sunscreen products contain either an organic chemical compound that absorbs UV light
Polymeric Nanoparticles	Polymeric nanoparticles (PNP) They are solid colloidal particles ranging in size from 10 to 1000 nm (1µm). Drug may be dissolved, entrapped, encapsulated or attached to a nanoparticle matrix. Because these systems have very high surface areas, drugs may also be adsorbed on their surface. Polymer-based nanoparticles effectively carry drugs, proteins and DNA to target cells and organs. Their nanometer-size promotes effective permeation through cell membranes and stability in the blood stream. Nanocapsules: They are the systems in which the drug is confined to a cavity surrounded by a unique polymer membrane. Nanospheres: They are the matrix systems in which the drug is physically and uniformly dispersed.

Emulsified Carriers	
Micro-emulsion	Emulsions (macro-emulsion) are dispersions made up of two immiscible liquid phases which are mixed using mechanical shear and surfactant. IUPAC defines micro-emulsion as dispersion made of water, oil, and surfactant(s) that is an isotropic and thermodynamically stable system with dispersed domain diameter varying approximately from 1 to 100 nm, usually 10 to 50 nm. The major components of micro emulsion system are:1) Oil phase 2) Surfactant (Primary surfactant) 3) Co-surfactant (Secondary surfactant) 4) Co-Solvent. **Phase titration method:** Micro emulsion was prepared by dispersing required quantity of drug in appropriate quantity of oil which is required for the solubilisation of drug. The mixture was homogenized and accurately weighed quantity of surfactant: co surfactant blends was added in small portion with stirring to it. The blends were mixed thoroughly using magnetic stirrer and drop wise double distilled water added to it with continuous stirring around 10 minute and rate of stirring was optimized as per requirement of particle size. **Phase inversion temperature method (PIT):** Phase inversion of micro emulsions means conversion of O/W to W/O system by adding excess of the dispersed phase or by rising temperature when non-ionic surfactant are used to change spontaneous curvature of the surfactant which brings system near to minimal surface tension and to form fine dispersed oil droplets. This method shows extreme changes in particle size which further leads to changes in in-vivo and in-vitro drug release pattern. • Evaluation parameters

Contd...

<table>
<tr><td></td><td>
<ul>
<li>Physical appearance</li>
<li>Globule size determination</li>
<li>Conductivity test</li>
<li>Dye-solubility test</li>
<li>Refractive index measurement</li>
<li>Filter paper test</li>
<li>Dilution test</li>
<li>Drug content determination</li>
<li>Polydispersity determination</li>
<li>pH determination</li>
<li>Viscosity determination</li>
<li>Scattering Techniques</li>
<li>Percent Transmittance (Limpidity Test) determination</li>
<li>Zeta potential determination</li>
<li>In-vitroand in-vivo drug release determination</li>
<li>Stability studies</li>
</ul>
</td></tr>
<tr><td>Nano-emulsion</td><td>
Nano-emulsions are very similar to microemulsions that are dispersions of nano-scale particles but obtained by mechanical force unlike to microemulsions which forms spontaneously. Microemulsions and nano-emulsions are promising delivery for poorly water soluble drugs.
Preparation Methods
High energy emulsification method: ultra sonication and high pressure homogenization
Low energy emulsification: Phase inversion temperature method, solvent displacement method and phase inversion composition method
High-Pressure Homogenization: specially designed high- pressure homogenization instrument is used to produce nanosized particles. At very high pressure (500 to 5000 psi), oil phase and water phase are allowed to force through small inlet orifice. Hence extremely small size particles are created due to strong turbulence and hydraulic shear. But this method requires high temperature and energy. Pressure, homogenization cycles are directly responsible for particle size. Higher the pressure and higher the homogenization cycles, smallest is particle size. This method is easy to scale up.
Microfluidization: In this method also specially designed device called as microfluidizer is used to create high-pressure (500 to 20000psi). Initially prepare coarse emulsion of by mixing oil and water phase. This device consists of interaction chamber of small micro channels through which coarse emulsion is forced to an impingement area to form nano size fine particles followed by filtration to obtain uniform particles.
Ultrasonication: This method is based on principle that when coarse emulsion is in ultrasonic field and external pressure is increased, cavitations threshold also increases to limit where fine nano size particles are formed.
Phase inversion method: This method uses principle of phase inversion temperature which is the temperature at which phase transition occurs. Low temperature favors O/W emulsions and high temperature favors W/O emulsion. Rapid cooling and heating cycles produces fine particles. Non-ionic surfactant like polyoxyethylene becomes lipophilic at high temperature and hydrophilic at low temperature due to dehydration of the polymer chain.
Spontaneous Emulsification: This method is simple and uses volatile
</td></tr>
</table>

Contd...

	organic solvent composition of oil, water, lipophilic and hydrophilic surfactant. This composition is allowed to mix homogenously by magnetic stirring. Then evaporate the water-miscible solvent under vacuum to obtain nano emulsion. **Solvent Evaporation Technique**: In this technique, initially mix drug with organic solvent using suitable surfactant and prepare O/W emulsion by mixing continuous phase. Then evaporate organic solvent under vacuum or heating or at atmospheric conditions to obtain microspheres loaded with drug followed by centrifugation or filtration. Hydrogel Method: This method shares similarity with solvent evaporation method. High shear forces are used to form nano emulsion of drug- solvent which is miscible with the drug anti-solvent. Evaluation parameters: Same as micro-emulsion

Other Novel NDDS

Oral Films

Fast dissolving film or oral dissolving films come in 1970[s] an alternative dosage form for disintegrating (compressed) tablet, syrup, capsule and other dosage form depending on patient compliance. This fast-dissolving film has more important in pharmaceutical industry because of their unique property and specific advantages like no need of water for take dose, accurate dosing, rapid onset of action, ease of transportability, ease of handling and good mouth feel. This fast-dissolving oral film undergoes rapid dissolution in salivary fluid and oral cavity within second and release active pharmaceutical medicament. these fast-dissolving films developed on the basis of transdermal patch technology, it has consisted of thin film or strips which is placed on patient tongue or any other mucosal tissue, hydrate and adhere on to site of application disintegrate rapidly dissolve and release medication for or mucosal absorption.

Types of Oral Films

1. Flash release wafer
2. Mucoadhesive melt away wafer
3. Mucoadhesive sustained release wafer

Types of oral films and their properties:

Property\ sub type	Flash release wafer	Mucoadhesive melt-away wafer	Mucoadhesive sustained release wafer
Area(cm^2)	2-8	2-7	2-4
Thickness (μm)	20-70	50-500	50-250
Structure	Film: single layer	Single or multiple system	Multi-layer or system
Excipient	Soluble, highly hydrophilic polymer	Soluble, hydrophilic polymer	Low / non soluble polymer
Drug phase	Solid solution	Solid solution or suspended drug particle	Suspension and solid solution

Contd...

Property\ sub type	Flash release wafer	Mucoadhesive melt-away wafer	Mucoadhesive sustained release wafer
Application	Tongue (upper palate)	Gingival or buccal region	Gingival (another region of oral cavity)
Dissolution	Maximum 60 sec	Disintegrations in a few minutes, foaming gel	Maximum 8-10 hr
Site of action	Systemic or local	Systemic or local	Systemic or local

Preparation Methods

1. Solvent casting method
2. Semisolid casting method
3. Hot melt extrusion method
4. Solid dispersion extrusion method
5. Rolling method

Evaluation Parameters	
Organoleptic evaluation	Organoleptic properties of film like colour, flavour and taste are studied by visual check or specialised designed apparatuses.
Thickness	Thickness of film is directly related to drug content uniformity and it is necessary to maintain thickness of film it can be measured by Micrometre screw gauge or calibrated Digital Vemier callipers.
Tensile strength	Tensile strength is the maximum stress applied to a point at which the strip specimen breaks. It is calculated by the applied load at rupture divided by the cross-sectional area of the strip as given in the equation below **Tensile strength = Strip thickness × Strip width/ Load at breakage**
Young's modulus	Young's modulus or elastic modulus is the measure of stiffness of strip. It is represented as the ratio of applied stress over strain in the region of elastic deformation.
Folding endurance	Folding endurance is determined by repeated folding of the strip at the same place till the strip breaks. The number of times the film is folded without breaking is computed as the folding endurance value
Disintegration time	For measurement of Disintegration of orally fast dissolving films requires U.S.P. disintegration apparatus. The disintegration time limit is 30 seconds or less than 30 sec for orally disintegrating films, described in C.D.E.R (The centre for drug evaluation and research.) guidance. Disintegration time will be changes depending on the formulation but typically the disintegration ranges from 5 to 30 seconds. Although, even no official guidance is available for oral fast disintegrating films.
Swelling property	Oral film in contact with saliva gets swollen, so swelling property of film can be measured by stimulated salivary solution method. Every film sample which will be measured is weighed and placed in a pre-weighed stainless steel wire mesh. The

Contd...

	mesh containing film sample is submerged into 15ml medium in a plastic container. Increase in the weight of the film was determined at pre-set time interval until a constant weight of film was observed. The degree of swelling was calculated using **parameters wt-w0/wo, wt** is weight of film at time t, and wo is weight of film at time zero.
Contact angle	A contact angle measurement is performed at room temperature with a goniometer. A drop of distilled water was placed on the surface of the dry oral film, and then Images of the water droplet were recorded within 10 seconds with the help of digital camera. The contact angle was measured on both sides of the drop.
Surface pH	This test is done to determine the pH of film. Films may cause irritation in buccal cavity, hence pH of the films should be close to neutral P^H.
Transparency	The transparency of the film can be determined by using a simple UV spectrophotometer. Cut the film sample into rectangles and place on the internal side of the spectrophotometer of the cell. The transmittance of the film is determined at 600 nm.

Transdermal Patch

The transdermal patch or transdermal drug delivery system (TDDS) is a medicated patch that can deliver drugs through skin portals directly to the bloodstream at a predetermined rate. This is the most comfortable dosage form – it is non-invasive, avoids the gastrointestinal tract and bypasses first-pass metabolism, can have multiday therapy, and can be terminated at any time. The site of application should be clean, not oily, and hairless, and the location may vary with the therapeutic category of drug, such as nitro-glycerine around the chest, oestradiol around the buttocks or abdomen, and nicotine around the upper torso or upper outer arm. The system consists of several layers:

- a backing layer to protect from the outside environment and water
- a drug reservoir on a semipermeable membrane to control the release of the drugan adhesive to glue onto skin
- a liner to protect the patch and adhesive.
- The liner has to be taken out before putting the patch on the skin surface. Figure 13.7 illustrates the makeup of a medicated patch.

Components of TDDS	
1. Polymer matrix / Drug reservoir These control the release rate of the drug from the device	*(a)* ***Natural Polymers***: e.g., cellulose derivatives, Zein, Gelatine, Shellac, Waxes, Proteins, Gums and their derivatives, Natural rubber, Starch etc. *(b)* ***Synthetic Elastomers***: e.g., polybutadiene, hydrin rubber, polyisobutylene, silicon rubber, nitrile, acrylonitrile, neoprene, butyl rubber etc. *(c)* ***Synthetic Polymers***: e.g., polyvinyl alcohol, polyvinylchloride, polyethylene, polypropylene, polyacrylate, polyamide, polyurea, polyvinylpyrrolidone, polymethylmethacrylate etc.

Contd...

2. Drug	Depending on disease
3. Permeation enhancers To increase permeability of stratum corneum so as to attain higher therapeutic levels of the drug candidate a	*(a)* ***Solvents-alcohols*** – methanol and ethanol; alkyl methyl sulfoxides – dimethyl sulfoxide, alkyl homologs of methyl sulfoxide dimethyl acetamide and dimethyl formamide; pyrrolic- ones- 2 pyrrolidone, N-methyl, 2-purrolidone; etc *(b)* ***Surfactants (for hydrophilic drug)-*** ***Anionic Surfactants:*** e.g., Decodecylmethylsulphoxide, Dioctylsulphosuccinate, Sodium lauryl sulphate etc. ***Non-ionic Surfactants:*** e.g., Pluronic F127, Pluronic F68, etc. Bile Salts: e.g., Sodiumtaurocholate, Sodium tauroglycocholate, Sodium deoxycholate ***Binary system:*** These systems open up the heterogeneous multilaminate pathway as well as the continuous pathways. Propylene glycol-oleic acid and 1, 4-butane diol-linoleic acid. *(c)* ***Miscellaneous agents*** - These include urea, a hydrating and keratolytic agent; N, N- dimethyl- toluamide; anticholinergic agent: calcium thioglycolate.
4. Pressure sensitive adhesives (PSA) maintains an intimate contact between transdermal system and the skin surface	Silicones based adhesives and polyacrylates, polyisobutylene
5. Backing Laminate Useful for backing layer.	Vinyl, polyethylene and polyester films
6. Release Liner It is a protective liner that is removed and discharged immediately before the application of the patch to skin during application of patch.	Base layer- non-occlusive (e.g. paper fabric) or occlusive (e.g. polyethylene, polyvinylchloride) and a release coating layer made up of silicon, Teflon, polyester foil and metallized laminates
7. Other excipients: to prepare drug reservoir or to provide plasticity to the transdermal patch	Chloroform, methanol, acetone, isopropanol and dichloromethane dibutylpthalate, triethylcitrate, polyethylene glycol and propylene glycol

Classification of Transdermal Drug Delivery System

Matrix System	**Adhesive Diffusion Controlled TDDS:** The drug reservoir is formed by dispersing the drug in an adhesive polymer and then spreading the medicated polymer adhesive by solvent casting or by melting the adhesive (in case of hot melt adhesives) onto an impervious backing layer. The drug reservoir layer is then covered by a non-medicated rate controlling adhesive polymer of constant thickness to produce an adhesive diffusion controlling drug delivery system. Deponit® (Nitroglycerine) for once-a-day medication of angina pectoris.

Contd...

Matrix System	**Matrix Diffusion Controlled System-** The drug is dispersed homogeneously in a hydrophilic or lipophilic polymer matrix. This drug containing polymer disk then is fixed onto an occlusive base plate in a compartment fabricated from a drug-impermeable backing layer. Instead of applying the adhesive on the face of the drug reservoir, it is spread along the circumference to form a strip of adhesive rim. Nitro Dur® (Nitroglycerine) used for once-a-day medication of angina pectoris.
Reservoir System	**Membrane Moderated TDDS-** In this system, the drug reservoir is embedded between an impervious backing layer and a rate controlling membrane. The drug releases only through the rate controlling membrane, which can be microporous or non-porous. In the drug reservoir compartment, the drug can be in the form of a solution, suspension, or gel or dispersed in solid polymer matrix. On the outer surface of the polymeric membrane a thin layer of drug-compatible, hypoallergenic adhesive polymer can be applied. The rate of drug release from this type of transdermal drug delivery system can be tailored by varying the polymer composition, permeability coefficient and thickness of the rate controlling membrane TransdermScop® (Scopolamine) for 3 days protection of motion sickness and TransdermNitro® (Nitroglycerine) for once-a-day medication of angina pectoris.
Reservoir System	**Micro reservoir System-** This drug delivery system is a combination of reservoir and matrix-dispersion systems. The drug reservoir is formed by first suspending the drug in an aqueous solution of water-soluble polymer and then dispersing the solution homogeneously in a lipophilic polymer to form thousands of unbleachable, microscopic spheres of drug reservoirs. The thermodynamically unstable dispersion is stabilized quickly by immediately cross-linking the polymer in situ. A transdermal system therapeutic system thus formed as a medicated disc positioned at the centre and surrounded by an adhesive rim. Nitro-dur® System (Nitro-glycerine) for once-a-day treatment of angina pectoris.

Methods for Preparation of TDDS	
Asymmetric TPX membrane method	A prototype patch can be fabricated for this a heat sealable polyester film (type 1009, 3m) with a concave of 1cm diameter will be used as the backing membrane. Drug sample is dispensed into the concave membrane, covered by a TPX {poly (4-methyl-1-pentene)} asymmetric membrane, and sealed by an adhesive.
Circular Teflon mould method	Solutions containing polymers in various ratios are used in an organic solvent. Calculated amount of drug is dissolved in half the quantity of same organic solvent. Enhancers in different concentrations are dissolved in the other half of the organic solvent and then added. Di-N-butylphthalate is added as a plasticizer into drug polymer solution. The total contents are to be stirred for 12 hrs and then poured into a circular Teflon mould. The moulds are to be placed on a leveled surface and covered with inverted funnel to control solvent vaporization in a laminar flow hood model with an air speed of 0.5 m/s. The solvent is allowed to evaporate for 24 hrs. The dried films are to be stored for another 24 hrs at 25±0.5°C in a desiccators containing silica gel before evaluation to eliminate aging effects. The type films are to be evaluated within one week of their preparation.

Contd...

Mercury substrate method	In this method drug is dissolved in polymer solution along with plasticizer. The above solution is to be stirred for 10-15 minutes to produce a homogenous dispersion and poured in to a levelled mercury surface, covered with inverted funnel to control solvent evaporation.
IPM membranes" method	In this method drug is dispersed in a mixture of water and propylene glycol containing carbomer 940 polymer and stirred for 12 hrs in magnetic stirrer. The dispersion is to be neutralized and made viscous by the addition of triethanolamine. Buffer pH 7.4 can be used in order to obtain solution gel, if the drug solubility in aqueous solution is very poor. The formed gel will be incorporated in the IPMmembrane.
EVAC membranes" method	In order to prepare the target transdermal therapeutic system, 1% Carbopol reservoir gel, polyethylene (PE), ethylene vinyl acetate copolymer (EVAC) membranes can be used as rate control membranes. If the drug is not soluble in water, propylene glycol is used for the preparation of gel. Drug is dissolved in propylene glycol; carbopol resin will be added to the above solution and neutralized by using 5% w/w sodium hydroxide solution. The drug (in gel form) is placed on a sheet of backing layer covering the specified area. A rate controlling membrane will be placed over the gel and the edges will be sealed by heat to obtain a leak proof device.
Aluminium backed adhesive film method	Transdermal drug delivery system may produce unstable matrices if the loading dose is greater than 10 mg. Aluminium backed adhesive film method is a suitable one. For preparation of same, chloroform is choice of solvent, because most of the drugs as well as adhesive are soluble in chloroform. The drug is dissolved in chloroform and adhesive material will be added to the drug solution and dissolved. A custom made aluminium former is lined with aluminium foil and the ends blanked off with tightly fitting cork blocks
Proliposomes Method	The proliposomes are prepared by carrier method using film deposition technique. From the earlier reference drug and lecithin in the ratio of 0.1:2.0 can be used as an optimized one. The proliposomes are prepared by taking 5mg of mannitol powder in a 100 ml round bottom flask which is kept at 60-70°c temperature and the flask is rotated at 80 90rpm and dried the mannitol at vacuum for 30 minutes. After drying, the temperature of the water bath is adjusted to 20-30°C. Drug and lecithin are dissolved in a suitable organic solvent mixture, a 0.5ml aliquot of the organic solution is introduced into the round bottomed flask at 37°C, after complete drying second aliquots (0.5ml) of the solution is to be added. After the last loading, the flask containing proliposomes are connected in a lyophilized and subsequently drug loaded mannitol powders proliposomes) are placed in a desiccator overnight and then sieved through 100 mesh. The collected powder is transferred into a glass bottle and stored at the freeze temperature until characterization.
Free film method	Free film of cellulose acetate is prepared by casting on mercury surface. A polymer solution 2% w/w is to be prepared by using chloroform. Plasticizers are to be incorporated at a concentration of 40% w/w of polymer weight. Five ml of polymer solution was poured in a glass ring which is placed over the mercury surface in a glass Petri dish. The rate of evaporation of the solvent is controlled by placing an inverted funnel over the Petri dish. The film formation is noted by observing the mercury surface after complete evaporation of the solvent. The dry film will be separated out and stored between the sheets of wax paper in a desiccator until use. Free films of different thickness can be prepared by changing the volume of the polymer solution.

Evaluation of Transdermal Patches	
Thickness	The thickness of transdermal film is determined by, dial gauge, screw gauge or micrometer, travelling microscope at different points of the film.
Uniformity of weight	Weight variation is studied through individually weighing 10 randomly selected patches and calculating the average weight. The individual weight should not deviate significantly from the average weight.
Flatness	For flatness determination, one narrow piece is cut from the centre and two from each side of patches. The length of each strip is measured and variation in length is measured by determining percent constriction. Zero percent constriction is equivalent to 100 percent flatness.
Tensile Strength	To determine tensile strength of the transdermal patches. The polymeric films in the transdermal patch are sandwiched individually by corked linear iron plates. One end of the films is kept fixed with the help of an iron screen and other end is connected to a freely movable thread over a pulley. The weights are added gradually to the pan close with the hanging end of the thread. A pointer on the thread is used to measure the elongation of the film. The weight just sufficient to break the film is noted. The tensile strength can be calculated using the following equation. Tensile strength= F/a. b (1+L/l) F is the force required to break, a is width of film, b is thickness of film, L is length of film, l is elongation of film at break point.
Moisture content	The prepared films are weighed individually and put in a desiccators containing calcium chloride at room temperature for 24 h. The films are weighed again after a specified interval until they show a constant weight. The percent moisture content is calculated using following formula. %Moisture content =Initial weight –Final weight X 100/ Final weight
Drug content determination	Accurately weighed portion of film (about 100 mg) is dissolved in 100 ml of suitable solvent in which drug is soluble and then the solution is shaken continuously for 24 h in shaker incubator. Then the whole solution is sonicated. After sonication and subsequent filtration, drug in solution is estimated spectrophotometrically by appropriate dilution.
Content uniformity test	10 patches are selected and content is determined for individual patches. If 9 out of 10 patches have content between 85% to 115% of the specified value and one has content not less than 75% to 125% of the specified value, then transdermal patches pass the test of content uniformity. But if 3 patches have content in the range of 75% to 125%, then additional 20 patches are tested for drug content. If these 20 patches have range from 85% to 115%, then the transdermal patches pass the test
Moisture Uptake	Weighed films are put in a desiccator at room temperature for 24 h. These are then taken out and exposed to 84% relative humidity using saturated solution of Potassium chloride in a desiccator until a constant weight is achieved. % moisture uptake is calculated as given below. % moisture uptake = Final weight – Initial weight X 100/Initial weight
Folding Endurance	Evaluation of folding endurance involves determining the folding capacity of the films subjected to frequent extreme conditions of folding. Folding endurance is determined by repeatedly folding the film at the same place until it break. The number of times the films could be folded at the same place without breaking is folding endurance value.

Contd...

Microscopic studies	Microscopic evaluation is used to determine the sharing of drug and polymer in the film can be studied using scanning electron microscope. For this study, the sections of each sample are cut and then mounted onto stubs using double sided adhesive tape. The sections are then coated with gold palladium alloy using fine coat ion sputter to render them electrically conductive. Then the sections are examined under scanning electron microscope.
Adhesive studies	The adhesive studies are used to determine the adhesive properties of TDDS. The therapeutic performance of TDDS can be affected by the quality of contact between the patch and the skin. The adhesion of a TDDS to the skin is obtained by using PSAs, which are defined as adhesives capable of bonding to surfaces with the application of light pressure. The adhesive properties of a TDDS can be characterized by considering the following factors. *Peel Adhesion properties:* It is the force necessary to remove adhesive coating from test substrate. It is tested by measuring the force required to pull a single coated tape, applied to substrate at 180° angle. The test is passed if there is no residue on the substrate. *Tack properties:* It is the ability of the polymer to adhere to substrate with little contact pressure. Tack is dependent on molecular weight and composition of polymer as well as on the use of testifying resins in polymer. Thumb tack test: The force necessary to remove thumb from adhesive is a measure of tack. *Rolling ball test:* This test involves measurement of the distance that stainless steel ball travels along an upward facing adhesive. The less tacky the adhesive, the further the ball will travel. *Quick stick (Peel tack) test:* The peel force required breaking the bond between an adhesive and substrate is measured by pulling the tape away from the substrate at 90° at the speed of 12 inch/min. Probe tack test: Force required to pull a probe away from an adhesive at a fixed rate is recorded as tack.
***In vitro* release studies**	In vitro release studies performed outside the body. This is used to determine the drug release mechanism and kinetics are two characteristics of the dosage forms which play an important role in describing the drug dissolution profile from a controlled release dosage form. The dissolution data explain the release mechanism of the drug. There are different methods available for determination of drug release rate of TDDS. *Paddle over disc:* In this method is identical to the USP paddle dissolution apparatus is used, except that the transdermal system is attached to a disc or cell resting at the bottom of the vessel which contains medium at 32 ±5°C. (USP apparatus 5) *Cylinder modified USP Basket:* This method is like to the USP basket type dissolution apparatus, except that the system is attached to the surface of a hollow cylinder immersed in medium at 32 ±5°C. (USP apparatus 6) *Reciprocating disc:* In this method patches attached to holders are oscillated in small volumes of medium, allowing the apparatus to be useful for systems delivering low concentration of drug. In addition, paddle over extraction cell method may be used. (USP apparatus 7) *Diffusion cells:* E.g. Franz Diffusion Cell and its modification Keshary- Chien Cell. These are used for determine the release rate of drug from transdermal dosage forms.
***In vitro* permeation studies**	It is used to determine the permeation of the drug from the transdermal dosage form. The amount of drug available for absorption to the systemic pool is greatly dependent on drug released from the polymeric transdermal films. The drug reached

Contd...

	at skin surface is then passed to the dermal microcirculation by penetration through cells of epidermis, between the cells of epidermis through skin appendages. Usually, permeation studies are performed by placing the fabricated transdermal patch with rat skin or synthetic membrane in between receptor and donor compartment in a vertical diffusion cell such as Franz diffusion cellorkeshary-chien diffusion cell.
***In vivo* evaluation**	In vivo evaluation of the transdermal dosage form performed in site the body. Invivo evaluations are the true description of the drug performance. The variables which cannot be taken during in vitro studies can be fully explored during in vivo studies. In vivo evaluation of TDDS can be carried out using: *(a) Animal models*: The most common animal species used for evaluating transdermal drug deliverysystem are mouse, hairless rhesus monkey, hairless rat, hairless dog, rabbit, guinea pig etc.Various experiments conducted lead us to a conclusion that hairless animals are preferred overhairy animals in both in vitro and in vivo experiments. Rhesus monkey is one of the most reliablemodels for in vivo evaluation of transdermal drug delivery in man. *(b) Human volunteers*: Human models are used for gathering of pharmacokinetic and pharmacodynamicperformance data of the transdermal dosage forms Clinical trials have been conducted toevaluate the efficacy, risk involved, side effects, patient compliance etc. Phase I clinical trials are conducted to find out mainly safety in volunteers and phase II clinical trials find out short term safety and mainly effectiveness in patients. Phase III trials indicate the safety and effectiveness in large number of patient population and Phase IV trials at post marketing surveillance are done for marketed patches to detect adverse drug reactions. Though human studies require significant resources but they are the best to assess the performance of the drug.
Stability studies	The stability studies are conducted to find out the effect of temperature and relative humidity on the drug content in different formulations. The transdermal formulations are subjected to stability studies as per ICH guidelines.
Skin irritation studies	White albino rats, mice or white rabbits are used to study any hypersensitivity reaction on the skin. Mutalik and Udupa (2005) carried out skin irritation test using mice.

Marketed TDDS Formulations					
Active Ingredient	**Mol. Wt. (Daltons)**	**Trade Name(s)**	**Daily Dose**	**Frequency of Application**	**Type of System**
Clonidine	230	Catapres-TTS®	0.1–0.3 mg	Weekly	Reservoir
Estradiol	272	Esclim®	0.025–0.1 mg	Weekly	Drug-in-adhesive
Lidocaine	234	Lidoderm®	Not stated	Daily	Drug-in-adhesive
Nicotine	162	Nicoderm CQ®	7–21 mg	Daily	Drug-in-adhesive
Fentanyl	337	Duragesic	0.6 mg	Once every three days	Reservoir
EthinylEstradiol	296	Ortho-Evra®	0.15 mg	Weekly	Drug-in-adhesive
Nitro-glycerine	227	Nitro-Dur®	1.4–11.2 mg	Daily	Drug-in-adhesive

Conclusion

Most of the Traditional dosage forms are replaced with conventional dosage forms to improve solubility, bioavaibility, reduce toxicity and dose. NDDS dosage forms are recently developed for herbal extracts, phytochemical fractions and or pure phytochemicals. With the advancement of technology, evaluation and packaging of dosage forms also evolve. Recently 3D printing of pharmaceuticals especially oral dosage forms developed to provide personalised medicines but regulatory framework is yet to establish for same. This chapter has summarised traditional, conventional and NDDS dosage forms so that readers are able to acquire general idea of past, present and future market potential of various herbal dosage forms.

Further Reading

1. Idson B, Lazarus J; Semisolids in the Theory and Practice of Industrial Pharmacy. In Lachman L, Lieberman HA, Kanig JL editors; Varghese Publishing House, Bombay, India, 1991: 534–563.
2. Block LH; Medicated Applications. In Gennaro AR; Remington: The Science and Practice of Pharmacy. Mack Publishing Company, Easton, Pennsylvania, 1995:1577–1597.
3. Lieberman HA, Rieger MM, Banker GS; Pharmaceutical Dosage Forms: Disperse System, 2nd edition, Volume 3, 473-511
4. FDA; Guidance for Industry, Non-sterile Semisolid Dosage Forms, Scale-Up and Postapproval Changes: Chemistry, Manufacturing, and Controls, in vitro Release Testing and in vivo Bioequivalence Documentation, Rockville, MD, May 1997.
5. Nash RA, Wachter AH; Pharmaceutical Process Validation; 3rd edition, 2003.
6. Agalloco JP, Carleton FJ; Validation of Pharmaceutical Processes; 3rd edition, 2007: 417-428.
7. Idson B, Lazarus J; Semisolids. In The Theory and Practice of Industrial Pharmacy. In Lachman L, Lieberman HA, Kanig JL editors, Varghese Publishing House, Bombay, India, 1991: 534–563.
8. Block LH; Medicated Applications. In Gennaro AR editor; Remington: The Science and Practice of Pharmacy. 19th edition, Mack Publishing Company, Easton, Pennsylvania, 1995: 1590–1597.
9. Zatz JL, Kushla P; Gels. In In: Lieberman HA, Rieger MM, Banker GS, editors; Pharmaceutical Dosage Forms: Disperse Systems. Voume 2, New York: Marcel Dekker, 1988: : 495-510.
10. Collett M, Aulton EA; Text Book of Pharmaceutical Practice. 2nd edition, 2002.
11. Lachman L, Lieberman HA, Kenig JL; The Theory & Practice of Industrial Pharmacy. 3rd edition, Varghese Publishing house, 1987.
12. Rafiee TM, Mehramizi A; In vitro release studies of piroxicam from oil-in-water creams and hydroalcoholic gel topical formulations. Drug Devlnd Pharm., 2000; 64: 409–414.
13. Ahmed M.Faheem, Dalia H.Abdelkader.Novel drug delivery systems. Engineering Drug Delivery Systems. 2020, Pages 1-16
14. Sahoo SK, Labhasetwar V. Nanotech approaches to drug delivery and imaging. Drug Discov Today. 2003;8:1112–20.

15. Amit J, Sunil C, Vimal K, Anupam P. The Pharma Review. New Delhi: Kongposh Publications Pvt. Ltd; 2008. Phytosomes: A revolution in herbal drugs; pp. 24–8.
16. Mukherjee, S et al. "Solid lipid nanoparticles: a modern formulation approach in drug delivery system." Indian journal of pharmaceutical sciences vol. 71,4 (2009): 349-58.
17. Singhal P, Singhal R, Kumar V, Goel KK, Jangra AK, Yadav R. Transdermal Drug Delivery System: A Novel Technique To Enhance Therapeutic Efficacy And Safety Of Drugs. Am J Pharm tech Res. 2012; 2: 106-125.
18. Yie Chien. Novel Drug Delivery Systems. CRC Press LLC, 2019.
19. Durgesh Nandini Chauhan, Madhu Gupta, Nagendra Singh Chauhan, Vikas Sharma. Novel Drug Delivery Systems for Phytoconstituents. CRC Press, 2019.
20. Ryan F. Donnelly, Thakur Raghu Raj Singh. Novel Delivery Systems for Transdermal and Intradermal Drug Delivery. Willey, 2015.

Scan QR code to view the website/guidelines

- General Guidelines for Drug Development of Ayurvedic Formulations- CCRS_Guidline of Drug_Book-7_CD MATTER.pdf (ccras.nic.in)

CHAPTER 4

Herbal Cosmetics and Regulations

Introduction

Cosmetic Ingredients/Raw Materials

Surfactants [Anionic, Amphoteric, Nonionic, Cationics]
Conditioning Ingredients [Cationic Surfactants, Occlusives, Emollients, Humectants], Lipids/Fats/Waxes/Non-volatile Oil, Gums/Mucilages/Carbohydrates/Polysaccharides
Volatile oils-Perfumes and Fragrances, Colorants
Protective agents or Antioxidants in products such as skin care, hair care and oral hygiene products
Skin whitening (Bleaching) Agents.

Classification of Cosmetics:

Cosmetic preparations for Skin, Hair, Mouth, Shaving, Nail

Cosmeceuticals for Skin

Cream, Lip Balm, Powder, Lotion, Face Pack, Suntan and Sunburn Preparations, Bath Preparation, Deodorants and Antiperspirants

Cosmeceuticals for Hair

Shampoo, Hair Oil/Hair Tonic, Hair Colorants, Shaving Preparation, After Shave Lotion

Dental Products

Dentifrices, Toothpaste and Mouthwash

Nail Products

Nail polish and enamels, Nail polish and enamel removers

Eye Makeup Products

Mascara, Eye shadow, Eyeliner, Eyebrow Pencil, Eye Makeup Remover

Baby Products

Baby Shampoos, Baby Lotions, Oils, Powders and Creams

Quality Control/Standardization of Herbal Cosmetics

Quality Control Analytical Methods

Cream/Lotion, Moisturizing cream/lotion, Sunscreen, Shampoo, Tooth paste, Face powder, Lip cosmetics- lipsticks, Lip Balm, Lip Liner)

Cosmetic Safety and Toxicity Screening

Cosmetic Regulations in Various Countries

Europe Cosmetics Regulations, ASEAN Cosmetics Regulations, Australian Cosmetics Regulations, USA Cosmetics Regulations, Indian Cosmetics Regulations, Good Manufacturing Practices (GMP)

BIS Regulations for Cosmetics

Introduction, Standards for Heavy metals, Standards for Colouring Agent, Standards for Preservatives, ANNEX D (Clauses 1 and 3) List of Permitted UV Filters Which Cosmetic Products May Contain

Cosmetic Evaluation Instruments

Instruments to Evaluate Skin Products

Sebumeter, Visioscope, Corneometer CM 825, Trans-Epidermal Water Loss Measurement (TEWL), Skin color measurement by Minolta CR-300 colorimeter

Instruments to Evaluate Hair Products

Hair Physical/Mechanical Proprieties, Hair Combing Properties, Hair Stretching Resistance Property, Scanning Electron Microscopy (SEM), Atomic Force Microscopy (AFM), Mechanical Assays, Piezoelectric Sensors, Glossmeters, Optical Coherence Tomography, Subjective Tests

Further Reading

Introduction

Cosmetics are defined as "items with mild action on the human body for the purpose of cleaning, beautifying, adding to the attractiveness, altering the appearance, or keeping or promoting the skin or hair in good condition" while functional cosmetics, even if falling under the cosmetic definition, are designated as "items fulfilling specific actions like skin whitening, minimizing the appearance of lines in the face and body, protecting from the sun and sun tanning".

Cosmeceuticals are cosmetic products having some specific therapeutic effects. Cosmeceuticals are cosmetic products that are claimed, primarily by those within the cosmetic industry, to have drug-like benefits. Cosmeceuticals represent a marriage between cosmetics and pharmaceuticals. Like cosmetics, cosmeceuticals are topically applied, but they contain ingredients that influence the biological function of the skin. Cosmeceuticals improve appearance, but they do so by delivering nutrients necessary for healthy skin. Cosmeceuticals are the fastest-growing segment of the natural personal care industry.

Cosmeceuticals are not subject to review by the Food and Drug Administration (FDA), and the term cosmeceutical is not recognized by the Federal Food, Drug, and Cosmetic Act. Although cosmetics and cosmeceuticals are tested for safety, testing to determine whether beneficial ingredients actually live up to a manufacturer's claims is not mandatory. Cosmeceuticals may contain purported active ingredients such as vitamins, phytochemicals, enzymes, antioxidants, and essential oils, but the manufacturer may not claim that these products penetrate beyond the skin's surface layers or that they have drug like or therapeutic effects. For cosmetic labels, no division between active ingredients and other ingredients is required; they are all listed together.

What are cosmetics?

It is not simple to define the term "cosmetic" as its scope and application to the care of different body part is very wide. According to definition these are

1. The articles intended to be rubbed, poured, sprinkled or sprayed on, introduced into , or otherwise applied to the human body or any part thereof for cleansing, beautifying, promoting attractiveness or altering the appearance, and
2. Articles intended for use as a component of any such articles; except that such term shall not include soap.

Objectives

- To enhance the general appearance of face and other body parts to minimize the skin defects to a considerable extent.
- To look more impressive, beautiful and smart to a considerable extent.
- Psychological, social
- Clinical benefits: cracking, wrinkles, ageing and minimizing effects of wind burn, sunburn, skin infection etc.

What are herbal cosmeceuticals?

Herbal cosmeceuticals are the preparations, which represent cosmetics associated with active bioactive ingredients or pharmaceuticals. The use of phytochemicals from a variety of botanicals has dual function,

1. They serve as cosmetics for the care of body and its pats and
2. The botanical ingredients present influence biological functions of skin and provide nutrient necessary for the healthy skin or hair.

Design of Herbal Cosmetic Formulation

Design of herbal cosmetics should involve following pre-formulation study parameters

- Selection of appropriate herbs or herbal extract/s, phytochemical fractions
- Quantity and Proportion of herbs or herbal extract/s, phytochemical fractions
- Nature of the Phytoconstituents
- Purpose of preparation
- Stability, compatibility and shelf-life Testing

Cosmetic Ingredients/Raw Materials

Surfactants

Surfactants are perhaps the most important of all cosmetic ingredients due to its cleansing, foaming, thickening, emulsifying, solubilizing, penetration enhancement, antimicrobial effects, and other special effects. Compatibility with both water and oil is key property of surfactants.

- ***Detergency:*** Surfactants in cosmetics are useful for cleansing skin and hair having presence of solid particulates of dust as well as oily deposits from natural sebum. The lipophilic part of surfactant removes fats on the surface of hair and skin while the hydrophilic ends of the molecules align toward the surface of these deposits, thereby increasing the hydrophilicity. That allows the lipid deposits to lift off the surface of skin or hair where the rinse water washes them away.
- ***Wetting:*** Wetting property of surfactants reduces the contact angle between a cosmetic and the surface which makes the product (creams and lotions) easier to spread.
- ***Foam:*** Foam characteristic relates to cleansing action in spite the fact that foam doesn't really contribute much to the removal of dirt and or lipids. Air bubbles surrounded by liquid and surfactants create foam.
- ***Thickening:*** thickening agent creates micelles where lipophilic tails of surfactant orient inwards and the polar heads orient outwards toward the water. Packed micelles useful for thickness while charged surfactants incorporated micelles forms cleansing thinner solution by repelling other micelles. Salt is frequently added to initiate packing of micelles to get desired thickness.

- ***Emulsification:*** Emulsions can be creams and lotions in the form of oil-in-water or water-in-oil emulsions or more complex multiple emulsions and mostly prefer to deliver active lipophilic ingredients to the surface of skin and hair.

Types of Surfactants

Surfactants can be classified according to the charge of their counterion or whether they form ions in solution or not. There are anionic surfactants, which have a negatively charged ion. There are amphoteric surfactants, which are capable of both positive and negative charges depending on the pH conditions of the solution they are in. There are cationic surfactants, which are positively charged. And, finally, there are nonionic surfactants, which have no charge at all. All four of these surfactant types are used in cosmetics for different reasons.

Anionic (positively charged surfactant ions)	Potent cleanser, good amounts of foam forming capacity and inexpensive but more irritating	Alkyl sulfates: sodium lauryl sulfate and ammonium lauryl sulfate (ALS), sulfosuccinates, alkyl benzene sulfanate, acyl methyl taurates, acyl sarcocinates, the isethionates, propyl peptide condensates, monoglyceride sulfates and fatty glycerol, ether sulfanates.
Amphoteric (have both a negative charge and a positive charge, depending on the pH)	Good detergency, less irritating but more expensive and less foam forming capacity	cocamidopropyl betaine, cocoamphopropionate, and sodium lauraminopropionate
Nonionic (do not have any charge)	Gentle cleansers (hence preferable in baby shampoos), good foam forming capacity, less irritating but more expensive	fatty alcohols and fatty alkanolamides, PEG-80, sorbitan laurate, including lauramide diethanolamine (DEA) and cocamide DEA, amine oxides such as lauramine oxide or stearamine oxide
Cationics (positively charged molecules)	Poor clean, rinse, or foam capacity, more irritating but useful as conditioning agents	Quaternary ammonium compounds, quaternized compounds, stearalkonium chloride, dicetyldimonium chloride, and behentrimonium chloride

Conditioning Ingredients

Conditioning and moisturizing ingredients like cationic surfactants, occlusive, emollients and humectants being "oily" in nature improve the feel or condition of skin or hair.

Cationic Surfactants

- It used for conditioning are also known as quaternary ammonium compounds, quaternized compounds, or just simply "quats." They contain at least one nitrogen atom bonded to four other hydrocarbon groups. Some common examples include stearalkonium chloride, dicetyldimonium chloride, and behentrimonium chloride.
- Although cationic surfactants don't make good cleansing products, they are excellent conditioning ingredients, particularly for hair care products. The main reason is because they are substantive to the damaged, negatively charged protein sites on hair and skin. When a quat is put on hair or skin, the positive portion of the molecule is attracted to the

negatively charged damaged site creating an electrostatic bond. While water rinses most things away, the cationic surfactant remains.

- Since these are hydrocarbon molecules, the longer the hydrocarbon chain is, the more conditioning they will do. So, all things being equal, a material such as behentrimonium chloride, which is a C22 carbon chain, will be more conditioning than a shorter chain molecule such as cetrimonium chloride, which is a C16 carbon chain.

Occlusives

- Perhaps the most effective skin moisturizing ingredients are occlusive agents. These are oily materials that can create a thin coating on the skin or hair. The most common types of occlusive agents used in cosmetics include petrolatum, mineral oil, and dimethicone.
- When occlusive agents are put on the skin (or hair) they form a thin, continuous film on the surface. This film is flexible but feels slightly greasy to the touch, which is why only a small amount is used in formulations. The occlusive film is also resistant to water, which helps explain its moisturizing effect.
- The body naturally loses water through skin. When atmospheric humidity is low, more moisture is lost and skin feels dryer. Occlusive agents create a film on the skin which slows the water loss. As water tries to leave the body, it hits this barrier and starts to accumulate in the outer layers of the skin (the epidermis). This extra moisture improves the way the skin looks and feels and also can reduce itching and redness. Occlusives such as petrolatum are so effective they can actually be used as OTC drugs for skin protection.

Emollients

- Emollients were some of the first ingredients used as cosmetics. They are not typically compatible with water and include ingredients such as oils, butters, waxes, and esters. Emollients are similar to occlusive agents, except that they tend to be lower-molecular-weight molecules and don't have the ability to form a continuous film to block water. But, emollients are important ingredients for improving the way the surface of the hair and skin feel, and they impart shine, which is the primary reason they are used.
- When creating skin creams, lotions, and even hair products, emollients are used to modify the way formulations feel, how they rub into the skin, the ease at which they spread, and the length of time they remain “workable.”
- Common examples of emollients include natural oils such as coconut oil, argan oil, almond oil, or olive oil. There are also a number of excellent esters that are emollients, including myristyl myristate, cetyl palmitate, and lauryl laurate. Each of these feels slightly different and has different abilities to absorb into the skin. In addition, many silicones make excellent emollients, as they provide great slickness and shine.

Humectants

- Humectants have been used as cosmetic compounds for as long as cosmetics have existed. They include natural materials such as honey, aloe, or glycerin, and are typically mild. The property that makes humectants useful is their ability to attract and hold water like a sponge. In fact, glycerin can hold as much as three times its weight in water. Such humectants are especially useful for surfaces that tend to dry out, such as skin or hair.

- The most common humectants used in cosmetics include glycerin, propylene glycol, sorbitol, sodium pca, hyaluronic acid, and various hydrolyzed proteins.
- Humectants have few significant negatives: They feel sticky and are easily rinsed away. This limits their use to cosmetic products that will be left on, making them great for skin lotions and leave-on hair conditioners but not so great for shampoos, body washes, or rinse-out hair conditioners.

Other ingredients as per type of cosmetic are summarized in classification section.

Lipids/Fats/Waxes/Non-volatile Oil

- Fatty acids are important in maintaining the structure and function of the outer layer or epidermis (stratum corneum, SC) which contains glycolipids, intercellular lipids (cement), and a lipid coat of the skin called the natural moisturizing factor. Lipids in intercellular matrix connect the SC, ensuring its cohesiveness, ability to protect the skin from xenobiotics, and forming a barrier against water loss.
- Chronologically aged skin is characterized by an inherent reduction in epidermal lipid content, resulting in dehydration and altered skin barrier function. Epidermal keratinocyte differentiation and desquamation slows with age, leaving skin dry and flaky.
- Dryness of the skin further accumulates into a reduction of elasticity andwrinkles of the skin consequently as evidenced by biomechanical properties ofthe skin. Therefore, application of skin hydrating cosmetics isnot only to hydrate the skin, but their pleiotropic skin benefits ultimately enhanceaesthetic preference of the skin. That is recently known as corneotherapy.
- Classification of lipids

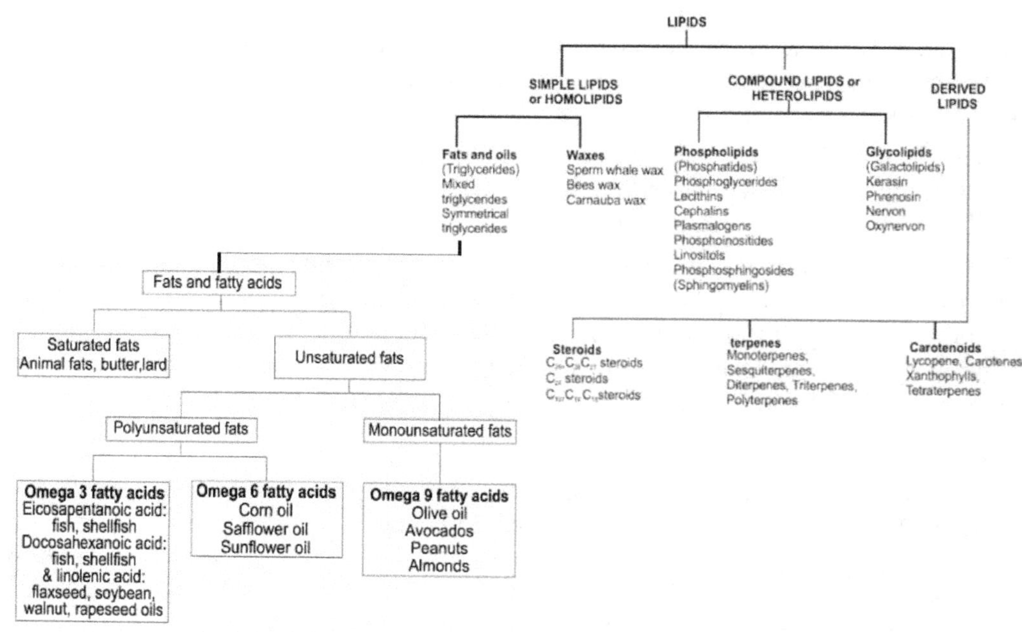

- Vegetable oils are used as a emulsifiers in detergents, creams, lotions, ointments, and makeup to acts a skin moisturizing, smoothing and lubrication, anti-eczema, anti-inflammation and arthritis, soothing of sunburn, and the healing of wounds, ulcers, and burns
- The oils incorporate into the cell membranes and regenerate the damaged lipid barrier of epidermis restricting water loss. The unsaturated fatty acids show pronounced healing effects on dermatoses such as atopic skin inflammation and are used in creams, emulsions, cosmetic milks, ointments, hair conditioners, cosmetic masks, lipsticks, bath fluids, nail polishes, etc
- Fatty acids, triglycerides, and glycerol are used as emollient and hydrating components, acts as a waterproof barrier
- Omega-9 fatty acid like ricinoleic acid from castor oil is found to be very useful for skin dryness, acne, and baldness.
- Omega-6 fatty acid like linoleic acid is found to be very useful in eczema, hair loss, reduced wound healing, and circulatory defects.
- Monounsaturated oleic acid, and also the saturated palmitic and stearic acids present in Cocoa butter are very good emollients, moisturizers, and in the treatment of dry skin.
- Polyunsaturated linoleic acid in Sunflower oil is useful for scaly lesions due to essential fatty acid deficiency, or for psoriasis and burns.
- Jojoba waxy oil (seeds of the desert shrub Simmondsia chinensis) is very useful in extrinsic skin aging and hair strengthening due to high penetrability and deliverability to deep skin layers through hydration, antioxidant and anti-inflammatory effects. It reduces wrinkles.
- Ceramides like sphingolipids containing linoleic acyl esters are extremely useful in skin rehydration.
- Oil-free moisturizers without vegetable oils use silicone derivatives such as dimethicone and cyclomethicone to retard moisture loss without the greasy feel.
- Vegetable oils commonly used in facial care are Almond, apricot, hazelnut, borage, jojoba, avocado, olive, wheat germ, macadamia, grapeseed
- Vegetable oils commonly used in hair care are Almond, borage, avocado, cocoa butter, jojoba, sesame, macadamia.

Type	**Biological source**	**Family**	**Chemical composition**
			PUFA/MUFA
Plant			
Almond oil	*Prunus dulcis (Mill.)*	Rosaceae	Aldobionic acid, Vit A, E, stearic and palmitic acid,
Apricot oil	*Prunus armeniaca*	Rosaceae	Amygdalin, oleic and linoleic acid, Vit A, C, and Vit E, stearic and palmitic acid,

Contd...

Type	Biological source	Family	Chemical composition
			PUFA/MUFA
Avocado oil	*Persea ameriana*	Lauraceae	Oleic acid(65%), linoleic acid(14%), palmitic acid(6%), high content of ω-3,6,9 fatty acids.
Borage oil	*Borago officinalis*	Boraginaceae	Palmitoleic acid (11%), oleic acid (20%), stearic acid (4.5%), Linolenic acid (38%), nervonic acid(1.5%), eicosenoic acid(5.5%).
Brazil nut oil	*Bertholletia excelsa*	Lecythidaceae	Beta sitosterol(54%), monounsaturated fat (24%), polyunsaturated fat(20%), satureted fat(15%).
Canola oil	*Brassica rapa*	Brassicaceae	Arachidic (5%), eicosenoic (5%), lignoceric(8%), oleic(40%), linolenic(8%), linoleic acids.
Cashew oil	*Anacardium occidentale*	Anacardiaceae	Anacardiac acid (71%), saturated fat (7%), unsaturated fat(0.2%), polysaturated fat (7%), monounsaturated fat(23.79%).
Chia seeds oil	*Salvia hispanica*	Lamiaceae	Omega -3- fatty acids, palmitic acid, linolenic acid.
Cocoa butter oil	*Theobroma cacao*	sterculiaceae	Stearic (34%), palmitic (25%), oleic (37%) acids and small amount of arachidic and linolenic acid.
Coconut oil	*Cocos nucifera*	Palmae	95% saturated fatty acid, caprylic acid, capric acid, myristic acid.
Corn oil	*Zea mays*	Gramineae	Stearic(4.5%), palmitic(13%), oleic(24%), linolenic(62%), linoleic acids(1.5%). Beta-sitosterol, compesterol.
Castor oil	*Ricinus communis*	Euphorbiaceae	Ricinoleic acid, Ricicine, ricin, phytin
Cottonseed oil	*Gossypium harbaceum*	Malvaceae	Glycerides like palmitooleolinoleins (35-40%), palmitodioleins (20%). Stearic(2.7%), palmitic(33%), oleic(29%), arachidic acid(1%).
Evening Primrose Oil	*Oenothera biennis*	Oenothera	Linoleic acid(74%), linolenic acid(10%).sterols.
Flaxseed/Linseed oil	*Linum usitatissimum*	linaceae	Glycerides of Stearic, palmitic, oleic, linolenic, linoleic acids. Squalene and tocopherol, linamarin and 5% of mucilage.
Grape seed oil	*Vitis vinifera*	Vitaceae	Palmitoleic acid (<1%), oleic acid (15.8%), polyunsaturated fatty acid (69.9%), Linolenic acid (69.6%)
Hazelnut oil	*Carylus avellana*	Betulaceae	palmitic, oleic, linolenic, linoleic acids. Arachidonic acid
Hemp seed oil	*Cannabis sativa*	cannabinaceae	Cannabidilic acid and transterahydrocanabinol.
Jojoba oil	*Simmondsia chimensis*	Simmonodsiaceae	Triglycerides, ionomycin, oleosin

Contd...

Type	Biological source	Family	Chemical composition
			PUFA/MUFA
Mustard oil	*Brassica nigra*	Brassicaceae	Arachidic(0.5%), behenic(3%), eicosenoic(8%), erusic(60%), lignoceric(18%), oleic(22%), linolenic(7%), linoleic acids.
Macadamia oil	*Macadamia integrifolia*	Proteaceae	Myristic acid(1.6%), Stearic(6.1%), palmitic(13.1%), oleic(51%), linoleic acids(3.7%), Gadoleic acid(3.7%), behenic acid (1.7%).
Olive oil	*Olea europoea*	Oleaceae	Glycerides of Stearic, palmitic, oleic, linolenic, linoleic acids. Arachidonic acid
Palm oil	*Elaeis guineensis*	Arecaceae	Olein, 3-monochloropropanediol MPCD, little amount f linoleic acid.
Peanut oil	*Arachia hypogaea*	Papilionaceae	Fatty acids like Stearic(3.1%), palmitic(8.3%), linolenic(26%), arachidic acid(24%), eicosenoic acid(3.1%).
Pecan oil	*Carya illinoinesis*	Juglandaceae	Oleic acid(57%), linoleic acid (30%), polyunsaturated fat (21%)
Perilla oil	*Perilla frutescens*	Lamiaceae	Limonene, linalool, alpha-pinene
Rice bran oil	*Oryza sativa*	Gramineae	Oleic (40-50%), linoleic (30-40%), palmitic acid (12-18%)
Safflower oil	*Carthamus tinctorius*	Composites	Glycerides of Stearic(3%), palmitic(6.5%), oleic(13%), linolenic(76%), linoleic acids(90%).
Sesame oil	*Sesamum indicum Linn.*	Pedaliaceae	Sesamolin oleic acid, linoleic acid.
Soybean oil Partially hydrogenated	*Glycine max*	Leguminosae	Saturated fatty acid (14.9), Oleic (42.4), linoleic (2.6), linolenic acid (34.9), palmitic acid, arachidic acid
Soybean oil	*Glycine max*	Leguminosae	Saturated fatty acid (15.5), Oleic (22.6), linoleic (7), linolenic acid (51), palmitic acid, arachidic acid
Sunflower oil (<60% linolenic acid)	*Carthamus tinctorius*	Compositae	Saturated fatty acid (10.1), Oleic (82.6), linoleic (0.2), linolenic acid(39.8), palmitic acid, arachidic acid
Sunflower oil (>70% oleic acid)	*Carthamus tinctorius*	Compositae	Saturated fatty acid (9.9), Oleic (82.6), linoleic (0.2), linolenic acid (3.6), palmitic acid, arachidic acid

Contd...

Type	Biological source	Family	Chemical composition
			PUFA/MUFA
Sunflower (standard)	*Carthamus tinctorius*	Compositae	Saturated fatty acid (10.3), oleic acid(19.5), linolenic acid(0.9), linoleic acid(65.7),
Tomato seed oil	*Solanum lycopersicum*	Solanaceae	High content of linoleic acid(54%), oleic acid(22%), palmitic acid(14%), stearic acid (6%).
Vigna mungo oil	*Vigna mungo*	Fabaceae	Total 1.64 gm of saturated and unsaturated fat in 100 gm contain Oleic, linoleic, linolenic acid, palmitic acid, arachidic acid
Walnut oil	*Juglans regia*	Juglandaceae	Ferulic acid, myricetin, vanillic acid, coumaric acid, syringic acid, sitosterol, ellagitannin.
Wheat germ Oil	*Triticum aestivum*	Gramineae	Saturated fatty acid (4.7%), linoleic acid (44.1%), linolenic acid (10.8%), vit E, unsaponifiable matter.
Animal Sources			
Beeswax	*Apis mellifeca*	Apidae	Myricin, melissic acid, cerolein, cero
Cocca butter	*Theobroma cacao*	sterculiaceae	Stearic (34%), palmitic (25%), oleic (37%) acids and small amount of arachidic and linolenic acid.
Shea butter	*Vitellaria paradoxa*	sapotaceae	Five principal of fatty acid Stearic, palmitic, oleic, linoleic and arachidic acids. Phenolic compound catechin.
Lanolin	*Ovis aries*	Bovidae	Complex mixture of ester and polystyrene 33 high molecular weight alcohol and 36 fatty acids. Ester of cholesterol and isocholesterol with oleic, linoleic, caranubic, linopalmatic acid.
Lecithin	*Glycine max (soyabean 33-35%)*	Leguminosae	Sterols, phosphatidyl choline.
Ceramides	*Triticum aestivum (wheat germ)*	Gramineae	Sphingosine and fatty acids.

Gums/Mucilages/ Carbohydrates/Polysaccharides

- Polysaccharides are macromolecules based on glycosidically linked combinations of up to 40 different monosaccharides, sometimes substituted by nonsugar groups such as alcohols, organic acids, or sulfates. Those from animals, terrestrial plants, marine macroalgae, and nonphotosynthetic microorganisms are widely exploited by industry as biological agents in various fields including agronomy, medicine, cosmetic, nutrition, and others.

- Gums/Mucilages/ Carbohydrates/Polysaccharides serve a variety of functions, such as thickening, emulsifying (keeping ingredients mixed together), creating protective films or barriers, and making products feel either "drier" or more moist, smoother, or more pleasant overall. Another advantage of Polysaccharides is that they are "high molecular weight," which means they do not easily penetrate the skin and are less likely than traditional alternatives to cause stinging, burning or redness.
- Water-based formulations are thin by nature, and polymers are used to thicken them or turn them into gels. When used to increase thickness in products like shampoos, conditioners, creams, and lotions, for example, the formulas feel more rich, smooth, and creamy. Polysaccharides such as starch, xanthan or guar gum, carrageenan, alginates, polysaccharides, pectin, gelatin, agar, and cellulose derivatives can be used as a thickener in cosmetics. More recent developments include combining hydrophobic and hydrophilic polymers into "copolymers" that stabilize products so that they don't get thin under high heat – for example, sunscreens.
- Hair sprays, lotions, gels, and foams containing polysaccharides, including starch and cellulose derivatives, natural gums, and mucilages as hair styling agents.
- Polysaccharides acts as"carrier" for active ingredients in cosmetics, such as antioxidants and antimicrobials or encapsulation of ingredients such as vitamins and peptides so that they are able to work when applied to hair and skin during use.
- Conditioning Polysaccharides deposits, adhere, or absorb into the proteins of the skin and hair. They improve skin feel and hair manageability, reduce static and make the skin and hair softer and smoother.
- Major plant polysaccharides are cellulose, pectins, and β-glucans. Gums/mucilages can be calssified based on source as follows:
    - marine origin/algal (seaweed) gums: agar, carrageenans, alginic acid, and laminarin;
    - plant origin:
        - shrubs/tree exudates: gum arabic, gum ghatti, gum karaya, gum tragacanth, and khaya and albizia gums;
        - seed gums: guar gum, locust bean gum, starch, amylose, and cellulose;
        - extracts: pectin, larch gum;
        - tuber and roots: potato starch;
    - animal origin: chitin and chitosan, chondroitin sulfate, and hyaluronic acid;
    - microbial origin (bacterial and fungal): xanthan, dextran, curdian, pullulan, zanflo, emulsan, Baker's yeast glycan, schizophyllan, lentinan, krestin, and scleroglucan.
- Glucans if combined with polysaccharides and proteins acts as a tissue matrix proteoglycans which enables to retain water and acts as a film formers, humectants, and skin moisturizers and helps in tissue regeneration and wound healing.
- β-glucan (Saccharomyces strains) useful in tissue regeneration which behaves like hyaluronic acid in stimulating collagen synthesis by fibroblasts.
- Carragenans from various red algae are used as emulsifiers in the preparation of creams, gels, pastes, and emulsions.

- Oat β-glucan (Avena sativa) is an un-branched polysaccharide that has been claimed to alleviate the signs of aging, protect against UV, activate collagen synthesis, and strengthen the hairs.
- β-glucan and hydrolyzed oat protein is also used to moisturize and soothe irritated skin.
- Gums and mucilages are employed as additives as well as acts as a antioxidant and emollient properties.

Volatile oils-Perfumes and Fragrance

Volatile oils or essential oils are major part of perfumes as well as flavours. Flavors affect both the sense of taste and smell, whereas fragrances affect only smell. The Fragrance wheel created in 1983 by Michael Edwards is classification method that is widely used in retail and in the fragrance industry.

Various terpenes from mono-terpenoid and sesquiterpenoid class (linear, cyclic, aromatic) with different functional groups (alcohol, aldehyde, ester, ether) are major constituents of natural perfumes. Example: Geraniol (Nerol), linalool, citronellol, citral, pinene, carvone, muskone

Different perfume sources	
Natural	**Example**
Flowers	Rose, jasmine, osmanthus, plumeria, mimosa, tuberose, narcissus, scented geranium, cassie, ambrette, blossoms of citrus
Wood	Sandalwood, rosewood, agarwood, birch, cedar, juniper, pine
Bark	Cinnamon, cascarilla, sassafras
Fruits	Apples, strawberries, cherries, oranges, lemons, limes
Leaves	Lavender leaf, patchouli, sage, violets, rosemary, citrus leaves
Roots	Vetiver, iris, ginger
Resins	Labdanum, olibanum, myrrh, balsam of peru, benzoin, pine, fir
Animal	Musk, ambergris, civet, hyraceum, castoreum
Synthetic	Synthetic derivatives of benzene, toluene, phenol, naphthalene, cyclopentanone or complete synthetic form of natural perfume chemicals

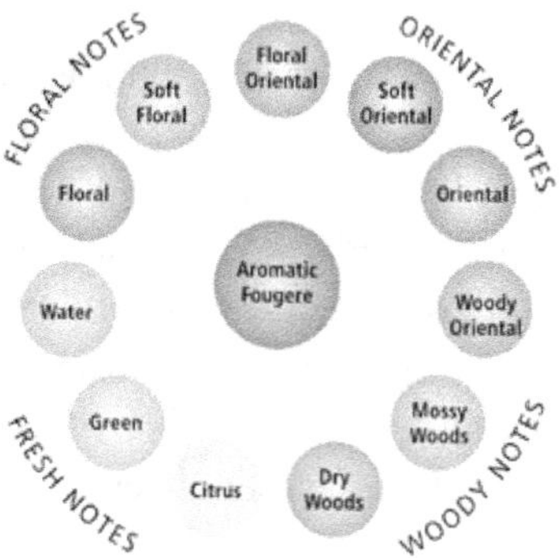

Figure 4.1 Fragrance wheel.

Plant	Biological source	Family	Volatile Chemical composition
Plants			
Agarwood	*Aquilaria malaccencis*	Thymelaeceae	Terpenes, sequiterpenes and oxygenated compound
Ambrette	*Abelmoschus moschatus*	Macalvaceae	Ambrettolide, Farnesol acetate,
Apples	*Malus domestica*	Rosaceae	Vitamin K, B6, Hydroxycinnamic acid, coumarolylquinic acid
Balsam of peru	*Myroxylonbalsamum*	Leguminosae	Styrene, vanillin, coumarin, benzyl alcohol, benzyl cinnamate, cinnamic acid, cinnamyl cinnamate
Benzoin	*Styrax tonkinensis*	Styracaceae	Benzoic acid, cinnamic acid, esters
Birch	*Betula nigra*	Betulaceae	Eugenol, linalool, palmitic acid
Cascarilla	*Croton eluteria*	Euphorbiacea	Cascarillins, lignins, tannins and resins
Cassie	*Acacia farnesiana*	Fabaceae	Essential oil cassie, ellagic acid, naringin, kaempferol
Cedar	*Cedrus deodara*	Pinaceae	Taxifolin, cedeodarin, ampelopsin, cedrin, cedrinoside, deodarin
Cherries	*Prunus avium*	Rosaceae	3-caffeoylquinic, p-coumaric acid, catechin
Cinnamon	*Cinnamomum zeylanicum*	Lauraceae	Eugenol, benzaldehyde cuminaldehyde
Citrus	*Citrus species*	Rutaceae	Lipids, vitamins & minerals, flavonoids-limonoids
Fir	*Firs species*	Pinaceae	Camphene, bornyl acetate, santene
Geranium	*Pelargonium graveolens*	Geraniaceae	Geraneol, citronellol
Ginger	*Zingiber officinalis*	Zingiberaceae	Zingiberene, curcumene
Iris	*Iris gemanica*	Iridaceae	Caprylic acid, capric, lauric, tridcanoic palmitic acid
Jasmine	*Jasminum offficinale*	Oleaceae	3-hexanol, linalool, benzyl alcohol
Juniper	*Juniperus communis*	Cupressaseae	A-pinene, camphor, thymol methyl ether
Labdanum	*Cistus ladanifer*	Cistaceae	Tricycline, α-thujene, Sabinene, Terpenilene
Lavender	*Lavendula officinalis*	Labiateae	Esters linalyl acetate linalool, pinene, geraniol, cineol
Lemons	*Citrus limonis*	Rutaceae	Limonene, citral geranyl acetate terpineol
Limes	*Citrus aurantifolia*	Rutaceae	Vitamin C, citric acid

Contd...

Plant	Biological source	Family	Volatile Chemical composition
Mimosa	*Mimosa pudica*	Fabaceae	Palmitic acid
Myrrh	*Commiphoramolmol*	Burseraceae	α,β,γ-commiphoric acid, α,β-heerabomyrrholic acid, cuminic aldehyde, eugenol
Narcissus	*Narcissus poeticus*	Amaryllidaceae	β-ocimene, 1,8-cineole, linalool
Olibanum	*Boswellia serrata*	Burseraceae	α-pinene, Sabinene, Limonene, α-Thujene
Oranges	*Citrus species*	Rutaceae	Vitami C, Limonene, citronellal
Osmanthus	*Osmanthus heterophullus*	Oleaceae	Linalool, Terpenoids-Te3, Te5, Te6
Patchouli	*Pogostemoncablin*	Lamiaceae	Germecrene, Patchoulol, Narpatchoulenol
Pine	*Pinus sylvestris*	Pinaceae	Hydrocarbens, terpenoids, phenols, resinous substance, terpentine
Plumeria	*Plumeria rubra*	Apocynaceae	Geraniol, linalool,
Rose	*Rosa alba*	Rosaceae	Geraniol, citronellol, nerol, linalool,
Rosemary	*Rosmarinus officinalis*	Lamiaceae	β-caryophyllene, limonene, α-pinene, 1,8-cineole, carnosol, ursolic acid
Rosewood	*Anibarosaeodora*	Meliaceae	Linalool,
Sage	*Salvia officinalis*	Lamiaceae	Thujones, camphor, α-pinene
Sandalwood	*Santalam album*	Santalaceae	α,β-santalol, santene, santenone, teresantol, standalone, santalene
Sassafras	*Sassafras albidum*	Lauraceae	Safrole, camphor, methyleugenol
Strawberries	*Fragaria ananassa*	Rosaceae	Ethyl esters, Palmitic acid,
Tuberose	*Palianthes tuberosa*	Asparagaceae	Methyl benzoate, butyric acid, augenol, nerol, farnesol, geraneol
Vetiver	*Chrysipogon zizanoides*	Poaceae	Citral, geraniol, α and β v
Animal			
Ambergris	*Physeter catoden*	Physeteridae	Ambrene, epicoprostemolcoprostemone
Musk	*Moschus moschiferus*	Cervidae	Musckone, Cholesterine, Albuminoids, Resin
Castoreum	*Caster faber*	Castoridae	Volatile oil, Resin, Castorin, benzyl alcohol, methyl phenol, l-borneol.
Civet	*Viverrazibetha*	Viverridae	Civetone, Indole civetole ethylamine, propylamine.

Colorants

Generally, plant pigments are classified as chlorophylls, carotenoids, flavonoids, phytochromes, betalains and naphthaquinones. These pigments are of great value in the preparation of cosmetics, foods and drugs in the form of colour additives. As compared to synthetic pigments, natural pigments have lower intensity and require large quantities of raw materials. But due to their low toxicity and no carcinogenic effects, natural pigments are always fascinating to mankind. Example:

Source	Color	Use
Flavonoid namely, brazilin from sappanwood (*Caesalpinia sappan*, Leguminosae)	Red	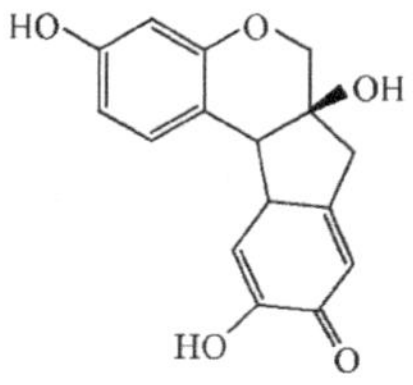 Color cosmetics
Tricyclic anthraquinone Alizarin from Madder (*Rubia tinctorium*) roots	Red	Hair 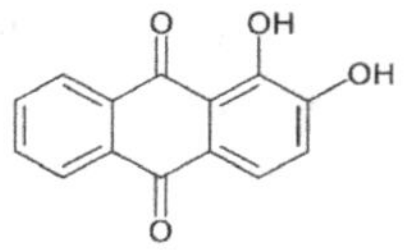
Napthquinone Juglon form walnut (Juglans nigra, Juglandaceae) shells and leaves	Brown [C.I. Natural Brown 7 and C.I. 75500]	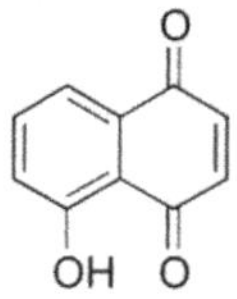 Hair
Napthquinone Lawsone from Henna (Lawsonia inermis) leaves	Orange yellow	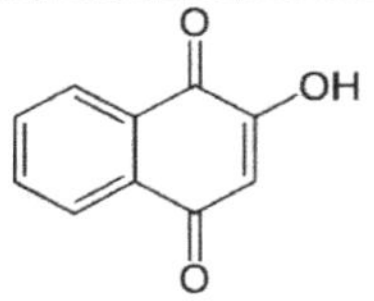 Hair
Carmine with the main component carminic acid is an approved food colorant E 120. It is obtained from scales of Dactylopius coccus (or cochineals). Carminic acid (C22H20O13) is a red glucosidal hydroxyanthrapurin.	Orange, red	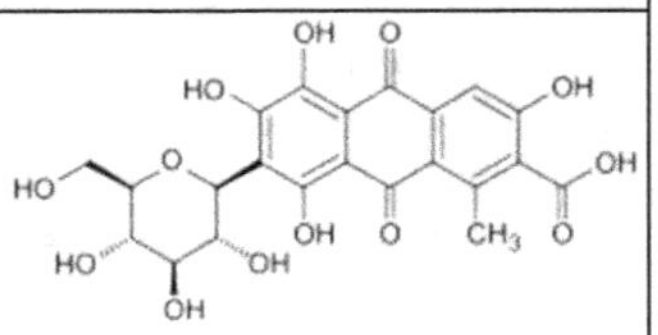 Color cosmetics
Carotenoid- Bixin from Annatto (Bixa orellana) seeds	Orange yellow	Lipstick 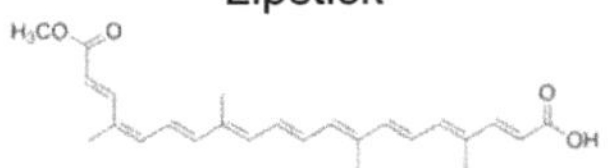

Contd...

Source	Color	Use
Indigo from *Indigofera tinctoria* and other species leaves	Blue	Lipstick 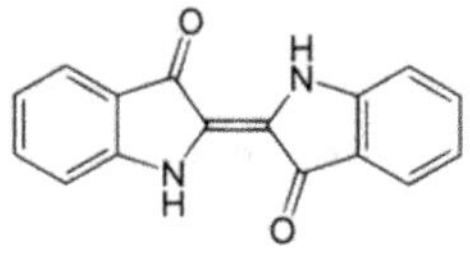
Sesquiterpene Guaiazulene from Guaiacum oil (Guaiacum officinale, Zygophyllaceae) and Chammomile (Matricaria chamomilla, Asteraceae)	Dark blue	Hair, color cosmetics 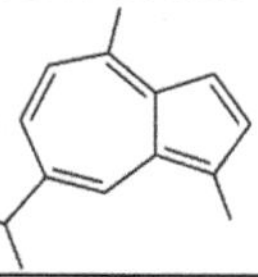
Curcumin a principle Curcuminoids from turmeric (Curcuma longa, Zingiberaceae) rhizomes	Ornage, yellow	Color cosmetics 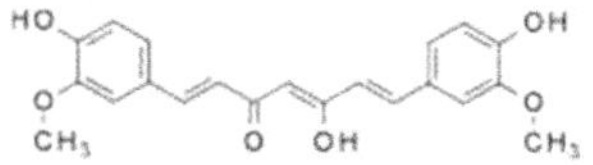
Betalains from beet (*Beta vulagris*) roots. **Betalains** are water-soluble nitrogen-containing pigments, which provide red-violet (betacyanins) and the yellow (betaxanthins) colors to some fruits and vegetables	Red–purple betacyanidins and the yellow betaxanthins	Color cosmetics 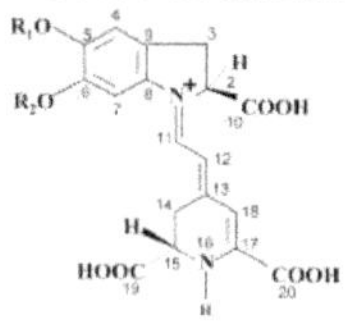 Betacyanins R_1 = glucosyl or derivatives R_2 = glucosyl, glucuronyl, derivatives or H
		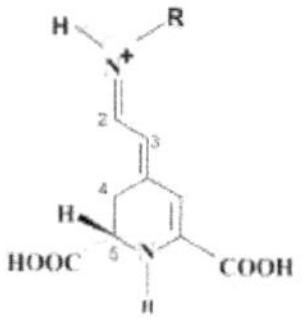 Betaxanthins R= amino acid, amine or derivatives
Tannins from barks and leaves of many sources	Yellow, brown, black	Hair
"**Carotenoids**" is a generic term used to designate the majority of pigments naturally found in animal and plant kingdoms. Two classes of carotenoids are found in nature: (a) the carotenes such as β-carotene, which consist of linear hydrocarbons that can be cyclized at one end or both ends of the molecule, and (b) the oxygenated derivatives of carotenes such as **lutein, lycopene, violaxanthin, neoxanthin,** and **zeaxanthin**, known as xanthophylls.	Red, orange, yellow	Color cosmetics 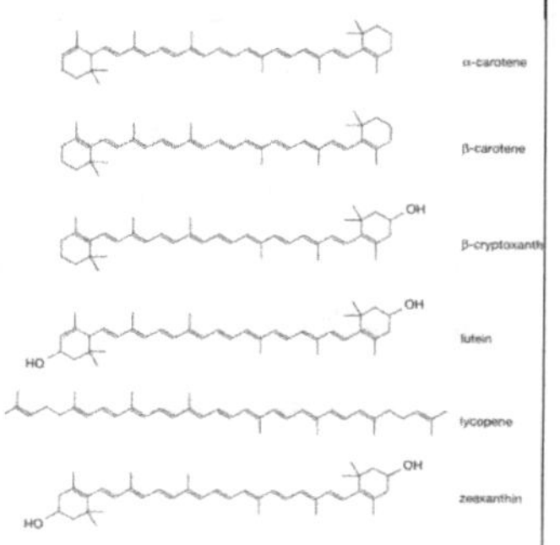 α-carotene β-carotene β-cryptoxanth lutein lycopene zeaxanthin

Contd...

Source	Color	Use
Anthocyanins Anthocyanins are colored water-soluble pigments belonging to the phenolic group. The pigments are in glycosylated forms. Anthocyanins responsible for the colors, red, purple, and blue, are in fruits and vegetables. Berries, currants, grapes, and some tropical fruits have high anthocyanins content. Red to purplish blue-colored leafy vegetables, grains, roots, and tubers are the edible vegetables that contain a high level of anthocyanins. Anthocyanin is in the form of glycoside while anthocyanidin is known as the aglycone. Anthocyanidins are grouped into 3-hydroxyanthocyanidins, 3-deoxyanthocyanidins, and O-methylated anthocyanidins, while anthocyanins are in the forms of anthocyanidin glycosides and acylated anthocyanins. The most common types of anthocyanidins are cyanidin, delphinidin, pelargonidin, peonidin, petunidin, and malvidin. Acylated anthocyanins are also detected in plants besides the typical anthocyanins. Acylated anthocyanin is further divided into acrylated anthocyanin, coumaroylated anthocyanin, caffeoylated anthocyanin, and malonylated anthocyanin.	Orange, red, purple, blue	Color cosmetics Anthocyanins have anti-oxidant, anti-inflammatory, and anti-cancer properties making them useful to protect health in general, but particularly suited to protecting skin from sun damage that contributes to skin aging and cancer. 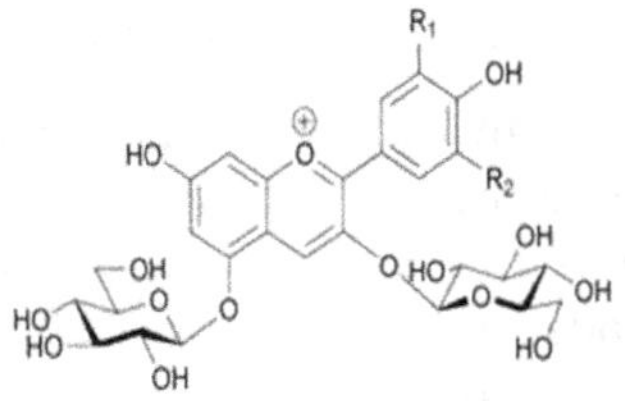 R_1 / R_2 / anthocyanin / aglycon H / H / pelargonin / pelargonidin OH / H / cyanin / cyanidin OCH_3 / H / peonin / peonidin OH / OH / delphin / delphinidin OCH_3 / OH / petunin / petunidin OCH_3 / OCH_3 / malvin / malvidin
Chlorophyll and copper-chlorophyll complex from green plant parts- *Piper betel* leaves, Eucalyptus leaves. Chlorophylls are numerous in types, but all are defined by the presence of a fifth ring beyond the four pyrrole-like rings. Most chlorophylls are classified as chlorins, which are reduced relatives of porphyrins (found in hemoglobin).	Bright green	Color cosmetics 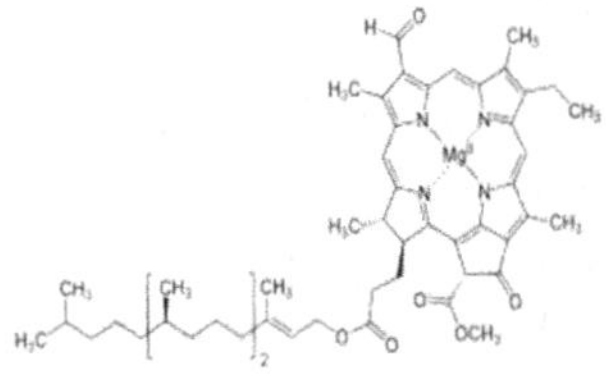

Protective agents or Antioxidants in products such as skin care, hair care and oral hygiene products

Free radicals are highly reactive molecules with an odd number of electrons that are generated from oxygen, they can damage various cellular structures, such as DNA, proteins, and cellular membranes. In addition, free radicals may lead to inflammation, which seems to play an additional role in skin aging. The body possesses endogenous defense mechanisms, such as antioxidative enzymes (superoxide dismutase, catalase, glutathione peroxidase) and nonenzymatic antioxidative molecules (vitamin E, vitamin C, glutathione, ubiquinone), protecting it from free radicals by reducing and neutralizing them.

Some of these antioxidant defense mechanisms can be inhibited by ultraviolet (UV) light. Moreover, as part of the natural aging process endogenous defense mechanisms decrease, while the production of reactive oxygen species increases, resulting in accelerated skin and hair aging.

Hence topical application of antioxidants may neutralize some of the resulting free radicals, and consequently lessen or prevent the signs of aging skin. In addition to their antioxidant activity, most of them possess numerous other biologic properties like wound healing, anti-inflammatory and anticancer. At present, topical antioxidants are marketed to prevent aging and UV-induced skin damage, as well as to treat wrinkles and erythema due to inflammation. For topically administered antioxidants to be effective in preventing skin aging, a couple of considerations should be made when formulating them:

- Product stabilization is crucial. Because antioxidants are very unstable, they may become oxidized and inactive before reaching the target.
- They must be properly absorbed into the skin, reach their target tissue in the active form, and remain there long enough to exert the desired effects.

In the oral cavity, oxidative stress is associated with gingivitis and other periodontitis. Nevertheless, factors including alcohol consumption, exposure to nicotine, dental procedures, bleaching agents, dental cements, composite fillings and metals used in dentistry also leads to oxidative stress. Periodontal pathogens can induce over production of ROS and leads to collagen and periodontal tissue breakdown. Recently, it has been affirmed that the onset and development of dental caries is due to imbalances in levels of free radicals, reactive oxygen species, and antioxidants in saliva. Most recently, dental manufacturers and distributors have incorporated antioxidant supplements due to their anti-angiogenic, anti-inflammatory, antiviral, and/or anti-tumor properties into toothpastes, mouth rinses/mouthwashes, lozenges, fluoride gels and dentifrices, oral sprays, breath fresheners, and other dental products for the control of gingival and periodontal diseases.

Hair is exposed every day to a range of harmful effects such as sunlight, pollution, cosmetic treatments, grooming practices and cleansing. The UV components of sunlight damage human hair, causing fibre degradation. UV-B attacks the melanin pigments and the protein fractions (keratin) of hair and UV-A produces free radical/reactive oxygen species (ROS) through the interaction of endogenous photosensitizers. UV radiations causes increase in protein and lipid degradation, changes in colour and shine and in adverse consequences for the mechanical properties. Natural antioxidants applications can improve hair mechanical properties and preserve colour and shine of fibres, coats and protects them against UV, reduces lipid peroxidation of the protein degradation and finally improves fiber integrity.

Following are commonly useful antioxidants in skin care, hair care and oral hygiene products	
Vitamin E (tocopherol)	Exerts photoprotective effects, inhibit human macrophage metalloelastase and thus inhibits degradation of elastin, but cuases contact dermatitis
Vitamin C (ascorbic acid)	Potent antioxidant, Ascorbate is required for collagen synthesis and hence reduces production of elastin, topical application cuases stinging and mild irritation
Vitamin B3 (Niacinamide, or nicotinamide)	Antiaging, anti-inflammatory, depigmenting, and immunomodulant,
Coenzyme Q10 (CoQ10)	Suppresses expression of collagenase without any side effect
Idebenone (synthetic analog of coenzyme Q10)	Stronger antioxidant than CoQ10, reduces in skin roughness/dryness, reduction in fine lines/wrinkles, but cuases contact dermatitis

Contd...

Lycopene	Powerful antioxidant carotenoid, photoprotective , less clinical data available
Green tea polyphenols	Antioxidant, anti-inflammatory, anticarcinogenic, suppress chemo- and photocarcinogenesis
Silymarin polyphenolic flavonoid from milk thistle plant, Silybum marianum	Antioxidant, photoprotective effects
Resveratrol	Antiaging, antioxidant, protects against UVB-mediated cutaneous damage and inhibits UVB-mediated oxidative stress.
Proanthocyanidins from Grape (Vitis vinifera)seed is extract	Stronger scavenger of free radicals than vitamins C and E, Antiaging, antioxidant
Genistein isoflavone from soybeans	Antiaging, antioxidant, photoprotective
Pycnogenol (Phenolic compound)	Antiaging, antioxidant, photoprotective, anti-inflammatory

Skin Whitening (Bleaching) Agents

Skin whitening agents are required to lighten skin in conditions like melasma or postinflammatory hyperpigmentation. They suppress melanin production eiher through competitive inhibition of melanogenesis enzyme tyrosinase or inhibition of the maturation of this enzyme or inhibition of transport of pigment granules (melanosomes) from melanocytes to surrounding keratinocytes. Bearberry, Licorice, Sophora and Peonia plant extracts are found to tyrosinase inhibitors. Following are various plants useful as skin whitening agents:

Tyrosinase inhibition is shown by following natural compounds

Artocarpus lakoocha heartwood	Oxyresveratrol
Astragalus taschkendicus	Askendoside B
Citrus fruit peel	3′,4′,5,6,7,8-hexamethoxy-flavone (nobiletin)
Morus alba Rheum undulatum	1. Oxyresveratrol; 2. Hydroxystilbene
Aloe vera	Aloesin; C-glycosylated chromone
Longan seed	Corilagin, gallic acid and ellagic acid or other phenolic/flavonoid glycosides and ellagitannins

Tyrosinase inhibition as well as pigmentation inhibition is shown by following natural compounds:

Source	Compounds (type)
Alpinia galanga and *Curcuma aromatica* medicinal plants	Eugenol and curcuminoids possible active ingredients
Angelica dahurica	Isoimperatorin imperatorin
Artocarpus incisus (best of) 23 heart wood species from Papua New Guinea.	(+)-Dihydromorin, chlorophorin, (+)-norartocarpanone, 4-prenyl-oxyresveratrol, artocarbene, artocarpesin and isoarto-carpesin
Aspergillus fumigatus and *Saccharomyces cerevisiae*	Melanin Degrading Enzymes

Contd...

Source	Compounds (type)
Carthamus tinctorius safflower seeds	*N*-feruloylserotonin, *N*-(*p*-coumaroyl)serotonin, and 3) acacetin
Cucumis sativus	Lutein
Erigeron breviscapus Chinese herb	(2Z,8Z)-matricaria acid methyl ester
Galla Chinensis Radix Clematidis out of 90 Chinese Herbs	Unknown
Gastrodia elata Blume Orchidaceae	(Synthetic) *p*-hydroxybenzyl alcohol
Glycyrrhiza glabra Licorice extract	Glabrene and 2′,4′,4-tri-hydroxychalcone
Glycyrrhiza uralensis	Glycyrrhisoflavone and glyasperin C
Grape seed	Oligomeric proanthocyanidins
Grape seed	Proanthocyanidin
Kaempferia pandurata	Chalcone compounds, isopanduratin A and 4-hydroxypanduratin A
Lespedeza cyrtobotrya	Haginin A
Malpighia emarginata Acerola fruit	Cyanidin-3-alpha-*O*-rhamnoside. pelargonidin-3-α-*O*-rhamnoside
Morus alba	Mulberroside F (moracin M-6, 3′-di-O-beta-d-glucopyranoside
Piper longum	Piperlonguminine
Pityrosporum ovale	Azelaic acid; C9-dicarboxylic acid
Podocarpus macrophyllus	2,3-dihydro-4′,4‴-di-*O*-methylamentoflavone
Polygonum cuspidatum. *Paris polyphylla* *Vitex negundo*	Physcion (anthraquinone + anthraquinone analog) (+)-Lyoniresinol
Punica granatum Pomegranate	Ellagic acid
Ramulus mori (young twigs of *Morus alba*)	2,3′,4,5′-tetrahydroxy-stilbene (2-oxyresveratrol)
Raspberry	Tiliroside
Rhus Ghinensis; Chinese galls	3 Gallotannins; 2,3,4,6-tetra-*O*-galloyl-d-glucopyranose, 1,2,3,6-tetra-*O*-galloyl-β-d-glucopyranose, and 1,2,3,4,6-penta-*O*-galloyl-β-d-glucopyranose
Rhus succedanea	10′(Z)-heptadecenyl-hydroquinone
Sophora flavescens	Kurarinol, kuraridinol, and trifolirhizin
Sophora japonica and *Spatholobus suberectus* out of 25 Chinese Herbs	High phenolic content, e.g., gallic acid
Spatholobus suberectus Dunn (Leguminosae) Chinese herb	Butin

Classification of Cosmetics

There is a wide variety of cosmeceutical preparation. They are classified on the basis of application on body parts which include:

1. **Cosmeceutical preparation for SKIN**
   - Cream
   - Lip bam
   - Powder
   - Lotion
   - Sunscreen and sunburn preparation
   - Face pack
   - Deodorant and antiperspirant
   - Bath preparation
2. **Cosmeceutical preparation for HAIR**
   - Shampoo
   - Hair oil/Hair tonic
   - Hair colorants
3. **Cosmeceutical preparation for MOUTH**
   - Dentifrices
4. **Cosmeceutical preparation for SHAVING**
   - Shaving preparation
   - After shave preparation
5. **Cosmeceutical preparation for NAIL**
   - Nail polish
   - Enamels
   - Nail polish removers
   - Enamel removers

Cosmeceuticals for Skin

The surface of the body is covered entirely by the skin. The main function of this covering is to protect body, eliminate waste material and regulate body temperature. It is possible to suffer skin ailments and infections through the external penetration of dirt, irritants, fungi and bacteria into the parts of the skin. Protection against these conditions is obtained through proper cleanings, and use of external applications. The cosmeceuticals used for the skin mainly depends on the type of skin i.e. oily, dry and normal skin.

Cream

Introduction	Creams are viscous liquid or semisolid emulsions of either the oil in water or water in oil. ➢ Oil in water type cream: Shaving cream, Foundation cream, Vanishing cream ➢ Water in oil type cream: Cold cream, Emollient cream
Properties	1. It should be non-toxic 2. It is easily spreads 3. It should remains stable in the presence of most other chemical agent 4. It should not too hygroscopic 5. It should be able to prevent heat insulating effects by providing low surface tension and a capacity to mix with water 6. It should be easy to remove without use of scrubber, brusher or a detergent other than soap
Common ingredients:	Purified Water, Stearic Acid, Glycerin, Isoparaffin, Liquid Paraffin, Cetearyl Octanoate, Glyceryl Stearate, Ceresin, Cetyl Alcohol, Cetearyl Alcohol, Triethanolamine, Polyethoxylated Alcohol, Glyceryl Stearate, PEG-1000 Stearate, Isopropyl Myristate, Sorbitan Stearate, Sucrose Cocoate, Dimethicone, Polysorbate 60, Cetyl Palmitate, Propylene Glycol, Polysorbate 80, Xanthan Gum, Processed Alum, .Fragrance, Phenoxyethanol, Mehtylparaben, Propylparaben, Sodium EDTA, BHT
Base formulation	The selection of ingredients depends very much on the final purpose and the desired consistency (creamy, hard, soft, greasy or dry) of the product. Changing one ingredient may require changes in many others if the physical characteristics of the product are to be maintained. The diversity of applications and the choice of ingredients (mostly synthetic or modified natural products) is simply too large and too complex. As a general guideline, the different oils, fats and waxes are chosen for their consistency and absorption characteristics, their mixability with other ingredients and for their function in protecting and providing moisture to the skin. Some oils may also be nourishing for the skin, give it special elasticity and readily absorbed. Different types of applications often require only slight changes in the proportions of ingredients, but sometimes, more specific ingredients have to be added to achieve the desired effect.
Ingredients and their uses	➢ Water soluble ingredients: Propylene glycol, Glycerol, sorbitol. They reduce evaporation of water in case of oil-in-water type of emulsion. The activity of retaining water in external Phase is known as emollient activity, which in turn provides water to stratum corneum ➢ Fat soluble ingredients: mineral oil, petroleum jelly, Paraffin, ceresin, dimethyl polysiloxanes, Methyl phenyl polysiloxanes etc. They help in reducing evaporation of water from the surface of the skin by forming a thin film.
Types	1. Cleansing cream 2. Cold cream 3. Night or massage cream 4. Nourishing cream 5. All-purpose or general cream

Contd...

Cold cream	It is an emulsion in which the proportion of fatty and oily material predominates, although when applied to the skin, a cooling effect is produced due to slow evaporation of the water contained in the emulsion.	**Herbal Ingredient**: Almond oil, White bees wax, Borax, Rose water **Method of formulation:** Here, almond oil and white bees wax is used to ensure whiteness and uniformity of the finished product. Borax is used as emulsifier. Dissolve borax in hot rose water. Melt various waxes together keeping the temperature about 70°C. Mix both the oil and water phase at same temperature with constant stirring. Mix without heat for about one hour and when cool (45-50°C), add perfume.
Moisturizing cream	It helps to retain moisture in the skin by preventing its loss by evaporation. Thus they preserve the skin in a soft, supple condition and allay formation of lines and wrinkles. In this type of cream oil content is low and it is easy to spread	**Herbal Ingredients**: *Aloe vera* gel, Cereus *grandiflorus* (Cactus), *Cucumis sativus* (Khira), *Matricaria recutita* (Chamomile), Vitamine E oil, Coconut oil, Beeswax **Method of formulation:** Heat first coconut oil and beeswax in a water bath until the wax is melted. Stir well, remove from the heat and while cooling, slowly add the aloe vera gel a drop at a time. Continue stirring and when the mixture thickens, add the vitamin oil and chamomile extract.
Nourishing cream	This type of cream is non-greasy and provides nourishment and protection to the skin	**Herbal Ingredients:** Aloe vera, Citrus limon, Centella asiatica, Indian Kino, Ashwaganda Here, Aloe vera nourishes and moisturizes the skin. Ashwaganda and Indian Kino Tree extracts protects skin from pollution and dry weather. Gotu Kola significantly increases the production of collagen
Night cream	Nourishes the skin all night with revitalizers, nutrients and moisturizers. It provide moisture to the skin by preventing evaporation.	**Herbal Ingredients:** Lemon, Tomato, Pommelo, Crab Apple, Wheat Germ, White Lily. Here, Tomato is antioxidant and a rich source of natural Alpha Hydroxy Acids (AHAs) that nourish the skin. Crab Apple and White Lily helps in cooling and soothing the skin. Wheat Germ is natural vitamin E source protects and moisturizes the skin.
Anti-acne cream	Acne is characterized as a superficial disease that affects the hair follicles and oil secreting glands of the skin. It manifests as blackheads, whiteheads and inflammation(redness).	**Herbal Ingredients:** *Allium sativum*(garlic), *Azadirachta indica* (Neem), *Butea frondosa* (Dhak), *Arnica montana* (Arnica), *Lavendula vera* (Lavender), Aloe Vera, Lentil, Silk Cotton Tree, Five-leaved Chaste Tree

Lip Bam

Introduction	It protects lips from drying by providing moisturizing effect. It is useful in cracking of lips.
Properties	1. It should be completely free from grittiness and be non-drying 2. It should have a desirable degree of plasticity 3. It should have pleasant odour and flavuor
Method of formulation	1. The preparation of fatty components i.e. of the oil and wax. 2. The addition of flavouring and colouring agents to this semisolid mass. 3. The molding of the mass into sticks.
Ingredients	***Common ingredients*:** Oil, wax, flavouring agent and sometimes colouring agent ***Herbal Ingredients*:** Carrot, Wheat Germ Oil, Coconut, Sweet Indrajao, Castor Plant ***Other Ingredients*:** Petrolatum, Ceresin, Liquid Paraffin, Isoprpyl Myristate, BHT, Cetyl Palmitate, Dimethicone, Black Currant Fragrance.

Powder

Introduction	The function of a face powder is to impart a smooth velvet-like finish to the skin by masking any shine due to the secretions of the sebaceous and sweat glands. It gives cooling effect.
Properties	1. Powder must not be too transparent to mask the shine neither must it be sufficiently opaque to give a 'clown-like' appearance. 2. It must have reasonable lasting properties. 3. It should possess desired properties like covering power, slip, absorbency, adhesiveness and bloom.
Types of powder	1. Face powders a. Compact powders b. Cake make-up powders c. Liquid and cream powders 2. Toilet powders a. Talcum powders b. Dusting powders c. After-shave powders d. Baby powder
Ingredients	***Common ingredients*:** Zinc stearate, Zinc oxide, Light calcium carbonate, Talc, Perfume, Colour ***Herbal Ingredients*:** Sandalwood powder, plant derived perfumes, starch powder Here, **zinc oxide** is used due to good covering power. Also it is mildly astringent, antiseptic and has soothing properties. Other ingredients having covering property are titanium dioxide, chalk, talc etc. **Calcium carbonate** and **Zinc stearate** has excellent absorption and grease resistant characteristics. Other examples include starch, magnesium carbonate, microcrystalline cellulose etc. **Talc** has slippery property and good adhesive power.
Method of formulation	• Mixing of the ingredients in face powder is usually carried out in a horizontal mixer with a screw agitator. • Perfume and colours are mixed with a small quantity of one of the constituents i.e. chalk, zinc oxide or talk and colour concentrate so formed mixed with the main bulk. • The bulk of powder is passed through 160 mesh and pack in a suitable container.

Lotion

Introduction	Lotion is a liquid application mainly for the skin to produce a beautifying effect. The main characteristic sought of lotions is an emollient and soothing effect. A lotion is a fairly liquid, i.e. aqueous, formulation with a high water or alcohol content. In general, lotions are used for cleaning and for adding moisture to the skin. Lotions may also contain substantial amounts of emulsified oil, fat or wax. Gums and similar substances are added to lotions to add body, lubrication and to produce emollient effects.
Types	1. Hand and body lotions 2. Skin toning lotions 3. Astringent lotions 4. Medicated lotions
Ingredients	➢ ***Common ingredients:*** Water, Alcohol, Vitamine E Acetate, Glycerin and other humectants, Glycerin, Isopropyl palmitate, Paraffinum Liquidum, Glycol Stearate, Methyl or Propyl Paraben. ➢ ***Herbal ingredients:*** Aloe vera gel, Cucumber extract, Apple Cider, Extract of Hamamelis, Aloe Vera, Sea Mineral Algae, Extracts of Yarrow leaf, Persimmon Leaf, Green Tea, Grapeseed and Chamomile, Vegetable Glycerin, Vegetable Sorbitol, Grapefruit Essential Oil, ➢ ***Natural gums and thickeners:*** Gum acacia (*Acacia Arabica),* Guar gum(*Cyamopsis tetragonolobus*), Tragacanth (*Astragalus gummifer*) ➢ ***Natural astringents:*** Witch hazel(*Hamamelis virginiana*), Rosemary oil (*Rosmarinus officinalis*), Yarrow (*Achillea millefolium)* ➢ ***Natural antiseptic:*** Haldi (*Curcuma longa*), Eucalyptus oil (*Eucalyptus globules*), Neem ➢ ***Cooling agents*** **:**Menthol (*Mentha piperita*) ➢ ***Perfume (Volatile oils)*** ➢ ***Natural preservatives:*** *Artemisia afra, Pteronia incana, Lavandula officinalis, Rosmarinus officinalis*
Method of formulation	Mix the gum with alcohol and stir into half the water. When dissolved strain through muslin cloth. Heat the rest of the water and dissolve in it the remaining ingredients (astringents, antiseptics etc), glycerin and agitate until cool. Then add mucilage, preservatives and the perfume.

Face Pack

Introduction	These preparation are applied to the face in the form of liquid or paste. They are then allowed to dry or to set with the object of improving the appearance of the skin, by producing a transient tightening effect as well as by cleansing the skin. The **warmth and tightening** effect resulting from their application produce the stimulating sensation of a rejuvenated face, while the colloidal and adsorptive clays and earth which are present in some packs will absorb grease and dirt from the facial skin. When they are eventually removed from the skin, skin debris and blackheads may be removed simultaneously.
Properties	1. It should be a smooth paste without gritty particles 2. After applied to face it should dry out rapidly, to form an adherent coating

Contd...

	3. It should removed by gentle washing without producing any pain 4. It should produce a definite sensation of tightening of skin after application 5. It should possess a significant cleansing of the skin 6. It must be dermatologically innocuous and non-toxic
Ingredients	Sandalwood, Orange peel, Rose petal, Chironji seed, Neem leaves, Tankana, Multani mitti, Excipients

Suntan and Sunburn Preparations

Introduction	Exposure to sunlight can have both beneficial as well as harmful effects on the human body, depending on the length and the frequency of exposure, the intensity of sunlight and the sensitivity of the individual concerned. The symptoms of sunburns are the direct result of damage or destruction of cells in the prickle cell layer of the skin, possibly through denaturing of its protein constituents.
Types	1. **Sunscreen:** They are designed to allow tanning with the minimum of sunburn. 2. **Palliative:** They are designed to alleviate the pain and irritation resulting from excessive exposure to sunlight. 3. **Simulative:** They are designed to stain the skin brown or promote the synthesis of melanoid materials in the skin.
Properties	1. They should either scatter the incident light effectively, or they should absorb the erythemal portion of the sun's radiant energy. 2. It must be non-toxic 3. It must be dermatologically innocuous 4. It must not be photo labile 5. It must be non volatile
Formulation	Effective base to formulate sunscreen cream is prepared by using mixtures of natural oils and mineral oils, or by blending these with fatty acid esters.
Ingredients	***Herbal Ingredients:*** *Aloe vera,* Badam (*Prunus amygdalus*), Cucumber (*Cucumis sativus*), Chameli (*Jasminum grandiflorum*), Lal gulab (*Rosa damascene*), Chandan (*Santalum album*), walnut extract, hydrogenated ricinus oil

Bath Preparation

Introduction	Bath preparation aid is useful in cleansing and beautifying the entire surface of the body. The purpose of such products is to cleanse the skin, to perfume the bath, to soften the bath, to form bubbles or foam in the bath water or to leave the skin in a pliable rejuvenated and cool after feeling condition.
Ingredients	***Herbal***: Aloe vera gel, Chamomile extract, Calendula extract, pollen or propolis extract, Neem leaf, Neem oil, Tulsi (Holy basil) leaf, essential oils of Coriander Seed, Camphor, lemongrass ***Common:*** Glycerol, Vitamin E, Liquid castile soap, Honey, Saponified oils of coconut, palm and olive
Properties	It protects against germs and bacteria and also helpful in skin irritation
Method of formulation	Combine all the ingredients except the soap and stir or shake well in ajar. Then add the liquid soap. Pour into a soap dispenser or storage vessel. Honey, lipid pollen extract and EEP propolis extract can be added in small percentages, as well as special herb extracts.

Contd...

Medimix soap	Acorus Calamus 2mg, Andropogan Muricatus 2mg, Mukul 1.75mg, Berberis Aristata 2mg, Cedrus Deodara 2mg, Celastrus 2mg, Paniculatus 2mg, Coriandrum Sativam 2mg, Cuminum Cyminum 2mg, Embelia Ribes 2mg, Glycyrrhiza Glabba 2mg, Hemidesmus Indicus 12mg, Holarrhena Anti Dysentrica 2mg, Melia Azadirachta 4mg, Nigella Sativa 2mg, Plumbago Rosea 225mg, Psoralea Corylifolia 2mg, Smilax China 6mg, Zingiber Zerumbet 108mg.

Deodorants and Antiperspirants

Introduction	Both deodorants and antiperspirants are designed to absorb, change, mask or prevent any unpleasant odours. Those used for cosmetic purposes are presented in soap, aerosol, cream and roll-on gel forms.
Types	➢ Deodorants act by deodorize the perspiration without checking its flow to any appreciable extent. ➢ Antiperspirants act by decreasing the sweat production, forming blockage or plug in the sweat duct, by altering the sweat duct permeability to fluids.
Properties	A deodorant should dry quickly without leaving a greasy film. The solvents and thickening agents are selected for the method of application.
Ingredients	The active ingredients comprise fragrances (or aromatic extracts), astringents, antibacterial agents and drying agents which interrupt the normal functions of sweat glands. Herbal ingredients: *Citrullus vulgaris* (Water melon), *Foeniculum vulgare* (Fennel), *Mentha arvevsis* (Mint), Essential oils of lavender, thyme, lemongrass, bergamot

Cosmeceuticals for Hair

If, on one hand, hair texture and shine are usually related to hair surface properties, on the other hand, the integrity of hair is due to the hair cortex. For this purpose, hair products that improve the structural integrity of hair fibers and increase tensile strength are available, along with products that increase hair volume, reduce frizz, improve hair manageability, and stimulate new hair growth. Interestingly, modern cosmetic products are formulated to clean hair from detritus, and to restore and improve hair physiology. For example, intensive conditioning agents can temporarily "replace" the f-layer, improving the moisture retention in the cortex and rebuilding some of the reduced physical properties of hair. Therefore, the boost in hair shine is a key benefit of modern products

Hair has several useful function in the animal world: It forms a protection cushion around the head and other delicate parts of the body. Whatever protective or other biological function hair may have played in past, there is little doubt that its main function today is decorative. By changing its shape, its colour, and its style.

Recent dermocosmetic developments include topical hair growth stimulants, photoprotectors of hair and scalp, and anti-aging compounds. The rational basis for the development of topical hair growth stimulants are: effect on androgen metabolism, effect on sebum production and microbial flora, effect on microinflammation and fibrosis, and effect on vascularization and vascular epidermal growth factor. Various cosmetics for hair are as follows:

Shampoo

Introduction	Shampoos are liquid, creamy or gel-like, depending on the inclusion of traditional soaps saturated with glycerides and natural or synthetic fatty alcohols or on the thickening agents (e.g. gum, resins and PEG) that are used. Its primary function is the cleansing of hair due to accumulated sebum, dust, scalp debris etc.
Properties	1. It must clean hair and scalp without leaving the hair greasy or dry and unmanageable. 2. It should have desirable hair conditioning action. 3. It should not produce irritation in eye and scalp. 4. In case of anti dandruff shampoo it should contain an effective germicide, fungicide or antiseptic material to counteract increased bacterial growth and prevent infection for a period after the shampoo. 5. By virtue of the above ingredients it should reduce the degree of itching, scaling and inflammation associated with the disease. 6. It should be easy to remove from the hair
Types	1. Protein shampoo: This preparation is used to provide natural proteins and nourishment to the hair. It cleans the excess oil, dust from the hair. 2. Anti-dandruff shampoo 3. Conditioning shampoo
Hair Cleansing Herbal Drugs	
Herbal Ingredient	**Uses**
Acacia concinna (Shikakai) Family:Mimisaceae	Pods extract is used as hair cleanser and for control of dandruff
Sapindus mukorossi (Ritha) Family:Sapindaceae	Extract of fruit coat works as natural shampoo as hair conditioner
Betula pendula (Birch) Family:Betulaceae	Extract of leaves is used as anti-dandruff
Salvia officinalis (Sage) Family:Lamiaceae	Aqueous extract is used as hair conditioner
Aloe vera (Ghikanwar) Family:Liliaceae	Leaves juice is used as conditioner and to clean the hair

Protein shampoo (Himalaya)		**Anti-dandruff shampoo (Ayush)**		**Conditioning shampoo**	
Herbal Ingredient	**Quantity**	**Herbal Ingredient**	**Quantity**	**Herbal Ingredient**	**Quantity**
Acacia concinna (Shikakai	47.60mg	Rosmarinus officinalis (Rosemary)	103mg	Cicer arietinum(Chickpea)	60mg

Contd...

Protein shampoo (Himalaya)		Anti-dandruff shampoo (Ayush)		Conditioning shampoo	
Herbal Ingredient	Quantity	Herbal Ingredient	Quantity	Herbal Ingredient	Quantity
Vetiveria zizanioids (Ushira	6.95mg	Azadirachta indica (Neem)	5.15mg	Sapindus mukorossi(ritha)	60mg
Nardostachys jatamansi (Musk roof	6.95mg	Ocimum sanctum (Tulsi)	5.15mg	Jasminum officinale(Jasmine)	40mg
Sapindus mukorossi (Soapnut)	2.08mg	Acacia concinna (Shikakai)	5.15mg	Eclipta alba(Thistle)	15mg
Trigonella foenum-graecum (Fenugreek	2.08mg	Phylsanthus emblica (Amla)	5.15mg		
Water	to 1ml	Lawsonia inermis(Henna)	5.15mg		
		Water	to 5ml		

Hair Oil/Hair Tonic

Introduction	Hair oils are formulated to give the hair a good shine and gloss, without the use of a heavy oil or grease. This is achieved by applying a thin continuous film of an oily material on the hair surface without causing greasiness or stickiness. They are mainly oils of low viscosity.
Common Herbal Ingredients	*Brassica campestris* (Toontubh) oil, *Azadirachta indica* (Neem) oil, *Pongamia pinnata* (Karanja) oil, *Psorelea corylifolia* (Bavchi) oil, Mahatrunak oil, *Camphora officinarum* (Karpoor) oil, Oive oil, Hydnocarpus laurifolia oil, With a base of Til oil
Herbal Ingredient	**Uses**
Arnica Montana (Arnica) Family:Asteraceae	Flowers extract is used in hair oil as a tonic
Brassica spp.(Mustard) Family:Brassicaceae	Seed oil is used as hair tonic and useful for hair nourishment
Carthamus tinctorius (Safflower) Family:Asteraceae	Alcoholic extract is used as hair tonic
Cocos nucifera (Nariyal) Family:Arecaceae	Well established hair oil and as a tonic
Nardostachys jatamansi (Jatamansi) Family:Valerianaceae	Extract of rhizome is used in hair tonics for their growth
Phyllanthus emblica (Amla) Family:Euphorbiaceae	Fruit extract is used in oil for promotion of hair growth
Sesamum indicum (Til) Family:Pedaliaceae	Seed oil is one of the major source of hair oils

Hair Colorants

Introduction	Hair Color Preparations are products that either reduces the color of hair, such as hair bleaches, or products that add color to attain a desirable effect. This can be achieved either with materials that are temporary and only last a few days, to products that last several weeks. The colouring of hair is one of the most important action of today's fashion. The usual reasons for colouring the hair are to change the natural colour of the hair, to colour the white hairs which begin to appear with age and to change the colour of hair temporarily on a particular occasion.
Properties	1. It should be non-injurious to the hair shaft 2. It should possess no systemic toxic effect or irritation when applied to the hair 3. It should have affinity for hair keratin
Method of formulation	All ingredients are dried and powdered and paste is made in decoction of tea leaves. This paste is applied on hair for required time and then it is removed.
Herbal Ingredient	**Uses**
Eclipta alba (Bhangra) Family:Asteraceae	Whole plant extract is useful for hair nourishment and dyeing
Juglans regia (Akroot) Family:Juglandaceae	Leaves and hull of fruits is used for hair dyeing
Lawsonia inermis (Henna) Family:Lythraceae	Leaves paste is used for hair dyeing and nourishment
Saussurea lappa (Kuth) Family:Asteraceae	Root extract is used in hair dyeing
Hair Bleaches	
Introduction	Hair Bleaches are products that lighten the color of the hair by alteration of the coloring components in the hair. They also work through diffusion of the natural color pigment or artificial color from the hair. The Hair Bleaching process is central to both permanent hair color and hair lighteners. Hair Bleaching ingredients have been extensively tested over many years and have been found to be safe. Their safety is established through the testing of the individual ingredients as well the other ingredients that are used to formulate the product.
Common ingredients	Glycerin, Sodium Lauryl Sulfate, Ammonium Persulfate, Potassium Persulfate, Sodium Persulfate, Laureth-4Hydrogen Peroxide, Stearyl Alcohol, Cetyl Alcohol, Disodium EDTA, Nonoxynol-4, Nonoxynol-9, Silica, Fragrance, Lauramide DEA, Water

Contd...

Hair Tints, Rinses and Shampoos	
Introduction	Hair Tints, Rinses and Shampoos are products intended to shade the existing color of the hair. Tints may be used also for applying highlighting effects to the hair. Hair Tints, Rinses and Shampoos contain ingredients that have been extensively tested over many years and have been found to be safe. Their safety is established through the testing of individual dying ingredients as well the other ingredients that are used to formulate the product.
Common ingredients	Dimethicone, Propylene Glycol, Ammonium Lauryl Sulfate, Cocamidopropyl Betaine, Citric Acid, Isopropyl Alcohol, Erythorbic Acid, Polyquaternium-10, Cetearyl Alcohol, Ceteareth-20, Ceteareth-25PEG-2 Cocamine, Fragrance, Hydroxyethylcellulose, Hair Dye Ingredients, Water
Hair Dyes and Colors	
Introduction	Hair Dyes and Hair Colors are products intended to impart color to the hair. Hair dye ingredients have been extensively tested over many years and have been found to be safe. This is established through the testing of individual dying ingredients as well the other ingredients that are used to formulate the products. In addition to ensuring the safety of the individual ingredients, hair dyes are assessed to make sure that are not irritating or cause an unusual incidence of allergic reactions.
Common ingredients:	Aminomethyl Propanol, Ammonium Hydroxide, Ascorbic Acid, Ceteareth-25Cetearyl Alcohol, Ceteth-2Cetyl Alcohol, Cocamide DEA, Cocamidopropyl Betaine, EDTA, Ethanolamine, Ethoxydiglycol, Hair Dye Ingredients, Hexylene Glycol, Isopropyl Alcohol, Lauramide DEA, Nonoxynol-2Oleic Acid, Oleyl Alcohol, Propylene Glycol, Sodium Lauryl Sulfate, Stearyl Alcohol, Water

Shaving Preparation

Introduction	Shaving preparation mainly include shaving cream and after shaving preparation. Menthol is mainly used in shaving preparation due to its cooling effect.
Properties	1. A small quantity must give an abundant lather. 2. When applied to the face there must no any astringent effect on the skin. 3. The cream must remain soft in the tube. 4. It must be sufficiently tacky to adhere to both brush and face and yet be easily washed off the razor.
Ingredients	Stearic acid, Mineral oil, Beeswax, Menthol, Soap flakes, Water
Method of formulation	Heat the water to 70^{0}C and dissolve the soap. Melt the stearic acid and beeswax in a water bath to 75 ^{0}C and menthol is dissolved in soapy water then melted wax is stirred into the soapy water and emulsify. Stir and mix well. When homogeneous, stir in the mineral oil

After Shave Lotion

Introduction	They are intended to cool and refresh the skin, allay irritation, be mildly astringent. They are also used to relieve the feeling of tautness and soreness and to promote healing of skin which has become damaged during shaving operation.

Contd...

Ingredients	Ethanol (96%), Sorbitol, Fragrance (aromatic oil), Menthol, Methyl paraben, Witch hazel extract, Propolis extract, Water
Method of formulation	Dissolve all the ingredients completely in the alcohol and dilute with the water, mix thoroughly. Leave to stand for 1 to 2 days with adequate chilling or 1 week without chilling, then filter to clear bottle.

Dental Products

Introduction	Dental product are orientated to prevent and control of teeth disorders. Which include Dentifrices. It includes toothpaste and mouthwash.
Dentifrices	They are used to clean and give shine to the teeth. The basic requirements of a dentifrice; ➢ When used properly with an efficient toothbrush, it should clean the teeth adequately, that is, remove food debris, plaque and stain. ➢ It should leave the mouth with a fresh, clean sensation. ➢ Its cost should be such that as to encourage regular and frequent use by all. ➢ It should be harmless, pleasant and convenient to use. ➢ Packing should be economically.

Herbal Dentifrices	**Uses**
Azadirachta indica(Neem) Family: Meliaceae	Protects gums from bacteria
Eugenia caryophyllus(Laung) Family: Myrtaceae	Clove oil is used as analgesic in toothpain
Glycyrrhiza glabra(Mulethi) Family:Leguminosae	It cures mouth ulcers
Cinnamomum zeylanicum(Dalchini) Family: Lauraceae	Cinnamon oil is used as flavouring agent
Mentha piperita(Pudina) Family: Labiatae	Mentha oil is used as flavouring agent and has mild antiseptic properties

Toothpaste	The primary function of toothpaste is to remove adherent soiling matter from a hard surface with minimal damage to that surface. Herbal ingredients useful to prevent bleeding gums, strengthens or tightens gums, cures toothache, prevents pyorrhea and helps to cure mouth ulcers
	Ingredients • **Abrasives:** It should have ability to clean the surface and to avoid damage to the teeth surface. • **Detergents:** Tooth cleaning is essentially a detergent process. The detergent must be tasteless, non-toxic and non-irritant to the oral mucosa. For example sodium lauryl sulphate. • **Humectants:** They are used to prevent dentifrices from drying out. E.g. glycerin, sorbitol • **Gelling agents:** They are used to maintain a high-solids suspension in a stable form. They are hydrophilic which disperse in aqueous media which include natural gums, silica, synthetic cellulosic products etc.

Contd...

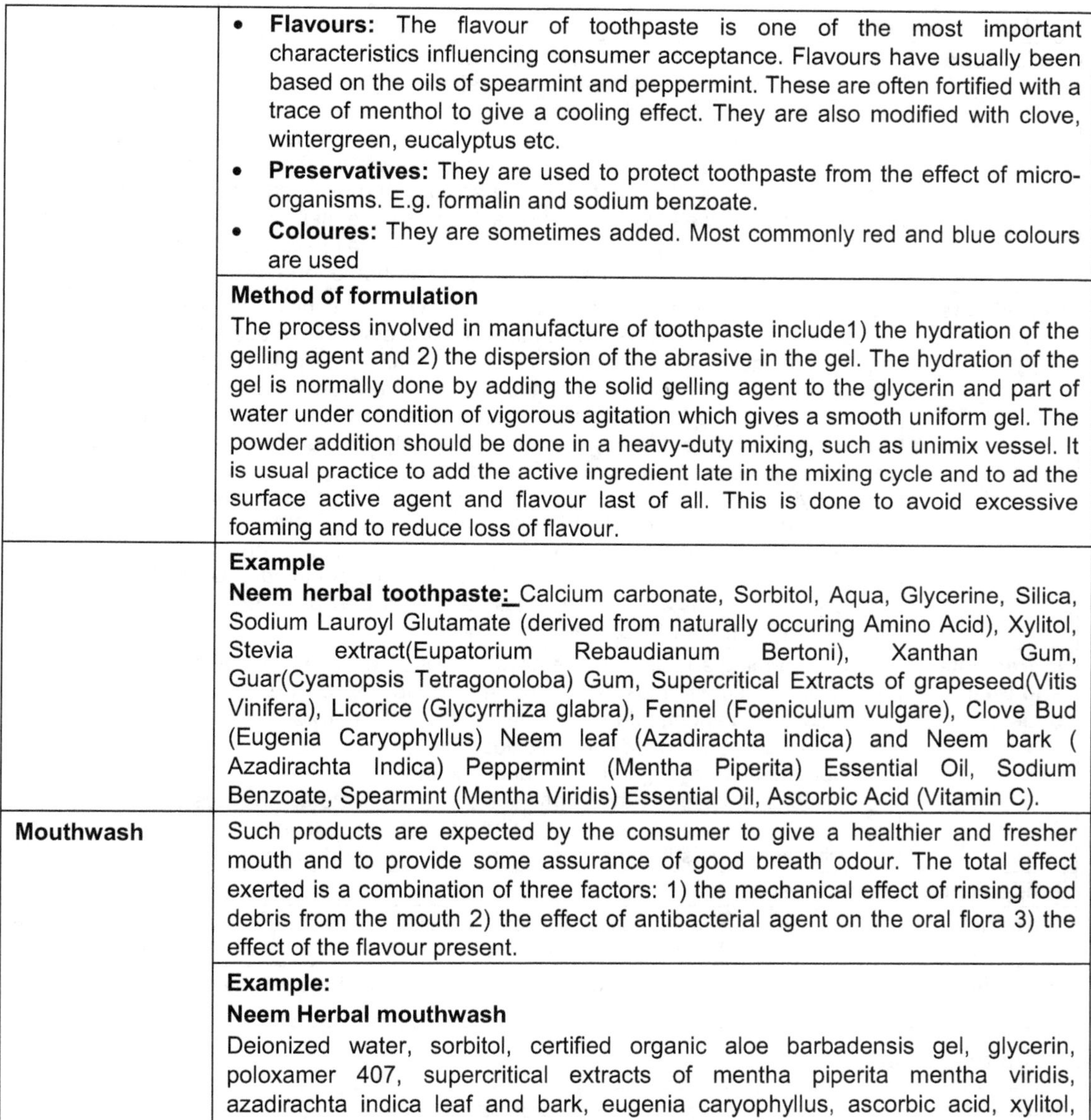

	• **Flavours:** The flavour of toothpaste is one of the most important characteristics influencing consumer acceptance. Flavours have usually been based on the oils of spearmint and peppermint. These are often fortified with a trace of menthol to give a cooling effect. They are also modified with clove, wintergreen, eucalyptus etc. • **Preservatives:** They are used to protect toothpaste from the effect of micro-organisms. E.g. formalin and sodium benzoate. • **Coloures:** They are sometimes added. Most commonly red and blue colours are used
	Method of formulation The process involved in manufacture of toothpaste include1) the hydration of the gelling agent and 2) the dispersion of the abrasive in the gel. The hydration of the gel is normally done by adding the solid gelling agent to the glycerin and part of water under condition of vigorous agitation which gives a smooth uniform gel. The powder addition should be done in a heavy-duty mixing, such as unimix vessel. It is usual practice to add the active ingredient late in the mixing cycle and to ad the surface active agent and flavour last of all. This is done to avoid excessive foaming and to reduce loss of flavour.
	Example **Neem herbal toothpaste:** Calcium carbonate, Sorbitol, Aqua, Glycerine, Silica, Sodium Lauroyl Glutamate (derived from naturally occuring Amino Acid), Xylitol, Stevia extract(Eupatorium Rebaudianum Bertoni), Xanthan Gum, Guar(Cyamopsis Tetragonoloba) Gum, Supercritical Extracts of grapeseed(Vitis Vinifera), Licorice (Glycyrrhiza glabra), Fennel (Foeniculum vulgare), Clove Bud (Eugenia Caryophyllus) Neem leaf (Azadirachta indica) and Neem bark (Azadirachta Indica) Peppermint (Mentha Piperita) Essential Oil, Sodium Benzoate, Spearmint (Mentha Viridis) Essential Oil, Ascorbic Acid (Vitamin C).
Mouthwash	Such products are expected by the consumer to give a healthier and fresher mouth and to provide some assurance of good breath odour. The total effect exerted is a combination of three factors: 1) the mechanical effect of rinsing food debris from the mouth 2) the effect of antibacterial agent on the oral flora 3) the effect of the flavour present.
	Example: **Neem Herbal mouthwash** Deionized water, sorbitol, certified organic aloe barbadensis gel, glycerin, poloxamer 407, supercritical extracts of mentha piperita mentha viridis, azadirachta indica leaf and bark, eugenia caryophyllus, ascorbic acid, xylitol, potassium sorbate, thymus serpyllum essential oil.

Nail Products

Introduction	Nail Products are products that are used to color the nails, to protect them against damage, to soften and condition cuticles, and to supplement the nails.
Types	➢ Nail polish and enamels ➢ Nail polish and enamel removers
Common ingredients:	Acetone, Acetyl Tributyl Citrate, Acrylates Copolymer, Benzophenone-1Butyl Acetate, Camphor, Color Additives, Dimethicone, Dimethyl Phthalate, Diethyl Phthalate and Dibutyl Phthalate, Ethyl Acetate, Isopropyl Alcohol, Nitrocellulose, Stearalkonium Hectorite, Titanium Dioxide, Tosylamide/Formaldehyde Resin

Contd...

Nail polish and enamels	
Introduction	Nail polishes (also called lacquers or enamels), base coats, top coats, nail hardeners, and nail treatments are coatings applied to the nail plate to provide a pleasing look and to address specific nail plate conditions, such as soft, peeling or brittle nails. Upon application of the polish, treatment, or hardener, the solvents in the product quickly evaporate, leaving a coating of film behind. Nail treatments are coatings applied to the nail plate for a specific purpose and include 1) base coats to increase polish wear, 2) ridge fillers to make the nail smooth, and 3) top coats designed to increase polish longevity and gloss. Nail hardeners or strengtheners, as their name imply, are designed to harden or strengthen the nail.
Ingredients	Nail polishes, treatments and hardeners have very similar formulation composition. All contain a film-former, such as nitrocellulose or cellulose acetate butyrate, to make the product hard and shiny when it dries. To make the film tough and resilient, a resin or secondary film-former such as tosylamide/formaldehyde resin or tosylamide/epoxy resin is used. To prevent chips and cracks, one or more plasticizers, including triphenyl phosphate, trimethyl pentanyl diisobutyrate, camphor, and dibutyl phthalate may be included. Low levels of solvents, including ethyl acetate, butyl acetate, isopropyl alcohol, and toluene, are used to help products flow smoothly. Colored polishes or products contain FDA-approved colorants or pigments which are evenly distributed in the product due to the inclusion of a suspension agent or clay, such as stearalkonium hectorite or bentonite. To prevent color fading, a UV stabilizer, such as benzophenone-1, is often added. Nail hardeners may also contain a small amount of formaldehyde to harden or strengthen the nail.
Ingredients and their uses	➢ Film forming agents: Nitro cellulose, ethyl cellulose, vinyl polymers ➢ Resinous substances: Aryl sulphonamide-formaldehyde ➢ Plasticizing agents: d-butyl phthalate, n-butyl stearate ➢ Coloring agent: 5% titanium dioxide (TiQ2) ➢ Nacreous/pearly pigments: Guanine crystal ➢ Dissolving solvent: Ether, ethyl acetate, amyl acetate, butyl acetate ➢ Dissolving solvent/co-solvent: Ethyl alcohol, butyl alcohol ➢ Miscellaneous substances: suspending agent, perfumes
Nail polish and enamel removers	
Introduction	Polish removers are designed to soften polishes, treatments, or hardeners so that the coating on the nail can be easily removed.
Ingredients	Ingredients used in polish removers can include acetone, ethyl acetate, and isopropyl alcohol.

Eye Makeup Products

Introduction	Eye Makeup Products include products that are used around the eye to enhance the appearance of the eyes and to emphazise the beauty of the eyes.
Types	➢ Mascara ➢ Eye-shadow ➢ Eye-liner ➢ Eye-brow products ➢ Eye Makeup Remover
Mascara	
Introduction	Mascaras are products intended to enhance the appearance of the eyes by thickening, lengthening, and usually darkening the eyelashes. Mascaras are usually applied with a brush. Mascaras contain special ingredients that apply the product where it is needed in a precise and controlled manner. The products are specially

Contd...

	formulated to ensure that potentially harmful microorganisms cannot grow and multiply. The safety of Mascaras is established by selection of ingredients that are safe and suitable for this purpose.
Common ingredients	Glycerin, Propylene Glycol, TEA-Stearate, Isopropyl Myristate, Copernicia Cerifera (Carnauba) Wax, Cyclomethicone, Magnesium Silicate, Ammonium Acrylates, Copolymer, Fragrance, Color Additives, Water
Eye shadow (Eye Color products)	
Introduction	Eye Color products are intended to apply color in the area of the eye to enhance and accent the appearance of the eyes. Eye Color products such as Eye shadow are applied on the eyelids and under the eyebrows. Eyeshadow adds depth and dimension to the eyes. They contain ingredients that apply color where it is needed in a precise and controlled manner. Eye Makeup Products are formulated to ensure that potentially harmful microorganisms cannot grow and multiply. The safety of Eye Color Products is established by selection of ingredients that are safe and suitable for this purpose.
Common ingredients	Dimethicone, Petrolatum, Ethylhexyl Palmitate, Ascorbyl Palmitate, Squalane, Tocopheryl Acetate, Zinc Oxide, Kaolin, Sorbitan Sesquiisostearate, Mineral Oil, Zinc Stearate, Silica, Fragrance, Color Additives
Eyeliner	
Introduction	Eyeliners are products that apply color to the area around the eyes to accent and highlight appearance of the eyes. Eyeliners are used to emphasize the eyelids and/or to change the perceived shape of the eyes. They contain special ingredients that apply color where it is needed in a precise and controlled manner. The products are specially formulated to ensure that potentially harmful microorganisms cannot grow and multiply. The safety of Eyeliners is established by selection of ingredients that are safe and suitable for this purpose.
Common ingredients	Ammonium Acrylates Copolymer, Carbomer, Color Additives, Dimethicone, Fragrance, Glycerin, Magnesium Silicate, Mineral Oil, PEG-6 Sorbitan Oleate, Polysorbate 20, Propylene Glyco
Eyebrow Pencil	
Introduction	Eyebrow Pencils are products that apply color to the eyebrows. They are used to fill in and define the eyebrows. They contain special ingredients that apply color where it is needed in a precise and controlled manner. The products are specially formulated to ensure that potentially harmful microorganisms cannot grow and multiply. The safety of Eyebrow Pencils is established by selection of ingredients that are safe and suitable for this purpose. In addition, Eyebrow Pencils are assessed for their potential to cause skin irritation or cause allergic reactions.
Common ingredients	Dimethicone, Glycerin, Talc, Ozokerite, Polysorbate-60, Copernicia Cerifera (Carnauba) Wax, PEG-6 Sorbitan Stearate, Fragrance, Color Additives
Eye Makeup Remover	
Introduction	Eye Makeup Remover products are intended to help easily remove makeup that has been applied. They help to remove the applied color and to make sure it easily wipes off using a tissue or other cloth. They contain special ingredients that apply color where it is needed in a precise and controlled manner. The products are specially formulated to ensure that potentially harmful microorganisms cannot grow and multiply. The safety of Eye Makeup Remover is established by selection of ingredients that are safe and suitable for this purpose.
Common ingredients	Glycerin, Propylene Glycol, Sodium Lauryl Sulfate, Polysorbate-20, Butylene Glycol, Poloxamer-184, Cyclomethicone, Triethanolamine, Benzyl Alcohol, Mineral Oil, Allantoin, Disodium Cocoamphodiacetate, Fragrance, Sodium Chloride, Botanical Ingredients, Color Additives

Baby Products

Introduction	Baby Products are products intended to be used on infants and children under the age of three. Baby products are specially formulated to be mild and non-irritating and use ingredients that are selected for these properties.
Types	baby shampoos and baby lotions, oils, powders and creams
Baby Shampoos	
Introduction	Baby Shampoos are products that are intended to be used to cleanse the hair of infants and children under the age of three. These products are specially formulated to be non-irritating and mild to the eyes. Often, these products contain non-ionic ingredients which tend to be milder than ionic ingredients which carry a slight negative charge. Adults that have sensitive hair or that are very sensitive to ordinary products may also use Baby Shampoos. Manufacturers conduct extensive safety tests to ensure that these products are safe for use on young children.
Common ingredients	Cocamidopropyl Betaine, Citric Acid, Polyquaternium-10, Tetrasodium EDTA, PEG-80 Sorbitan Laurate, PEG-150, Distearate, Fragrance, Botanical Ingredients, Color Additives, Water
Baby Lotions, Oils, Powders and Creams	
Introduction	Baby Lotions, Oils, Powders and Creams are products that are intended to be used to moisturize and soften the skin of infants and children under the age of three. These products are specially formulated to be mild and non-irritating. Many Baby Lotions, Creams and Oils contain mineral oil. Adults that have sensitive skin or that are very sensitive to ordinary products may also use Baby Lotions, Oils, Powders and Creams. Manufacturers conduct extensive safety tests to ensure that these products are safe for use on young children.
Common ingredients	Botanical Ingredients, Carbomer, Cetyl Alcohol, Color Additives, Dimethicone, Dipropylene Glycol, Fragrance, Glycerin, Glyceryl Stearate, Isopropyl Palmitate, Mineral Oil, Myristyl Myristate, PEG-100 Stearate, Sorbitan Stearate, Stearic Acid, Stearyl Alcohol, Synthetic Beeswax, Talc, Tocopheryl Acetate, Water

Quality Control/Standardization of Herbal Cosmetics

Quality Control Analytical Methods

Cream/Lotion	➢ **P^H:** Prepare 10% solution of lotion measure pH with a digital pH meter. ➢ **Viscosity:** evaluate viscosity using Brookfield viscometer using LV-64 spindle at rotation rate to 25 RPM. Immerse the spindle into formulated lotion and measure the viscosity. ➢ **Spreadability:** Determine the spreadability of lotion by the parallel plate method. Select two glass slides of 20/20 cm. Place about 1 g of the lotion formulation over one of the slides. Place the other slide upon the top of the lotion such that the lotion is sandwiched between the slides and 125 g weight is placed upon the upper slide so that lotion between the two slides is pressed uniformly to form a thin layer. Remove the weight and measure the spread diameter. ➢ **Stability Test:** Store the formulated lotion at different temperatures and humidity conditions of 25±2°C / 60±5% RH (at room temperature), 40±2°C/ 75±5% RH (accelerated temperature) for a period of three months and studied for pH, viscosity and spreadability.

Contd...

	➢ **Sensitivity Test:** Apply a portion of lotion on the forearms of 6 volunteers and keep for 20 minutes. After 20 minutes, note if any kind of irritation or redness occurs. ➢ **Washability Test:** Apply a portion of lotion over the skin of hand and allow to flow under the force of flowing tap water for 10 minutes. Note the time when the lotion is completely removed. ➢ **Appearance:** Determine the color, odor and homogeneity of the lotion visually. ➢ **Type of emulsion test:** Conduct dye solubility and dilution test t determine the type of emulsion formed • ***In vitro* skin permeation studies:** *In vitro* skin penetration studies can be performed with human cadaver skin, using Keshary-Chien cells or Franz diffusion cells. Remove the hair and subcutaneous fat tissue from the human cadaver skin and mount on the diffusion cell containing PBS as a receptor fluid. Apply the small quantity (0.5 g) of product to the skin surface. After 24 hours, extract the amount of drug in the receptor compartment, the drug remaining on the skin, and the drug concentration in the skin into a suitable solvent and determine the amount by spectrophotometric analysis.
Moisturizing cream/lotion	• ***In-vitro* occlusion studies:** This determines the occlusivity of formulations by Vringer's in vitro model. Take a beaker of water covered with filter paper. Spread 200 mg of the product on a filter surface. Similarly, prepare the beaker having filter paper without product as a reference control. If the occlusion factor is zero, it means that there is no occlusion effect as compared to the reference. The maximum occlusion factor is 100. Calculate the occlusion factor by the given formula : $$F = 100\left[\frac{(A - B)}{A}\right]$$ where, A = water loss without sample (reference), B = water loss with sample. • ***In vivo* skin hydration studies:** This study is useful to determine the skin hydrating effect of the product which is also responsible for the increased drug penetration into the skin. Select healthy female rats. Apply the cosmetic product to the shaved skin of rats. After 24 hours, kill the animals and isolate the skin. Prepare the slices and stain with haematoxylin and eosin. Observe the stained skin under a microscope and measure the thickness of stratum corneum. Due to improved hydration, the thickness of stratum corneum should be increased.
Sunscreen	• ***In vitro* sun protection factor determination by UV spectrophotometer:** Use this method to determine the SPF (sun protection factor). It measures the spectral transmittance at UV wavelengths from 290 to 320 nm, at interval of 5 nm, and thus, the reduction of the irradiation after passing through a film of the product. Calculate the SPF factor by following formula: $$SPF = CF \times \sum_{290}^{320} FE(\lambda) \times I(\lambda) \times Abs(\lambda)$$ where, CF = Correction factor, i.e. 10, EE (λ) = Erythemogenic effect of radiation with wavelength λ, I (λ) = solar intensity spectrum; Abs (λ) = Spectrophotometric absorbance values at wavelength λ. Note: The values of EE (λ) x I (λ) are constants. They were determined by Sayre et al. (1979) which are given in below table:

Contd...

	<table><tr><th>Wavelength (λ nm)</th><th>EE × I (normalized)</th></tr><tr><td>290</td><td>0.0150</td></tr><tr><td>295</td><td>0.0817</td></tr><tr><td>300</td><td>0.2874</td></tr><tr><td>305</td><td>0.3278</td></tr><tr><td>310</td><td>0.1864</td></tr><tr><td>315</td><td>0.0839</td></tr><tr><td>320</td><td>0.0180</td></tr><tr><td>Total</td><td>1</td></tr></table>
Shampoo	➢ **Physical appearance/visual inspection:** Evaluate the shampoo for the clarity, color, odor and foam producing ability. ➢ **Determination of pH:** Measure the pH of 10% v/v shampoo solution in distilled water by using pH meter at room temperature. ➢ **Determination of % of solid contents:** Place 4 grams of shampoo in a previously clean, dry and weighed evaporating dish. Weigh the dish and shampoo again to confirm the exact weight of the shampoo. Evaporate the liquid portion of the shampoo by placing the evaporating dish on the hot plate. Calculate the weight and thus % of the solid contents of shampoo left after complete drying. ➢ **Dirt dispersion test:** Add two drops of shampoo to 10 mL of distilled taken in a large test tube. To this solution, add one drop of India ink added and the stoppered the test tube and shake ten times. The amount of ink in the foam will be indicated by the rubric such as None, Light, Moderate or Heavy. ➢ **Surface tension measurement:** Measure the surface tension of 10% w/v shampoo in distilled water using Stalagmometer at room temperature. ➢ **Cleansing power of shampoo:** This method is developed by Barnet and Powers. Take 5 g of soiled human hair sample and keep in 200 cc (cubic centimeter) of water containing 1 g of shampoo. Shake the flask for 50 times within 4 minutes and wash. Dry and weigh the hair to calculate the amount of soil cleaned by shampoo. ➢ **Foaming ability and foam stability:** Determine foaming ability by using cylinder shake method. Place 50 mL of the 1% commercial or formulated shampoo solution into a 250 mL graduated cylinder; cover with one hand and shake 10 times. Record the total volume of the foam content after 1 min of shaking. Evaluate foam stability by recording the foam volume after 1 min and 4 min of shake test. ➢ **Wetting time test:** Cut a canvas paper into 1-inch diameter discs having an average weight of 0.44 g. Place the smooth surface of disc on the surface of 1% v/v shampoo solution and start the stopwatch. The time required for the disc to begin to sink is noted down as the wetting time. ➢ **Evaluation of conditioning performance:** Take the hair tress of an Asian woman from a local salon. Cut it into four swatches of the tresses with approximately the length of 10 cm and the weight of 5 g. A swatch without washing served as the control. Wash other three tresses with the formulated shampoos in an identical manner. For each cycle, shake each tress with the mixture of 10 g of a sample and 15 g of water in a conical flask for 2 min and then rinse with 50 mL water. Afterward, dry each tress at room temperature. Wash the tresses for maximum ten cycles. Evaluate the conditioning performance of the shampoos i.e. smoothness and softness, by a blind touch test, by twenty randomly selected student volunteers. All the students should blind folded and asked to touch and rate the four tresses for conditioning performance from score 1 to 4 (1 = poor; 2 = satisfactory; 3 = good; 4 = excellent).

Contd...

Tooth Paste	➢ **Determination of abrasive particles**: Extrude the paste about 15 to 20 cm length from collapsible tube of each sample on a butter paper. Then test all the samples by pressing it along its entire length by a finger for the presence of hard and sharp edged abrasive particles for all samples. Hard and sharp edged abrasive particles should be absent. ➢ **Determination of spreadability:** Weigh and place about 1 gm of each sample at the centre of the glass plate (10X10 cm) and place another glass plate over it carefully. Place 2 kilogram weight above the glass plates at the centre of the plate. Avoid sliding of the plate. After 30 minutes, measure the diameter of the paste in centimeters for all samples. Repeat the experiment three times and calculate the averages for all samples. Spread ability (cms) should be 8.5 ➢ **Determination of fineness:** Weigh accurately 10gm of each sample and place in a 100ml beaker. Add 50ml of water and allow standing for 30 mins with occasional stirring until the toothpaste is completely dispersed. Pass this solution through 150 micron Indian Standard sieve. Wash the sieve with running tap water. Continue washing until all the matters passed by through the sieve. After washing collect the residue remains on sieves and dry in an oven at 105°C. Calculation: Percentage by mass = 100 M1 / M M1 - Mass in grams of residue retained on sieve M - Mass in grams of material taken for the test Fineness (% by mass) should be 0.5 ➢ **Determination of pH:** Weigh accurately 5 gm of all samples and place in a 150 ml beaker. To this add 45 ml of freshly boiled and cooled water at 27°C. Stir it well to make a thorough suspension. Determine the pH for all samples within 5 minutes by using pH meter. pH should be 5.5-10.5 (Max.) ➢ **Determination of foaming power:** Weigh and place about 5gm of each sample in a 100ml glass beaker. To this add 10ml of water and covere the beaker with a watch glass and allow to stand for 30 minutes to disperse the toothpaste in water. Stir the contents of the beaker with a glass rod and transfer slurry to a 250ml graduated measuring cylinder, during this transfer ensure that no foam is produced and no lump paste pass into the measuring cylinder. Transfer the residue left in the beaker with further portion of 5-6 ml of water to the cylinder. Adjust the content of cylinder to 50ml by adding sufficient water and the content has to be maintained at 30°C. Stir the contents of the cylinder with a glass rod to ensure a uniform suspension. As soon as the temperature of the content reach to 30°C, stopper the cylinder and shake. Allow to stand the cylinder for 5 minutes and note the volume of foam with water and water content only of all samples. Foaming power = V1 – V2 V1 - Volume in ml of foam with water V2 - Volume in ml of water only. Foam formation (ml) should be Min 50
Face Powder	➢ **Determination of matter insoluble in boiling water**: weigh and transfer 1gm of each sample to a 500ml beaker. Wet each sample with little rectified spirit. To this add 200ml of water and boil. Allow to settle and filter the supernatant liquid through Gooch crucible. Wash the residue with water and transfer completely to the filter. Dry the residue remains in the crucible at 105°C to obtain a constant mass. Calculation: Mater insoluble in boiling water, percent by mass = 100 M1 / M M1 - Mass in grams of the residue, M - Mass in grams of the material taken for the test. Matter insoluble in boiling water (mg) should be (Max) 90 ➢ **Test for solubility of colors:** Take 1gm of each sample. To this add 50 ml of water and boil for 15 minutes and filter. Take out 10ml of sample from this filtered solution and add 15ml of rectified spirit. Reflux for 15 minutes and filter. The filtrate should be colorless or faintly colored. Solubility of colors should be Colorless

Contd...

	➢ **Determination of fineness:** Place about 10gm of each sample material in specified (standard sieve 150 micron) sieve. Wash it by means of slow stream of running tap water and finally with fine stream from a wash bottle until as much material is passed through the sieve. In case the material is not easily wetted by water, the washing should be started with slow stream of filtered denatured spirit. The water should be completely drained from the sieve and it should be dried on steam bath. Then transfer the residue carefully to a tarred watch glass and dry at 105°C for constant mass. Calculation: The fineness of all samples is calculated by using the following formula. Material retained on the specified sieve, percent by mass =100 M1 / M M1 - Mass in grams of the residue retained on the specified sieve, M - Mass in grams of the material taken for the test Fineness (% by mass) should be (Max) 0.5 ➢ **Determination of pH of aqueous suspension:** Take 10gm of each sample face powder in a 150ml beaker. To this add 90ml of freshly boiled and cooled water. Stir well to make a thorough suspension. Determine the pH within 5 minutes for all samples using pH meter. Standard Value should be pH: 5.5-8 ➢ **Determination of moisture and volatile matter:** Weigh accurately about 5gm of each sample material and place in a porcelain or glass dish, about 6-8cm in diameter and about 2- 4cm in depth. Dry it in an air oven at a temperature of 105°C to a constant mass. Calculation: The moisture and volatile matter of all samples is calculated by using the following formula. : Moisture and volatile matter, percent by mass =100 M1 / M M1 - loss in mass in g on drying and, M - Mass in grams of the material taken for the test. Moisture and volatile matter (% by mass) should be (Max) 2
Lip Cosmetics- Lipsticks, Lip Balm, Lip Liner	• **Melting point:** Determination of melting Point & is determined by capillary tube method by keeping the size of capillary length of fill & rate of heating constant. • **Breaking point**: The maximum weight at which the lipstick breaks, is its breaking point. Breaking point is done to determine the strength of lipstick. The lipstick is held horizontally in a socket, ½ inch away from the edge of support. The weight is gradually increased by a specific value (10 g) at specific interval of 30 seconds and weight at which it breaks up is considered as the breaking point. • **Force of application**: This test is done for comparative measurement of the force to be applied for application. A piece of coarse brown paper can be kept on a shadow graph balance and lipstick can be applied at 45° angle to cover 1 inch area until fully covered. The pressure reading is an indication of force of application and it depends on the operator. • **Thixotropy**: This is done by using penetrometer. Standard needle of specific diameter is allow to penetrate for 5 sec. under a 50 gm load at 25?c. the depth of penetration is a measurement of the thixotropic structure. Penetration of 9 to 10.5 mm is indicative of a soft and thixotropic structure.

Cosmetic Safety and Toxicity Screening

Microbial test	As herbal products are sensitive to microbial growth, microbial assay has to be carried out by agar well diffusion method or turbidometric method.
Stability studies	It is carried out at elevated temperatures (like 45^{0}C, 90^{0}C, and 120^{0}C), relative humidity, and pH level for a period of 6 months and all above parameters are evaluated periodically to confirm changes in product.
Sensitivity test	It is also called as patch test. Apply product on 1 cm^2 of animal (preferably rabbit) skin or human epidermis. If there is no inflammation or rashes, then it

Contd...

	is free from sensitivity. Cell viability can be assessed with the use of 3-(4,5-dimethylthiazol-2-yl)-2,5-diphenyltetrazolium bromide (MTT) assay too. This study should be carried out in accordance with the guidelines of the CPSC (Consumer Product Safety Commission). The study has to be approved by the Institutional Ethics Committee.
Irritation test	Apply the product on 1 cm^2 of animal (preferably rabbit) skin or human epidermis and observe for erythema and edema at 24 and 72 hours respectively. Calculate the primary irritation index (PII) based on the sum of the scored reactions divided by 24 (2 scoring intervals multiplied by 2 test parameters multiplied by 6 rabbits). If there are no signs of erythema or edema on the intact and abraded rabbit skin, the PII of the formulation is supposed to be 0.00. Thus, the product is nonirritant to rabbit skin.
Toxicity test	It is carried out on animals to calculate lethal dose 50% (LD/50), It is the amount of the substance required (usually per body weight) to kill 50% of the test population, values and acute, chronic toxicity parameters using mice preferably. Carry out these studies as per the Guidelines of OECD (Organization for Economic Co-operation and Development) for acute and chronic toxicity. It also requires the approval of CPCSEA (Committee For The Purpose Of Control and Supervision on Experiments on Animals).
Eye irritation test for shampoo or eye cosmetics	This is the test which should be carried out using rabbits. Drop the 0.1 ml of shampoo to the conjunctiva sac of one eye of rabbit, while other eye serves as control. Prepare 3 groups of animals on the basis of washing of eye with water. Thus, first group of animals without any washing; second washing with water after 2 seconds; and third washing after instillation. Observe for seven days for any irritation, and if irritation occurs, then observe the effect of water on irritation removal.

Cosmetic Regulations in Various Countries

Europe Cosmetics Regulations

The EU Cosmetic Regulation 1223/2009 came into force in 2013 and concerns 31 European countries (28 countries of the EU + Norway + Iceland + Lichtenstein)

The regulation is based on three principles:

1. Safety of Raw Materials and Ingredients
2. Good manufacturing practices
3. Invigilating of cosmetic market

These principles translate into requirements for the cosmetic brand (non-exhaustive list):

- Designate a Responsible Person (RP)
- Prepare a Product Information file (PIF) including a Safety Assessment
- Respect the Good manufacturing practices (GMP) for cosmetics
- Comply with Labeling and Packaging requirements
- Ensure notification via the Cosmetic Products Notification Portal (CPNP)

ASEAN Cosmetics Regulations

ASEAN with its 10 member countries (Brunei, Darussalam, Cambodia, Indonesia, Malaysia, Myanmar, Lao PDR, Philippines, Singapore, Thailand and Viet Nam) has always focused on its economic and social growth. Certain cosmetics products (e.g. anti-dandruff shampoos) are classified as cosmetics in some countries (e.g. in EU and China), whereas they may be regulated as over-the-counter drugs in other countries (as in USA) or quasi-drugs (as in Japan). These guidelines require information of Product Types, Product Presentation, Product Notification, Sample Testing, Adverse Event Reporting, List of Annexes (detailed Information about product presentation type, Labeling requirements, PIF guidelines) and Electronic Submission of Notification.

Australian Cosmetics Regulations

In Australia, TGA is main regulatory authority and there are also interlinked authorities which are and regulating the cosmetic products. Ingredients in cosmetic products are classified as industrial chemicals, and new cosmetic ingredients are subject to notification to the National Industrial Chemicals Notification Assessment Scheme (NICNAS) for assessment unless they qualify for an exemption, Manufacturers and importers can check the conditions or restrictions of chemicals which are available for use in Australia, using the Australian Inventory of Chemical Substances (AICS) and the NICNAS Cosmetics Guidelines. Several factors influence whether a product is a cosmetic or therapeutic good, including:- • the primary use or purpose of the product, • the ingredients in the product and their effects on the body, • how the product is applied and/or administered, and • How the product is promoted, represented, presented or labelled.

USA Cosmetics Regulations

Cosmetic products are regulated by the FDA through different laws like: "Federal Food Drugs and Cosmetic Act (FD&C 1938)" and "Fair Packaging and Labeling Act". USFDA states that a product can be both drug and cosmetic, the classification of products are arranged & simple and depending upon the product claim.

Indian Cosmetics Regulations

Manufacture of cosmetics of cosmetics for sale / distribution licence is issued by the state regulatory authorities (State Drugs Control Department or state Food & Drug Administration). Cosmetics appearing under Schedule "S" should conform to the Indian Standards framed by the Bureau of Indian Standards (BIS). Particulars to be shown in the manufacturing records as per schedule U(I). As per D&C Rules, 1945 labelling requirements must be full fill such as Product name along with site address on both the inner and the outer labels.

Good Manufacturing Practices (GMP)

The Good Manufacturing Practices are prescribed to ensure that raw materials used in the manufacture of drugs are authentic of prescribed quality and are free from contamination. The manufacturing process is as has been prescribed to maintain the standards. Adequate quality control measures are adopted. The manufactured drug which is released for sale is of acceptable quality. The manufacturing plant should have adequate space for: Receiving & storing raw material, manufacturing process areas, quality control section, finished goods store, office, rejected goods/drugs store. General Requirements of location & surroundings, buildings, water supply, containers cleaning, stores, working space, health clothing sanitation & hygiene of workers, medical services, machinery & equipments, batch manufacturing records, distribution records, record of market complaints, quality control should be as per GMP norms.

There should be 150 sq.feet area for quality control section. For identification of raw drugs, reference books & reference samples should be maintained. Manufacturing record should be maintained for the various processes. To verify the finished products, controlled samples of finished products of each batch will be kept foe 3 years. To supervise & monitor adequacy of conditions under which raw materials, semi-finished products & finished products are stored. Keep record in establishing shelf life & storage requirements for the drugs. Manufacturers who are manufacturing patent, proprietary Ayurvedic, Siddha & Unani medicines shall provide their own specification & control references in respect of such formulated drugs.

Offences and Penalties for misbranded cosmetic and spurious cosmetic or for offences relating to import, manufacture for sale /distribution & sale of cosmetics have been mention in sections 13, 18& 27A of the Drugs & Cosmetics Act. Import of certain cosmetics is prohibited under section 10 of the Act & rule 134A,135,135A of the Drugs & Cosmetics Rules ,145.

Cosmetics can be imported into India only through ports of entry prescribed under Rule 43A & are:

Firozepur Cantonment & Amritsar Railway Stations (through Pakistan border),Ranaghat, Bongaon & mohiassan Railway Stations (through Bangladesh border) Raxaul (by road/railways lines connecting Raxaul in India & Birganj in Nepal),Chennai, Kolkata, Mumbai, cochin, Nhava Sheya & Kandla, Ahmedabad, Chennai, Delhi, Hyderabad, Kolkata & Mumbai(by Air).

Now there are 28 Cosmetic which are Placed under Schedule S to the rule which are imported in India only after compliance with the Indian standards. They are: 1.Skin Powder 2. Skin Powder for infants 3. Tooth powders 4. Toothpastes 5. Skin Creams 6. Hair oils 7. Shampoos soap based 8. Shampoos synthetic detergent based 9. Hair creams 10. Oxidation hair dyes, liquid 11. Cologne 12. Nail Polish 13. Aftershave Lotion 14. Pomades and Brilliantine's 15. Depilatories 16. Shaving Creams 17. Cosmetic Pencils 18. Lipstick 19. Toilet soap 20. Liquid Toilet soap 21. Baby Toilet soap 22. Transparent toilet soap 23. Shaving soap 24. Lipslave 25. Powder Hair dye 26. Bindi 27. Kumkum Powder 28. Henna Powder.

Rule 134A also prescribes that no cosmetic shall be imported which contains a coal tar color other than one prescribed in schedule Q and Indian standards (IS: 4707 Part I) to the above rules and coal tar color used in cosmetic should not contain more than – Two ppm of arsenic as arsenic trioxide, 20 ppm of Lead, 100 ppm of heavy metals other than lead calculated as total of the respective metals.

BIS Regulations for Cosmetics

Introduction

The Bureau of Indian Standards is the National Standards Body of India under Department of Consumer affairs, Ministry of Consumer Affairs, Food & Public Distribution, Government of

India. It is established by the Bureau of Indian Standards Act, 2016 which came into effect on 12 October 2017. Cosmetics products in India are regulated under the Drugs and cosmetics Act 1940 and Rules 1945 and Labeling Declarations by Bureau of Indian Standards (BIS). BIS sets the standards for cosmetics for the products listed under Schedule 'S' of the Drugs and cosmetics Rules 1945. List of Indian Standards referred in Schedule S of the Drugs and Cosmetics Rules, 1945:

(i) Skin powders (IS 3959)
(ii) Skin powders for infants (IS 5339)
(iii) Tooth Powder (IS 5383)
(iv) Tooth paste (IS 6356)
(v) Skin Creams (IS 6608)
(vi) Hair Oils (IS 7123)
(vii) Shampoo, Soap-based (IS 7669)
(viii) Shampoo, Synthetic-Detergent based (IS 7884)
(ix) Hair Creams (IS 7679)
(x) Oxidation hair dyes, Liquid (IS 8481)
(xi) Cologne (IS 8482)
(xii) Nail polish (IS 9245)
(xiii) After shave lotion (IS 9255)
(xiv) Pomades and Brilliantines (IS 9339)
(xv) Depilatories chemicals (IS 9636)
(xvi) Shaving creams (IS 9740)
(xvii) Cosmetic Pencils (IS 9832)
(xviii) Lipstick (IS 9875)
(xix) Lipsalve (IS 10284)
(xx) Powder hair dyes (IS 10350)
(xxi) Bindi (Liquid) (IS 10998)
(xxii) Kum kum powder (IS 10999)
(xxiii) Henna powder (IS 11142)
(xxiv) Sindoor (IS 14649)
(xxv) Liquid foundation make-up (IS 14318)
(xxvi) Cold Wax-Hair remover (IS 15152)
(xxvii) Face pack (IS 15153)
(xxviii) Kajal (IS 15154)
(xxix) Oxidation Hair Dyes (Emulsion type) (IS 15205)
(xxx) Cream Bleach (IS 15608)

Cosmetics Sectional Committee has published two Indian Standards for raw materials/ingredients for use in cosmetics, namely, IS 4707 (Part 1) : 2017 Classification for cosmetic raw materials and adjuncts : Part 1 Colourants and 4707 (Part 2) : 2017 Classification for cosmetic raw materials and adjuncts : Part 2 List of raw materials generally not recognized as safe for use in cosmetics which are widely used by Central Drugs Standard Control Organization (CDSCO) and Food and Drug Administrations (FDAs). Moreover, IS 4707 (Part 1) is referred in the Drugs and Cosmetics Rules, 1945 for colourants to be used in cosmetics.

Standards for Heavy metals

According to IS 6608:200, if all the raw materials requiring a test for heavy metals have been so tested and comply with the requirements, then the manufacturer may not test the finished cosmetic for heavy metals and arsenic. There should be a declaration for Heavy Metal and Hexachlorophene content for registration of cosmetics products. The test report including result of lead, arsenic, mercury, other heavy metals and if any microbiological test. Undertaking from the manufacturer stating compliance of all raw materials/pigments used, heavy metals (with specified limits) and Hexachlorophene contents in products with BIS and Drugs & Cosmetic Rules, 1945.

Standards for Colouring Agent

While manufacturing skin creams and lipstick if dyes colour (pigments lakes) are used then they shall comply with IS 4707 (Part I). It should be according to the Schedule Q of Drugs and Cosmetics Act and Rules by CDSCO and as amended from time to time. The other ingredients shall comply with the provisions of IS 4707 (Part 2).

Rule 134 of Drugs and Cosmetics Rules prohibited on use of cosmetics containing Dyes, Colours, and Pigments other than those specified by the Bureau of Indian Standards (IS: 4707 Part 1 as amended) and Schedule Q. According to Rule 145 of the Drugs and Cosmetics Rules, the use of lead and arsenic compounds in cosmetics for the purpose of colouring is prohibited. The import of cosmetics in which a lead or arsenic compound has been used for the colouring purpose is not allowed under Rule 135. Cosmetics containing mercury compounds are not manufactured and imported under Rule 145 D and 135 A.

Bureau of Indian Standards (BIS) has provided the specification for Skin Creams and Lipstick in the Indian Standards (IS) 6608:2004 and 9875:1990 respectively. IS 6608:2004 says that if all the raw materials requiring test for heavy metals have been so tested and comply with the requirements, then the manufacturer may not test the finished cosmetic for heavy metals and arsenic.

The Dyes colors (pigments lakes) if used in the manufacture of skin creams and lipstick shall comply with IS 4707 (Part I) subject to the provision of Schedule Q of Drugs and Cosmetics Act and Rules, issued by the Government of India, and as amended from time to time. Other ingredients shall comply with the provisions of IS 4707 (Part 2).

Rule 134 of Drugs and Cosmetics Rules has laid down restrictions on use of cosmetics containing Dyes, Colors and Pigments other than those specified by the Bureau of Indian Standards (IS: 4707 Part 1 as amended) and Schedule Q. The permitted Synthetic Organic Colors and Natural Organic Colors used in the Cosmetic shall not contain more than:

- 2 ppm (parts per million) of Arsenic calculated as Arsenic Trioxide.
- 20 ppm of lead calculated as lead.
- 100 ppm of heavy metals other than lead calculated as the total of the respective metals.

These coloring agents are generally recognized as safe (GRAS). For some of these, purity requirements are mentioned as laid down in the EEC directive of 1962. Maximum concentration in finished products is mentioned in some. Rule 145 of the Drugs and Cosmetics Rules prohibits use of lead and arsenic compounds in cosmetics for the purpose of coloring. Rule 135 prohibits import of cosmetics in which a lead or arsenic compound has been used for the coloring purpose. Rule 145 D and 135 A prohibits manufacture and import respectively of cosmetics containing mercury compounds

Standards for Preservatives

1. Preservatives are substances which may be added to cosmetic products for the primary purpose of inhibiting the development of micro-organisms in such products.
2. The substances marked with the symbol (*) may also be added to cosmetic products in concentration other than those laid down in this Annex for other specific purposes apparent from the presentation of the products, e.g.; deodorants in soaps or as and-dandruff agents in shampoos.
3. Other substances used in the formulation of cosmetic products may also have anti-microbial properties and thus help in the preservation of the products, as, for instance, many essential oils and some alcohols. These substances are not included in this Annex.
4. For the purposes of this list:
5. (a) 'Salts' is taken to mean: salts of the cations sodium, potassium, calcium, magnesium, ammonium and ethanolamines; salts of the anions chloride, bromide, sulphate, acetate.
6. (b) 'Esters' is taken to mean: esters of methyl; ethyl, propyl, isopropyl, butyl, isobutyl, phenyl'
7. All finished products containing formaldehyde or substances in this Annex and which release formaldehyde must be labelled with the warning 'contains formaldehyde where, the concentration of formaldehyde in the finished product exceeds 0.05 percent.

ANNEX D (Clauses 1 and 3) List of Permitted UV Filters Which Cosmetic Products May Contain

For the purpose of this Directive. UV Filters are substances, which contained in cosmetic sunscreen products, are specifically intended to filter certain UV rays in order to protect the skin from certain harmful effects of these rays. These UV filters may bee added to other cosmetic products within the limits and under the condition laid down in this Annex. Other UV filters used in cosmetic products solely for the purpose of protecting the product against UV rays are not included in the list.

Cosmetic Evaluation Instruments

Instruments to Evaluate Skin Products

Sebumeter: Sebaceous gland activity has four distinct components which are sebum production (a secretion rate function), storage (a volume function), surface output (a delivery rate function) and stratum corneum permeation (an influx rate function). The oily appearance of skin results from an excess of sebum excretion and spreading over the body surface and its interaction with the skin surface. A multi-pronged approach is often useful to assess skin greasiness with precision. The clinical evaluation of skin greasiness and its shiny appearance should be further complemented by quantifying the large pores, follicular plugs and comedones. The sebum amount present at the skin surface can be measured non-invasively using one of several methods based on solvent extraction, cigarette paper pads, photometric assessment, bentonite clay and lipid-sensitive tapes. Quantitative parameters include the sebum casual level, the sebum excretion rate, the sebum replacement time, the instant sebum delivery, the follicular excretion rate, the density in sebum-enriched reservoirs and the sustainable rate of sebum excretion. A series of environmental and biological features influence the data. Hence rigorous methodological designs are mandatory to support claims. As a rule, accuracy of the methods is adversely affected by skin temperature, degree of hydration and surface roughness. An additional confounding factor is the inherent difficulty of collecting the surface lipids without a contribution from the follicular reservoir. A better understanding of factors that alter the sebum amount at the skin surface may well assist in the development of sebosuppressive agents to help the reduction of the skin greasiness and improve acne.

The Sebumeter(®) is widely used in both cosmetic and medical research, for measuring changes in sebum levels from skin, hair and scalp. It is commonly reported that the units correlated to a mass of sebum on the skin in μg cm(-2). The Sebumeter(®) is a precise analytical instrument capable of quantitative measurement of deposition of oily materials onto skin from topical products (down to the μg cm(-2) level), as well as its traditional use of measuring sebum levels. However, the output values do not directly correlate with the mass of oil present, and generation of a calibration curve is necessary for any ingredient of interest to produce quantitative data for claim support and formulation development.

Principle: The measurement is based on grease-spot photometry. The measuring is generally taken with a parchment like foil which becomes transparent after contact with lipid substances. The foil is pressed on the skin for a defined period. The change in transparency is then measured with the help of a source of light (photometric method). This method is insensitive to humidity. It is recommended to take sebumeter® readings before any product application.

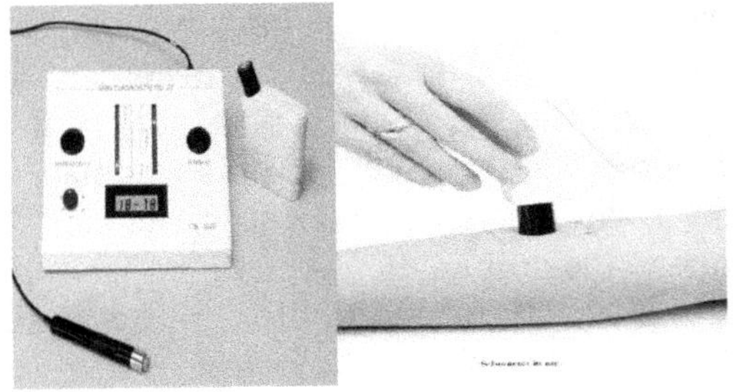

Visioscope® PC 35: USB camera with normal and cross polarized light

The camera enables the visualization of skin structure, hair, scalp as well as pigmentation and blood flow. Showing lines and wrinkles, skin impurities, pores, facial erythrosis and hair structure are some of the manifold applications.

Dermaviduals® corneotherapy

It is a basic device for the skin diagnosis. Determining the skin hydration, the lipid content and further significant parameters is of extreme importance for a safe and accurate skin diagnosis, for qualified product consultation and the following monitoring of the efficacy of cosmetic and dermatological products. The device comes with a comprehensive software package adapted to the products of the dermaviduals® system and includes additional measuring and consultation data and information. dermaviduals®-corneotherapy is a modular basic device, which contains the following probes:

- Measurement of sebum
- Measurement of skin moisture
- Measurement of skin elasticity
- dermaviduals® corneotherapy can be equipped with further specific probes like: Cosmetic probes, Lab probes (calibrated)

Visiopor® PP 34-camera for determination of porphyrines

The camera uses UVA light (375 nm) to detect acne lesions. The porphyrines generated by propionibacterium acnes show fluorescence from orange to reddish.

Corneometer® CM 825

It is a device to determine the hydration level of the skin surface. The accuracy of other hydration measurement instrumentation on the market is always assessed against the standard of the Corneometer®.

Principle: The measurement is based on capacitance measurement of a dielectric medium. The Corneometer® CM 825 measures the change in the dielectric constant due to skin surface hydration changing the capacitance of a precision capacitor. The reproducibility of the measurement is very high and the measurement time is very short (1 s).

Trans-Epidermal Water Loss Measurement (TEWL)

The measurement of transepidermal water loss or skin surface vapor loss is a good indicator of the integrity of the skin barrier function which inherently refers to the skin's ability to retain moisture. An increase in the TEWL indicates an impaired barrier function. Transepidermal water loss (TEWL) is the amount of water that passively evaporates through skin to the external environment due to water vapor pressure gradient on both sides of the skin barrier and is used to characterize skin barrier function. The average TEWL in human is about 300–400 mL/day; however, it can be affected by environmental and intrinsic factors. In high humidity, the amount of water loss will decrease due to the drop in the water vapor pressure gradient. TEWL varies in different anatomic sites and is inversely related to the corneocyte size. Skin sites with smaller corneocytes have higher TEWL values. Multiple instruments are commercially available to measure TEWL, providing valuable data with applications in clinical settings, toxicology, and product development. TEWL is a sensitive indicator of skin irritation and is widely used in objective analysis of irritancy potential or protective properties of topical products. The accuracy of TEWL measurements can be influenced by environmental factors such as humidity, temperature, ventilation, and intrinsic factors. It is essential that these measurements be conducted under standard conditions.

Skin color measurement by Minolta CR-300 colorimeter (Minolta Company Ltd., Osaka, Japan)

This instrument is a reflectance spectrophotometer that measures reflected light in the visible spectrum (range, 400–700 nm). It also works as a tristimulus chromameter, recording colors in a three-dimensional space known as Commission International d'Eclairge 1976 L*a*b* (CIELAB) color space. Every color in the CIELAB colorimetric system can be described by a combination of three coordinates, L*, a*, and b*, where L* is the total quantity of light reflected or skin brightness (described as light, dark, etc.), a* represents color ranging from red (positive values) to green (negative values), and b* represents color ranging from blue (negative values) to yellow (positive values). The a* and b* coordinates can be converted into polar coordinates defined as hue angle (h° = arctan(b*/a*)) and chroma, often referred to as saturation of color (C = [(a*)2 + (b*)2]1/2). Hue refers to the basic color of an object, where 0° represents red and 90° represents yellow. The hue angle in our population ranged from 43° to 82°. Chroma describes the intensity of color, with higher chroma indicating greater intensity.

Instruments to Evaluate Hair Products

Characterization of the structure and physical and mechanical properties of hair are essential to develop better cosmetic products. Some of the most used methods for evaluating hair products are listed below.

Hair physical/ mechanical proprieties: Physical proprieties of hair depend mostly on its geometry like oval (Caucasian hair), circular (Asian hair), elliptic (Afro hair). Hair is surprisingly strong still flexible. Several mechanical proprieties like stretching, elasticity and hydrophilic power are directly related with fibers diameter. Combability, Surface properties of hair, Hair surface porosity, Friction, Static load, Isoelectric point and Shine (reflects and diffuses the incident light beam) are other important evaluation parameters.

Hair Combing Properties: It is well known that conditioning shampoos and hair conditioners are used to provide a variety of benefits to hair: they reduce the combing force, enhance the gloss, confer smoothness and antistatic properties and improve the manageability of the hair. One of the methods that is used to determine conditioning efficiency is combability. Combability measurement is a method used to assess any alteration of the hair cuticle due to improvement or degradation sources. These include: mechanical sources such as brushing and friction; chemical sources, for example perms, oxidative colouring, lipid-depleting surfactants; and environmental sources like solar radiation, heat from hot blow drying or chlorine from swimming pools. Many haircare products are marketed on their ability to de-tangle hair and eliminate the difficulties associated with brushing and combing. Advertising and sales promotion will encourage consumers to try a product, but to ensure repeat purchase the product must live up to its claims. Using Stable Micro Systems' Hair Combing Rig, manufacturers can perform 'before and after' tests that will accurately assess the effectiveness of their products, to allow product optimisation

Hair Stretching Resistance Property: In general, the weight needed to produce a natural hair thread rupture is 50-100 g. An average head has about 120,000 threads of hair and would support about 12 tons. The resistance to breakage is a function of the diameter of the thread, of the cortex condition, and it is negatively affected by chemical treatments. When a certain load is applied on a hair and its elongation is measured we obtain the graphic representation of its several characteristic regions:

- Hookean's region or pre-recovering: during the stretching between 0 and 2% the elongation is proportional to the load applied.
- Recovering region: between 25-30% of stretching, the elongation considerably increases without a relationship with the load applied.
- After-recovering region: from 30% stretching load and fiber extension are proportional again.

Scanning Electron Microscopy (SEM): The scanning electron microscopy (SEM) is very used for analyzing hair threads. This technique allows observations of thick and not transparent samples under an electron beam. It also allows determining the shape of a material, the size of its component particles, and its layout. SEM is very used for big magnification of a given sample, generally to evaluate hair surface morphological conditions. The sample is coated with a carbon/gold film in order to lead electric current; then, under high vacuum, an electron beam is directed over it and the scattering is assessed by a detector, thus the image is generated.

Atomic force microscopy (AFM): This equipment allows observing sample images through the microscope, in environment conditions or even when we have a solution. The image is captured by a probe which has physical contact with the sample, and follows a parallel plan to the surface while acquires each point of the topographic component. The probe deflection is then measured by a computer program (software) which generates the image. Through this equipment it is also possible to have quantitative data on electric loads distribution and sensor force to travel the sample.

Mechanical Assays: The hair, when considered as a physical body, is a very resistant fiber. The rupture load of a healthy hair thread ranges from 50 to 100 g. The relative value is directly proportional to the thread length. To perform this assay a dynamometer is used – this is equipment frequently used for evaluating: hair rupture tension, elasticity, combability and detangling. The device exerts a tension on the hair thread and measures the needed force versus elongation. The hair lock is tied with a support, and then two combs pass through it as well as the needed force for this action.

Piezoelectric Sensors: This analysis is very close to the sensorial perception. The piezoelectric principle is based on the deformation of a crystal by a mechanical action. When this occurs, a load displacement is induced – so creating a voltage signal. In hair, it is possible applying this technique to the tactile perceptions of hair proprieties, as: conditioning, cleanliness and surface roughness. During the evaluation, the sensor is placed on a mechanical arm which touches the hair lock and afterwards it is released. This is repeated several times. Results are expressed as voltage arbitrary values.

Glossmeters: Glossmeter is a piece of equipment designed to measure the hair shine. The regularity of the hair surface helps to determine the light reflection. When the light follows a uniform surface, as in a mirror, the incidence angle is exactly equals to the reflection angle. However the hair is not totally uniform and at some points the light beam is reflected forming different angles (0 to 75o) and this kind of reflectance is known as diffuse reflectance.

Optical Coherence Tomography: Optical coherence tomography (OCT) is a diagnostic imaging technology based on low length coherence interferometry in which the coherence features of photons are exploited, leading to an imaging technology that is capable of producing non-contact, non-destructive, high-resolution cross-sectional images of the internal microstructure of living tissue such as: retina, skin and teeth. Its applications in medicine were reported less than a decade ago, but its roots lie in early works on white-light interferometry. The OCT image is based mainly in an optical property of sample, the backscattering coefficient. The false color in the image represents the backscattering coefficient, where white color represents high scattering and black color low scattering.

Subjective Tests

This kind of test aims to have a response through a trained panel or a specialized technician, or a group of trained volunteers' subjective assessment, after their evaluation of a test-product, in a way to mimic the final consumers' opinion. These assays allow non-parametric results and the protocols used in them search after standardizing some procedures in order to extrapolate a small group opinion to the target public. The main tests are: salon test and test under normal use conditions.

Further Reading

1. Ralph Gordon Harry, John Bernard Wilkinson, Raymond Jack Moore. Harry's Cosmeticology. Chemical Publications. 1982
2. Gubitosa J, Rizzi V, Fini P, Cosma P. Hair Care Cosmetics: From Traditional Shampoo to Solid Clay and Herbal Shampoo, A Review. Cosmetics. 2019; 6(1):13. https://doi.org/10.3390/cosmetics6010013
3. Tiwari, M. V. Dubey, A. Lahiri. "Comparative study of various herbal cosmetics: a survey". Asian Journal of Pharmaceutical and Clinical Research, Vol. 13, no. 10, Oct. 2020, pp. 31-34.
4. Rabasco AA, Gonzalez RM. Lipids in pharmaceutical and cosmetic preparations. Grasasy Aceites 2000;51:74-96.
5. Bruno Burlando, Luisella Verotta, Laura Cornara, Elisa Bottini-Massa. Herbal Principles in Cosmetics Properties and Mechanisms of Action. CRC Press, 2010.
6. Jared R. Jagdeo, Peter Elsner, Howard I. Maibach Cosmeceuticals and Active Cosmetics. CR C Press, 2015
7. P. K. Chattopadhyay. Herbal Cosmetics & Ayurvedic Medicines (EOU) (3rd Revised Edition). NIIR Project Consultancy Services. 2013

8. H. Panda. Perfumes and Flavours Technology Handbook. NIIR Project Consultancy Services. 2010
9. The Complete Technology Book on Flavours, Fragrances And Perfumes. NIIR Project Consultancy Services. 2007
10. Amritpal Singh Saroya. Contemporary Phytomedicines. CRC Press. 2017
11. Neelesh Malviya, Sapna Malviya. Herbal Drug Technology. CBS India. 2018
12. Ashok Katdare, Mahesh Chaubal. Excipient Development for Pharmaceutical, Biotechnology, and Drug Delivery Systems. CRC Press. 2006

Scan QR code to view the website/guidelines

- Indian Standards Referred In Government Regulations-
Indian standards referred in government regulations - Bureau of Indian Standards (bis.gov.in)

- FDA Small Businesses & Homemade Cosmetics: Fact Sheet-
Small Businesses & Homemade Cosmetics: Fact Sheet | FDA

- The Drugs And Cosmetics Act, 1940 –
2016DrugsandCosmeticsAct1940Rules1945.pdf (cdsco.gov.in)

CHAPTER 5

Nutraceuticals and Regulations

Introduction

Nutraceutical is word coined by Dr. Stephen in 1989, a combination of the words "nutrition" and "pharmaceutical", is a food or food product that reportedly provides health and medical benefits, including the prevention and treatment of disease. It is defined as food stuff (as a fortified food or a dietary supplement) that provides health benefits. Nutraceuticals are non-specific biological therapies used to promote wellness, prevent malignant processes and control symptoms. Nutraceutical foods are not subject to the same testing and regulations as pharmaceutical drugs. As per the Food Safety Standard Act, 2006 (Chapter 4, Section 22) it has been recommended that Food should be classified as follows:

- Novel foods
- Genetically modified food
- Irradiated food
- Organic foods
- Foods for special dietary use
- Functional foods
- Nutraceuticals
- Health Supplements

This makes it very clear that Nutraceuticals are a part of the food segment and it should not be considered as a form of pharmaceutical or drug formulation.

Why Nutraceutical?

- Awareness that prevention is better than cure
- People especially of younger generation are becoming progressively more health-conscious
- Gradual shift toward natural ingredients
- Unnourished population
- Increased work stress, busy schedule and Agricultural pollution unable to provide proper nutrition
- High cost of health care with the expensive disease-treatment approach
- Chronic diseases without effective medicines

So there is great demand of alternative beneficial products like dietary supplement, functional food and nutraceuticals by people as well as researchers to explore therapeutic values.

Nutraceuticals have numerous health and nutritional benefits which helps in immunity enhancement, reduction of disease risk and also have anti-ageing effect.

But, unrealistic claims, poor packaging and labeling, poor stability and poor taste masking are few of challenges in the field of nutraceuticals.

Market Scenario of Nutraceutical

Globally, the US and Japan are the most developed markets for nutraceuticals, due to the consumer acceptability achieved in these regions. India, China and Brazil are developing nations which show huge potential for the nutraceuticals market, India and China have emerged as a key sourcing destination for natural ingredients. The global market for Nutraceuticals is projected to reach US$ 250 billion by 2018, driven primarily by the growing affinity among the general populace towards adopting a healthy lifestyle. Nutraceutical foods were the largest market segment in 2007, worth $39.9 billion. This is expected to increase $56.7 billion in 2013. Nutraceutical supplements have the second largest market share, generating $39.0 billion in 2007. This segment should reach $48.8 billion in 2013. The nutraceutical beverages segment represents the fastest growing segment and is expected to have the largest share of the market by 2013. This segment was worth $38.4 billion in 2007 and is expected to increase to and $71.3 billion in 2013.

Types of Nutraceutical products available in market

Functional Food

- Probiotics Fortified Food
- Omega Fatty Acid Fortified Food
- Branded Ionized Salt
- Branded Wheat Flour Market
- Other Functional Food

Functional Beverages

- Fruit & Vegetable Juices and Drinks
- Dairy & Dairy Alternative Drinks
- Noncarbonated Drinks
- Other

Dietary Supplements

- Proteins & Peptides
- Vitamins & Minerals
- Herbals
- Other

Personal Care and pharmaceuticals

Major Key players:

- GlaxoSmithKline: Horlicks, Boost, and Viva.
- Britania: Nutraceutical biscuits and juices
- Parle: Nutraceutical biscuits and juices

- Kellogg: Vitamin and mineral fortifies breakfast options
- Amway: Nutrilite
- Baidyanath: Chyawanprash
- Nestle: ActiPlus
- Danone: Yakult
- Coca-Cola: Minute Maid juices
- PepsiCo: Tropicana juices
- Abott: Pediasure, Ensure or Glucerna

Segments wise Key players in India

- **Functional/ fortified foods**: Cargill, Britannia, Kelloggs, Nestle, PepsiCo, Heinz, Baggrys, GlaxoSmithKline Consumer Healthcare, Patanjali, Mother Dairy, General Mills, Ruchi Soya
- **Functional beverages**: Redbull, Coca-cola, PepsiCo, Goldwin Healthcare, GlaxoSmithKline, Hector Beverages
- **Dietary supplements**: Amway, Dabur, Herbalife International, Danone, Novartis

Future Scope

Globalization of the nutraceutical and functional food industries presents significant challenges, not the least of which is the regulatory variance between countries active in the marketplace. Next issue is that the claims of medicinal benefits of the product should require to be complied by company. Insight on quality manufacturing techniques, cGMP and standardized analytical techniques with respect to safety, efficacy and quality testing and marketing authorisation procedures should be explored.

- Cognitive health
- Anti-aging
- Bone and joint health
- Teeth health
- Muscle development
- Cardiovascular health
- Blood pressure control
- Cholesterol control
- General cardiovascular health
- Weight control
- Restorative products
- Immune system

Classification

Generally nutraceutical are grouped as follows:

- Substances with established nutritional functions, such as vitamins, minerals, amino acids and fatty acids, also defined nutrients;
- Herbs or botanical products as concentrates and extracts, often called herbals; and
- Reagents derived from other sources (e.g., pyruvate, chondroitin sulphate, steroid hormone precursors) serving specific functions, such as sports nutrition, weight-loss supplements and meal replacements, also indicated as dietary supplements

Nutraceuticals can be classified on the basis of their nomenclature which is as follows:

Dietary supplements	Vitamins, minerals, herbs or other botanicals, amino acids, and substances such as enzymes, organ tissues, and metabolites.
Functional foods	It can be any ordinary food that has components or ingredients added to give it a specific medical or physiological benefit, other than a purely nutritional effect
Medical foods	It covers probiotics, antioxidants manufactured in liquids, tablets, capsule form
Farmaceuticals	It is a melding of the words farm and pharmaceuticals. It refers to medically valuable compounds produced from modified agricultural crops or animals (usually through biotechnology).

Nutraceuticals can be classified on the basis of their market which is as follows:

Dietary supplements	Vitamins, minerals, extracts, protein supplements, ayurvedic supplements (Chyawanprash, honey), powders
Functional foods	Fortified food, prebiotics, probiotics, iodinated food, gluten free food,
Functional Beverages	Energy drinks, nutritional drinks, fortified juices, sport drinks

Nutraceuticals are commonly classified on the basis of ingredients which is as follows

Minerals	Over twenty dietary minerals are necessary for human being and each have its specific role in maintain health ➢ Calcium: maintaining bone strength important in nerve, muscle and glandular functions. ➢ Iron: Metabolism and energy production. ➢ Magnesium: for nerve and muscle function ➢ Phosphorous: Part of genetic material. ➢ Chromium: With insulin helps to convert carbohydrates and fats into energy. ➢ Cobalt: Essential component of vitamin B12 ➢ Copper: Part of hemoglobin and collagen production ➢ Iodine: Essential for proper functioning of the thyroid. ➢ Zinc: Essential for immune function, would healing, blood clotting ➢ Selenium: Essential for fertility and sperm motility

Contd...

Vitamins	Vitamin is an organic compound required by an organism as a vital nutrient in limited amounts and cannot be synthesized in sufficient quantities by an organism, and must be obtained from the diet. Dietary supplements, often containing vitamins, are used to ensure that adequate amounts of nutrients are obtained on a daily basis, if optimal amounts of the nutrients cannot be obtained through a varied diet. ➢ Vitamin A: Antioxidant, essential, for growth and development and in the treatment of certain skin disorders. ➢ Vitamin E: Antioxidant, helps form blood cells, muscles, lung and nerve tissue, boosts the immune system. ➢ Vitamin K: Essential for blood clotting. ➢ Vitamin C: Antioxidant, for healthy bones, gums, teeth and skin, in wound healing, prevent common cold and attenuate its symptoms. ➢ Vitamin B_1 (Thiamine), B_2 (Riboflavin), B_3 (Niacin), B_5 (Panthothenic acid), B_6 (Pyridoxol), B_7 (Biotin): energy production, essential in nerve functions, healthy eyes, skin. ➢ Vitamin B_9 (Folic acid): Produce the genetic materials of cells, in pregnancy for preventing birth defects, RBCs formation, protects against heart disease. ➢ Vitamin B12 (Cobalamine): Proper functioning of nervous system
Antioxidants	Antioxidants are widely used in dietary supplements and have been investigated for the prevention of diseases such as cancer, coronary heart disease and even altitude sickness. An antioxidant is a molecule that inhibits the oxidation of other molecules. Oxidation is a chemical reaction that transfers electrons or hydrogen from a substance to an oxidizing agent. Oxidation reactions can produce free radicals. In turn, these radicals can start chain reactions. When the chain reaction occurs in a cell, it can cause damage or death to the cell. Antioxidants terminate these chain reactions by removing free radical intermediates, and inhibit other oxidation reactions. They do this by being oxidized themselves, so antioxidants are often reducing agents such as thiols, ascorbic acid, or polyphenols, vitamins, minerals.
PUFA	Polyunsaturated fatty acids (PUFAs) are fatty acids that contain more than one double bond in their backbone. This class includes many important compounds, such as essential fatty acids. Essential fatty acids, or EFAs, are fatty acids that humans and other animals must ingest because the body requires them for good health but cannot synthesize them. The term "essential fatty acid" refers to fatty acids required for biological processes, and not those that only act as fuel. Only two EFAs are known for humans: alpha-linolenic acid (an omega-3 fatty acid) and linoleic acid (an omega-6 fatty acid). Other fatty acids that are only "conditionally essential" include gamma-linolenic acid (an omega-6 fatty acid), lauric acid (a saturated fatty acid), and palmitoleic acid (a monounsaturated fatty acid). Essential fatty acids play a part in many metabolic processes, and there is evidence to suggest that low levels of essential fatty acids, or the wrong balance of types among the essential fatty acids, may be a factor in a number of illnesses, including osteoporosis
Prebiotics	Prebiotics (Oligofructose, galacto-olig sachharides, lactulose) are non-digestible food ingredients that stimulate the growth and/or activity of bacteria in the digestive system in ways claimed to be beneficial to health. Traditional dietary sources of prebiotics include soybeans, inulin sources, raw oats, unrefined wheat, unrefined barley, and yacon. Some of the oligosaccharides that naturally occur in breast milk are believed to play an important role in the development of a healthy immune system in infants.

Contd...

Probiotics	Probiotic are Live microorganisms which when administered in adequate amounts confer a health benefit on the host. Lactic acid bacteria (LAB) and bifidobacteria are the most common types of microbes used as probiotics; but certain yeasts and bacilli may also be used. Probiotics are commonly consumed as part of fermented foods with specially added active live cultures; such as in yogurt, soy yogurt, or as dietary supplements.
Fibers	Dietary fiber (roughage or ruffage) is the indigestible portion of plant foods having two main components: soluble (may be prebiotic and/or viscous) fiber that is readily fermented in the colon into gases and physiologically active byproducts, and insoluble fiber (may be metabolically inert and provide bulking or metabolically fermented in the large intestine as a prebiotic fiber). Bulking fibers absorb water as they move through the digestive system, easing defecation. Fermentable insoluble fibers mildly promote regularity, although not to the extent that bulking fibers do, but they can be readily fermented in the colon into gases and physiologically active byproducts.
Health drinks	Health drinks are either just water fortified with some kind of flavor or teas, milk, juices enriched with healthy ingredients. Dairy drinks (19%), general health drinks (13.4%), ready-to-drink (RTD) tea and coffee (11.2%) and sports and energy drinks (10.%) are famous types of health drinks. Claims like "rich "or "free" needs scientific evidences.
Digestive enzymes	Digestive enzymes are produced and secreted by the gastrointestinal system to degrade fats, proteins, and carbohydrates, to accomplish the digestion and, afterwards, the absorption of nutrients. Their supplementation, when indicated, may provide a reliable help as an adjuvant treatment of several disorders characterized by an impairment of digestive functions. To date, various formulations of enzyme supplementation are available on the market, and they are currently used in clinical practice for the management of several digestive diseases, especially those involving organs designated to the production of digestive enzymes, including the exocrine pancreas (which produces pancreatic enzymes) and the small intestinal brush border (which produces lactase). Pancreatic enzyme supplementation is the therapy of choice for the management of exocrine pancreatic insufficiency (EPI) in chronic pancreatitis, pancreatic cancer, cystic fibrosis (CF) or diabetes. Another relevant application of enzyme supplementation in the clinical practice is the management of lactose intolerance. It is estimated that 75 percent of individuals worldwide experience hypolactasia, or some decrease of lactase activity, especially during adulthood. Recent evidence suggests that digestive enzymes may be useful also in celiac disease, but they are far from being used in the routine management of the disease. In celiac disease a lifelong gluten-free diet may bring about difficulties as avoiding gluten completely is problematic owing to the contamination with gluten of presumably gluten free foods. New therapeutic approaches include enzyme supplementation, correction of the intestinal barrier defect against gluten entry, blocking of gliadin presentation by human leukocyte antigen blockers and tissue transglutaminase inhibitors. Pancreatic enzymes can be divided into three groups, according to their respective function: proteolytic enzymes (mainly trypsinogen and chymotripsinogen and their active forms trypsin and chymotripsin), amylolitic enzymes (pancreatic amylase), and lipolitic enzymes (principally lipase).

Contd...

<table>
<tr><td></td><td>Exogenous pancreatic enzymes are primarily extracted from porcine or bovine sources. Lipase may also be synthesized from microbial sources, such as Aspergillus oryzae and Rhizopus arrhizus.
Replacement of native lactase through the use of exogenous enzymes, derived from yeast or fungi, with microbial exogenous lactase (obtained from yeasts or fungi) may be considered a reliable therapeutic option. Exogenous lactase can be administered with milk, or as capsules/tablets before eating dairy products.</td></tr>
<tr><td>Cereals and grains</td><td>In recent years, cereals and its ingredients are accepted as functional foods and nutraceuticals because of providing dietary fibre, proteins, energy, minerals, vitamins and antioxidants required for human health.
Cereals include dietary fibre such as β-glucan and arabinoxylan, carbohydrates such as resistant starch and oligosaccharides. Also, cereals can be used as fermentable substrates or the growth of probiotic microorganisms. Common cereals are wheat, rice, oat, barley, flaxseed, psyllium, brown rice, and their products are notified the most common cereal based functional foods and nutracuticals. Preventing cancer and CVD, reducing tumor incidence, lowering blood pressure, risk of heart disease, cholesterol and rate of fat absorption, delaying gastric emptying and supplying gastrointestinal are the protective effect of the cereals. Several of the nutrients in cereals have known potential for reducing risk factors for CHD; the linoleic acid, fiber, vitamin-E, Selenium and folate. Cereals also contain phytoestrogens of the lignin family and several phenolic acids with antioxidant properties.
Composition of different varieties of cereals expressed as 100 g of edible portion
<table>
<tr><th>Parameter</th><th>Rice</th><th>Wheat</th><th>Maize</th><th>Sorghum</th><th>Millets</th></tr>
<tr><td>Water (%)</td><td>12</td><td>12</td><td>13.8</td><td>11</td><td>11.8</td></tr>
<tr><td>Protein (g)</td><td>7.5</td><td>13.3</td><td>8.9</td><td>11</td><td>9.9</td></tr>
<tr><td>Fat (g)</td><td>1.9</td><td>2.0</td><td>3.9</td><td>3.3</td><td>2.9</td></tr>
<tr><td>Carbohydrates (g)</td><td>77.4</td><td>71.0</td><td>72.2</td><td>73.0</td><td>72.9</td></tr>
<tr><td>Fibre (g)</td><td>0.9</td><td>2.3</td><td>2.0</td><td>1.7</td><td>3.2</td></tr>
<tr><td>Ca (mg)</td><td>32</td><td>41</td><td>22</td><td>28</td><td>20</td></tr>
<tr><td>P (mg)</td><td>221</td><td>372</td><td>268</td><td>287</td><td>311</td></tr>
<tr><td>Fe (mg)</td><td>1.6</td><td>3.3</td><td>2.1</td><td>4.4</td><td>68</td></tr>
<tr><td>K (mg)</td><td>214</td><td>370</td><td>284</td><td>350</td><td>430</td></tr>
<tr><td>Mg (mg)</td><td>88</td><td>113</td><td>147</td><td>n.d.</td><td>162</td></tr>
<tr><td>Riboflavin (mg)</td><td>0.05</td><td>0.12</td><td>0.12</td><td>0.15</td><td>0.38</td></tr>
<tr><td>Niacin (mg)</td><td>1.7</td><td>4.3</td><td>2.2</td><td>3.9</td><td>2.3</td></tr>
<tr><td>Thiamin (mg)</td><td>0.34</td><td>0.55</td><td>0.37</td><td>0.38</td><td>0.73</td></tr>
</table>
SOURCE: Adapted from Severson (1998)</td></tr>
<tr><td>Phytochemicals</td><td>Polyphenols useful to prevent and control arterial diseases. Flavonoids useful to block the Angiotensin converting enzyme inhibitors (ACE) and strengthen the tiny capillaries that carry oxygen and essential nutrients to all cells. Glucosamine and chondroitin sulfate obtained from fish and animals are used against osteoarthritis and regulate gene expression and synthesis of NO and PGE2.</td></tr>
</table>

Nutraceutically Valuable Plants

Acacia: *Acacia Senegal* *Leguminoseae*	Arabin oxidase, salt of arabic acid, L-arabinose, L-rhamnose, L-galactose. oxidase	Emulsifying agent, suspending agent, demulcent
Broccoli (*Brassica oleracea* var. italica) Crucifereae	Vitamins, flavonoid, phenolic compounds, carotenoids, quercetin, and ascorbic acids	antioxidants, anti-carcinogenic compounds, and health-promoting
Green Tea (*Camellia sinensis*) Theaceae	Flavanols, epigallocatechin gallate (EGCG) and epigallocatechin (EGC	Cancer prevention, amelioration of diabetes side-effects, cardiovascular safety, cognitive boost, promotion of weight loss, skin care, allergy suppression, protection from osteoarthritis, prebiotics
Herbal Tea- Black tea, Green tea, Chamomile tea, Ginger tea, Ginseng tea, Peppermint tea, Cinnamon tea etc.	Vitamins, flavonoid, phenolic compounds,	Cancer prevention, amelioration of diabetes side-effects, cardiovascular safety, cognitive boost, promotion of weight loss, skin care, allergy suppression, protection from osteoarthritis, prebiotics
Black cohosh *Actaea racemosa* (formerly named *Cimicifuga racemosa*) Ranunculaceae	Triterpene glycosides, phenolic constituents, and formononetin	Treatment of symptoms related to menopause
Soybeans (*Glycine max*) Leguminosae	saponins, protease inhibitors, phytic acid, and isoflavones (genistein; daidzein and glycitein)	Treatment and prevention of cardiovascular diseases, cholesterol lowering, osteoporosis, diabetes, cancer, cognitive decline, and menopausal symptoms.
Turmeric *Curcuma longa, Zingiberaceae.*	Volatile oil, curcuminoids, curcumin, pinene, camphor, zingiberene.	Spices, coloring agent, anti inflammatory, anti arthritic, cervical cancer.
Garlic: *Allium sativum,* Liliaceae	Diallyl disulphide, allin, allicin, polysulphides, volatile oils, proteins, vitamins, lipids, amino acids	Food supplement, treatment of cough, cold, bronchitis, hypertension, cancer, atherosclerosis, antifungal, hypoglycemic.
Spirulina (type of blue-green algae) *Arthrospira platensis* and *A. maxima.*	It is a biomass of cyanobacteria and rich in protein, vitamins, minerals, and carotenoids	Antioxidant, potent dietary support in malnourishment
Ginseng: Asian or Korean ginseng (*Panax ginseng*) and American ginseng (*Panax quinquefolius*), Araliaceae	Steroidal saponins, phytosterols	Immunomodulatory, Antistress
Linseed/Flaxseed: *Linum usitatissimum,* Linaceae	Rich source of omega-3 fatty acids, natural phenolic glucosides, secoisolariciresinol diglucoside, p-coumaric acid glucoside, and ferulic acid glucoside	Reduces total and LDL-cholesterol in the blood

Regulatory Aspects

Different countries have different Nutraceutical terminologies and their regulations which are as follows

Country	Body Known as	Body Governed by	Definition covers
Canada	Natural health products in 2004	FDA	Vitamins, mineral, homeo-pathic, Chinese medicine, amino acids, essential fatty acids
EU	Food supplements in 2002	Food safety authority	Concentrated sources of nutrients, substances with nutritional or physiological effects
Russia	Biologically active food in 1997	Ministry of health and social development	Vitamins, amino acids, dietary fibers, para-pharmaceuticals (bioflavonoid, polysaccharides)
USA	Dietary supplement in 1994	FDA	Vitamins, minerals, bota-nicals, amino acids, extract
Australia	Complementary medicines in 1991	Department of health and ageing	Herbal medicines, vita-mins, minerals, nutritional supplements.
Japan	Foods for specific health use in 1991	Japan health and nutrition food association	Functional foods that can have three functions: nutrition, sensory satis-faction, physiological improvement
India	Foods for special dietary use in 2005	Food safety and standards act passes in 2006 yet to be implemented	Vitamins, minerals, botanicals, extracts
China	Health Food	State Food and Drug Administration (SFDA) in 2003	Any finished product or raw material intended for people to eat or drink, as well as any product that has traditionally served as both food and medication, with the exception of products used solely for medical purposes.

USFDA Regulations for Nutraceuticals

The guidance document released by the FDA for nutraceuticals contains the following components:

Current Good Manufacturing Practice (CGMP): The CGMP guidelines for the nutraceuticals are defined for all the areas of the production. CGMP includes the sanitation standards that a company needs to follow in its processing and storage locations while guiding it the process of implementation for the process and production control systems to maintain a consistent flow of quality for every batch.

Warning Letters & Safety Alerts: Similarly, like CGMP guidelines, there are certain warning letters and safety alerts that shall be specified by the manufacturers. They also need to provide all the information that backs up the safety component of the product for human consumption. The FDA requires all such information at the time of reviewing the findings to ensure they are consistently maintained and make an informed decision on approval of the product to be further distributed in the market and being sold.

Labeling and Regulation: Providing correct information on product labeling is one of the critical requirements defined under regulations for the nutraceuticals. The manufacturers need to continuously demonstrate compliance for the FDA requirements. Nutraceuticals aka dietary supplements are intended to serve health benefits to buyers, and this must be reflected through package labeling. The labeling information should also include the claims that if the supplement's dosage is taken in a higher amount than what is prescribed, it may induce risks.

The FDA strictly recommends the labeling and regulation for information to make consumers aware of the safe consumption limits for the particular dietary supplements they take. Hence, nutraceutical manufacturers need to follow the guidelines of labeling for consumer's health as well as their regulatory benefits.

Correspondence, Statements, and Agreements Related to Policy: This FDA regulation for the nutraceuticals implies that nutraceuticals manufacturers must upgrade the relevant information about the products, safety consumptions, and much more as soon as new statements or agreements issued by the regulatory. It involves informing consumers about the new ingredients being introduced, new policies to state the nutritional facts that make dietary supplements different from the other beverages, and their improved health significance.

Health Claims: With the consumers getting more aware of what they eat in the name of natural health foods and functional foods, it has become important for companies to do bountiful of research to develop the improved quality food products. Most of research results into new findings and health claims that should be included in labeling to communicate all the critical information to the consumers. This makes them even more aware of the nutraceutical products they are investing in.

Qualified Health Claims: Qualified health claims are the ones that are backed by some scientific evidence, but do not necessarily meet the standard requirements that one needs for an authorized health claim. Nutraceuticals manufacturers must ensure that these claims are not misleading by providing their information through disclaimer or any other valid communicating label. This also ensures that consumers understand the scientific evidence required for qualified health claims.

Adverse Events Reporting: The manufacturers who adhere to all the compliance requirements specified by FDA must follow a practice of creating and maintaining the records of all systems, processes, and events including the ones that may adversely affect them to meet compliance. A well-defined record-tracking and reporting system help nutraceutical manufacturers to demonstrate that they have an established set of processes and procedures to manage the adverse events tactfully.

General Compliance and Inspection Information for Industry: The general compliance and inspection information is required to ensure that a consistent approach is implemented for maintaining the environmental regulatory framework. This is intended for the entire nutraceutical industry to demonstrate the regulated processes that every company needs to follow so that they market only the safe health and dietary supplements to the consumers.

Food Safety and Security Act of India [FSSAI] guidelines 2006, Rules and Regulations, 2011

Introduction: The Nutraceutical is an emerging business and the growth of the business in the forthcoming years is huge. In India, Food Safety Standards Act 2006, and Food Safety Standard Rules and Regulations 2011, are implemented to avoid the grouping of Nutraceutical product either into food or drug. The new regulations would benefit the industry by expanding the scope for new product innovation and imports. The new regulations cover supplement guidelines for kids above two years old. Previously, the regulations only stated the supplement guidelines for individuals above the age of five. The additional formats covered under the new regulations are drops, gummies, chewable and mouth-dissolving strips, bars, biscuits, and candies. This is an expansion from tablets, capsules, liquids, semi-solids, pills, jelly or gel, and sachets allowed in the 2016 regulations.

Food and Nutraceuticals Regulations in India	
1990s	Prevention of Food adulteration act to prevent food adulteration
2006-2008	Food safety and standard (FSS) Act and Establishment of Food safety and standard authority of India (FSSAI)
2011-2015	Implementation of regulations and mandatory FSSAI Logo with license number on food labels
2016	Introduction of regulation of functional food and nutraceuticals
2017-2018	Implementation of regulation of functional food and nutraceuticals Introduction of import regulations and organic food

Nutraceuticals are considered as foods by the FSS Act, 2006, Rules and Regulations, 2011.

The Food Safety and Standards Authority of India (FSSAI) has issued regulations with respect to licensing and registration of food business, manufacturing, packing and labelling, food product standard and so on. In FSSA in India (FSSAI) has defined regulatory guidelines for approval of nutraceuticals in the Indian market. This Act consists of 21 chapters and in that the 4th Article that means 22 of the Act says about nutraceuticals, dietary supplements and various functional foods, and these products can be produced/manufactured, marketed that means sold or distributed that means import can be done by any of the company. In the Nutraceuticals Regulations, 2016, under the 'General Requirements,' the FSSAI has stated that mere combination of vitamins and minerals formulated in tablets, capsules, syrup formats shall not be covered in any of the categories of these regulations except when vitamins and minerals are added.

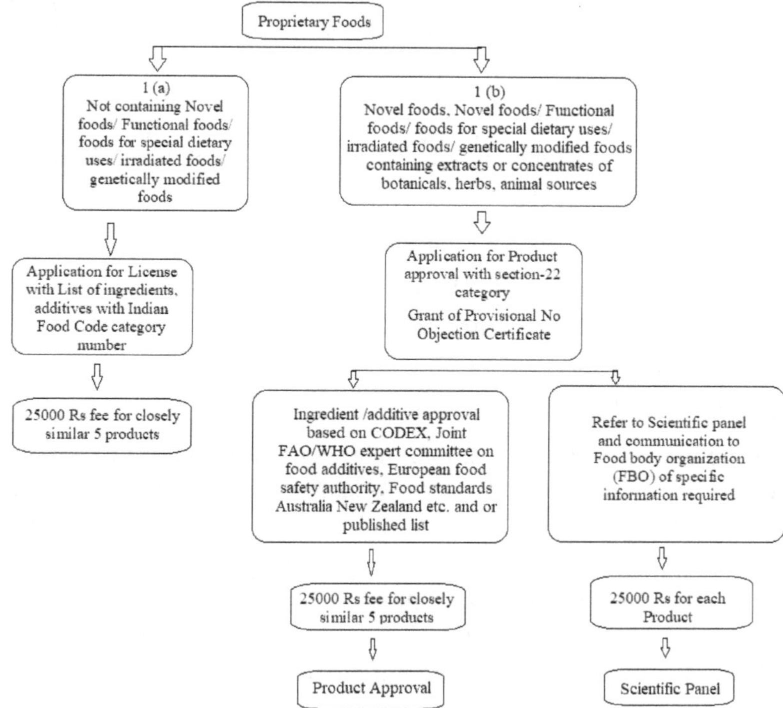

Figure 5.1 Nutraceutical Product registration process.

As per FFSAI Food supplements include:

(a) Health Supplements
(b) Nutraceuticals
(c) Food for special dietary use, other than infants, and those products intended to be taken under medical advice.
(d) Food for Special Medical Purpose
(e) Functional Food
(f) Novel Food
(g) Food with added probiotic ingredients
(h) Food with added prebiotic ingredients
(i) Specialty food containing plant or botanical ingredients with safe history of usage

FSSAI Regulations, 2011, has issued guidance for licensing and registration of food businesses; packaging and labelling; food product standards and food additives; prohibition and restriction on sales; contaminants, toxins and residues; laboratory and sampling analysis. FSS issued regulations for food or health supplements, nutraceuticals, foods for special dietary uses, foods for special medical purpose, functional foods, and novel food in 2015. The following information shall be included in any claimed novel foods - (a) chemical composition of the engineered food; (b) surface modification/ surface chemistry; (c) primary particle size; (d) solubility; (e) digestibility; (f) amount of nanomaterial if any in the food product; (g) specific claim, if applicable.

Ingredients

Nutraceuticals shall contain any of the ingredients specified in Food Act Schedule

Schedule I- Vitamins and minerals

Schedule II- Essential amino acids and other nutrients

Schedule IV- List of plants and botanical ingredients

Schedule VI- List of ingredients as nutraceuticals

Schedule VII- List of strains as probiotics

Schedule VIII- List of prebiotic compounds

The FSSAI issued notice on Dec 31, 2018, that disallowed the use of several ingredients in nutraceutical foods. FSSAI has directed Nutraceutical Regulations to stop using 14 ingredients lacking scientific data for safe usage.

The label of nutraceuticals products should mention "Nutraceuticals" Recommended Usage Warning for the risk of excess consumption. Prohibitions on labelling claims must mention for Nutraceuticals Products Cure of disease claims, e.g. "Prevents bone fragility in post menopausal women," implied cures for disease claims through pictures, vignettes or symbols.

Comparison of Regulatory Guidelines of USA (DSHEA) and India (FSSAI)

	USA	India
Regulation for licensing and registration	By United States Food, and Drug Administration (USFDA)	By Food Safety and Standard Authority of India (FSSAI)
Definition	USFDA defines Nutraceuticals as "Dietary Supplements" Under DSHEA	FSSAI defines Nutraceuticals as "Foods for special dietary uses". Act/Regulatory authority for registration of nutraceuticals Dietary Safety and Health Education Act Food Safety and Standard Authority of India Regulations w.e.f 1994 2011
Regulatory requirements for registration	Product licensing, evidence requirements for safety & efficacy, labeling, health claims, GMP, adverse reaction reporting and clinical trials	Product evaluations, licenses, health and label claims
Form for registration	Form 3537	Form A, B. and C

Dietary Supplement Health and Education Act of 1994 [DSHEA]

Background

DSHEA defines the term "dietary supplement" to mean a product (other than tobacco) intended to supplement the diet that bears or contains one or more dietary ingredients, including a vitamin, a mineral, an herb or other botanical, an amino acid, a dietary substance for use by man to supplement the diet by increasing the total dietary intake, or a concentrate, metabolite, constituent, extract, or combination of any of the aforementioned ingredients. Furthermore, a dietary supplement must be labeled as a dietary supplement and be intended for ingestion and must not be represented for use as conventional food or as a sole item of a meal or of the diet. In addition, a dietary supplement cannot be approved or authorized for investigation as a new drug, antibiotic, or biologic, unless it was marketed as a food or a dietary supplement before such approval or authorization. Under DSHEA, dietary supplements are deemed to be food, except for purposes of the drug definition.

Safety of Dietary Supplements under Section 402 (21 U.S.C. 342) is applicable if dietary supplement or contains a dietary ingredient that - presents a significant or unreasonable risk of illness or injury under conditions of use recommended or suggested in labeling, or under ordinary conditions of use and or inadequate information of new drug. to provide reasonable assurance that such ingredient does not present a significant or unreasonable risk of illness or injury; **and Burden of Proof on FDA** under sections 554 and 556 of title 5in case **Dietary Supplements are** adulterated under paragraph (a)(1), the United States shall bear the burden of proof on each element to show that a dietary supplement is adulterated.

Dietary Supplement Claims

Dietary Supplement Labeling Exemptions under Sec. 403B involves a publication (article, a chapter in a book, or an abstract prepared by the author or the editors of the publication) are not considered as labeling when used in connection with the sale of a dietary supplement to consumers when it is not false or misleading, does not promote a particular manufacturer or brand of a dietary supplement and when it is balanced view of the available scientific information on a similar or other type of dietary supplements.

In any proceeding brought under subsection (a), the burden of proof shall be on the United States to establish that an article or other such matter is false or misleading.".

Statements of Nutritional Support

Section 403(r) (21 U.S.C. 343(r)) is amended that nutritional support of dietary supplement may be made if nutrient or dietary ingredient/s are beneficial to a classical nutrient deficiency disease with exact role and mechanism as well as general well-being from consumption of a nutrient or dietary ingredient. The manufacturer of the dietary supplement has substantiation that such statement is truthful and not misleading, andthe statement contains, prominently displayed and in boldface type, the following: "This statement has not been evaluated by the Food and Drug Administration. This product is not intended to diagnose, treat, cure, or prevent any disease.".

Dietary Supplement Ingredient Labeling and Nutrition Information Labeling

Dietary supplements must include list including the name, source, quantity of each ingredient or total quantity of all ingredients in the blend, quality (including tablet or capsule disintegration), purity, or compositional specifications, based on validated assay or other appropriate methods, nutritional benefits charts.

New Dietary Ingredients

The term "new dietary ingredient" means a dietary ingredient that was not marketed in the United States before October 15, 1994. The dietary supplement should be an article be in food supply or there is history of use or other evidence (any citation to published articles) of safety for recommended conditions based on labeling at least 75 days before being introduced into commerce. The Secretary shall keep confidential any information provided under paragraph (2) for 90 days following its receipt. After the expiration of such 90 days, the Secretary shall place such information on public display, except matters in the information which are trade secrets or otherwise confidential, commercial information. Any person may file with the Secretary a petition proposing the issuance of an order prescribing the conditions under which a new dietary ingredient under its intended conditions of use will reasonably be expected to be safe. The Secretary shall make a decision on such petition within 180 days of the date the petition is filed with the Secretary.

Good Manufacturing Practices

Under Section 402 (21 U.S.C. 342), dietary supplement should be prepared, packed, or follow conditions for expiration date labeling according to current good manufacturing practice regulations. Such regulations may not impose standards for which there is no current and generally available analytical methodology.

To read in detail short title, reference, table of contents, findings, definitions, conforming amendments, withdrawal of the regulations and notice and commission on dietary supplement labels and office of dietary supplements click-..................,

New Dietary Ingredient [NDI]

The term "new dietary ingredient" means a dietary ingredient that was not marketed in the United States in a dietary supplement before October 15, 1994. (See section 413(d) of the Federal Food, Drug, and Cosmetic Act (the FD&C Act), 21 U.S.C. 350b(d)). There is no authoritative list of dietary ingredients that were marketed in dietary supplements before October 15, 1994. Therefore, manufacturers and distributors are responsible for determining if an ingredient is a "new dietary ingredient" and, if not, for documenting either that a dietary supplement that contained the dietary ingredient was marketed before October 15, 1994, or that the dietary ingredient was marketed for use in dietary supplements before that date. A dietary ingredient is a vitamin; a mineral; an herb or other botanical; an amino acid; a dietary substance for use by man to supplement the diet by increasing total dietary intake; or a concentrate, metabolite, constituent, extract, or combination of any of the above dietary ingredients.

NDI Dossier information

If a dietary supplement that contains a new dietary ingredient then following information need to be submited to FDA, at least 75 days before the dietary ingredient is introduced or delivered for introduction into interstate commerce:

- Name and complete address of company
- The name of the new dietary ingredient. If the new dietary ingredient is an herb or other botanical, include the Latin binomial name (including the author).
- A description of the dietary supplement or dietary supplements that contain the new dietary ingredient, including the:
    - level of the new dietary ingredient in the product;
    - conditions of use of the product recommended or suggested in the labeling or if no conditions of use are recommended or suggested, the ordinary conditions of use; and
    - history of use or other evidence of safety establishing that the dietary ingredient, when used under the conditions recommended or suggested in the labeling of the dietary supplement, will reasonably be expected to be safe.
        - Any reference to published materials must be accompanied by reprints or photocopies.
        - Any material in a foreign language must be accompanied by a translation.
- The signature of a person you designate who is responsible for the content of the notification and can be contacted if we have questions.

Generally Recognized as Safe (GRAS) Dossier Information

"GRAS" is an acronym for the phrase "**G**enerally **R**ecognized **as** **S**afe". Under sections 201(s) and 409 of the Federal Food, Drug, and Cosmetic Act (the Act), any substance that is intentionally added to food is a food additive, that is subject to premarket review and approval by FDA, unless the substance is generally recognized, among qualified experts, as having been adequately shown to be safe under the conditions of its intended use, or unless the use of the substance is otherwise excepted from the definition of a food additive.

Under sections 201(s) and 409 of the Act, and FDA's implementing regulations in 21 CFR 170.3 and 21 CFR 170.30, the use of a food substance may be GRAS either through scientific procedures or, for a substance used in food before 1958, through experience based on common use in food Under 21 CFR 170.30(b), general recognition of safety through scientific procedures requires the same quantity and quality of scientific evidence as is required to obtain approval of the substance as a food additive. General recognition of safety through scientific procedures is based upon the application of generally available and accepted scientific data, information, or methods, which ordinarily are published, as well as the application of scientific principles, and may be corroborated by the application of unpublished scientific data, information, or methods.

Under 21 CFR 170.30(c) and 170.3(f), general recognition of safety through experience based on common use in foods requires a substantial history of consumption for food use by a significant number of consumers.

Specific chemical identity (including, but not limited to scientific and common names, Chemical Abstracts Service Number, empirical and structural formula) or if derived from a natural substance, the genus and species; specifications and stability information; food categories in which the ingredient would be used (for example, baked goods, hard candy, snack foods – for a full list, refer to 21 CFR 170.3(n)) and the amount used in each category (from this information the exposure information may be calculated); proposed technical effect (for example, will it be used as a buffer, preservative, texturizer – for a full list, refer to 21 CFR 170.3(o)); manufacturing or processing procedures and; safety data, from which a (safe) Acceptable Daily Intake (ADI) is derived with core information including, but not limited to in vitro genotoxicity and cytoxicity data and in vivo genotoxicity data and; other in vivo toxicity information, which will include performance of a 28-day or 90-day safety study in rats.

Further Reading

1. "FDA Statement: Statement from FDA Commissioner Scott Gottlieb, MD, on the agency's new efforts to strengthen regulation of dietary supplements by modernizing and reforming FDA's oversight." US Food and Drug Administration, 11 February 2019. FDA website. www.fda.gov/news-events/press-announcements/statement-fda-commissioner-scott-gottlieb-md-agencys-new-efforts-strengthen-regulation-dietary. Accessed Dec. 2020.
2. Adom KK, Liu RH. Antioxidant activity of grains. J Agric Food Chem., 2002; 50: 6182-6187.
3. Alasalvar C, Shahidi F, Quantick P. Food and health applications of marine nutraceuticals: a review. In: Alasalvar C, Taylor D, editors. Seafoods-Quality,technology and nutraceutical applications. New York: Springer-Verlag. 2002. PP 175-204.
4. Allen LV., Nutritional products, In: Covington TR, Berardi RR, Young LL, Kendall SC, Hickey MJ, editors. Handbook of Nonprescription Drugs. Washington DC: American Pharmaceutical Association, 1997
5. Aronson JK. Defining 'nutraceuticals': neither nutritious nor pharmaceutical. Br J Clin Pharmacol. 2017 Jan;83(1):8-19.
6. Austin B. "Kim Kardashian-Jameela Jamil Feud has Done More to Expose Detox tea Lies Than the FDA." NBC News, 7 April 2019. www.nbcnews.com/think/opinion/kim-kardashian-jameela-jamil-feud-has-done-more-expose-detox-ncna991816. Accessed Dec. 2020.
7. Bickford PC, Tan J, Shytle RD, Sanberg CD, El-Badri N, Sanberg PR., Nutraceuticals synergistically promote proliferation of human stem cells. Stem Cells Dev., 2006; 15:118-23.
8. Brower V., Nutraceuticals: poised for a healthy slice of the healthcare market? Nat Biotechnol., 1998; 16 :728-731.
9. Burdock GA, Carabin IG. Generally recognized as safe (GRAS): history and description. Toxicol Lett. 2004 Apr 15;150(1):3-18. doi: 10.1016/j.toxlet.2003.07.004. PMID: 15068820.

10. Charis M. Galanakis. Nutraceuticals and Natural Product Pharmaceuticals. Elsevier Science.
11. Cohen P. "How America's Flawed Supplement Law Creates the Mirage of Weight Lost Cures." Harvard Public Health Review. Vol. 2, 2014. harvardpublichealthreview.org/how-americas-flawed-supplement-law-creates-the-mirage-of-weight-loss-cures. Accessed Dec. 2020.
12. Debasis Bagchi, Sreejayan Nair. Developing New Functional Food and Nutraceutical Products. Elsevier Science. 2016
13. DeFelice SL. FIM, Rationale and Proposed Guidelines for the Nutraceutical Research & Education Act NREA, Foundation for Innovation in Medicine. Available at: http://www.fimdefelice.org/archives/arc.researchact.html, November 10 2002.
14. Devi V.K. and Rehman F., Nutraceutical antioxidants-An overview, Indian journal of pharmaceutical education,. 2002; 36 (1):3-8.
15. Dossett ML, Cohen EM, Cohen J. Integrative Medicine for Gastrointestinal Disease. Prim Care. 2017 Jun;44(2):265-280.
16. Dwyer JT, Coates PM, Smith MJ. Dietary Supplements: Regulatory Challenges and Research Resources. Nutrients. 2018 Jan 4;10(1):41.
17. Elizabeth AC,. Over-the-counter products: nonprescription medications, nutraceuticals, and herbal agents. Clin Obstet Gynecol. 2002; 45(1):89-98.
18. FDA 2012. Code of Federal Regulations Title 21, Part 111. Current Good Manufacturing Practice in Manufacturing, Packaging, Labeling, or Holding Operations for Dietary Supplements. Food and Drug Administration.
19. Frasher P.D. Phytosterols as functional food components and nutraceuticals, Phytochemistry. 2006; 67: 212-214 .
20. Halliwell B., Antioxidants in human health and disease. Ann Rev Nutr, 1996;16: 33-50.
21. Hamid AA and Luan YS., Functional properties of dietary fiber prepared from defatted rice bran. Food Chemistry. 2000;68: 15-19.
22. https://www.fda.gov/food/dietary-supplements Accessed Dec. 2020
23. https://www.fda.gov/food/generally-recognized-safe-gras/fdas-approach-gras-provision-history-processes Accessed Dec. 2020
24. Inti M and Faoro F., Grape phytochemicals: a bouquet of old and new nutraceuticals for human health Medical Hypotheses. 2006;67: 833-838.
25. Kasbia GS.,Functional foods and nutraceuticals in the management of obesity. Nutrition and Food Science.2005;35: 344-351.
26. Lipson P. "DSHEA: a Travesty of a Mockery of a Sham." Science-Based Medicine. 20 July 2009, sciencebasedmedicine.org/dshea-a-travesty-of-a-mockery-of-a-sham. Accessed Dec. 2020.
27. Nordvisk E, Salomonsson AC, Aman P., Distribution of insoluble bound phenolic acids in barley grains. J Sci Food Agric. 1984;35: 657-661.
28. Rajesh K. Kesharwani. Anil K. Sharma. Nutraceuticals and Dietary Supplements-Applications in Health Improvement and Disease Management. Apple Academic Press. 2020
29. Ramesh Gupta. Nutraceuticals-Efficacy, Safety and Toxicity. Elsevier Science. 2016
30. Ravi Subbiah M. T., Nutrigenetics and nutraceuticals: the next wave riding on personalized medicine. Translational Research. 2007; 149: 55-61.

31. Sagar B.P.S., Zafar R., Tyagi K., Kumar V., Kumar S. and Panwar R., 'Antioxidants', The Indian Pharmacist, 2004; 29-35.
32. Santini A, Cammarata SM, Capone G, Ianaro A, Tenore GC, Pani L, Novellino E. Nutraceuticals: opening the debate for a regulatory framework. Br J Clin Pharmacol. 2018;84(4):659-672.
33. Serna-Thomé G, Castro-Eguiluz D, Fuchs-Tarlovsky V, Sánchez-López M, Delgado-Olivares L, Coronel-Martínez J, Molina-Trinidad EM, de la Torre M, Cetina-Pérez L. Use of Functional Foods and Oral Supplements as Adjuvants in Cancer Treatment. Rev Invest Clin. 2018;70(3):136-146.
34. Sharpless N. Public Meeting to Discuss Responsible Innovation in Dietary Supplements, Food and Drug Administration, 16 May 2019, Center for Food Safety and Applied Nutrition, College Park, MD. Opening Remarks. Ibid.
35. Shukla Y and Singh M., Cancer preventive properties of ginger: a brief review. Food and Chemical Toxicology, 2007;45: 683-690.
36. Swathi , FSSAI guidance and notification on nutraceuticals – An insight. Monday, 08 June, 2020 Puttahttps://fssai.gov.in/upload/media/FSSAI_News_Guidance_FNB_09_06_2020.pdf
37. Tucker G., Nutritional enhancement of plants. Current Opinion in Biotechnology, 14: 221-225 (2003). 16. Sirtori C R and Galli C., Fatty acids and the Omega3. Biomedecine and Pharmacotherapy. 2002;56: 397-406.
38. Whitman M., Understanding the perceived need for complementary and alternative nutraceuticals: lifestyle issues. Clin J Oncol Nurs., 2001;5:190-194.
39. Yashwant Pathak. Handbook of Nutraceuticals Volume I.Ingredients, Formulations, and Applications. CRC Press.2010

Scan QR code to view the website/guidelines

- Food Safety and Standards (Health Supplements, Nutraceuticals, Food for Special Dietary Use, Food for Special Medical Purpose, Functional Food And Novel Food) Regulations, 2016-

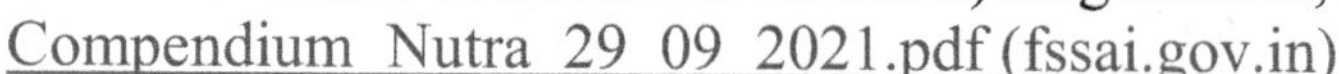
Compendium_Nutra_29_09_2021.pdf (fssai.gov.in)

- US-FDA Dietary supplements guidance-
Dietary Supplements | FDA

- Dietary Supplement Health & Education Act (DSHEA)-
Dietary Supplement Health & Education Act (DSHEA) | Council for Responsible Nutrition (crnusa.org)

CHAPTER 6

Labeling and Packaging of Herbal Products

Labeling of Herbal Products

- General Guidelines of labeling
- Name and Address of Manufacturer, Packer or Distributor
- No Reference to International Bodies etc.
- Declaration of ingredients
- Identification Number assigned by the Agency
  - Identification Mark on Tablets, Capsules etc
  - Adequate Labeling for Herbal Medicines and Related Products
  - Labeling of Bulk Package
  - Labelling Information for Practitioners
  - Adequate Information on the Insert
  - Prohibition of Labelling of Herbal Medicines or Related Products for Certain
- Treatments

Packaging of Herbal Products

- Introduction
- Types of Packaging
- Materials for Packaging
- Choice of Primary and/or Secondary Packaging Materials
- Functions of Packaging
  - Containment, Stability, Containers, Closures

Further Reading

Labeling of Herbal Products

General Guidelines of labeling:

- All information on a label shall be - (a) clearly and prominently displayed thereon; and (b) readily discernible to the consumer.
- All labelling information shall be in English language and may include other languages.
- Herbal medicines and related products labeling shall be informative and accurate and neither promotional in tone nor false or misleading.
- The labeling shall be based whenever possible on data derived from human experience.
- No implied claims or suggestions of herbal medicines or related products may be made, if there is inadequate evidence of safety or a lack of substantial evidence of effectiveness.
- Where a claim of effectiveness or therapeutic indication labelling is made by a herbal medicine or related product, it shall carry boldly and in close proximity to the claim, a statement to the fact that such claim have not been evaluated by the Agency, unless such claims has been clinically proven and deemed satisfactory by the Agency.

Name and Address of Manufacturer, Packer or Distributor

- The label of herbal medicines and related products in package form shall specify conspicuously the name and place of business of the manufacturer, and may include the distributor or packer.
- Where a herbal medicine or related product is not manufactured by a person whose name appears on the label, the name shall reveal the connection between the person and the manufacturer, such as "Manufactured for _.._.", Distributed by____..", or any other wording that expresses the facts.

No Reference to International Bodies etc.

No reference, direct or indirect to international bodies shall be made upon any label of herbal medicine or related product, except as prescribed by the Agency.

Declaration of ingredients

- Name or index number of colour used in the preparation shall be declared on the label. (2) A quantitative list of ingredients of the herbal medicines by their botanical names or, by their common names, shall be declared quantitatively on the label. Trade mark 7. (1) Where a herbal medicine or related product have a trade mark displayed on the label, the trade mark shall not give a wrong impression of the nature, quality or substance of the herbal medicine or related product.
- Where the trade mark registration is in conflict with any regulations or requirements of the Agency, the latter shall supersede.

Identification Number assigned by the Agency

The inner and outer labels of a herbal medicine or related product shall show, in a clear terms, the Agency registration number (NAFDAC REG. NO.) assigned to it as indicated on the certificate of registration in a manner prescribed by the Agency.

Identification Mark on Tablets, Capsules etc.

- All tablets, capsule, caplets and similar dosage forms of herbal medicines and related products shall bear identification marks traceable to the manufacturer or holder of a certificate of registration of the herbal medicine or related product unless otherwise exempted by the Agency.

- Exemptions request shall be made in writing to the Agency giving reasons why a waiver is justified.

Adequate Labelling for Herbal Medicines and Related Products

Herbal medicines and related products shall be properly labelled with the following information on the inner and outer labels:

- The brand name, botanical or common name if any shall be qualified as herbal, homeopathic, animal or mineral medicinal product and or admixture there of.
- The name shall not be suggestive of therapeutic claim.
- Each product shall have a distinct design.
- A quantitative list of all ingredients of the product by their botanical or common names.
- The net content of the product in terms of weight, measure, or numerical count and shall be in metric unit.
- The name and address of the manufacturer.
- Adequate directions for safe use of the product, including amount for use in specific age groups
- The lot or batch number of the product.
- The manufacture and expiration dates.
- The storage conditions.
- Dosage, route and frequency of administration.
- Indication for the product.
- Throughout manufacturing, a succession of specific outer labels is applied to the container of the herbal product. The level of processing is indicated by the following words:• Quarantine, Storage and Distribution.

Labeling of Bulk Package

Where a herbal medicine or related product is sold in bulk for further manufacturing, provisions of this regulation shall not apply, provided that, the label of the bulk product contains the following information:

- The proprietary or brand name of the herbal medicines.
- The botanical or common name of the herbal medicines.
- A statement of net contents.
- An identifying lot or batch number.
- The manufacture and expiration dates.
- Statement of caution e.g. "manufacturing purpose only".

Labelling Information for Practitioners

All herbal medicines or related products may be accompanied by an outer label and package insert with relevant information to practitioners for the safe use of the products.

Adequate Information on the Insert

- Relevant information required to appear on the package insert for Practitioners shall include: (a) Description; (b) Clinical Pharmacology; (c) Indications and usage; (d) Contraindications; (e) Warnings against misuse; (f) Precautions; (g) Dosage and administration; (h) Adverse reactions; (i) Drug abuse and dependence; (j) Symptoms of over dosage and antidote; (k) How supplied; (l) Animal Pharmacology and/or Animal; (m) Toxicology; (n) Clinical studies; (o) Storage conditions; (p) References.

- The labeling shall contain a "Product Title" section preceding the "Description" section.

Prohibition of Labelling of Herbal Medicines or Related Products for Certain Treatments

- No person shall label a herbal medicine or related product as a treatment, preventive or cure for any of the diseases, disorders or abnormal states as identified in schedule 1 to the Food and Drug Act 1990 (as amended.)
- No person shall sell, advertise, display or orally present any herbal medicine or related product to the general public whose label contains such words as "for vitality".

Packaging of Herbal Products

Introduction

Every medicinal product has to be contained in a container & the basic purpose of a container is to successfully contain the medicated preparation. Closures most often have a separate identity of their own but should be generally looked upon as part and parcel of the containers. They are the devices by means of which the containers can be 'opened' and 'closed' at will. Container is the device that holds the article. The immediate container is that which is in direct contact with the article at all times. Most of the containers are such that they necessitate opening at different periods of time for withdrawal of doses and hence have to have closures which can facilitate this operation. Packaging is an multiple user means provide presentation, protection, identification information, about a product during storage, carriage, display and until the product is consumed. The quality of the packaging of herbal products plays a very important role in the quality of such products. It must carry the correct information and identification of the product as well as protect against all adverse external influences that can alter the properties of the product, e.g. moisture, light, oxygen and temperature variations; biological contamination; physical damage.

Types of packaging

1. Primary packaging: It is in immediate contact with the product. Example: vials, bottle, rubber closure etc.
2. Secondary packaging: It is not in immediate contact with the product. . Example: label on bottle, aluminium caps, corrugated box.

Materials for packaging: The container and closure used for herbal products are constructed from the basic materials such as: Glass, Plastics, Rubber, Paper and Aluminum

Choice of primary and/or secondary packaging materials

It depends on the degree of protection required, compatibility with the contents, the filling method and cost, but also the presentation for over-the-counter (OTC) drugs and the convenience of the packaging for the user (e.g. size, weight, method of opening/reclosing (if appropriate), legibility of printing).Containers may be referred to as primary or secondary, depending on whether they are for immediate use after production of the finished product or not.

Both single-dose and multi-dose containers exist. Containers may be well-closed, tightly closed, hermetically closed or light-resistant, airtight.

Functions of Packaging

Containment: The containment of the product is the most fundamental function of packaging for medicinal products. The design of high-quality packaging must take into account both the needs of the product and of the manufacturing and distribution system. This requires the packaging should provide protection as well as should not to leak, nor allow diffusion and permeation of the product. It must be strong enough to hold the contents when subjected to normal handling. It should not be altered by the ingredients of the formulation in its final dosage form. The packaging must protect the product against all adverse external influences that may affect its quality or potency, such as: light, moisture, oxygen, biological contamination and mechanical damage.

Stability: Information on stability is given in the guidelines for stability testing of pharmaceutical products containing well-established drug substances in conventional dosage forms. For primary packaging, it is necessary to know the possible interactions between the container and the contents. Normally, product/component stability and compatibility are confirmed during the primary research and development stage. There are numerous possibilities of interactions between (primary) packaging materials and pharmaceutical products, such as: release of chemicals from components of the packaging materials; release of visible and/or sub visible particles; absorption or adsorption of phytochemical components by the packaging materials; Chemical reactions between the herbal product and the packaging materials; The degradation of packaging components in contact with the herbal products and influence of the manufacturing process (e.g. sterilization) on the container.

Containers: The materials selected must have the following characteristics-

1. They must protect the preparation from environmental conditions and must be non-toxic.
2. The container must be rigid enough to prevent damage to the contents
3. E.g. fracture of the tablets and crushing of tablets.
4. The material of construction must not react physically or chemically with the contents placed in it so as to alter the strength, quality or purity of the contents beyond the official requirement.
5. The closure must prevent-
   (a) Access of moisture .e, g. to moisture sensitive tablets and because their shells are hygroscopic to capsules.
   (b) Loss of moisture from creams and from water containing ointments and pastes.
   (c) unintentional escape of the contents &
   (d) Entry of dirt or other contaminants such as odours, vapours that might cause tainting.
   1. The closure must be easily removed and replaced.
   2. For many products, protection from light must be given.
   3. Medicament or adjuncts must not be absorbed by the container materials nor must diffusion through the walls be possible.
   4. It must be easy to label the container correctly.

5. They must be FDA approved.
6. It must have pharmaceutical elegant appearance.
7. They must be adaptable to commonly employed high speed packaging equipments.

Types of containers

With respect to method of closure, the B.P.C. defines four types of the container-

1. ***Well closed container***: This container protects the contents from contamination with extraneous, solid and under normal conditions of handling, storage and transport, prevents unintentional release of the contents.
2. ***Air tight container / tightly closed container***: This container gives protection from extraneous, solids, liquids and vapours and under normal conditions of handling, storage and transport, prevents changes due to efflorescence, deliquescence and evaporation. A tightly closed container must be capable of being tightly reclosed after use.
3. ***Securely closed container:*** This is an air tight container with a means of preventing unintentional displacement of the closure.
4. ***Hermetically sealed container:*** This container is impervious to air and other gases under normal conditions of handling, storage and transport. the most common example is a glass ampoule sealed by fusion.

Closures: The closure is normally the most vulnerable and critical component of a container in so far as stability and compatibility with the product are concerned. An effective closure must prevent the contents from escaping and allow no substance to enter the container. The adequacy of the seal depends on a number of things, such as the resiliency of the liner, the flatness of the sealing surface on the container and most important, the tightness or torque with which it is applied. In evaluating an effective closure system, the major considerations are the type of the containers the physical and chemical properties of the product and the stability –compatibility requirements for a given period under certain conditions.

Closure liners: A liner may be defined as any material that is inserted in a cap to affect a seal between the closure and the container.

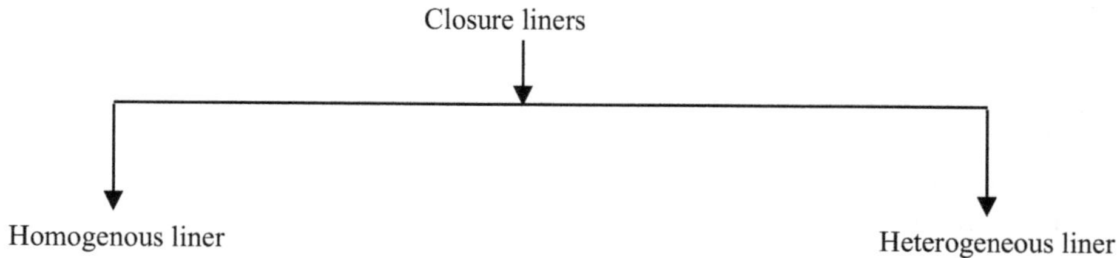

Homogenous liner: These one piece liners are available either as a disk or as a ring of rubber or plastic. Although they are more expensive and more complicated to apply, they are widely used for pharmaceuticals because their properties are uniform and they can withstand high temperature sterilization.

Heterogeneous or composite liners: These are composed layers of different materials chosen for specific requirements. In general the composite liner consists of two parts, a facing and a backing. Usually the facing is in contact with the product & the backing provides the cushioning and sealing properties required.

Dosage forms	Packing type
Solid dosage forms	General packing-Film wrappers, Blister package, Strip package, Child Resistant Containers- Bubble pack, Shrink seal and bands, Foil paper or plastic pouches, Bottle seals, Tape seals, Breakable caps and Sealed tubes
Semi solid dosage forms like ointments, creams, jell, emulsions, lotions, pastes, poultices.	Collapsible Metal and Plastic Tubes, Glass Plastic Pots, Aerosols
Suppositories package	Bottle packing, Strip packing, UPVC FILM- (Unplasticised Polyvinyl Chloride)
Containers for liquids Parentrals	Ampoules, syringes, vials, bottles, cartridges, bags
	Hermetically sealed borosilicate glass ampoules, Narrow-mouth borosilicate glass bottles, Wide-mouth borosilicate glass bottles, Screw Cap Storage Vial
Transdermal patches	Backing Film, Adhesives, Release Liner:

Labeling & Packing of ASU Medicines in India as per D & C Act, 1970	
Rule 161	1. Name of the drug has given in API / UPI or mentioned in the authoritative books included in the First Schedule. 2. Quantity of the drugs in metric system. 3. Name and address of manufacturer. 4. Manufacturing License No. or "M.L.". 5. Batch No. or Lot Number. 6. Date of Manufacture. 7. The word "Ayurvedic medicine or Siddha medicine or Unani medicine. 8. The words for external uses only if the medicine is for external application. 9. Physicians sample not to be sold if it is for distribution to the medical profession as a free sample.
Rule 161-A	1. Labeling and packing to meet the requirement of the law of the country to which exported. (a) Name of the ASU drugs (Single or compound formulation). (b) Name and address of Manufacturer with Mfg. No. (c) Batch No. or Lot No. (d) Date of Mfg. along with date for "Best for uses before". (e) Main ingredients with quantity, if required by the importing country

Further Reading

1. Bhalerao S, Munshi R, Tilve P, Kumbhar D. A survey of the labeling information provided for ayurvedic drugs marketed in India. Int J Ayurveda Res. 2010;1:220–2.
2. Carter SJ. Copper and Gunn's Packaging in Tutorial Pharmacy. 2005:133–41.
3. CDSCO [Homepage on the Internet]. India: Ministry of Health and Family Welfare the Drugs and Cosmetic Act, 1940 (as Amended Upto 30th June, 2005). Schedule D (II) 2005.
4. Devi KV, Burande M, Deepak H, Jobanputra SB. Packaging solutions to the changing pharma market needs. Pharma Times. 2007; 39:29–34.
5. European Commission [Homepage on the Internet]. Guideline on the packaging information of medicinal products for human use authorised by the Union. London: European Medicines Agency.

6. Good manufacturing practices for pharmaceutical products. In: WHO Expert Committee on Specifications for Pharmaceutical Preparations. Thirty-second report. Geneva, World Health Organization, 1992, Annex 1 (WHO Technical Report Series, No. 823).
7. Jain UK, Nayak S. 1st ed. Hyderabad: Pharma Med Press; 2008. Pharmaceutical Packaging Technology; pp. 1–273.
8. Kumar MR, Janagam D. Export and import pattern of medicinal plants in India. Indian J Sci Technol. 2011;4:245–8.
9. M.E. Aulton. The Science of Dosage Form Design. Secondedition.pageno:554-570
10. Mallick A, Roy A, Bose A, De K. Assessment on the label of ayurvedic classical and proprietary medicines in accordance with the drugs and cosmetics act, 1940. IJPRBS. 2012;1:67–74.
11. Manoi, Shekhawati College of pharmacy, Dundlod. Pharmatutor. Review on: the pharmaceutical packaging
12. Matthew S. Thomas Associate Senior Consultant Engineer, Pharmaceutical Packaging Development, Eli Lilly and Company October 2nd, 2010
13. Mehta Kunal C, Akhilesh. D and Shyam Kumar. B, Recent Trends in Pharmaceutical Packaging: A review. International journal of pharmaceutical and chemical sciences .2012; 1:3. pg no: 932-944
14. Michael J. Akers, PhD. http://www.pharmpress.com/files/docs/Remington_Ch_26.pdf, Sample chapter from Remington: Essentials of Pharmaceutics, Parenteral Preparations pg no 495-532
15. US Department of Health and Human Services [Homepage on the Internet]. United States: Food and Drug Administration. Prescription Drug Advertising.
16. WHO [Homepage on the Internet]. Quality Assurance of Pharmaceuticals. Geneva: Headquarters; c2015.
17. WHO [Homepage on the Internet]. Regulatory Situation of Herbal Medicines – A Worldwide Review. Geneva: Headquarters; c2015.
18. World Health Organization. Annex 9, Guidelines on packaging for pharmaceutical products, WHO Technical Report Series, No. 902, 2002.

Scan QR code to view the website/guidelines

- ASEAN Guidelines On Labelling Requirements For Traditional Medicines-

ASEAN Guidelines for Minimizing the Risk of Transmission of Transmissible Spongiform Encephalopathies in Traditional Medicines and Health Supplements

- Herbal Medicine and Related Products Labelling Regulations 2021-

Herbal Medicine and Related Products Labelling Regulations 2021. S.I. no. 76 of 2021. | UNEP Law and Environment Assistance Platform

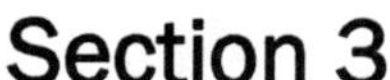

Section 3

Traditional Medicines Regulations

CHAPTER 7

Indian Systems of Medicines, Regulations and Related Guidelines

Indian System of Medicines (AYUSH)

Introduction

In India, herbal drug products constitute a major share of all the officially recognized systems of health viz. Ayurveda, Yoga and Naturopathy, Unani, Siddha, Homeopathy (AYUSH).The Ministry of AYUSH was formed in 2014 to ensure the optimal development and propagation of AYUSH systems of health care. Herbal remedies and medicinal plants which are to be incorporated in the modern system (Allopathic) must follow Drug Controller General of India (DCGI's) regulations. In spite of number of hurdles, the traditional medicine of India in acknowledged widely around the world and the demand is increasing continuously.

Basic Principles Involved in Ayurveda, Siddha, Unani and Homeopathy

Ayurveda System

It is about 5000 year old system of medicine native to India. It is holistic system of medicine which considers whole body while treating disease and not just a diseased part of body. Ayurveda has thousands year's evidence based history so it can be just complete system rather alternative system or complementary system. Ayurveda is a Sanskrit word which means (*Ayur*-life and *veda* – to gain knowledge or science) science of life. Ayurveda deals with different types of plants, minerals and animal products. Charak samhita by Charak includes the principle components or theory of Ayurveda. Sushrut samhita edited by Sushrut is about the surgical treatments in Ayurveda.

It is assumed that Sushruta was born in the Eastern part of India near Bihar (which was famous for sacred schools and universities at that time). Sushruta was a physician by occupation. In Mahabharata, he is represented as a son of Rishi Visvamitra. His Samhita, divided into six volumes, compromises all aspects of general medicine. However, due to an extraordinary accuracy and detail of surgery in his work, he is also considered as the father of surgery. These six volumes contain 184 chapters describing 1120 illness, 700 medical plants, 64 drugs prepared from minerals, and 57 from animal sources. It also discusses different surgical techniques suitable for different body parts along with 14 different types of bandages. Mostly, the Samhita focuses on surgery and midwifery, but it also deals with topics such as genetics, mental illness, embryology, anatomy, geriatric illness, and diabetes. It has 300 surgical procedures and it classifies surgery into five subheadings such as

- Aharya (extraction of solid bodies),
- Bhedya (excising),
- Chhedya (incising),
- Eshya (probing),
- Lekhya (scarifying),
- Sivya (suturing),
- Vedhya (puncturing), and
- Visravaniya (evacuating fluids).

It describes more than 300 kinds of operations that call for 42 different surgical processes and 121 different types of instruments. For the purpose of anesthesia, he advised the use of wine with the incense of cannabis and this is the oldest form of anesthesia used with no world record before that. The instruments used for surgeries were constructed after the shape of beasts and birds and named after them like the crocodile forceps and hawk's bill forceps.

The Sushruta Samhita is best known for its approach and discussions of surgery. It was one of the first in human history to suggest that a student of surgery should learn about human body and its organs by dissecting a dead body. It describes haemorrhoidectomy, amputations, plastic, rhinoplastic, ophthalmic, lithotomic and obstetrical procedures.

***Theory and principles*:** Ayurveda involves following fundamental principles:

Pancha Mahabhuta	*Prithvi* (earth), *Apa* (water), *Tej* (fire), *Vayu* (air), *Akash* (sky)
Panchshil theory	*Rasa* : Therapeutically active substances *Guna* : Quality *Virya* : Active principle and potency *Vipaka* : The end product of digestion *Prabhava* : Actual effect of drug on body.
Sapta Dhatu theory	*Rasa* (Plasma), *Raktam* (Blood), *Mansa* (Muscles), *Meda* (Fat), *Asthi* (Bone), *Majja* (Bone marrow and nerves), *Shukra* (Reproductive fluid or Semen)
Tridosha theory	*Vatta* = *Vayu* + *akash* = respiration and mobility *Pitta* = *Agni* = digestion and metabolism *Kapha* = *Prithvi* + *apa* = lubrication of joints and stability.
Triguna	*Satva* (good), *Raja* (aggressive), *Toma* (dullness)
Ama	➢ (a Sanskrit word meaning "uncooked" or "undigested") is used to refer to the concept of anything that exists in a state of incomplete transformation.

Diagnosis: The non-equilibrium between any of above principles causes to person suffers from diseases. Mental, physical, social and spiritual welfare of human beings is considered by Ayurveda to cure the disease cause. Observation of body color, tongue, nail, eyes, pulse and investigation of blood, urine and fecal matter is criteria of diagnosing actual cause of disease.

Treatment: Panchkarma is an important treatment in Ayurveda which includes Snehan (massage), Swedan (steam), Vaman (vomit), Virechan (expulsion) and Basti (medicated enemas). The medicines are given in the form of powder (churna, bhasma), liquid (asava, arishta and taila), semisolid (leha or paka) and tablets (gutika, vati). Treatment of ayurveda involves use of drugs obtained from plant, animal and mineral sources. Ayurveda also focuses on exercise, yoga, and meditation. One type of prescription is a Sattvic diet. Dosage forms of Ayurveda are powders (churna), bhasma (metal oxides), asava and arishtha (alcohol containing liquids), quath (extracts), gutika (pills), lep (ointment) or taila (Medicated oils).

There are eight branches of Ayurveda:

1. Kayachikitsa (internal medicine)
2. Kumarbhritya (pediatrics)
3. Trachchikitsa (psychology medicine)
4. Shalakya Tantra [ear, nose and throat]
5. Shalya Tantra (surgery)
6. Agada tantra (toxicology)
7. Rasayana tantra (geriatrics)
8. Vajikaran tantra [gynecology]

Siddha System

Sidha system of medicine is one of the oldest medical systems known to mankind even before ayurvedic system which was flourished in Vedic culture, Dravidian culture and Indus Valley Civilization. Tamil traditional medicine is origin of Siddha system and hence most of literature of this system is given in Tamil Language. 18 "Siddhas" (Spiritual persons) developed this system so it is called as Sidha. Sage Agathiyar is considered the guru of all Sidhas.

According to Palm Leaf manuscript, it is believed that it was first described by Lord Shiva to his wife Parvathy and then to their son Lord Muruga. Then he passed this knowledge to his disciple sage Agasthya. Agasthya educated 18 Siddhars. Human beings got this knowledge from 18 Siddhars. Siddhars have to get Siddhi means attainment of supernatural powers.

Theory and principles: Generally the basic principles of Siddha and Ayurveda medicine are almost similar. But siddha system explains in detail about various basic treatments of diseases while surgery like modern treatments are practiced and written in detail in Ayurveda. Like Ayurveda, Siddha medicine also, classifies physiological components of the human beings as vata (air), pitta (fire) and kapha (earth and water). Siddha system is based on 96 principles and out of these Triguna theory, i.e., vatta, pitta and kapha is more prominent. Under normal conditions, the ratio between Vatta, Pitta, and Kapha is 4:2:1, respectively. Siddha deals with thousands of herbs, animal, mineral and metals. Siddha system believes that health is perfect state of physical, mental, social, moral and spiritual component. It is based on Andapinda Thathuvam means relationship between universe and human body. Siddhas are called as Vaithiyars.

Diagnosis: A Siddha physician studies eight important things of body i.e. nadi (pulse), varna (colour), na (tongue), mala (faeces) kan (eyes), swara (voice), sparisam (touch), and neer (urine).

Guna	Personalities	Complications
Vata	Stout, black, cold and inactive healthy	Increased *Vata* shows arrogant behaviour, paralysis, heart attack.
Pitta	Lean, whitish complexion and perfectionist	Increased *Pitta* shows graying of hair, anemia and instability.
Kapha	Well built, good complexion and well behaved	Increased *Kapha* causes jaundice, heart attack.

Treatment: Siddha medicines are divided into three categories: Thavaram (Herbal), Thadu (inorganic) and Janganam (animal). Internal as well as external medicines are divided into 32 categories each separately. Pressure or massage techniques are also part of treatment and called as Thokkanam. There are 108 varma points for pressure techniques.

Treatment is classified into three categories:

- **Devamaruthuvum (Divine method):** The medicines prepared from metals and minerals come under this topic. The specialty of these medicines is a very small dose brings quick recovery even from chronic ailments. These are highly potent. Most of these medicines has no expiry date that is they can be preserved life-long. In this method use of metals and minerals medicines like parpam, chendooram, guru, kuligai made of mercury, sulphur and pashanams recommended.
- **Manuda maruthuvum (Rational method):** In this method herbal medicines like churanam, kudineer, vadagam are used. They are herbal medicines which have short definite life span. Dose may vary accordingly. They comprise of 34 types – 22 Internal medicines and 12 External medicines
- **Internal medicines:** Charu (juice), Surasam (boiling the extracted juice), Kudineer (decoction), Karkam (Raw materials prepared into paste) etc.
- **External applications:** Vedhu (Steam- therapy), Pattru (Pasting processed raw drugs on diseased part), Ottradam (Fermentation), Kattu (Like Bandaging)
- **Asura maruthuvum (surgical method):** use of surgical method, incision, excisions, use of heat or leech

Treatment in this system emphasizes preparation of fresh medicine. It is then prepared and administered with some Pathya (some restriction). Example- Day time sleeping is not allowed or some food material is restricted like chicken, mango, coconut, mustard, groundnut, almond, tobacco etc. Medicine can be kashayam (extract), churnam (powder), tailams (medicated oil), gulligai (pills), chenduram (metal), bhasmam (calcination product) and or ghritam (medicated ghee).

Unani System

This system is also called asUnani-tibb or Yunani Medicine. Arab and Persian physicians such as Rhazes, Avicenna (Ibn Sena), Al-Zahrawi, and Ibn Nafis developed this system.

Book: Ibn Sina's the Canon of Medicine. First book, "On General Means of Treatment" describes that treatments are done in three ways: "one of them is regimen and nutrition; the second, application of drugs; and the third, manual treatment, i.e., surgery". The second book gives rather detailed pharmacological and pharmacotherapeutic characteristic of 811 drugs, among which those of vegetable kingdom constitute 594 (73.7%), of animal kingdom 118 (14.5%) and of mineral origin 99 (12.2%).

Theory and principles: Unani medicine involves concept of the four humours (akhlat) i.e. Phlegm (Balgham), Blood (Dam), Yellow bile (Safra) and Black bile (Sauda). These "humors" and a open air blood sedimentation test exhibits close relation where a dark clot at the bottom resembles black bile, a layer of unclotted erythrocytes resembles blood, a layer of white blood cells resembles phlegm and a layer of clear yellow serum resembles yellow bile. Abnormality in humor leads to disease condition in body.

***Diagnosis*:** The human body is considered to be made up of seven components i.e. 1. Elements (Arkan) 2. Temperament (Mijaz). 3. Humors (Aklat) 4. Organs (Aaza) 5. Faculties (Quwa) 6. Spirits (Arwah). 7. Functions (Afaal) which have direct bearing on the health status of a person and considered by the physician for diagnosis and treatment. In diagnosis Unani Physican (Hakim) asks a detail history and decides treatment.

Treatment: After diagnosing the disease, treatment involves either to eliminate cause (Izalae sabab), normalize humors (Tadeele akhlat) or to normalise tissues or organs (Tadeele aza). Method of treatment involves modification of essential pre-requisites of health (Ilaj- Bil-Tadbeer) or Panchkarma like in Ayurveda (Ilaj-Bil-Tadbeer) or pharmacotherapy (Ilaj bil advia) or surgery (Ilaj-Bil-Yad).

- Regimental therapy (Ilajbil tadbeer) – Use of exercise, climate change, massage, venesection, leaching, cupping, diet therapy etc.
- Pharmacotherapy (Ilajbil dava) – use of plant, animal and mineral origin drugs, either alone or in combination.
- Surgery (Ilajbil Yad) – Surgical intervention in treatment

As far as possible Unani medicine therapy attempts to use simple physical means to cure a disease. Some of the techniques used in Ilaj bil- Tadbir (Regimental therapy) include Hijamah (Cupping), Fasd (Venesection), Tareeq (Sweating), Idrar-e-Baul (Diuresis), Hamam (Turkish Bath), Dalak (Massage), Kai (Cauterization), Ishal (Purging), Qai (Vomiting), Riyazat (Exercise) and Taleeq (Leeching).

Unani dosage forms are-

- Solid dosage forms [Example: (Habb (pills), quers (tablet), safoof (powder)]
- Liquid dosage forms [Joshnda (decoction), Khisanda (Infusion), Arq (Distillate), Sharbat (Syrup), Qutur (Drops)]
- Semi-solid dosage forms [Huqna (enema) and tila (liniment)].

Homeopathy System

Homeo means similar and Pathos means suffering so homeopathy is the "system of similar suffering". German physician Samuel Hahnemann first stated the basic principle of homeopathy in 1796, known as the "law of similars" (let like be cured by like.")

This system was developed by Dr Samuel Hahnemann in Germany. Dr Samuel had written a book *The Curative Powers of Drugs and Some Examinations of Previous Principles* which was based on his study of effect of *cinchona* on his own body where he actually found "law of similars" which indicates similarity between drug and disease.

***Theory and principle*:** Homeopathy emphasises the root cause of the disease and the nature's law of its cure that is 'like cures like'. Thus, homeopathy deals with the following seven principles which are outlined below:

- ***Individualisation:*** No two individuals in the world are alike, i.e. the disease affecting two individuals cannot be similar though they may share common symptoms. So the medicines used to cure the same disease in different individuals are different.
- ***Principle of similiar*:** Use of the medicine will produce similar symptoms of disease in an healthy individual. For example, watery eyes and burning nose caused by an onion hence an attack of hay fever with watering eyes and a burning nose can be cured homeopathic remedy made from onion.
- ***Principle of simplex:*** Only one single simple medicine at one time and no combination is allowed.
- ***Minimum dose:*** Minimum medicine at a time
- ***Law of proving:*** Medicine should have the capacity to produce disease state in a healthy individual.
- ***Law of dynamisation:*** Medicine should preserve the normal state of healthy body.
- ***Vital force:*** Medicine should have the capacity to arouse sufficient energy to maintain a healthy body.

Diagnosis: It involves knowing of complete hereditary history as well as observation of moods, habits, skin, eyes, tongue, blood, urine etc of patients.

Treatment: Not considering imponderabilia, the source materials for homeopathic medicines may consist of the following:

- **plant material such** as: roots, stems, leaves, flowers, bark, pollen, lichen, moss, ferns and algae;
- **microorganisms** such as: fungi, bacteria, viruses and plant parasites;
- **animal materials** such as: whole animals, animal organs, tissues, secretions, cell lines, toxins, nosodes, blood products;
- **human materials such** as: tissues, secretions, cell lines and endogenous molecules such as hormones;
- **minerals and chemicals**.

When the symptoms picture matches with the drug picture, the physician always attempts to identify a single medicine. Homeopathic preparation involves "dynamisation" or "potentiation", whereby a substance is diluted with alcohol or distilled water and then vigorously shaken in a process called "succussion". Three logarithmic potency scales are in regular use in homeopathy for dilution. Hahnemann created the "centesimal" or "C scale", diluting a substance by a factor of 100 at each stage. Inert substance like sugars, typically lactose, is used to prepare homeopathic pills and then a drop of liquid homeopathic preparation is placed on pills. Hahnemann began to test what effects substances produced in humans, a procedure that would later become known as "homeopathic proving". Following are important terms in Homeopathy:

- ***Imponderabilia***: Homeopathic medicines prepared from energy, emanating from natural and physical reactions. It means "not weighable", i.e. which have no perceptible weights. They are energy forms such as sunlight (Sol), magnetic fields (Magnet is Polus Australis), radiation (X-ray).
- ***Mother solution (also called solution):*** the most concentrated solution prepared from a substance of mineral or chemical origin by dissolving it in alcohol or purified water. It may also be prepared by exposing alcohol or purified water to an energy source (see Imponderabilia).
- ***Mother tincture (also called tincture):*** The initial homeopathic preparation made from source material that can be further potentized (also called "liquid stock"), sometimes used as homeopathic medicines, is regarded as the most concentrated form of a finished homeopathic medicine. Mother tinctures are obtained classically by maceration or percolation (sometimes also by digestion, infusion, decoction or fermentation) techniques from source materials according to a procedure prescribed by a recognized homeopathic pharmacopoeia. Sometimes a mother tincture corresponds to the first decimal dilution, "1D" or "1X" (10-1), mostly when dry plant material is used as starting material.
- **Nosodes**: Homeopathic medicines prepared from disease products from humans or animals; from pathogenic organisms or their metabolic products; or from decomposition products of animal organs.
- **Sarcodes**: Homeopathic medicines made from healthy animal tissues or secretions. In Greek, sarcode means fleshly.
- **Potency**: The denominated degree of serial trituration or dilution and succession that is reached for each homeopathic medicine. The degrees of dilution or potencies are normally indicated by the letters D, DH or X for successive 1 to 10 (decimal) dilutions, the letters C, CH or K or CK for successive 1 to 100 (centesimal) dilutions while Q or LM denote successive 1 to 50 000 (Hahnemannian quinquagintamillesimal) dilutions.

  Dilution by 1 to 10 denotes 1 part processed with 9 parts of diluent (Hahnemannian decimal), dilution by 1 to 100, 1 part processed with 99 parts (Hahnemannian or Korsakovian centesimal), and so on.

  The number preceding the letters (e.g. D, C or LM) normally indicate the number of dilution steps employed.

As a consequence of different views in various approaches in homeotherapy and because the notion of these terms may depend on the nature of the starting materials, the terms "high potency" and "low potency" cannot be defined unambiguously.

- **Potentization (also called dinamization):** The combined process of serial dilution and succussion or trituration at each step in the manufacture of homeopathic medicines from stocks. (According to the tenet of homeopathy, potentization represents the process by which the activity of a homeopathic medicine is developed.) The potentisation steps in a potency row can be performed in different dilution ratios:

  D or X: 1:10

  C or CH: 1:100

  LM 1:50,000.

  So, for example, D4 means potentised four times in the ratio 1:10. The higher the number of potency, the lower the concentration.

Sowa – Rigpa or Amchi

Introduction

"Sowa-Rigpa" commonly known as Amchi system of medicine is one of the oldest, living and well documented medical tradition of the world. It has been popularly practiced in Tibet, Mongolia, Bhutan, some parts of China, Nepal, Himalayan regions of India and few parts of former Soviet Union etc. There are various schools of thought about the origin of this medical tradition. Some scholars believe that it originated from India, some say China and while others consider it to have originated from Tibet itself. The majority of theory and practice of Sowa-Rigpa is similar to "Ayurveda". The first Ayurvedic influence came to Tibet during 3rd century AD but it became popular only after 7th century with the approach of Buddhism to Tibet. Thereafter, this trend of exportation of Indian medical literature, along with Buddhism and other Indian art and sciences were continued till early 19th century. India being the birth place of Buddha, Buddhism has always been favorite place for learning Buddhist art and culture for Tibetan students; lots of Indian scholars were also invited to Tibet for prorogation of Buddhism and other Indian art and sciences. This long association with India had resulted in translation and preservation of thousands of Indian literature on various subjects like religion, sciences, arts, culture and language etc. in Tibetan language. Out of these around twenty-five text related to medicine are also preserved in both canonical and non-canonical forms of Tibetan literatures. Many of these knowledge were further enriched in Tibet with the knowledge and skills of neighboring countries and their own ethnic knowledge. "Sowa-Rigpa" (Science of healing) is one of the classic examples of it. Gyud-Zi (four tantra) the fundamental text book of this medicine was first translated from India and enriched in Tibet with its own folklore and other medical tradition like Chinese and Persian etc. The impact of Sowa-Rigpa along with Buddhism and other Tibetan arts and sciences were spread in neighbouring Himalayan regions. In India, this system has been practiced in Sikkim, Arunachal Pradesh, Darjeeling (West Bengal), Lahoul & Spiti (Himachal Pradesh) and Ladakh region of Jammu & Kashmir etc.

Theory and Practice

Sowa-Rigpa is based on the principles of Jung-wa-nga (Skt: panchamahabhutas) and Ngepa-Sum (Skt: Tridosa). Bodies of all the living beings and non living objects of the universe are composed of Jung-wa-nga; viz Sa, Chu, Me, Lung and Nam-kha (Skt: Prithvi, Jal, Agni, Vayu and Akash). The physiology, pathology Pharmacology and metria -medica of this system are established on these theories. Our body is composed of these five Cosmo physical elements of Jung-wa-nga; when the proportion of these elements is in imbalance in our body disorder results. The medicine and diet used for the treatment of disorders are also composed of the same five basic elements. In the body these elements are present in the form of Ngepa-Sum (Skt: Tri-dosa) Lus-sung-dun (Skt: Sapta Dhatu) and Dri-ma-Sum (Skt: Trimala). In drugs, diet and drinks they exist in the form of Ro-dug (Skt: Shast-rasa) Nus-pa (Virya) Yontan (Skt: Guna) and Zhu-jes (Skt: Vipaka). It is in context of this theory that a physician would use his knowledge, experience and skills in treating a patient, using the theory of similarity and dissimilarity (Skt: Samanaya and Vísesa) of five elements.The basic theory of Sowa-Rigpa may be adumbrated in terms of the following five points:

The body in disease as the locus of treatment

Antidote, i.e., the treatment

The method of treatment through antidote

Medicine that cures the disease

Materia Medica, Pharmacy & Pharmacology

Role of Indian Medicine Systems in Modern Drug Discovery

Drug discovery from medicinal plants used in different Indian medicinal systems is a hot spot of research. A number of drugs were obtained from the plant sources and several others have discovered by using natural substance as lead. Investigations in India and abroad became played a key role in such research.

In 1931, Sen and Bose reported two alkaloids from Rauwolfia serpentina, Siddiqui and Siddiqui in same year isolated five alkaloids which named as Ajmaline, Ajmalinine, Ajmalicine, Scrpentine, and Serpentinine.

Chopra and his colleagues in 1933 isolate an alkaloid from the plant and observed the hypotensive and CNS depressant activity. Several others investigations had also been made by the Indian researchers in subsequent years.

In 1949, a historical paper by Dr Vakil in British Heart Journal reported the antihypertensive activity of Rauwolfia in patients. During that time nearly 90% of doctors in India used it as a routine hypotensive drug and about 50 million tablets had been sold by a manufacturing agency alone.

Peruvoside, a cardiac glycoside was isolated from Thevetia peruviana at the Indian laboratory and developed in Germany. Taxol, potent anticancer drug discovered from Taxus brevifolia, the plant has been utilized by western Indian cultures as a medicine since long time.

A national/international research discovered a number of drugs from plant which has been used Indian traditional medicine since ancient time.

Novel semisynthetic derivatives of rohitukine (from the plant Amoora rohituka & D. binectariferum) named as flavopiridol and P-276-00 are in the advance clinical trial as anticancer drug. Guggulu, an oleo-gum resin obtained from the bark of Commiphora wightii has been used in Ayurveda for the treatment of inflammation, gout, rheumatism, obesity, and disorders of lipids metabolism. Several compounds namely Z-guggulsterone, E-guggulsterone, guggulsterol-I, guggulsterol-II etc. have been isolated from guggulu. CSIR and its constituents laboratories are involved in the development of new herbal drug or formulation.

Some of the key developments in Central Drug Research Institute (CDRI) in this area are,

(i) Standardized fraction of gugulipid was developed by CDRI and marketed (Guglip®, Cipla Ltd) as a drug for hyperlipidaemia and atherosclerosis,

(ii) Arteether (a semisynthetic derivative of artemisinin, the active constituent of Artemisia annua) as antimalarial drug which is marketed by Themis Chemicals Ltd., Mumbai under the trade name E-Mal,

(iii) Consap (a local spermicidal cream) contain saponins from Sapindus mukorossi,

(iv) Picroliv, an iridoid glycoside mixture containing 60% picroside I and kutoside obtained from Picrorhiza kurroa developed as hepatoprotective agent,

(v) A standardize herbal preparation derived from the plant B. monnieri as memory enhancer.

(vi) RRL Jammu has commercialized Boswellia serrata gum resin as NSAID (non-steroidal anti-inflammatory drug) (Sallaki® Gufic).

(vii) A number of herbal pain reliever, antifungal cream, anti-dandruff shampoo has been developed by different CSIR labs across the country.

(viii) Very recently, an antidiabetic drug (BGR-34) has developed jointly developed by scientist of CSIR-NBRI & CSIR-CIMAP. Under the 'Golden Triangle Partnership' project between AYUSH, Indian Council of Medical Research (ICMR), CSIR there is an attempt to find few formulations and developing new drugs.

In recent years research on these areas is increasing and lot more drug/formulations investigated by public or private sector in India are in queue or in under clinical trial. India has great pool of diverse medicinal plant sources, a long and well characterized traditional medicinal system which makes India a unique place of new drug discovery.

Regulations of Indian Traditional Medicines

In India herbal drugs are under the control of CDSCO (Central Drug Standard Control Organization) and Central authority under Central Government Ministry of Health and Family Welfare. Import, manufacturing, distribution and sale of herbal drugs are regulated by the following Acts and Rules in India.

- Drug and Cosmetics Act 1940.
- Drug and Cosmetics Rules 1945.

- Drug and Magic Remedies Act, 1954.
- Narcotic Drugs and Psychotropic Substances Act, 1985.
- Industries (Development Regulation) Act 1951.
- Trade and Merchandise Marks Act 1958.
- Indian Patents and Design Act 1970.
- Factories Act 1948.
- Indian Forest Act 1927
- Wild Life Protection act, 1972
- Biodiversity Act, 2002
- Food safety and standards act, 2006

Different Administrative Departments of AYUSH-ISM & H

Ministry of AYUSH

The Ministry of AYUSH was formed on 9th November 2014 to ensure the optimal development and propagation of AYUSH systems of health care. Earlier it was known as the Department of Indian System of Medicine and Homeopathy (ISM&H) which was created in March 1995 and renamed as Department of Ayurveda, Yoga and Naturopathy, Unani, Siddha and Homoeopathy (AYUSH) in November 2003, with focused attention for development of Education and Research in Ayurveda, Yoga and Naturopathy, Unani, Siddha and Homoeopathy. AYUSH has published list of 277 essential drug s in 2013.

CCRAS

The Central Council for Research in Ayurvedic Sciences (CCRAS) is an autonomous body of the Ministry of AYUSH (Ayurveda, Yoga & Naturopathy, Unani, Siddha and Homeopathy), Government of India. It is an apex body in India for the formulation, coordination, development and promotion of research on scientific lines in Ayurveda and Sowa-Rigpa system of medicine.

CCRS

For the development of Siddha system of Medicine, Govt. of India, by bifurcating the erstwhile CCRAS, formed CCRS (Central Council for Research in Siddha) with its headquarters in Chennai and six Research Institutes/Units in four states namely, Tamil Nadu (Chennai, Mettur & Palayamkottai), Puducherry (Puducherry), New Delhi and Kerala (Thiruvananthapuram). Siddha is a science of holistic health emphasising both drug and diet for human health care.Central Council for Research in SiddhaThe Council has the vision of preservation and transmission of Knowledge and enhancement of the quality of research for developing drugs with quality, safety and efficacy through well-established preclinical and clinical research facilities --- to prevent / manage /cure the diseases of varied aetiology. To undertake scientific research works in Siddha in a time-bound and cost-effective manner, to coordinate, aid, promote and collaborate research with different units of sister Councils and Research Organizations.

CCRUM

The Central Council for Research in Unani Medicine (CCRUM) is an autonomous organization under the Ministry of AYUSH, Government of India. Since its establishment in 1978, the CCRUM as the apex government organization for research in Unani Medicine has been engaged in conducting scientific research on the applied as well as fundamental aspects of Unani system of medicine with the efforts of over 300 scientists and technical manpower at its 23 research centres spread across the country. The Central Research Institute of Unani Medicine (CRIUM), Hyderabad is the most celebrated institute of the Council which has earned fame for treatment of vitiligo (Baraṣ) and other chronic and stubborn diseases. The CRIUM, Lucknow has attained good repute for research and development of treatment for musculoskeletal disorders. The Regional Research Institute of Unani Medicine (RRIUM), Chennai is the major research centre known for treatment of infective hepatitis and other chronic liver diseases. The RRIUM, Bhadrak has developed safe and effective treatment of filariasis (Dā' al-Fīl). The RRIUM, Srinagar has conducted research on respiratory disorders and has been awarded a patent for development of drug for bronchial asthma. In the area of drug standardization, the Council has developed pharmacopoeial standards for 298 single drugs and 100 compound formulations which have been published in Unani pharmacopoeia of India. Besides, six volumes of National Formulary of Unani Medicine have also been revisited recently for bringing out their revised addition. Under the literary research programme, translation of over 56 classical books have been translated into Urdu and other languages and published. Besides, reprinting of out of print 72 classical books had also been undertaken.

PLIM

Pharmacopoeial Laboratory for Indian Medicine (PLIM) is a subordinate office of the Ministry of Health & Family Welfare, (Deptt. of AYUSH), Govt. of India. This laboratory is a Standards Setting cum Drugs Testing Laboratory at National Level for Indian Medicines which include drugs of Ayurveda, Unani and Siddha systems.

Historical developments in Regulations of Indian Traditional Medicines	
1940	Drug and Cosmetic Act 1940 and Drug and Cosmetic Rule
1959	Govt of India recognized traditional Indian System of Medicine (ISM) and updated Drug and Cosmetic Act
1962	Several expert committees for different ISM
1969	separate chapter related to Ayurveda, Siddha and Unani drugs was inserted by act 13 of 1964 in the Act
1970	Central Council of Indian Medicine (CCIM) is constituted
1970	Pharmacopoeial Laboratory of Indian Medicine was formed to ensure standardization and testing of ASU drugs
1983, 1987, 1994 and 2002	Drug and Cosmetic Act 1940 modified again with some substitutions
1995	Department of Indian Medicine and Homeopathy (ISM & H) was formed
2001	Launched- Traditional Knowledge Digital Library (TKDL) (http://www.tkdl.res.in-collaborative project between Council of Scientific and CSIR, Ministry of

Contd...

	Science and Technology and Department of AYUSH, Ministry of Health and Family Welfare) is a database containing codified literature from Indian Systems of Medicine. TKDL contains more than 2.23 lakh formulations from the texts of traditional medicine systems of India viz. Ayurveda, Unani and Siddha. TKDL prevent misappropriation of Indian traditional knowledge by making it accessible for search and examination.
2002	National Policy on Indian Systems of Medicine & Homoeopathy
2003	Department of Indian Medicine and Homeopathy (ISM & H) was renamed as Department of Ayurveda, Yoga and Naturopathy, Unani, Siddha and Homoeopathy (AYUSH)
2006 and 2008	Guideline for evaluation and analysis of drugs under ISM was given under Drug and Cosmetic Rule 1945
2008	Manufacturing units to maintain record of the raw material in the Performa schedule TA by 30th June of the succeeding financial year
2009	AYUSH department in collaboration with Quality Council of India (QCI) introduced certification scheme for AYUSH drug products
2009	NMPB Guidelines and standard for Good Field Collection Practices for Indian Medicinal Plants
2012	Sowa Rigpa system of medicine is incorporated in the CCIM
2013	Good clinical practice guidelines for clinical trials to have a well-programmed clinical study Siddha and Unani Medicine (GCP-ASU).
2014	Separate ministry on AYUSH was formed
2018	General guidelines for Drug development of Ayurvedic formulations
2018	AYUSH General Guidelines for Safety/Toxicity Evaluation Of Ayurvedic Formulations 2018
2018	Central Sector Scheme of Pharmacovigilance of Ayurveda, Siddha, Unani and Homoeopathy Drugs to facilitate the establishment of three-tier network of National Pharmacovigilance Centre (NPvCC), Intermediary Pharmacovigilance Centres (IPvCCs) and Peripheral Pharmacovigilance Centres (PPvCC).

Quality Regulations for ASU Drugs in India	
Manufacturing, packaging, labelling and sale of ASU drugs.	Chapter IVA in the Drugs & Cosmetics Act, 1940 describe the provisions for regulation 1. Rule 151 - 155 B - Manufacture and regulate licensing of ASU herbal medicines. 2. Rule 156 – 160 – Conditions of Licensing. 3. Rule 160 A – 160 J – Approval of testing laboratory and regulate testing and quality control.
GMP for ASU drugs	Schedule 'T' of the Indian Drugs & Cosmetics Act, 1940 and Rules, 1945 was notified in 2000.
Advice to attain the uniformity in the administration of Drugs & Cosmetics Act, 1940 (related to ASU drugs) throughout India	Ayurveda, Siddha and Unani Drugs Consultative Committee (ASUDCC)
Good Manufacturing Drugs (GMP) for ASU drugs	Schedule 'T' of the Indian Drugs & Cosmetics Act, 1940 and Rules, 1945 notified in 2000.

Contd...

Rule regarding the maintenance of records of raw materials, guideline of permitted excipients along with their standards, law to test heavy metals, stipulation of expiry date for Ayurvedic medicines.	Schedule E(1) of the Drugs and Cosmetics Rules 1945

Guidelines for ASU Drugs

Quality related guidelines for ASU drugs	• Quality control methods for medicinal plant materials(WHO, 1998) • Quality control methods for herbal materials (WHO 2011) • Laboratory Manual for the Analysis of Ayurveda and Siddha formulations (CCRAS, 2010) • Quality Control Manual for Ayurvedic, Siddha & Unani Medicine, Pharmacopoeial Laboratory for Indian Medicine (PLIM, 2008) • Protocol for Testing of ASU Medicines, (PLIM, 2007) • General Guidelines for Drug Development Of Ayurvedic Formulations (CCRAS, 2016) • ASU Pharmacopoeias
Safety and Toxicity Study guideline for ASU drugs	• General Methodologies & Research evaluation Traditional Medicines (WHO, 2000) • OECD guidelines, 2001 • Schedule Y of Drug and Cosmetic Act, 1945 • GCP Guidelines for ASU Medicines, 2013, Ministry of AYUSH • General Guidelines of Safety/Toxicity Evaluation of Ayurvedic Formulations (CCRAS, 2016)
Good Clinical practice guideline for ASU drugs	• General Guidelines for Clinical Evaluation of Ayurvedic Interventions (CCRAS, 2016)

ASU Drugs Manufacturing License Requirements

- ***Application and Fees***- FORM-24D and 1000/- (renewal 1200+600=1800/-)
- ***For Manufacturing*** FORM-25D: Follow rule 157
- ***Certificate of Renewal*** FORM-26D
- The certificate of GMP to manufacturers of ASU drugs shall be issued to licensees who comply the GMP requirements of ASU drugs as per the schedule T.-FORM-26E-I (valid for 5 years)
- ***Duration of License***: 5 years from the date of issue
- ***Conditions after Approval***: Licensee should maintain proper records, Licensee should allow inspector to inspect the premises, Inspection book – Form-35
- ***Labeling, Packaging, and Limit of Alcohol***: Language in both English and Hindi; The following particulars should be on the label are: Name of the drug, Correct statement of the net content, Name and address of the manufacturer, Manufacturing licenses, Batch number, Date of Manufacturing, For External Use Only [if applicable]

- ***Schedule T requirements:*** General requirements Location and surrounding Buildings Water supply Stores Raw materials Packaging materials Health, clothing, sanitation, and hygiene of workers Machineries and equipment Distribution records Record of market complaints
- ***Documents Required-***
    - Plan and layout of the premises showing the installation of machinery and equipment.
    - Attested copies of documents relating to the ownership/rent/lease
    - Appointment letter to full-time technical supervisor
    - Declaration of the partnership deed/memorandum
    - Detailed list of manufacturing and analytical equipment as required for formulations applied.
    - Attested copies of certificates of academic qualification, experience certificate from
    - Ayurveda/Unani, and declarations of technical Staff in the prescribed pro forma with photo duly attested
    - Draft labels of the product
    - Self-addressed envelope with sufficient postal Stamps for registered post
    - Drug information a. Name of the product b. Formula shall contain Shastric/Tibbi name, part used and quantity c. Detailed method of preparation d. Purification of drugs wherever required e. Indications f. Dosage schedule in detail g. Side effects h. Anti-doses i. Diet restrictions, if any"

ASU Drugs Loan License Requirements

- Application and fees: FORM-24E and 600/- (renewal 600+300=900/-)
- For manufacturing: FORM-25E
- Certificate of renewal: FORM-26E
- Duration of license: December 31 of the year, the request for the renewal of a loan license shall be made pursuant to Rule 153-A.
- Conditions of authorization: Licensee should maintain proper records and Licensee should allow inspector to inspect the premises Inspection book – Form-35

Import and Export of Herbs and Derived Drugs in India

The process of Import Export of Drugs in any country including India is a lengthy process involving the various reviewing and registration processes. The requirements for any drug to be approved for Import/Export as a New Drug for the first time are more stringent & informative than the requirements for an already approved Drug which are considerably relaxed. There are following categories of herbal drugs:

- **Category 1: Indigenous herbal medicines:** These can be used freely by the local community or region, and no safety data would be required. However, if the medicines in this category are introduced into the market or moved beyond the local community or region, their safety has to be reviewed by the established national drug control agency. If the medicines belong to safety category 1, safety data are not needed. If the medicines belong to safety category 2, they have to meet the usual requirements for safety of herbal medicines. Medicines belonging to safety category 3, i.e. 'herbal medicines of uncertain safety', will be identical to that of any new substance.

- **Category 2: Herbal medicines in systems:** The medicines in this category have been used for a long time and have been officially documented. Review of the safety category is necessary. If the medicines are in safety categories 1 or 2, safety data would not be needed. If the medicines belong to safety category 3, they have to meet the requirements for safety of 'herbal medicines of uncertain safety'.
- **Category 3: Modified herbal medicines:** The medicines in this category can be modified in any way including dose, dosage form, mode of administration, herbal medicinal ingredients, methods of preparation, or medical indications based on categories 1 and 2. The medicines have to meet the requirements of safety of herbal medicines or requirements for the safety of 'herbal medicines of uncertain safety', depending on the modification.
- **Category 4: Imported/exported products with a herbal medicine base:** Exported products shall require safety data, which have to meet the requirements for safety of herbal medicines or requirements for safety of 'herbal medicines of uncertain safety', depending on the safety requirement of the importing/recipient countries.

Procedure for Import of Herbal Drugs: Applications for grant of permission to import or manufacture new phytopharmaceutical drug are to be made in Form 44 prescribed in D&C Rule to Drugs Controller General (India), Central Drugs Standard Control Organization, Directorate General of Health Services, Ministry of Health and Family Welfare, Government of India, FDA Bhawan, ITO, Kotla Road, New Delhi -110002. Applicant shall submit all the documents specified under Appendix IB of Schedule Y of D&C Rules. (Checklist for submission is available on CDSCO website). Applications as per checklist can be mailed by Post to Drugs Controller General (India).

Various forms required for manufacture, loan license for sale, analysis testing of ASU drugs as per drugs & cosmetics act, 1940	
Form Number	**Details of Application**
1-A	Memorandum to the Pharmacopoeial Laboratory for Indian Medicine (PLIM)
2-A	Certificate of Test or Analysis from the Pharmacopoeial Laboratory for Indian Medicine or Government Analyst
8 & 8 A	Application for License to Import Drugs Form 8 (drugs excluding Schedule X) or 8-A (Schedule X drugs)
9	Form of Undertaking to Accompany an Application for an Import License
10	License to Import Drugs Form 10 (drugs excluding Schedule X) or 10-A (Schedule X drugs)to the Drugs and Cosmetics Rules, 1945
11	License to Import Drugs for the Purpose of Examination, Test or Analysis

Contd...

Various forms required for manufacture, loan license for sale, analysis testing of ASU drugs as per drugs & cosmetics act, 1940	
Form Number	**Details of Application**
11-A	License to Import Drugs by a Government Hospital or Autonomous Medical Institution for the Treatment of Patients
12	Application for License to Import Drugs for Purpose of Examination, Test or Analysis
12-A	Application for the Issue of a Permit to Import Small Quantities of Drugs for Personal Use
13-A	Certificate of Tests or Analysis by Government Analyst under Section 33-H of the Drugs and Cosmetics Act, 1940
18-A	Memorandum to Government Analyst
24-D	Application for the Grant/Renewal of License to Manufacture for Sale of Ayurvedic/Siddha or Unani Drugs
24-E	Application for Grant or Renewal of a Loan License to Manufacture for Sale Ayurvedic (including Siddha) or Unani Drugs
25-D	License to Manufacture for the Sale of Ayurvedic (including Siddha) or Unani Drugs
25-E	Loan License to Manufacture for Sale Ayurvedic (including Siddha) or Unani Drugs
26-D	Certificate of Renewal of License to Manufacture for Sale Ayurvedic (including Siddha) or Unani Drugs
26-E	Certificate of Renewal of Loan License to Manufacture for Sale Ayurvedic (including Siddha) or Unani Drugs
26-E1	Certificate, of Good Manufacturing Practices (GMP) to Manufacturer of Ayurvedic (including Siddha) or Unani Drugs
41	A single application in Form 41 for issuance of a single Registration Certificate for the import of more than one drug or class of drugs, manufactured by the same manufacturer.
47	Application for grant or renewal of approval for carrying out tests on Ayurvedic, Siddha and Unani drugs or raw materials used in the manufacture thereof on behalf of licensees for manufacture for sale of Ayurvedic, Siddha and Unani drugs
48	Approval for carrying out tests or analysis on Ayurvedic, Siddha and Unani drugs or raw Materials used in the manufacture thereof on behalf of licensees for manufacture for sale of Ayurvedic, Siddha and Unani drugs
49	Certificate of renewal for carrying out tests or analysis on Ayurvedic, Siddha or Unani drugs or raw materials used in the manufacture thereof on behalf of licensees for manufacture for sale of Ayurvedic, Siddha or Unani drugs
50	Report of Test or Analysis by Approved Laboratory

Further Reading

1. Anonymous. Amendments and Notifications Drugs and Cosmetics Rules (1945) Accessed from: www.drugscontrol.org/amendments.asp?act=Drugs%20and%20Cosmetics%20Rules,%201945
2. Anonymous. AYUSH, About the System (2015) Accessed from: http://www.indianmedicine.nic.in
3. Anonymous. Section 1: Summary of All-India AYUSH Infrastructure Facilities (2015) Accessed from: http://indianmedicine.nic.in/writereaddata/linkimages/0913923524-Summary.pdf
4. B.V. Subbarayappa. Siddha medicine: an overview. Lancet, 350 (1997), pp. 1841-1844
5. Central Council for Research in Unani Medicine. Unani Pharmacopeial Committee. (2015) Accessed from: http://www.ccrum.net/research/upc/
6. K. Joshi. Indian Herbal Sector. (2008) Accessed from: http://www.nistads.res.in/indiasnt2008/t4industry/t4ind19.htm
7. K. Mangathayaru. Pharmacognosy: An Indian Perspective. Pearson, Chennai (2013)
8. Ministry of AYUSH. AYUSH for Holistic Healthcare & Healthy Living (2015) Accessed from: http://www.indianmedicine.nic.in
9. Ministry of Health and Family Welfare, Govt. of India Regulation of Manufacture and Sale of ASU Drugs (2006) Accessed from: http://www.pib.nic.in/newsite/erelcontent.aspx?relid=14876
10. National Medicinal Plants Board. Standard for Good Field Collection Practices of Medicinal Plants [DOC: NMPB-GFCP-01(FD)] (2015) Accessed from: http://www.nmpb.nic.in/WriteReadData/links/9695357829Standard%20for%20Good%20Field%20Collection%20Practices.pdf
11. P. Gurmet. "Sowa-Rigpa": Himalayan art of healing. Indian J Tradit Know, 3 (2004), pp. 212-218
12. P. Patel. Global Resurgence and International Recognition of Ayurveda. (2003) Accessed from: http://iaf ngo.org/pdf/GLOBAL%20RESURGENCE%20&%20INTL.%20RECOGNITION%20OF%20AYURVEDA%20(No.%2010).pdf
13. Pharmacopoeial Laboratory for Indian Medicine. Publications (2015) Accessed from: http://www.plimism.nic.in/index.html
14. S. Sen, R. Chakraborty. Toward the integration and advancement of herbal medicine: a focus on Traditional Indian medicine. Bot Target Ther, 5 (2015), pp. 33-44
15. S. Sen, R. Chakraborty. Traditional knowledge digital library: a distinctive approach to protect and promote Indian indigenous medicinal treasure. Curr Sci, 106 (2014), pp. 1340-1343
16. S. Thillaivanan, K. Samraj. Challenges, constraints and opportunities in herbal medicines – a review Int J Herb Med, 2 (2014), pp. 21-24
17. S.C. Mandal, M. Mandal. Quality, safety, and efficacy of herbal products through regulatory harmonization. Drug Info J, 45 (2011), pp. 45-53
18. S.K. Sharma, D.C. Katoch. Current Status & Infrastructure of Ayurveda (2006) Accessed from: http://herbalnet.healthrepository.org/bitstream/123456789/2075/6/3.%20Ayur53-65.pdf
19. T. Siddiqi. Unani medicine in India. Indian J Hist Sci, 16 (1981), pp. 22-25
20. V.N. Kasagana, S.S. Karumuri. Conservation of medicinal plants (past, present & future trends). J Pharm Sci Res, 3 (2011), pp. 1378-1386

21. W.M. Bandaranayake. Quality control, screening, toxicity and regulations of herbal drugs. I. Ahmad, F. Aquil, M. Owais (Eds.), Modern Phytomedicine: Turning Medicinal Plants into Drugs, Wiley-VCH Verlag GmbH & Co, Germany (2006), pp. 25-27
22. World Health Organization. National Policy on Traditional Medicine and Regulation of Herbal Medicines – Report of a WHO Global Survey. WHO, Geneva (2005)
23. World Health Organization. Traditional Medicine (2013) Accessed from: http://www.who.int/mediacentre/factsheets/2003/fs134/en/
24. World Health Organization. WHO Traditional Medicine Strategy 2002–2005. World Health Organization, Geneva (2002)
25. B. S. Kuchekar (8 January 2008). Pharmaceutical Jurisprudence. Pragati Books Pvt. Ltd. pp. 5.0–5.2. ISBN 978-81-85790-28-2. Retrieved 26 December 2014.
26. https://cdsco.gov.in/opencms/opencms/en/Home/
27. Lily Srivastava. Law & Medicine. Universal Law Publishing. pp. 216–. ISBN 978-81-7534-949-0.
28. Malik, Surendra (2014). Supreme Court on Drugs, Medical Laws and Medical Negligence (1st ed.). Lucknow: Eastern Book Company. ISBN 978-93-5028-850-4.
29. Malik, Surendra (2016). Supreme Court on Narcotics and Drugs (2nd ed.). Lucknow: Eastern Book Company. ISBN 978-93-5145-318-5.
30. Malik, Vijay (2014). Law Relating to Drugs and Cosmetics (24th ed.). Lucknow: Eastern Book Company. ISBN 978-93-5145-313-0.
31. National Centre for Biological Sciences. Overview of Indian Healing Traditions. (2015)
32. Pillay (30 November 2012). Modern Medical Toxicology. Jaypee Brothers Publishers. p. 30. ISBN 978-93-5025-965-8. Retrieved 22 February 2015.
33. R.R. Chaudhury, U.M. Rafei. Traditional Medicine in Asia. World Health Organization (Regional Office for South-East Asia), New Delhi (2001)
34. V. Naswamy. Origin and development of Ayurveda. Anc Sci Life, 1 (1981), pp. 1-7
35. World Health Organization. WHO Traditional Medicine Strategy 2014–2023. World Health Organization, Geneva (2013)

Scan QR code to view the website/guidelines

- Related links for AYUSH Medicine systems-
Related links | CCRAS | Ministry of AYUSH (Govt. of India)

CHAPTER 8

WHO - General Guidelines for Methodologies on Research and Evaluation of Traditional Medicine-2000

Introduction

Practices of traditional medicine vary greatly from country to country, and from region to region, as they are influenced by factors such as culture, history, personal attitudes and philosophy. The quantity and quality of the safety and efficacy data on traditional medicine are far from sufficient to meet the criteria needed to support its use worldwide. The term complementary and alternative medicine is used in some countries to refer to a broad set of health care practices that are not part of the country's own tradition and are not integrated into the dominant health care system.

Research and evaluation of traditional medicine is divided into two parts: herbal medicines and traditional procedure-based therapies. However, successful treatment is often the consequence of both types of treatment acting synergistically and should be evaluated in an integrated manner. As traditional medicine relies on a holistic approach, conventional efficacy assessment measures may not be adequate.

Purpose of the Guidelines

To promote the proper harmonized use, summarize key issues, improve the quality and value, provide appropriate evaluation methods to facilitate the development of regulation and registration in traditional medicine.

Definitions: Following are important definitions to understand concept of traditional medicines and scope of guideline:

Methodologies for Research and Evaluation of Herbal Medicines

Traditional medicine: Traditional medicine has a long history. It is the sum total of the knowledge, skills and practices based on the theories, beliefs and experiences indigenous to different cultures, whether explicable or not, used in the maintenance of health, as well as in the prevention, diagnosis, improvement or treatment of physical and mental illnesses. The terms complementary/alternative/non-conventional medicine are used interchangeably with traditional medicine in some countries.

Herbs: Herbs include crude plant material such as leaves, flowers, fruit, seed, stems, wood, bark, roots, rhizomes or other plant parts, which may be entire, fragmented or powdered.

Herbal materials: Herbal materials include, in addition to herbs, fresh juices, gums, fixed oils, essential oils, resins and dry powders of herbs. In some countries, these materials may be processed by various local procedures, such as steaming, roasting, or stir, baking with honey, alcoholic beverages or other materials.

Herbal preparations: Herbal preparations are the basis for finished herbal products and may include comminuted or powdered herbal materials, or extracts, tinctures and fatty oils of herbal materials. They are produced by extraction, fractionation, purification, concentration, or other physical or biological processes. They also include preparations made by steeping or heating herbal materials in alcoholic beverages and/or honey, or in other materials.

Finished herbal products: Finished herbal products consist of herbal preparations made from one or more herbs. If more than one herb is used, the term mixture herbal product can also be used. Finished herbal products and mixture herbal products may contain excipients in addition to the active ingredients.

Contd...

However, finished products or mixture products to which chemically defined active substances have been added, including synthetic compounds and/or isolated constituents from herbal materials, are not considered to be herbal.

Herbal medicines include herbs, herbal materials, herbal preparations and finished herbal products that contain as active ingredients parts of plants, or other plant materials, or combinations.

Traditional use of herbal medicines: Traditional use of herbal medicines refers to the long historical use of these medicines. Their use is well established and widely acknowledged to be safe and effective, and may be accepted by national authorities.

Therapeutic activity: Therapeutic activity refers to the successful prevention, diagnosis and treatment of physical and mental illnesses; improvement of symptoms of illnesses; as well as beneficial alteration or regulation of the physical and mental status of the body.

Active ingredients: Active ingredients refer to ingredients of herbal medicines with therapeutic activity. In herbal medicines where the active ingredients have been identified, the preparation of these medicines should be standardized to contain a defined amount of the active ingredients, if adequate analytical methods are available. In cases where it is not possible to identify the active ingredients, the whole herbal medicine may be considered as one active ingredient.

Botanical Verification and Quality Considerations: The correct botanical verification includes binomial name and synonyms, vernacular names, the parts of the plant used for each preparation, and detailed instructions for agricultural production and collection conditions according to the each country's good agricultural practice.

Research and Evaluation of Safety and Efficacy: For herbal medicines with a well-documented history of traditional use, the following procedures for conducting research and evaluating safety and efficacy may be followed:

Literature Review: The literature search should include reference books, review articles, systematic surveillance of primary sources, and/or database searches. To evaluate inaccurate information if any, literature search should then be extended to gather information on closely related plant species for chemotaxonomic correlation. In vitro (biochemical or cellular) and in vivo data from animal studies serves as indicators of potential toxicity but not necessarily applicable to humans. Hence well-documented reports of pharmacological activity in animals and clinical studies in humans (number of patients, specific diagnosis, authoritative national documents (such as pharmacopoeias or official guidelines of national authorities) or in highly respected scientific publications) may be viewed as having scientific rationale.

Review of Theories and Concepts of Systems of Traditional Medicine: When reviewing the literature on traditional medicine, holistic approach based on the physical, emotional, mental, spiritual and environmental levels simultaneously along with certain behavioural rules promoting healthy diets and habits must be taken into account.

Review of Safety: New preparative methods may alter the chemical, toxicological and even pharmacological profiles of traditionally used herbal medicines. Reported and documented side-effects are required to take decisions about the need for new pharmacological or toxicological studies. The absence of any reported or documented side-effects is not an absolute assurance of safety for herbal medicines. Suggested tests include immunotoxicity (e.g. tests for allergic reactions), genotoxicity, carcinogenicity and reproductive toxicity. Only when there is no documentation of long historical use of a herbal medicine, or when doubts exist about its safety, should additional toxicity studies be performed. Where possible, such studies should be carried out in vitro. Using in vitro tests can reduce the number of in vivo experiments. If in vivo studies are needed, they are to be conducted humanely, with respect for the animals' welfare and rights.

Review of Efficacy: A therapeutic or scientific rationale must exist for the presence of each herb in the mixture. The proof of efficacy, including the documentation required to support the indicated claims, should depend on the nature and level of the indications. Definitions of levels of evidence and the grading of recommendations of Annex IV or Annex V could also be used for reference.

Clinical Trials: Relevant authenticate literature is sufficient for traditional use claims. But, in the case of a new herbal medicine, a new indication for an existing herbal medicine, or a significantly different dosage form or route of administration, the general principles and requirements for a clinical trial should be very similar to those which apply to conventional drugs (see Annex VI). In some cases, however, the design of such studies must be adapted to deal with the particularities of herbal medicines.

Well-established, randomized controlled clinical trials provide the highest level of evidence for efficacy. Such studies facilitate the acceptance of herbal medicines in different regions and in people with different cultural traditions. However, methods such as randomization and use of a placebo may not always be possible as they may involve ethical issues as well as technical problems. For example, it may be not possible to have a placebo control if the herbal medicine has characteristic organoleptic property like a strong or prominent smell or taste, as is the case for products containing certain essential oils. Observational studies involving large numbers of patients may also be a very valuable tool for the evaluation of herbal medicines. Single-case studies for the evaluation of efficacy of a herbal medicine should not be ignored.

Methodologies for Research and Evaluation of Traditional Procedure-based Therapies

Types of Traditional Procedure-based Therapies: Traditional procedure-based therapies are acupuncture and related techniques, chiropractic, osteopathy, manual therapies, qigong, tai ji, yoga, naturopathy, thermal medicine, and other physical, mental, spiritual and mind–body therapies.

Evaluation of Safety and Efficacy: Traditional procedure-based therapies are relatively safe, but accidents occur when

- practitioners are not fully trained to parameters and equipments.
- Therapies are not performed within accepted parameters,
- incompetent examination of patients, incorrect diagnoses and errors of technique,
- improper selection of patients for traditional procedure-based therapy

Non-specific effects of the therapy can also contribute to efficacy, but these are difficult to measure or quantify. Therefore, clinical trials and other research methodologies are extremely important in the evaluation of the efficacy of traditional procedure-based therapies (see Part 3).

Clinical Research

General Considerations: In addition to evaluating the safety and efficacy of traditional medicine through clinical trials, there may be a number of different objectives when evaluating traditional medicine through clinical research, as when using clinical research to evaluate conventional medicine. Some of the objectives specific to the assessment of traditional medicine through clinical research are to: ¨ evaluate traditional medicine in its own theoretical framework (e.g. mechanistic studies); ¨ evaluate traditional medicine in the theoretical framework of conventional medicine (e.g. mechanistic studies); ¨ compare the efficacy of different systems of traditional medicine and/or conventional medicine; and ¨ compare the efficacy of different traditional practices within a system of traditional medicine.

Literature Review: Literature review, including the traditional use, existing scientific research and if little or no literature then oral tradition and the source of this tradition need to be evidently specified by well-established and accepted guidelines. Due to the lack of large clinical trials of good quality, meta-analysis in traditional medicine may be difficult.

Selection of Study Design: Conventional concepts of clinical research design (like randomized controlled trials or observational studies) may be difficult to apply when using clinical research to evaluate various systems and practices of traditional medicine, depending on the goal of the assessment. In such circumstances, the choice of study design should be discussed on a case-by case basis with experienced traditional medical practitioners as follows:

- Single-case design
- Black-box design
- Ethnographic design
- Observational design
- Parameters like study outcome measures (quantitative and qualitative outcomes; primary and/or secondary outcomes; and generic and/or highly specific outcomes), selection of patients (clear description of the patients using both traditional and conventional terms), sample size (adequate), Control groups, randomization, blind assessment are also need to be considered while selecting study design.

In both the development of a study protocol to assess traditional medicine and in its submission for publication or for health-authority approval, the following information regarding study outcomes should be clearly provided:

- description and reasons for the selection of the therapeutic intervention either herbal medicines (composition and manufacturing) or therapy (tools and equipment used).;
- description of the rationale for the choice of the study outcomes, measurements (validity and reliability) and statistical method used
- The type of intervention must be clearly defined. In treatment using
- The training, skills and experience of the traditional medical practitioner
- description of the dose, frequency duration of a treatment, duration of follow-up [In acupuncture, for example, "dose" includes the force of a physical manipulation, duration

of each episode of therapy, duration of needled manipulation, the number of repetitions of a procedure, the number of needles used, the depth of stimulation, the needle sensation if elicited, the details of any electrical stimulation including stimulus, frequency, intensity, etc.]

Other Issues and Considerations

- **Pragmatic Research Issues:** Appropriate infrastructure, funding, facilities including laboratories and equipment, involvement of properly trained research personnel and traditional medical practitioners and adequate safety for the subjects are also equally important in traditional medicine research.
- **Ethics:** Clinical trials must always be conducted within the framework of the prevailing ethical guidelines and law in a given country or state. Ethical committee of institute should guide each clinical studies case by case. Whenever applicable, rescue treatment may be provided to patients involved in a clinical trial involving the use of a placebo or unproven treatment. Use of the rescue treatment may be a secondary outcome measure. In some countries and hospitals, there are ethical issues that restrict the use of clinical trials. In some cases, the use of a placebo is even illegal, particularly for patients suffering from certain illnesses, such as cancer.
- **Education and Training:** The practitioners' knowledge and skills need to be continuously upgraded to enable them to engage in clinical research within their own individual specialty, if necessary.
- **Surveillance Systems:** There is need of national surveillance systems at different levels of the health sector to monitor and evaluate any adverse effects of traditional medicine where comprehensive evaluation of any adverse effect is documented.

Annexures

1. Annex I. Guidelines for the Assessment of Herbal Medicines is related to assessment of quality, safety, efficacy and intended use as well as utilization of these guidelines
2. Annex II. Research guidelines for evaluating the safety and efficacy of herbal medicines is about toxicity investigation of herbal medicines (acute toxicity test, long-term toxicity test)
3. Annex III. Report of a WHO consultation on traditional medicine and AIDS: clinical evaluation of traditional medicines and Natural Products explain preclinical & clinical considerations and further recommendations.
4. Annex IV. Definition of levels of evidence and grading of recommendations explains levels of evidence and grading of recommendations.
5. Annex V. A guideline for levels and kinds of evidence to support claims for therapeutic goods explains claims based on evidence of traditional use, What Kinds of Claims Does the Evidence Support?, registrable diseases list and claims based on evidence of traditional use.

6. Annex VI. Guidelines for good clinical practice (GCP) for trials on pharmaceutical products and explains ethical principles of clinical trials.
7. Annex VII is related to Guidance for Industry: Significant Scientific Agreement in the Review of Health Claims for Conventional Foods and Dietary Supplements which explores concept of identifying Data for Review.
8. Annex VIII. Guideline for Good Clinical Practice is about Clinical Trial Protocol and Protocol Amendment(s).
9. ANNEX IX. WHO QOL (Quality of Life) User Manual: Facet Definitions and Response Scales Introduction discusses overall Quality of Life and Health under six domains (Domain I - Physical Domain, Domain II – Psychological, Domain III - Level of Independence, Domain IV - Social Relationships, Domain V – Environment, Domain VI - Spirituality/Religion/Personal Beliefs Response Scales).
10. Annex X is related to Participants in the WHO Consultation on Methodologies for Research and Evaluation of Traditional Medicine.

Further Reading

1. World Health Organization. Quality control methods for medicinal plant materials. Geneva, World Health Organization, 1998.
2. World Health Organization. WHO monographs on selected medicinal plants. Vol. I. Geneva, World Health Organization, 1999.
3. World Health Organization Regional Office for the Western Pacific. Research guidelines for evaluating the safety and efficacy of herbal medicines. Manila, World Health Organization Regional Office for the Western Pacific, 1993.
4. World Health Organization. Regulatory situation of herbal medicines: a worldwide review. Geneva, World Health Organization, 1998 (unpublished document WHO/TRM/98.1; available on request from Traditional Medicine (TRM/EDM/HTP), World Health Organization, 1211 Geneva 27, Switzerland).
5. World Health Organization. Guidelines on basic training and safety in acupuncture. Geneva, World Health Organization, 1999 (unpublished document WHO/EDM/TRM/99.1; available on request from Traditional Medicine (TRM/EDM/HTP), World Health Organization, 1211

Scan QR code to view the website/guidelines

- General guidelines for methodologies on research and evaluation of traditional medicine-

General guidelines for methodologies on research and evaluation of traditional medicine (who.int)

CHAPTER 9

Drug & Cosmetic Act, 1940 - Schedule T Good Manufacturing Practice of Indian Systems of Medicine

Introduction

Part I-Good Manufacturing Practices

General Requirements

(a) Location and Surroundings
(b) Buildings
(c) Water Supply
(d) Disposable of Waste
(e) Container's Cleaning
(f) Stores (a) Raw Materials (b) Packaging Materials (c) Finished Good Stores
(g) Working Space
(h) Health Clothing, Sanitation and Hygiene of Workers
(i) Medical Services
(j) Equipments
(k) Batch Manufacturing Record
(l) Distribution Records
(m) Record of Market Complaints
(n) Quality Control

Requirement for Sterile Product

(a) Manufacturing Areas
(b) Precautions against Contamination and Mix

Part II: List

(a) List of Machinery, Equipment and Minimum Manufacturing Premises Required for the Manufacturing
(b) List of Machinery, Equipment and Minimum Manufacturing Premises Required for the Manufacture of Various Categories of Unani System of Medicines

(c) List of Equipment Recommended for In-house Quality Control Section (Alternatively, unit can get testing done from the Government approved laboratory)

(d) Supplementary Guidelines for Manufacturing of Rasaushadhies or Rasamarunthukal and Kushtajat (Herbomineral-metallic Compounds) of Ayurveda, Siddha and Unani Medicines

Schedule TA (Rule 157A)

Further Reading

Introduction

Good Manufacturing Practices for Ayurvedic, Siddha and Unani Medicines are prescribed to ensure that:

- Raw materials used in the manufacture of drugs are authentic, of prescribed quality and are free from contamination.
- The manufacturing process is as has been prescribed to maintain the standards.
- Adequate quality control measures are adopted.
- The manufactured drug which is released for sale is of acceptable quality.
- To achieve the objective listed above, each licensee shall evolve methodology and procedures for following the prescribed process of manufacturer of drugs which should be documented as a manual and kept for reference and inspection.
- However teaching institutions and registered qualified Vaidyas, Siddha and Hakeems who prepare medicines on their own to dispense to their patients and not selling such drugs in the market are exempted from the purview of G.M.P.

Part-I Good Manufacturing Practices

Factory Premises: The manufacturing plant should have adequate space for:–

(i) Receiving and storing raw material

(ii) Manufacturing process areas

(iii) Quality control section

(iv) Finished goods store

(v) Office

(vi) Rejected goods/drugs store

General Requirements

(A) Location and surroundings: The factory building: for manufacture of Ayurvedic, Siddha and Unani medicines shall be so situated and shall have such constructions as to avoid contamination from open sewerage, drain, public lavatory or any factory which produces disagreeable or obnoxious odour or fumes or excessive soot, dust or smoke.

(B) Buildings: The building used for factory shall be such as to permit production of drugs under hygienic conditions and should be free from cobwebs and insects/rodents. It should have adequate provision of light and ventilation. The floor and the walls should not be damp or moist. The premises used for manufacturing, processing, packaging and labeling will be in conformity with the provisions of the Factory Act. It shall be located so as to be:

(i) Compatible with other manufacturing operations that may be carried out in the same or adjacent premises.

(ii) Adequately provided with working space to allow orderly and logical placement of equipment and materials to avoid the risk of mix up S between different drugs or components thereof and avoid the risk of omission of any manufacturing or control step.

(iii) Designed, constructed and maintained to prevent entry of insects and rodents. Interior surface (walls, floors and ceilings) shall be smooth and free from cracks and permit easy cleaning and disinfection. The walls of the room in which the manufacturing operations are carried out shall be impervious to and be capable of being kept clean. The flooring shall be smooth and even and shall be such as not to permit retention or accumulation of dust or waste products.

(iv) Provide with proper drainage system in the processing area. The sanitary fitting and electrical fixtures in the manufacturing area shall be proper and safe.

(v) Furnace Bhatti section could be covered with tin roof and proper ventilation, but sufficient care should be taken to prevent flies and dust.

(vi) There should be fire safety measures and proper exits should be there.

(C) Water Supply: The water used in manufacture shall be pure and of potable quality. Adequate provision of water for washing the premises shall be made.

(D) Disposal of Waste: From the manufacturing sections and laboratories the waste water and the residues which might be prejudicial to the workers or public health shall be disposed off after suitable treatment as per guidelines of pollution control authorities to render them harmless.

(E) Container's Cleaning: In factories where operations involving the use of containers such as bottles, vials and jars are conducted, there shall be adequate arrangements separated from the manufacturing operations for washing, cleaning and drying of such containers.

(F) Stores: Storage should have proper ventilation and shall be free from dampness. It should provide independent adequate space for storage of different types of material, such as raw material, packaging material and finished products.

(a) Raw Materials: All raw materials procured for manufacturing will be stored in the raw materials store. The manufacture based on the experience and the characteristics of the particular raw material used in Ayurveda, Siddha and Unani system shall decide the use of appropriate containers which would protect the quality of the raw material as well as prevent it from damage due to dampness, microbiological contamination or rodent and insect infestation, etc. If certain raw materials require such controlled environmental conditions, the raw materials stores may be sub-divide with proper enclosures to provide such conditions by suitable cabinization. While designing such containers, cabins or areas in the raw materials store, care may be taken to handle the following different categories of raw materials:

1. Raw material of metallic origin.
2. Raw material of mineral origin.
3. Raw material of animal source.

4. Fresh Herbs.
5. Dry Herbs or plant parts.
6. Excipients etc.
7. Volatile oils/perfumes & flavors.
8. Plant extracts and exudates/resins.

Each container used for raw material storage shall be properly identified with the label which indicates name of the raw material, source of supply and will also clearly state the status of raw material such as 'UNDER TEST' or 'APPROVED' or 'REJECTED' The labels shall further indicate the identity of the particular supply in the form of- Batch No. or Lot. No. and the date of receipt of the consignment. All the raw materials shall be sampled and got tested either by the in-house Ayurvedic, Siddha and Unani experts (Quality control technical person) or by the laboratories approved by the Government and shall be used only on approval after verifying. The rejected raw material should be removed from other raw material store and should be kept in a separate room. Procedure of 'First in first out' should be adopted for raw materials wherever necessary. Records of the receipt, testing and approval or rejection and use of raw material shall be maintained.

(b) Packaging Materials: All packaging materials such as bottles, jars, capsules etc. shall be stored properly. All containers and closure shall be adequately cleaned and dried before packing the products.

(c) Finished Goods Stores: The finished goods transferred from the production area after proper packaging shall be stored in the finished goods stores within an area marked "Quarantine" After the quality control laboratory and the experts have checked the correctness of finished goods with reference to its packing/labeling as well as the finished product quality as prescribed, then it will be moved to "Approved Finished Goods Stock" area. Only approved finished goods shall be dispatched as per marketing requirements. Distribution records shall be maintained as required. If any Ayurvedic, Siddha and Unani drug needs special storage conditions, finished goods store shall provide necessary environments requirements.

(G) Working Space: The manufacturing area shall provide adequate space (manufacture and quality control) for orderly placement of equipment and material used in any of the operations for which these are employed so as to facilitate easy and safe working and to minimize or to eliminate any risk of mix-up between different drugs, raw materials and to prevent the possibility of cross contamination of one drug by another drug that is manufactured, stored or handled in the same premises.

(H) Health Clothing, Sanitation and Hygiene of Workers: All works employed in the Factory shall be free from contagious diseases. The clothing of the workers shall consist of proper uniform suitable to the nature of work and the climate and shall be clean. The uniform shall also include cloth or synthetic covering for hands, feet and head wherever required. Adequate facilities for personal cleanliness such as clean towels, soap and scrubbing brushes shall be provided. Separate provision shall be made for lavatories to be used by men and women, and such lavatories shall be located at places separated from the processing rooms. Workers will also be provided facilities for changing their clothes and to keep their personal belongings.

(I) Medical Services: The manufacturer shall also provide:

- adequate facilities for first aid;
- medical examination of workers at the time of employment and periodical check up thereafter by a physician once a year, with particular attention being devoted to freedom from infections. Records thereof shall be maintained.

(J) Equipments: For carrying out manufacturing depending on the size of operation and the nature of product manufactured, suitable equipment either manually operated or operated semi-automatically (Electrical or steam based) or fully automatic machinery shall be made available. These may include machines for use in the process of manufacture such as crushing, grinding, powdering, boiling, mashing, burning, roasting, filtering, drying, filling, labeling and packing etc. To ensure ease in movement of workers and orderliness in operations a suitably adequate space will be ensured between two machines or rows of machines. These equipments have to be properly installed and maintained with proper cleaning. Proper standard operational procedures (SOPs) for cleaning, maintaining and performance of every machine should be laid down.

(K) Batch Manufacturing Records: The licencee shall maintain batch manufacturing record of each batch of Ayurvedic, Siddha and Unani drugs manufactured irrespective of the type of product manufactured (classical preparation or patent and proprietary medicines.) Manufacturing records are required to provide an account of the list of raw material and their quantities obtained from the store, tests conducted during the various stages of manufacture like taste, colour, physical characteristics and chemical tests as may be necessary or indicated in the approved books of Ayurveda, Siddha and Unani mentioned in the First Schedule of the Drugs and Cosmetics Act, 1940 (23 of 1940). These tests may include any in-house or pharmacopoeial test adopted by the manufacturer in the raw material or in the process material and in the finished product. These records shall be duly signed by Production and Quality Control Personnel respectively. Details or transfer of manufactured drug to the finished products store including dates and quantity of drugs transferred along with record of testing of the finished product, if any, and packaging, records shall be maintained. Only after the manufactured drugs have been verified and accepted quality shall be allowed to be cleared for sale. It should be essential to maintain the record of date, manpower, machine and equipments used and to keep in process record of various shodhana, Bhavana, burning in fire and specific grindings in terms of internal use.

(L) Distribution Records: Records of sale and distribution of each batch of Ayurvedic, Siddha and Unani Drugs shall be maintained in order to facilitate prompt and complete recall of the batch, if necessary.

(M) Record of Market Complaints: Manufactures shall maintain a register to record all reports of market complaints received regarding the products sold in the market. The manufacturer shall enter all data received on such market complaints investigations carried out by the manufacturers regarding the complaint as well as any corrective action initiated to prevent recurrence of such market complaints shall also submit the record of such complaints to the licensing authority. The Register shall also be available for inspection during any inspection of the premises. Reports of any adverse reaction resulting from the use of Ayurvedic, Siddha and Unani drugs shall also be maintained in a separate register by each manufacturer. The manufacturer shall investigate any of the adverse reaction to find if the same is due to any defect in the product, and whether such reactions are already reported in the literature or it is a new observation.

(N) Quality Control: Every licensee is required to provide facility for quality control section in his own premises or through Government approved testing laboratory. The test shall be as per the Ayurvedic, Siddha and Unani pharmacopoeial standard. Where the tests are not available, the test should be performed according to the manufacturers specification or other information available. The quality control section shall verify all the raw materials monitor in process, quality checks and control the quality of finished product being released to finished goods store/warehouse. Preferably for such quality control there will be a separate expert. The quality control section shall have the following facilities:

1. There should be 150 sq feet area for quality control section.
2. For identification of raw drugs, reference books and reference samples should be maintained.
3. Manufacturing records should be maintained for the various process.
4. To verify the finished products controlled samples of finished products of each batch will be kept for 3 years.
5. To supervise and monitor adequacy of conditions under which raw material, semi-finished products and finished products are stored.
6. Keep record in establishing shelf life and storage requirements for the drugs.
7. Manufactures who are manufacturing patent proprietary Ayurveda, Siddha and Unani medicines shall provide their own specification and control references in respect of such formulated drugs.
8. The record of specific method and procedure of preparation, that is "Bhavana", "Mardana" and "Puta" and the record of every process carried out by the manufacturer shall be maintained.
9. The standards for identity, purity and strength as given in respective pharmacopoeias of Ayurvedic, Siddha and Unani systems of medicines published by Government of India shall be complied with.
10. All raw materials will be monitored for fungal, bacterial contamination with a view to minimize such contamination.
11. Quality control section will have a minimum of
    (a) one person with Degree qualification in Ayurveda/ Siddha/Unani (A.S.U) as per Schedule II of Indian Medicine Central Council Act, 1970 (84 of 1970) of a recognized university of Board.

(b) Provided that Bachelor of Pharmacy, Pharmacognosy and Chemistry may be associated with the quality control section.

Requirement for Sterile Product

(A) Manufacturing Areas: For the manufacture of sterile Ayurvedic, Unani and Siddha drugs, separate enclosed areas specifically designed for the purpose shall be provided. These areas shall be provided with air locks for entry and shall be essentially dust free and ventilated with an air supply. For all areas where aseptic manufacture has to be carried out, air supply shall be filtered through bacteria retaining filters (HEPA Filters) and shall be at a pressure higher than in the adjacent areas. The filters shall be checked for performance on installation and periodically thereafter the record of checks shall be maintained. All the surfaces in sterile manufacturing areas shall be designed to facilitate cleaning and disinfection. For sterile manufacturing routine microbial counts of all Ayurvedic, Siddha and Unani drug manufacturing areas shall be carried out during operations. Result of such count shall be checked against established in-house standards and record maintained. Access to manufacturing areas shall be restricted to minimum number of authorized personnel. Special procedure to be followed for entering and leaving the manufacturing areas shall be written down and displayed. For the manufacture of Ayurvedic, Siddha and Unani drug that can be sterilized in their final containers, the design of the areas shall preclude the possibility of the products intended for sterilization being mixed with or taken to be products already sterilized. In case of terminally sterilized products, the design of the areas shall preclude the possibility of mix up between non-sterile and sterile products.

(B) Precautions against Contamination and Mix:

(a) Carrying out manufacturing operations in a separate block of adequately isolated building or operating in an isolated enclosure within the building.

(b) Using appropriate pressure differential in the process area.

(c) Providing a suitable exhaust system.

(d) Designing laminar flow sterile air systems for sterile products.

(e) The germicidal efficiency of UV lamps shall be checked and recorded indicating the burning hours or checked using intensity.

(f) Individual containers of liquids and ophthalmic solutions shall be examined against black-white background fitted with diffused light after filling to ensure freedom from contamination with foreign suspended matter.

(g) Expert technical staff approved by the Licensing Authority shall check and compare actual yield against theoretical yield before final distribution of the batch. All process controls as required under master formula including room temperature, relative humidity, volume filled, leakage and clarity shall be checked and recorded.

PART-II-List

A. List of Machinery, Equipment and Minimum Manufacturing Premises required for the Manufacturing

Sr. No	Category of Medicine	Minimum manufacturing Space required	Machinery/equipment recommended
		1200 square feet covered area with separate cabins, Partitions for each activity. If Unani medicines are manufactured in same premises and additional area of 400 sq. feet will be required.	
1	Anjana/Pisti	100 sq. feet	Karel/mechanized/ motorized, kharel. End runner/Ball – Mill Sieves/Shifter
2	Churan/Nasya/ Manjan Lepa/ Kwath Churn	200 sq. feet	Grinder/Disintegrator/ Pulverizer/Powder Mixer/sieves/shifter
3	Pills/Vatti/Gutika		Ball Mill, Mass Mixer Powder mixer Granulator drier. Tablet compressing machine pill/vati cutting machine, stainless steel trays/containers for storage and sugar coating, polishing pan in case of sugar coated tablets, mechanised chattoo (for mixing of guggul) where required.
4	Kupi pakva/Ksara/ Satva/Sindura Kapur/ Multani/Matti/Plaster Uppu Param	150 sq. feet	Bhatti, Karahi/Stainless Parpati/Lavana Bhasma steel Vessels/Patila Flask, of Paris, Copper Rod, Earthen container, Gaj Put Bhatti, Muffle furnace (Electrically operated) End/Edge Runner, Exhaust Fan, Wooden/S.S. Spatula.
5	Kajal	100 sq. feet	Earthen lamps for collection of Kajal, Tipple Roller Mill, End Runner, Sieves, S.S Patila, Filling/packing and manufacturing room should be provided with exhaust fan and ultra violet lamps
6	Capsules	100 sq. feet	Air Conditioner dehumidifier, hygrometer, Thermometer, Capsule filling machine and chemical balance
7	Ointment/Marham	100 sq. feet	Tube filling machine Passi Crimping Medicine/ Ointment Mixer, End Runner/Mill (Where required) S.S Storage Container S.S Patila

Contd...

Sr. No	Category of Medicine	Minimum manufacturing Space required	Machinery/equipment recommended
8	Pak/Avaleh/Khand/ Modak/Lakayam	100 sq. feet	Bhatti section fitted with Exhaust Fan and should be fly proof. Iron Kadahi/S.S Patila and S.S Storage Container
9	Panak Syrup/Pravahi Kwath Manapaku	150 sq. feet	Tinctum press, exhaust fan fitted and fly proof Bhatti section. Bottle washing machine, filter press Gravity filter Liquid filling machine, P.P. Capping Machine,
10	Asava/Aristha	200 sq. feet	Same as mentioned above. Fermentation tanks containers and Distillation plant where necessary, Filter Press.
11	Sura	100 sq. feet	Same as mentioned above plus Distillation plant and Transfer pump.
12	Ark Tinir	100 sq. feet	Maceration tank, Distillation plant, Liquid filling tank with tap/Gravity filter/Filter press, Visual inspection box.
13	Tail Ghrit Nev	100 sq. feet	Bhatti, Kadahi/S.S. Patila S.S. Storage Containers, Filtration Equipment filling tank with tap/Liquid filling machine
14	Aschyotan/Netra/ Malham Panir/ Karn bindu Nasa bindu	100 sq. feet	Hot air oven electrically heated with thermo, static control, cattle gas or electically heated with suitable mixing arrangement collation mill or ointment mill, tube filling equipment, mixing and storage tanks or stainless steel or of other suitable material sintered glass funnel, seitz filter or filter candle, liquid filling equipment, autoclave.
15	Each manufacturing unit will have a separate area for Bhatti, furnaces, boilers, puta, etc. This will have proper ventilation, removal of smoke, prevention of files, insects, dust etc. The furnace section could have tin roof.	200 sq. feet	

B. List of Machinery, Equipment and Minimum Manufacturing Premises Required for the Manufacture of Various Categories of Unani System of Medicines

One medicine indicated for one category of medicine could be used for the manufacturing of other category of medicine also. Similarly some of the manufacturing area like powdering, furnace, packing of liquids could also be shared for these items.

Sr. No	Category of Medicine	Minimum manufacturing Space required	Machinery/equipment recommended
		1200 square feet covered area with separate cabins, partitions for each activity. If Ayurveda/Siddha, Medicines are also Manufactured in same premises an additional area of 400 square feet will be required.	
1	Itrifal Tiryao majoon/Laooq/ Jawarish Khamiras	100 sq. feet	Grinder/Pulveriser, Sieves, powder mixer (if required), S.S Patilas, Bhatti and other accessories. Planter mixer for Khamiras
2	Arq	100 sq. feet	Distillation Plant (garembic) S.S Storage Tank, Boiling Vessel, Gravity filter, Bottle Filling machine. Bottle washing machine. Bottle drier
3	Habb (Pills) and Tablets	200 sq. feet	Ball Mill, Mass Mixer Powder mixer Granulator drier. Tablet compressing machine pill/vati cutting stainless steel trays/containers for storage and sugar coating, polishing pan in case of sugar coated tablets, mechanised chattoo (for mixing of guggul) where required.
4	Sufoof (Powder)	100 sq. feet	Grinder/Pulveriser, Sieves, Trays, Scoops, Powder mixer (Where required).
5	Raughan (oils)	100 sq. feet	Oil Expeller, S.S. Patilas (Crushing & boiling) oil Filter bottle, Filling machine, Bottle drier, Bhatti.
6	Shiyaf, Surma, Kajal	100 sq. feet	End runner, mixing S.S. Vessel
7	Marham, Zimad (Ointment)	100 sq. feet	Kharal, Bhatti, End runner, Grinder, Pulveriser, Tripple Roller Mill (if needed)
8	Qurs (Tab)	100 sq. feet	Grinder/Pulveriser, Sieves, Powder mixer (where needed), Granulator, Drier Tablet Compressing Machine, Die punches Trays, O.T. Apparatus, Balance with weights. Scoops, Sugar Coating Pan, polishing pan Heater.
9	Kushta	100 sq. feet	Bhatti, Kharal, Sil Batta, Earthen pots
10	Murabba	100 sq. feet	Aluminium Vessels 50- 100 kgs. Capacity, Gendna, Bhatti

Contd...

Sr. No	Category of Medicine	Minimum manufacturing Space required	Machinery/equipment recommended
11	Capsule	100 sq. feet	Pulveriser, Powder mixer (where needed), capsule filling machine. Air Conditioner, De humidifier Balance with weights, storage containers, glass.
12	Sharbat & Jushanda	100 sq. feet	Tinctum Press, exhaust fan fitted, Bhatti section, Bottle washing machine, Filter Press, Gravity filter, Liquid filling tank with tap/liquid filling machine, Hot air oven electrically heated with thermostatic control, Kettle. Hot air oven eclectically heated with thermostatic control, cettle.
13	Qutoor Chasm and Marham (Eye drops, eye ointment)	100 sq. feet	
14	Each manufacturing unit will have a separate area for Bhatti, furnaces, boilers, putta, etc. This will have proper ventilation, removal or smoke, prevention of files, insects, dust etc.	200 sq. feet	

C. List of Equipment Recommended for In-House Quality Control Section (Alternatively unit can get the testing done from the government approved laboratory)

(A) Chemistry section	(B) Pharmacognosy section
1. Alcohol Determination Apparatus 2. Volatile Oil Determination Apparatus 3. Boiling Point Determination Apparatus 4. Melting Point Determination Apparatus 5. Refractometer 6. Polarimeter 7. Viscometer 8. Tablet Disintegration Apparatus 9. Moisture Meter 10. Muffle Furnace 11. Electronic Balance	1. Microscope Binocular (complete set) 2. Dissecting Microscope 3. Microtome 4. Physical balance 5. Aluminium Slide trays 6. Stage Micrometer 7. Camera Lucida (Prism and Mirror Type) 8. Chemicals, Glass-ware etc.

Contd...

12. Magnetic Stirrer 13. Hot Air Oven 14. Refrigerator 15. Glass/Steel Distillation Apparatus 16. LPG Gas Cylinders with Burners 17. Water Bath (Temperature Controlled) 18. Heating Mantles/Hot Plates 19. TLC apparatus with all Accessories (Manual) 20. Paper Chromatography apparatus with accessories 21. Sieve Size 10 to 120 with Sieve shaker 22. Centrifuge machine 23. De-humidifier 24. pH Meter 25. Limit Test Apparatus	

Note: The above requirement of machinery, equipments, space, qualifications are made subject to the modification at the discretion of the Licensing Authority; if he is of the opinion that having regard to the nature and extent of the manufacturing operations it is necessary to relax or alter then in the circumstances in a particular case.

D. Supplementary Guidelines for Manufacturing of Rasaushadhies or Rasamarunthukal and Kushtajat (Herbomineral-metallic Compounds) of Ayurveda, Siddha and Unani Medicines:

These guidelines are intended to complement those provided above and should be read in conjunction with the parent guidelines. The supplementary guidelines are to provide general and minimum technical requirements for quality assurance and control in manufacturing Rasaushadhis or Rasamarunthukal and Kushtajat (Herbo-mineral-metallic formulations). These supplementary guidelines deal with Bhasmas, Sindura, Pishti, Kajjali, Khalviya Ras, Kupipakwa, Rasayan, Parpati, Potali Rasa, Satwa (of Metals and Minerals origin) Druti Parpam, Karpu, and Kushta etc. used in Ayurvedic, Siddha and Unani Systems of medicine. The supplementary GMP guidelines for Rasaushadhi or Rasamarunthukal and Kushtajat are needed to establish the authenticity of raw drug, minerals and metals, in process validation and quality control parameters to ensure that these formulations are processed and prepared in accordance with classical texts and for which safety measures are complied.

Only those manufacturing units which have Good Manufacturing Practices for ASU drugs and supplementary certificate for Rasaushadhi or Rasamarunthukal and Kushtajat formulations shall be allowed to manufacture the same. Supplementary Good Manufacturing practices Certificate for Rasaushadhies shall be issued by the State Licensing Authority only after thorough inspection by an expert team including Rasashastra experts nominated by the Department of AYUSH

1. Manufacturing Process Areas
2. Quality Control
3. In Process Control- Shodhan, Bhavana and Putta Register with details, Grinding Record Register, Packing details

4. Product Quality Control
5. Product recalls
6. Medical examination of the Employee
7. Self-Inspection
8. Dosage form of Rasaushadhis
9. Area Specifications/ requirement for an applicant companies only to have GMP of Rasaushadhis or Rasamarunthukal and Kushtajat (Herbomineral/metallic compounds) of Ayurveda, Siddha and Unani medicines

Schedule TA (Rule 157A)

Schedule TA describes the form for record of utilization of raw material by Ayurveda or Siddha or Unani licensed manufacturing units during the financial year.

Further Reading

1. A.K. Jain, B.K. Sharma. Developments in the field of Ayurveda – past to present. Ayushdhara, 1 (2014), pp. 51-64
2. Anonymous. Amendments and Notifications Drugs and Cosmetics Rules (1945) Accessed from: www.drugscontrol.org/amendments.asp
3. Anonymous. AYUSH, About the System (2015) Accessed from: http://www.indianmedicine.nic.in
4. Anonymous. Section 1: Summary of All-India AYUSH Infrastructure Facilities (2015) Accessed from: http://indianmedicine.nic.in/writereaddata/linkimages/0913923524-Summary.pdf
5. B.V. Subbarayappa. Siddha medicine: an overview. Lancet, 350 (1997), pp. 1841-1844
6. Central Council for Research in Unani Medicine. Unani Pharmacopeial Committee. (2015) Accessed from: http://www.ccrum.net/research/upc/
7. K. Joshi. Indian Herbal Sector. (2008) Accessed from: http://www.nistads.res.in/indiasnt2008/t4industry/t4ind19.htm
8. K. Mangathayaru. Pharmacognosy: An Indian Perspective. Pearson, Chennai (2013)
9. Ministry of AYUSH. AYUSH for Holistic Healthcare & Healthy Living (2015) Accessed from: http://www.indianmedicine.nic.in
10. Ministry of Health and Family Welfare, Govt. of India Regulation of Manufacture and Sale of ASU Drugs (2006) Accessed from: http://www.pib.nic.in
11. National Medicinal Plants Board. Standard for Good Field Collection Practices of Medicinal Plants [DOC: NMPB-GFCP-01(FD)] (2015) Accessed from: http://www.nmpb.nic.in
12. P. Gurmet. "Sowa-Rigpa": Himalayan art of healing. Indian J Tradit Know, 3 (2004), pp. 212-218
13. P. Patel. Global Resurgence and International Recognition of Ayurveda. (2003) Accessed from: http://iafngo.org/
14. Pharmacopoeial Laboratory for Indian Medicine. Publications (2015) Accessed from: http://www.plimism.nic.in/index.html

15. S. Sen, R. Chakraborty. Toward the integration and advancement of herbal medicine: a focus on Traditional Indian medicine. Bot Target Ther, 5 (2015), pp. 33-44
16. S. Sen, R. Chakraborty. Traditional knowledge digital library: a distinctive approach to protect and promote Indian indigenous medicinal treasure. Curr Sci, 106 (2014), pp. 1340-1343
17. S. Thillaivanan, K. Samraj. Challenges, constraints and opportunities in herbal medicines – a review Int J Herb Med, 2 (2014), pp. 21-24
18. S.C. Mandal, M. Mandal. Quality, safety, and efficacy of herbal products through regulatory harmonization. Drug Info J, 45 (2011), pp. 45-53
19. S.K. Sharma, D.C. Katoch. Current Status & Infrastructure of Ayurveda (2006) Accessed from: http://herbalnet.healthrepository.org
20. T. Siddiqi. Unani medicine in India. Indian J Hist Sci, 16 (1981), pp. 22-25
21. V.N. Kasagana, S.S. Karumuri. Conservation of medicinal plants (past, present & future trends). J Pharm Sci Res, 3 (2011), pp. 1378-1386
22. W.M. Bandaranayake. Quality control, screening, toxicity and regulations of herbal drugs. I. Ahmad, F. Aquil, M. Owais (Eds.), Modern Phytomedicine: Turning Medicinal Plants into Drugs, Wiley-VCH Verlag GmbH & Co, Germany (2006), pp. 25-27
23. World Health Organization. National Policy on Traditional Medicine and Regulation of Herbal Medicines – Report of a WHO Global Survey. WHO, Geneva (2005)
24. World Health Organization. Traditional Medicine (2013) Accessed from: http://www.who.int/mediacentre/factsheets/2003/fs134/en/
25. World Health Organization. WHO Traditional Medicine Strategy 2002–2005. World Health Organization, Geneva (2002)
26. https://cdsco.gov.in/opencms/export/sites/CDSCO_WEB/Pdf-documents/acts_rules/2016 DrugsandCosmeticsAct1940Rules1945.pdf

Scan QR code to view the website/guidelines

- The Drugs and Cosmetics Act, 1940- 2016DrugsandCosmeticsAct1940Rules1945.pdf (cdsco.gov.in)

Section 4

Quality Control, Standardisation, Regulations for Herbal Products

CHAPTER 10

WHO Good Agricultutal and Collection Practices [GAP, GCP, GACP] 2003

GACP Guidelines

Section 1: General Introduction and Glossary

Section 2: Good Agricultural Practices [GAP] for Medicinal Plants

1. Identification/Authentication of Cultivated Medicinal Plants
2. Seeds and Other Propagation Materials
3. Site selection
4. Personnel
5. Ecological Environment and Social Impact
6. Soil
7. Climate
8. Irrigation and Drainage
9. Cultivation
10. Plant Maintenance and Protection
11. Harvest

Section 3: Good Collection Practices [GCP] for Medicinal Plants

1. Permission to Collect
2. Technical Planning
3. Selection of Medicinal Plants for Collection
4. Collection
5. Personnel

Section 4: Common Technical Aspects of GACP

1. Post-harvest Processing
   (a) Inspection and Sorting
   (b) Primary Processing
   (c) Drying
   (d) Specific Processing
2. Bulk Packaging and Labelling
3. Storage and Transportation
4. Equipment
5. Quality Assurance
6. Documentation
7. Personnel (growers, collectors, producers, handlers, processors)

Section 5: Other Relevant Issues

1. Ethical and Legal Considerations
2. Intellectual Property Rights and Benefits-sharing
3. Threatened and Endangered Species

Further Reading

GACP Guidelines

Section 1: General Introduction and Glossary

This section involves following important descriptions.

Need of GACP Guidelines

1. Interest in herbal medicines risen the issues related to safety and quality of herbal medicines
2. Inadvertent use of the wrong plant species
3. Adulteration with undeclared other medicines and/or potent substances
4. Contamination with undeclared toxic and/or hazardous substances
5. Over dosage, inappropriate use by health-care providers or consumers
6. Interaction with other medicines
7. Use of inferior quality raw medicinal plant materials results in poor quality finished products
8. Collection from wild populations leads to global, regional and/or local over-harvesting
9. Protection of endangered species
10. Impact on environment and ecological processes
11. Impact on the welfare of local communities should be considered
12. Respect of intellectual property rights

Objectives

1. Supply of good quality raw material applicable to national and/or regional quality standards thus improve the quality, safety and efficacy of finished herbal products;
2. Guide the formulation of national and/or regional GACP guidelines and GACP monographs for medicinal plants and related standard operating procedures; and
3. Encourage and support the conservation of medicinal plants and the environment

Structure

The guidelines are divided into five sections:

- Section 1: Provides a general introduction and a glossary for relevant terms
- Section 2: Good Agricultural Practices for Medicinal Plants
- Section 3: Discuss Good Collection Practices for Medicinal Plants.
- Section 4: Outlines common technical aspects of good agricultural practices for medicinal plants and good collection practices for medicinal plants
- Section 5: Considers other relevant issues
- Annexure 1: National and regional documents on good agricultural practices for medicinal plants from the China
- Annexure 2: National and regional documents on good agricultural practices for medicinal plants from the European Agency

- Annexure 3: National and regional documents on good agricultural practices for medicinal plants from the Japan
- Annexure 4: Model structure for monographs on good agricultural practices for specific medicinal plants
- Annexure 5: Sample record for cultivated medicinal plants

Section 2: Good Agricultural Practices (GAP) for Medicinal Plants

1. **Identification/Authentication of Cultivated Medicinal Plants:** The botanical identity, scientific name (genus, species, subspecies/variety, author, and family) of each medicinal plant under cultivation should be verified and recorded. If available, the local and English common names should also be recorded. Documentation of the botanical identity should be included in the registration file as a specimen.
2. **Seeds and other propagation materials:** Propagation materials should be from any disease or contamination and provide all necessary information relating to the identity, quality and performance of their products, as well as their breeding history, where possible. Materials used for organic production should be certified as being organically derived.
3. **Site Selection:** Medicinal plant materials derived from the same species can show significant differences in quality when cultivated at different sites, owing to the influence of soil, climate and other factors. Risks of contamination as a result of pollution of the soil, air or water by hazardous chemicals should be avoided.
4. **Personnel:** Growers and producers should have formal or informal practical education and training of the medicinal plant concerned. This should include botanical identification, cultivation characteristics and environ-mental requirements (soil type, soil pH, fertility, plant spacing and light requirements), as well as the means of harvest, storage and personal hygiene, issues relevant to the protection of the environment, conservation of medicinal plant species, and proper agricultural stewardship. Smoking and eating should not be permitted in medicinal plant processing areas.
5. **Ecological Environment and Social Impact:** The introduction of non-indigenous medicinal plant species into cultivation may have a detrimental impact on the biological and ecological balance of the region. In terms of local income- earning opportunities, small-scale cultivation is often preferable so that local communities benefit directly from, for example, fair wages, equal employment opportunities and capital reinvestment.
6. **Soil:** Optimal soil conditions, including soil type, drainage, moisture retention, fertility and pH, will be dictated by the selected medicinal plant species and/or target medicinal plant part. Optimal soil conditions, including soil type, drainage, moisture retention, fertility and pH, will be dictated by the selected medicinal plant species and/or target medicinal plant part. Green manure should be preferred.
7. **Climate:** The duration of sunlight, average rainfall, average temperature, including daytime and night-time temperature differences, also influence the physiological and biochemical activities of plants, and prior knowledge should be considered.

8. **Irrigation and Drainage:** should be controlled and carried out in accordance with the needs of individual plant
9. **Cultivation:** The conditions and duration of cultivation required vary depending on the medicinal plant materials required. Scientific and if no scientific data available then traditional methods should be used to cultivate medicinal plant.
10. **Plant Maintenance and Protection:** timely application of measures such as topping, bud nipping, pruning and shading, Integrated pest management should be followed where appropriate
11. **Harvest:** The time of harvest depends on the plant part to be used. The best time for harvest (quality peak season/time of day) should be determined according to the quality and quantity of biologically active constituents rather than the total vegetative yield of the targeted medicinal plant parts. No foreign matter, weeds or toxic plants are mixed with the harvested medicinal plant materials. Avoid dew, rain or exceptionally high humidity. If harvesting occurs in wet conditions, the material should be transported immediately to an indoor drying. Use clean devices to harvest as well as to store. Material should be stored in dry and free from insects, rodents, birds and other pests, and inaccessible to livestock and domestic animals. If the underground parts (such as the roots) are used, any adhering soil should be removed from the medicinal plant materials as soon as they are harvested. Medicinal plants should not be collected in or near areas where high levels of pesticides or other possible contaminants are used or found, such as roadsides, drainage ditches, mine tailings, garbage dumps and industrial facilities which may produce toxic emissions.

Section 3: Good collection Practices (GCP) for Medicinal Plants

1. **Permission to Collect:** In some countries, collection permits and other documents from government authorities and landowners must be obtained prior to collecting any plants from the wild. Sufficient time for the processing and issuance of these permits must be allocated at the planning stage. For medicinal plant materials intended for export from the country of collection, export permits, phytosanitary certificates, Convention on International Trade in Endangered Species of Wild Fauna and Flora (CITES) permit(s) (for export and import), CITES certificates (for re-export), and other permits must be obtained, when required.
2. **Technical Planning:** Essential information on the target species (the geographical distribution and population Density, taxonomy, distribution, phenology, genetic diversity, reproductive biology and ethnobotany) should be obtained. Data about environmental conditions, including topography, geology, soil, climate and vegetation at the prospective collecting site(s), should be collated and presented in a collection management plan. Transport, personnel, equipments and storage facilities should be ready.
3. **Selection of Medicinal Plants for Collection:** select and authenticate plant species for collection.
4. **Collection:** same as above given in GAP
5. **Personnel:** same as above given in GAP

Section 4: Common Technical Aspects of GACP

1. **Post-harvest Processing:**
   - (a) **Inspection and Sorting:** Raw medicinal plant materials should be inspected and sorted for foreign matter, cross contamination and organoleptic characters prior to primary processing.
   - (b) **Primary Processing:** Harvested or collected raw medicinal plant materials, Prior to processing, should be protected from rain, moisture and any other conditions that might cause deterioration.
   - (c) **Drying:** Medicinal plants can be dried in a number of ways: in the open air (shaded from direct sunlight); placed in thin layers on drying frames, wire-screened rooms or buildings; by direct sunlight, if appropriate; in drying ovens/rooms and solar dryers; by indirect fire; baking; lyophilization; microwave; or infrared devices. When possible, temperature and humidity should be controlled to avoid damage to the active chemical constituents. The method and temperature used for drying may have a considerable impact on the quality of the resulting medicinal plant materials.
   - (d) **Specific Processing:** Common specific processing practices include pre-selection, peeling the skins of roots and rhizomes, boiling in water, steaming, soaking, pickling, distillation, fumigation, roasting, natural fermentation, treatment with lime and chopping. Processing procedures involving the formation of certain shapes, bundling and special drying may also have an impact on the quality of the medicinal plant materials.
   - (e) **Processing Facilities:** Facilities should preferably be located in areas that are free from objectionable odours, smoke, dust or other contaminants, and are not subject to flooding. Roadways should not be near vicinity, building ceilings, floors should be clean. Sufficient lighting, ventilation and water supply should be maintained.
2. **Bulk Packaging and Labelling:** immediate packing and labelling is necessary. Packaging material should be clean and stored in dry places. Appropriate labels should be affixed to each batch packing.
3. **Storage and Transportation:** Conveyances used for transporting bulk medicinal plant materials from the place of production to storage for processing should be cleaned between loads. Bulk transport, such as ship or rail cars, should be cleaned and, where appropriate, well ventilated to remove moisture from medicinal plant materials and to prevent condensation.
4. **Equipment:** All equipments should be clean and well labelled
5. **Quality Assurance:** regular auditing visits to cultivation or collection sites and processing facilities by expert representatives of producers and buyers and through inspection by national and/or local regulatory authorities.
6. **Documentation:** SOP should be prepared for each stage.
7. **Personnel (growers, collectors, producers, handlers, processors):** Same as GAP

Section 5: Other Relevant Issues

1. **Ethical and Legal Considerations**: must be carried out in accordance with legal and environmental requirements and with the ethical codes or norms of the community and country in which the activities take place. The provisions of the Convention on Biological Diversity must be respected.
2. **Intellectual Property Rights and Benefits-sharing:** Agreements on the return of immediate and/or long-term benefits and compensation for the use of source medicinal plant materials must be discussed and concluded, in writing, prior to collection or cultivation.
3. **Threatened and Endangered Species:** Medicinal plants that are protected by national and international laws, such as those listed in national "red" lists, may be collected only by relevant permission according to national and/or international laws.

Further Reading

1. WHO Guidelines on Good Agricultural and Collection Practices (GACP) for Medicinal Plants by World Health Organization, WHO · 2003 Accessed -htpps.who.int/iris/handle/10665/42783
2. H. Panda Medicinal Plants Cultivation & Their Uses. Asia Pacific Business Press. 2002
3. Cultivation and Utilization of Medicinal Plants. Regional Research Laboratory, Council of Scientific & Industrial Research. 1982
4. K. Chopra. Medicinal Plants-Conservation, Cultivation and Utilization. Daya Publishing House. 2007
5. Ravindra Sharma. Agro-Techniques of Medicinal Plants. Daya Publishing House. 2004.
6. Azhar Ali Farooqi, B. S. Sreeramu. Cultivation of Medicinal And Aromatic Crops. Universities Press (India) Pvt. Limited. 2004
7. J.C. Tarafdar, K.P. Tripathi, M. Kumar. Organic Agriculture. Scientific Publishers. 2012
8. S. S. Purohit, S. P. Vyas.A Scientific Approach: Including Processing and Financial Guidelines. Agrobios (India). 2004
9. Serdar Oztekin, Milan Martinov. Medicinal and Aromatic Crops-Harvesting, Drying, and Processing. CRC Press. 2014
10. Nirmal Joshee, Prahlad Parajuli, Sadanand A. Dhekney Medicinal Plants-From Farm to Pharmacy. Springer International Publishing. 2019

Scan QR code to view the website/guidelines

- WHO GACP Guidelines-
WHO guidelines on good agricultural and collection practices (GACP) for medicinal plants

CHAPTER 11

NMPB Guidelines and Standard for Good Field Collection Practices for Indian Medicinal Plants 2009

Guidelines on Good Field Collection Practices for Indian Medicinal Plants 2009

1. Introduction
2. Compliance to Regulatory Requirements
   - International Regulation and Guidelines
   - National Regulations
   - Local Regulations
   - Permission for Collections
3. Harvesting of Medicinal Plant Produce
   - Quality Considerations
   - Environmental Considerations
   - Social Considerations
4. Post-Harvest Management
   - Primary Processing
   - Drying
5. Packaging and Storage
   - Packaging of Medicinal Plant Produce
   - Storage of Medicinal Plant Produce
6. Guidelines for collection and Post-harvest Management of Various Categories of Medicinal Plant Produce
   - Underground parts
   - Annual herbs/ Whole plants
   - Stem Bark
   - Stem or wood
   - Leaves
   - Flower and floral parts
   - Fruits and seeds
   - Gums and resins
   - Others
7. Documentation

Guidelines on Good Field Collection Practices for Indian Medicinal Plants 2009

1. Introduction

The European Pharmacopoeia provides an official definition for the term "Herbal Drugs" as follows: Mainly whole, fragmented, or cut plants, parts of plants, algae, fungi or lichen, in an unprocessed state, usually in dried form but sometimes fresh and certain exudates. The most frequently encountered criticism about the herbal medicines and allied healthcare products relates to consistency of products in terms of quality, efficacy and safety, which can be summed-up as "minimum therapeutic guarantee". The demand-supply disparity resulted in the supply of sub-standard medicinal plant produce, lack of appropriate knowledge about the natural resources being used and techno- cultural variance in harvesting and post harvest practices - is one of major contributory factors for such poor-quality medicinal produce. Over-exploitation, habitat loss, threat to plant species and even local extinction in a few cases are increasing. The WHO guidelines on Good Agriculture and Collection Practices (GACPs) recommend that individual countries should develop their own national guidelines for collection of medicinal plants. Hence Government of India provides these guidelines on "Good field collection practices for Indian medicinal Plants" comprising eight sections in conjunction with the existing documents relating to quality of medicinal produce, for example, the "Good Manufacturing Practices (GMPs) for Ayurveda, Siddha and Unani Medicines" published in Schedule 'T' of the Drugs and Cosmetic Act and Rules (3) based on following **Objectives:**

- Encourage and support conservation and sustainable utilization of medicinal plants for inter generational equity.
- Ensure consistency in the quality of raw medicinal and thus safety and efficacy of herbal formulations.
- Ensure extraneous contaminants and toxic adulterants free medicinal plants produce
- Minimize direct and indirect negative impact on environment due to collection of medicinal plants from the wild sources
- Promote community involvement in management of medicinal plant resource including its quality and sustainability.
- Encourage training and benefit sharing to optimize the returns to the collectors, and other stakeholders.
- Encourage documentation of required information related to medicinal plant produce.
- Ensure equitable returns to collectors and other stakeholders.

2. Compliance to Regulatory Requirement

The collection, processing, storage and sale of medicinal plant produce must be carried out in accordance with the existing laws. Being a concurrent subject, forests in India are regulated by both Central as well as State Governments, concurrently. This needs compliance to laws enacted by both Central and local Governments. Further, India being a signatory to various international treaties and conventions related to conservation of biodiversity, provisions laid down in such and other regulations applicable from time to time must be respected while collecting any medicinal plant produce from the wild.

(a) **International Regulation and Guidelines:** Provisions laid down in the CITES regulations must be adhered to while collecting any medicinal plant produce from the wild. In case the medicinal plant produce is meant for export, existing laws of the importing country must be honoured. Besides the regulatory authorities in the country of import, local secretariats of CITES, IUCN and TRAFFIC International may be consulted for such laws and regulations.

(b) **National Regulations:** Collectors and collection managers must keep themselves updated about the provisions in various Acts from Government of India to ensure conservation and sustainable use of wild resources including medicinal plants. Indian Forest Act 1927, The Wildlife (Protection) Act 1972, The Forest (Conservation) Act 1980, The Biological Diversity Act 2002, The Scheduled Tribes and Other Traditional Forest-Dwellers (Recognition of Forest Rights) Act 200, export-import policy and the negative list of export contain provisions related to collection, transit and trade of medicinal plant produce.

(c) **Local Regulations:** Collectors/collection managers should be aware of modified Indian Forest Act 1927 in different States of India to accommodate the regional intricacies and necessities of conservation and utilization of wild resources. Some of the examples are – The Madhya Pradesh Sustainable Harvesting Act 2005, The Andhra Pradesh Red Sanders Wood Possession Rules 1989, The HP Forest Produce Transit (Land Routes) Rules, 1977, The Tamil Nadu Sandalwood Transit Rules, 1967, and The Maharashtra Forest Produce (Regulation of Trade) Act, 1969.

(d) **Permission for Collections:** Wherever the provision requires, collectors/collection managers should take prior written permission from the authorized agency for collection, possession, transit and sale of the medicinal plant produce.

3. Harvesting of Medicinal Plant Produce

Medicinal plants should be harvested in such ways and at such rates that the species perpetuates indefinitely in its natural habits. Collectors should adopt such practices that do not merely fulfill their commercial needs but also ensure that the produce the quality. Collectors/collection managers should adopt following guidelines for harvesting the medicinal plants produce.

Quality Considerations:

- Botanical authenticity of species (genus, species, sub-species, if any, along with author citation) must be verified, recorded and established before a plant species is collected from the wild based on AYUSH Pharmacopoeias of India or reference books in consultation with BSI or FRI or any recognized national or regional herbaria.
- Collection of healthy plants unless the medicinal value of the species comes from such associations as in the case of insect galls, agar wood and specified parts developed due to pathogens) should always be preferred

- Harvesting at right phenological stage should be done at appropriate developmental stage because concentration of biologically active substances varies with the stages of growth and development of plant. The collection time must be documented.
- Weather conditions like rain, mist or exceptionally high humid conditions for collection should be avoided
- collection should be always from Right places (clean and free from any possible exposure to insects, chemicals, toxic gases, sewage, automobiles etc.) and avoid collection from contaminated places (near anthills, industrial areas, sewage lines, crematoria, hospitals, mining sites, public utilities, automobile workshops and any other places like close to roadside as perpetual exposure to vehicular exhaust) as such material is unsuitable for human consumption.
- Sorting for various grades depending on color, size etc. may be done either immediately after the harvesting or after drying of the produce depending upon the ease of sorting.
- Foreign matter (soil particles, organic matters like leaves, stems, wood pieces or food articles, cross-contamination with other medicinal plant produce) should be removed during the harvesting and post-harvest management.
- Mixing of Toxic weeds should be avoided by careful harvesting.

Environmental Considerations

The over exploitation of any plant species may threaten the existence of the species in natural habitat. Application of the Principles and Criteria of the International Standard for Sustainable Collection of wild medicinal plants (ISSC – MAP) developed by the IUCN/WWF/BfN through an intensive consultation of various stakeholders. This application can be ensured through different paths such as a scientific resource management regime, legal and regulatory adherence or through a certification process.

- Regulators (e.g., forest and wild life field officials) as well as the collectors must be aware of the current conservation status or RET status of the desired plant species.
- Collection managers should be aware of the Sensitive species that are of increased threat.
- Collection of a species should start with knowledge of Distribution of species and only be done from areas where its frequency of occurrence is sustainable.:
- Certain percentage of the species population should be left as such so as to allow the natural regeneration and thus conservation of species.
- Frequency of collection cycle should synchronize with the regeneration cycle of the plant species or the produce, whichever is the case.
- Efforts should be made to minimize the harm to source plant While collecting the desired plant parts such as leaves, fruits, flowers, seeds etc.
- While harvesting the desired species, collectors should ensure that the minimum damage, avoid destruction of specialized habitats of the species to ensure its sustainability.
- Equipment used for digging, cutting, sorting, shearing, spilling, peeling and any other activity must be made of a non-toxic material, suitable for the purpose and thoroughly cleaned after use to avoid cross contamination.

Social Considerations

In case of organized large-scale collection, care should be taken that local inhabitants get the equitable employment opportunities and wages, should not affect the availability of species for use by local people, must have suitable fair price and equitable benefit sharing mechanism as per Biological Diversity Act, 2002 of India. Health Status of Collectors (allergies, open wounds, inflammations and skin infections etc) and wearing appropriate personal protective equipments like safety shoes, gloves, and eye and nose protection while collecting produce from wild habitats must be taken care. The harvesting as well as the post-harvest management of medicinal plant produce must be carried out in accordance with Cultural Considerations like ethical codes, holy practices (social and religious values) and norms of local community and the region in which the activities take place.

4. Post-Harvest Management

Primary Processing: To preserve the quality and enhance shelf life, timely and right primary processing of medicinal plant produce to remove any type of foreign matter, scraping, peeling, brushing or washing is required.

Drying: to achieve better drying, choice of method like open sun or air-drying, shade drying, artificial drying like oven or hot air depends upon plant parts. Fleshy plant parts require more attention and should be cut or sliced into small/ thin pieces and then spreading to ensure proper drying of the produce.

5. Packaging and Storage

Packaging of Medicinal Plant Produce: The storage containers of medicinal plant produce must provide protection from heat, humidity and temperature and at the same time should not contaminate the produce. Each category of produce requires specific packaging needs. Appendix 1 enlists a few packaging options for Indian medicinal plant produce, which can be adopted. Each container of medicinal plant produce should be labeled properly. The label should contain all the required information of medicinal plant produce. A prototype label is given as Appendix II.

Storage of Medicinal Plant Produce: Storage of produce is of utmost importance as inappropriate storage conditions may render the produce unusable, no matter with what care it has been harvested and processed. Medicinal plant produce (approved, rejected and untested lots separately) with appropriate signboards and label of valid shelf-life period should be stored in a dedicated cool and dry storehouse free from dampness, dirt and dust, entry of rodents, birds and other animals and should be. Medicinal plant produce should never be stored in open areas and in or near cattle sheds. To the greatest possible extent, the medicinal plant produce should be supplied/consumed on FIFO (First in first out) basis to minimize storage of old stock. FIFO system allows sequential use of produce, in order of the arrivals in the storehouse. Documentation of produce coming in and going out should be displayed at an appropriate place to know the exact availability of the medicinal plant produce in stock. There should be provision for separate climate (temperature and humidity) controlled facility to store hygroscopic material and volatile material. Inflammable produce like resins, gum-resins, oils etc. should be stored at isolated place in closed containers (flammable materials should be clearly labeled as such on each container).

6. Guidelines for Collection and Post-harvest Management of Various Categories of Medicinal Plant Produce:

It is recommended that a detailed SOP should be written for each category of produce in order to minimize the harm to nature and to optimize the quality of the produce. Some of the important points, which need to be taken care of while harvesting various categories, are given below.

- **Underground parts (**when the plants are well developed and mature, after the seed shedding)
- **Annual herbs/ Whole plants (**at flower bud or flowering stage)
- **Stem Bark (**from mature branches when the tree is under new growth like spring season)
- **Stem or wood (**mature branches of a tree or shrub and don't harvest same plant every year)
- **Leaves (**before their flowering, unless otherwise specified)
- **Flower and floral parts (**Flowers when just opened or shortly afterwards, flower buds before the buds open and floral parts like stigma, anthers, petals etc at appropriate time of their maturity to ensure the availability of desired active substance)
- **Fruits and seeds** (on maturity unless specified)
- **Gums and resins** (from mature trees or shrubs in clear and dry weather, only few small long sharp cut blazes or longitudinal incisions)
- **Others (Galls, Lac etc.) (**from stipulated species as specified)

7. Documentation

The documentation of following essential information related to collection of medicinal plant is recommended: Plant species, area of collection, time of collection, drying conditions, regulatory information, phenological stage of species at the time of collection, processes or events that could affect the quality of the produce, any extra-ordinary circumstances, agreements between collectors (e.g. co-operative society, village Panchayat etc.) with traders and manufacturers, permits from the authorities.

8. Training and Monitoring

Training and Capacity Building: Collectors should have received adequate botanical identity, regulatory, personal hygiene and safety training.

Baseline Assessment and Monitoring: To avoid unsustainable harvesting and quality degradation due to demand and supply mismatch, baseline assessment of availability of medicinal plant produce in wild should be done adopting mathematical approaches including computer softwares. Wherever it is not possible to arrive at sustainable level of harvesting, it can be carried out with reference to supply (for example setting of extraction quotas) or with reference to both supply and demand.

Standard for Good Field Collection Practices of Medicinal Plants

Background

India has a rich heritage of plant based healthcare systems like Ayurveda, Unani and Siddha with a very high degree of societal acceptance. Almost 90 percent of the raw materials of medicinal plants used by the manufacturing units are sourced from natural forests, often with little regard to environmental and social considerations, often resultingin harvest much in excess of sustainable limits. The major challenges facing growth and outreach of the traditional/herbal medicinal productsare their quality, safety and efficacy. The requirements given in this standard are subject to the following statutory and regulatory provisions:

- The Drugs and Cosmetics Act and Rules (as amended up through 30th June 2005. New Delhi: Department of Health. 2005.Schedule T: Good Manufacturing Practices (GMPs) for Ayurveda, Siddha and Unani Medicines.
- The Ayurvedic Pharmacopoeia of India, 5 Volumes, Ministry of Health and Family Welfare, Govt. of India, New Delhi, 1989-2005
- The Siddha Pharmacopoeia of India, Part I(1), Ministry of Health and Family Welfare, Govt. of India, New Delhi, 2007
- The Unani Pharmacopoeia of India, Part-I, Ministry of Health and Family Welfare, Govt. of India, New Delhi
- The Indian Forest Act, 1927
- Wild Life (Protection) Act, 1972
- Biological Diversity Act 2002

Scope

This standard has appraisal and assessment system based on control criteria, compliance criteria and level of compliance. The requirements stated in Table 01 shall be evaluated to establish that collectors comply with those requirements. On evaluation of deficiencies that may appear in evaluation need to be resolved to establish compliance to the requirements. These deficiencies have been classified as:

- **Critical**: When evidence shows that the grower has not complied with requirements in its documentation and implementation and which raises doubts on the operation and practice of GAP calling for an early correction and corrective actions within the time frame.
- **Major:** When evidence suggests major break down in the implementation in certain elements of the criteria calling for the early corrective actions within a time frame
- **Minor:** When evidence shows an isolated non-compliance to the GAP criteria and has negligible impact on the operation of the system and its results.

To develop a self-assessment against the criteria, a checklist has been developed and is given in Table 02. This will bring uniformity in evaluation of the system. This also indicates when a violation of a particular criteria leads to critical, major or minor nonconformities.

Table 11.1 Requirements and Evaluation Criteria.

No.	Control criteria	Compliance criteria	Level of compliance
1. Site Selection			
2. Compliance to Regulatory Requirement			
3. Harvest/Collection Management Guidelines given in Annex B must be kept in mind			
3.1	Quality Considerations		
3.2	Environmental Considerations		
3.3	Social Considerations:		
4. Post Harvest Management			
4.1	Cleaning		
4.3	Drying		
5. Packaging and Storage			
5.1	**Packaging**		
5.2	**Storage**		
6. Machinery and Equipment used in Different Operations			
7. Documentation for Identification and Traceability			
7.1	**Identification**		
7.2	**Traceability**		
7.3	Documentation		
8. Training and Monitoring			
9. Workers Health, Safety and Welfare			
9.1	**Risk Assessments**		
9.2	Training on health and safety		
9.3	Hazards and First Aid		
10. Record Keeping and Internal Self-assessment/Internal Inspection			

Table 11.2 Checklists for Self-Assessment.

No.	Control criteria	Level of compliance	Compliance		Remarks
			Yes	No	
1 Site Selection					
2 Compliance to Regulatory Requirement					
2.1	General				
2.2	International regulation andguidelines				
2.3	National regulations				
2.4	Local regulations				
2.5	Permission for collections				

Contd...

No.	Control criteria	Level of compliance	Compliance		Remarks
			Yes	No	
3 Harvest/Collection Management					
3.1	Quality Considerations				
3.1.1	Botanical authenticity of species:				
3.1.2	Botanical authenticity of new plants				
3.1.3	Is Field Collection Protocolavailable?				
3.1.4	Collection of healthy plants				
3.1.5	Harvesting at right phenological stage				
3.1.6	Weather conditions for collection:				
3.1.7	Sorting of produce:				
3.1.8	Foreign matter:				
3.1.9	Mixing of Toxic weeds:				
3.2	Environmental Considerations				
3.2.1	Conservation status of species:				
3.2.2	Sensitive species:				
3.2.3	Distribution of species:				
3.2.4	Regeneration of species:				
3.2.5	Baseline Assessment& Monitoring:				
3.2.6	Frequency of collection:				
3.2.7	Minimizing the harm to source plant:				
3.2.8	Habitat management:				
3.3	Social Considerations:				
3.3.1	Local use of the species:				
3.3.2	Equity				
3.3.4	Cultural Considerations:				
4 Post Harvest Management					
4.1	Cleaning				
4.2	Sorting				
5 Packaging and Storage					
5.2	Storage				
6 Machinery and Equipment used in Different Operations					
7 Documentation for Identification and Traceability					
7.1	Identification				
7.2	Traceability				
8 Training and Monitoring					
9 Workers Health, Safety and Welfare					
9.1	Risk Assessments				
9.2	Training on health and safety				
9.3	Hazards and First Aid				
9.4	Protective Clothing/Equipment				
10 Record keeping and internal Self-assessment/Internal Inspection					

Further Reading

1. WHO Traditional Medicines Strategy: 2002–2005. Geneva, World Health Organization, 2002 (document WHO/EDM/TRM/2002.1).
2. Good Manufacturing Practices for pharmaceutical products: main principles. In: WHO Expert Committee on Specifications for Pharmaceutical Preparations. Thirty-seventh report. Geneva, World Health Organization, 2003, Annex 4 (WHO Technical Report Series, No. 908).
3. Good manufacturing practices: supplementary guidelines for manufacture of herbal medicinal products. In: WHO Expert Committee on Specifications for Pharmaceutical Preparations. Thirty-fourth report. Geneva, World Health Organization, 1996, Annex 8 (WHO Technical Report Series, No. 863). (These guidelines are also included in Quality Assurance of Pharmaceuticals: A compendium of guidelines and related materials, Vol. 2: Good manufacturing practices and inspection. Geneva, World Health Organization, 1999.)
4. Quality control methods for medicinal plant materials. Geneva, World Health Organization, 1998.
5. Guide to good storage practices for pharmaceuticals. In: WHO Expert Committee on Specifications for Pharmaceutical Preparations. Thirty-seventh report. Geneva, World Health Organization, 2003, Annex 9 (WHO Technical Report Series, No. 908).
6. Good trade and distribution practices (GTDP) for pharmaceutical starting materials. In: WHO Expert Committee on Specifications for Pharmaceutical Preparations. Thirtyeighth report. Geneva, World Health Organization, in press, Annex 2 (WHO Technical Report Series).
7. General guidelines for methodologies on research and evaluation of traditional medicine. Geneva, World Health Organization, 2000 (document WHO/EDM/TRM/2000.1).
8. Guidelines for the assessment of herbal medicines. In: WHO Expert Committee on Specifications for Pharmaceutical Preparations. Thirty-fourth report. Geneva, World Health Organization, 1996, Annex 11 (WHO Technical Report Series, No. 863). (These guidelines are also included in Quality Assurance of Pharmaceuticals. A compendium of guidelines and related materials, Vol. 1. Geneva, World Health Organization, 1997.)
9. WHO monographs on selected medicinal plants, Vol. 1. Geneva, World Health Organization, 1999.
10. WHO monographs on selected medicinal plants, Vol. 2. Geneva, World Health Organization, 2002.
11. Report of the Inter-Regional Workshop on Intellectual Property Rights in the Context of Traditional Medicine, Bangkok, Thailand, 6−8 December 2000. Geneva, World Health Organization, 2001 (document reference WHO/EDM/TRM/2001.1).
12. WHO/IUCN/WWF Guidelines on the conservation of medicinal plants. Gland, Switzerland, IUCN - The World Conservation Union (formerly known as the International Union for Conservation of Nature and Natural Resources), 1993 (currently being updated).
13. Codex Alimentarius Code of Practice - General Principles of Food Hygiene, 2nd ed. Rome, Joint FAO/WHO Food Standards Programme, 2001 (document Codex Alimentarius GL 33).

14. Codex Alimentarius Guidelines on production, processing, labelling and marketing of organically produced foods. Rome, Joint FAO/WHO Food Standards Programme, 2001 (document Codex Alimentarius GL 32-1999, Rev. 1-2001).
15. Codex Alimentarius Code of hygienic practice for spices and dried aromatic plants. Rome, Joint FAO/WHO Food Standards Programme, 1995 (document Codex Alimentarius CAC/RCP 42-1995).
16. Youngken, HW. Textbook of Pharmacognosy, 6th ed. Philadelphia, Blakiston, 1950.
17. Cultivation of medicinal plants and quality control, Vols. 1–10. Tokyo, Ministry of Health, Labour and Welfare Ed. Yakuji Nippo, 1992–2001 (in Japanese).
18. Committee on Herbal Medicinal Products (HMPC) guidelines good agricultural and collection practice (GACP) for Starting materials of herbal origin. 2006. Available at https://www.ema.europa.eu/en/documents/scientific-guideline/guideline-good-agricultural-collection-practice-gacp-starting-materials-herbal-origin_en.pdf
19. Good Agricultural and Collection Practices and Good Manufacturing Practices For Botanical Materials. American Herbal Products Association. 2017

Scan QR code to view the website/guidelines

- NMPB-AYUSH Ministry GAP Guidelines-
Good_Agricultural_Practicies_GAPs_Standard_for_Medicinal_Plants.pdf (nmpb.nic.in)

- NMPB-AYUSH Ministry GFCP Guidelines-
Good_Field_Collection_Practicies_GFCPs_Standard_for_Medicinal_Plants.pdf (nmpb.nic.in)

CHAPTER 12

WHO Guidelines on Good Herbal Processing Practice for Herbal Medicine 2018

Technical Issues Supporting Good Herbal Processing Practices

Processing facilities

Packaging and labelling

Storage and transportation

Equipment

Quality assurance and quality control

Documentation

Personnel

Other Relevant Issues

Ethical and legal considerations

Research, research training and information sharing

Adoption of good herbal processing practices

Intellectual property rights and benefits-sharing

Threatened and endangered species

Safety management of toxic herbs

Further Reading

Introduction

The safety and quality at every stage of the of herbal medicines production process contribute to efficacy of herbal medicines. These guidelines will provide technical guidance on GHPP in the:

1. processing of herbs into herbal materials;
2. processing of herbal materials into herbal preparations; and
3. processing of herbal materials or herbal preparations into herbal dosage forms.

Under the overall context of quality assurance and control of herbal medicines, the main objectives of these guidelines are to:

- provide general and specific technical guidance on GHPP for herbal medicines;
- provide technical information on general as well as specific good herbal processing techniques and procedures applied to the preparation of herbal materials from herbs;
- provide technical information on good herbal processing techniques and procedures applied to the production of herbal preparations from herbal materials;
- provide supplemental technical information on good herbal processing techniques and procedures applied to the production of dosage forms of herbal medicines;
- provide a model for the formulation of national and/or regional good herbal processing practices guidelines and monographs for herbal materials, as well as for herbal preparations, and related standard operating procedures (SOP); and
- contribute to the quality assurance and control of herbal materials, herbal preparations and herbal dosage forms to promote safety, efficacy and sustainability of herbal medicines.

Definitions of Terms

- **Herbs:** Herbs include crude plant materials such as leaves, flowers, fruits, seed, stem wood, bark, roots, rhizomes or other plant parts, which may be entire, fragmented or powdered.
- **Herbal materials:** Herbal materials include, in addition to herbs, fresh juices, gums, fixed oils, essential oils, resins and dry powders of herbs. In some countries, these materials may be processed by various local procedures, such as steaming, roasting or stir- baking with honey, alcoholic beverages or other plant materials.
- **Herbal preparations:** Herbal preparations are the basis for finished herbal products and may include comminuted or powdered herbal materials, or extracts, tinctures and fatty oils of herbal materials. They are produced by extraction, fractionation, purification, concentration or other physical or biological processes. They also include preparations made by steeping or heating herbal materials in alcoholic beverages and/or honey, or in other materials.
- **Finished herbal products:** Finished herbal products consist of one or more herbal preparations made from one or more herbs (i.e. from different herbal preparations made of the same plant as well as herbal preparations from different plants. Products containing different plant materials are called “mixture herbal products”). Finished herbal products and mixture herbal products may contain excipients in addition to the active ingredients. However, finished products or mixture herbal products to which chemically defined active substances have been added, including synthetic compounds and/or isolated constituents from herbal materials, are not considered to be “herbal”.

Contd..

- **Herbal dosage forms:** Herbal dosage forms are the physical form (liquid, solid, semi-solid) of herbal products produced from herbs, with or without excipients, in a particular formulation (such as decoctions, tablets and ointments). They are produced either from herbal materials (such as dried roots or fresh juices) or herbal preparations (such as extracts).
- **Medicinal plants** are plants (wild or cultivated) used for medicinal purposes.
- **Medicinal plant materials:** see Herbal materials
- **Herbal processing:** Herbal processing refers to the overall treatment in the course of production of herbal materials, herbal preparations and herbal dosage forms. For the purpose of the present guidelines, herbal processing includes "post-harvest processing" described in the WHO guidelines on GACP for medicinal plants, as well as "processing" procedures and protocols set out in the WHO guidelines on GMP for herbal medicines.
- **Post-harvest processing:** Post-harvest processing covers any treatment procedures performed on the herbs after harvest or collection when they are being processed into herbal materials. It includes processes such as inspection, sorting and various primary processing and drying. Often, well-defined combined or serial procedures are applied to herbs before they can be used in therapeutic treatment or as intermediates for manufacturing finished herbal products. These treatment processes are considered important pharmaceutical techniques in the herbal industry, through which purity and/or quality of raw herbs is assured (such as prevention of microbial and insect infection or infestation), and the therapeutic properties of raw herbs are altered (such as enhancement of effectiveness or reduction of toxicity). These primary processing procedures may vary from one herbal material to another, depending on its chemical and pharmacological characteristics, as well as the intended therapeutic purposes.
- **Adjuvants:** Adjuvants are adjunctive substances added during the herbal processing procedures for the purpose of altering the pharmacological or therapeutic properties of the herbal materials, neutralizing or reducing toxicity, or masking the taste, assisting formulation into suitable herbal dosage forms, maintaining stability or extending the storage time. Common adjuvants include water, wine, vinegar, honey, milk and clarified butter, among other materials.
- **Active ingredients** refer to constituents with known therapeutic activity, when they have been identified.
- **Markers (marker substances)** reference substances that are chemically defined constituents of a herbal material. They may or may not contribute to their therapeutic activity. However, even when they contribute to the therapeutic activity, evidence that they are solely responsible for the clinical efficacy may not be available.
- **Master formula** is a document or set of documents specifying the starting materials with their quantities and the packaging materials, together with a description of the procedures and precautions required to produce a specified quantity of a finished product as well as the processing instructions, including the in-process controls.
- **Specification** is a list of defined requirements with which the products or materials used or obtained during manufacture have to conform. They serve as a basis for quality evaluation.
- **Standard operating procedure** is an authorized written procedure giving instructions for performing operations not necessarily specific to a given product or material (for example, equipment operation, maintenance and cleaning; validation; cleaning of premises and environmental control; sampling and inspection). Certain SOPs may be used to supplement product-specific master and batch production documentation.

Good Herbal Processing Practices for the Production of Herbal Materials

General information

Herbs obtained from field collection or cultivation should be subjected to a series of good practice post-harvest processing procedures set out in the GACP guidelines. In general, post-harvest processing of herbs includes inspection and sorting, primary processing and drying. The exact herbal processing procedures may vary from one herb to another. Thus, some procedures consist of only a few simple steps of primary processing such as cleaning, primary cutting and sectioning, before being dried. Others may require more complicated steps such as advanced cutting and sectioning (for example, decoction pieces processing), comminuting, ageing, sweating (fermentation), baking/roasting, boiling/steaming and stir-frying, for the purpose of improving the quality, preventing damage from mound and other microorganisms, detoxifying intrinsic toxic ingredients or enhancing therapeutic efficacy. The present GHPP guidelines elaborate and supplement the GACP guidance.

Purposes and functions of primary processing

Simple post-harvest processing (such as sorting, washing and leaching) serves to remove dirt and other unwanted materials, neutralization of toxicity and diminishing side-effects (raw aconite, Aconitum carmichaelii, Debeaux or related species root, containing significant amounts of toxic alkaloids such as aconitine, must be boiled or steamed for hours to hydrolyze aconitine into less toxic derivatives), modification of therapeutic properties (processed rhubarb can be used in reducing inflammation instead of purgative), enhancing efficacy and reinforcing therapeutic effects (pain-relieving property of corydalis (*Corydalis yanhusuo* W.T. Wang) rhizomes increases when they are stir-fried with rice vinegar)

Post-harvest processing procedures

Raw herbs are subjected to a series of on-site primary processes and exact processing methods may differ from one herb to another. An example of a model format for a GHPP monograph/SOP protocol is given in Appendix 1.

Sorting (garbling) to ensure the purity and cleanliness of the herbs by removing dirt and foreign substances; discarding damaged parts; peeling, sieving, trimming, singeing manually or by mechanical means

Primary processing

Washing, Leaching, Primary cutting, Ageing (storing for long period prior to use), Sweating (like fermentation by keeping the herbal materials at a temperature of 45–65 °C in conditions of high humidity for an extended period, from one week to two months, Example-vanilla beans to undergo repeated sweating between woollen blankets in the sun during the day and packed in wool-covered boxes at night for about two months), parboiling (blanching), boiling or steaming, baking or roasting, stir-frying, fumigation, irradiation, advanced cutting, sectioning and comminution and other primary processing procedures for gums or resins, crude essential oils and expression to obtain fresh juice.

Drying

Drying will also prevent tissue deterioration and phytochemical alteration caused by the actions of enzymes and microbial organisms. It will also facilitate grinding and milling, desired appearance of the final form, and converts the herbal materials into a convenient form for further processing. However, attention must be given to the potential loss of volatile (for example, essential oil) constituents present in the fresh material. The final moisture content for dried herbal materials varies depending on the tissue structure, but should ideally be below 12%. Information on the appropriate moisture content for a particular herbal material may be available from pharmacopoeias or other monographs.

Proper drying involves four major aspects: control of temperature, humidity, airflow and cleanliness of the air. The drying conditions are determined by the nature of the raw medicinal plant material to be dried (tissue structure and chemical composition) and by the. The drying method used may have considerable impact on the quality of the resulting herbal materials. Hence, the choice of a suitable procedure is crucial. Information on appropriate drying methods and procedures for particular herbal materials may be available from pharmacopoeias or other authoritative monographs. Raw herbal materials are most often dried by sun-drying, shade- drying or by artificial heat. The drying conditions chosen should be appropriate to the type of the herbal material. They are dependent on the characteristics (for example, volatility and stability) of the active ingredients and the texture of the plant part collected (for example, root, leaf or flower).

General issues

Selection of processing method: It is commonly found that different processing methods for same plant species show significant differences in quality and therapeutic properties. Hence, prior to processing, it is important to consult the national or regional regulatory standards and other literature sources to decide on the most appropriate method to use. Once a method has been adopted, adherence to the SOP is necessary to ensure batch-to-batch consistency.

Temperature parameters, duration of procedure/treatment and amounts and quality of adjuvants (water, wine, vinegar, honey, ginger juice, ghee, milk, cow's urine, coconut water, lemon juice and mineral materials) affect the quality, safety and contamination of the resulting materials.

Documentation

Written processing records should include, but not be limited to, the following information:

- Name of herbal material – botanical name (binomial – genus, species, with the authority (abbreviations, if used, should follow internationally accepted rules)) and the plant family name of the medicinal plant are essential. If required by national legislation, synonyms and applicable subspecies, variety, cultivar, ecotype or chemotype should be documented; if available, the local and English common names should also be recorded;
- Plant part(s) of the medicinal plant or herb; stage of vegetative development, for example, flowering and fruiting, vegetative maturation;
- Site/geographical location (if possible, based on GPS data,) and time of harvesting/collection;
- State of the medicinal plant or herb (for example, fresh or dried);
- Batch number, batch size and any other identification code;
- Name of supplier;
- Dates of receipt of the material, processing of the material, and completion of the process;

Contd..

- Name of person in charge of the processing, and person in charge of batch release;
- General processes that the plant material has already undergone (for example, drying, washing and cutting, including drying time and temperatures, and size of herbal material);
- Gross weight of the plant material before and after processing;
- Method used for special processing;
- Details of the procedures (master formula), including descriptions of the utensil and equipment used, steps of operation, manufacturer, specification, amount and quality grade of the adjuvant (for example, wine or vinegar) and/or other substances (for example, sand, bran) used, temperature control, length of processing time, after-process steps (for example, cooling, drying, cutting), and other relevant information;
- Details of animal-derived materials or adjuvants used and their microbiological certificates, if applicable;
- Batch production – detail deviations from or modifications of the master formula;
- In-process control, for example, organoleptic changes of the herbal material before and after processing (such as change in colour, shape, texture, odor and taste);
- Quality control parameters, grades and/or specifications, and assay results, where appropriate, of active ingredient(s), markers or chemical reference standard(s);
- Storage conditions and containers; and
- Shelf life/retest period.

Good Herbal Processing Practices for the Production of Herbal Preparations

General information

Herbal preparations are obtained by subjecting the herbal materials to treatments such as extraction, distillation, fractionation, concentration, fermentation, or other physicochemical or biological methods. The resulting preparations include extracts, decoctions, tinctures, essential oils and others.

Preparation of herbal materials for processing

- The quality of herbal materials should meet the requirements specified in the national pharmacopoeia or recommended by other documents of the end-user's country.
- Authentication of herbal materials should be performed prior to extraction. Purity (absence of contaminants) should also be ensured.
- Proper documentation on the herbal material should be available as recommended in section 2.5.
- The herbal material should be cleaned, dried (unless fresh material is required), and comminuted into an optimal size for extraction.
- The herbal materials should be processed as soon as possible after arrival at the processing facility. Otherwise, they must be properly stored to avoid contamination, damage and deterioration (for example, loss of active constituents).

- All operational steps should be reproducible and performed hygienically, in accordance with the processing SOP.

In general, for processes such as extraction, fractionation, purification and fermentation, the rationale for the guidelines should be established on a case- by-case basis. An example of a model format for a good herbal processing practice monograph/SOP protocol to produce a herbal preparation is given as Appendix 2. General guidance is provided below.

Extraction

Extraction is a process in which soluble plant chemical constituents (including those which have therapeutic activity) are separated from insoluble plant metabolites and cellular matrix, by the use of selective solvent (which is sometimes called the menstruum). The purpose of extraction of herbal material is to eliminate unwanted materials and to concentrate other chemical constituents in a soluble form. Herbal extracts include liquid (fluid) extracts, soft extracts, oleoresins, dry extracts and others. The herbal preparations so obtained may be ready for use as medicinal agents, or they may be further processed into herbal dosage forms such as tablets and capsules. Various techniques are used for extraction, including maceration, infusion, digestion, percolation – including hot continuous (Soxhlet) extraction – and decoction. Other extraction techniques can also be applied, for example, heat reflux extraction, counter-current extraction, microwave-assisted extraction, ultrasonic extraction (sonication) and supercritical fluid extraction.

Common methods of extraction (Maceration, Infusion, Percolation, Decoction and Supercritical fluid extraction): The use of appropriate extraction technology, extraction conditions, extraction solvents, ratio between herbal material and solvents, and type of equipment are crucial to produce quality herbal preparations.

Steps involved in the extraction of herbs and herbal materials are comminution, fragmentation, grinding or milling, Extraction (cold or hot), Separation techniques (filtration, decantation, centrifugation or straining), Concentration (evaporation under reduced pressure, freeze-drying or spray-drying)

Common herbal preparations obtained by extraction: The extraction process using suitable solvents can yield herbal extracts of liquid, semi-solid or solid consistency. There are four general categories of herbal extracts, i.e. liquid (fluid) extract, soft extract, oleoresin and dry extract.

1. **Liquid (fluid) extract:** Liquid (fluid) extract is a liquid preparation of herbal materials obtained using water, alcohol or other extraction solvents. Common preparations include:
   - ***Fluid extract***: Fluid extract is an alcoholic liquid extract produced by percolation of herbal material(s) so that 1 mL of the fluidextract contains the extractive obtained from 1 g of the herbal material(s).
   - ***Decoction***: Decoction is a water-based herbal preparation made by boiling herbal materials with water, and is commonly utilized in various traditional medicine contexts. In some cases, aqueous ethanol or glycerol can also be used to prepare decoctions.
   - ***Infusion***: Infusion is a dilute solution prepared by steeping the herbal materials in boiling water for a short time. Infusions prepared in edible oil or vinegar are also available.
   - ***Tincture***: As a general rule, a "tincture" is an alcoholic or hydroalcoholic extract of a herbal material, typically made up of 1 part herbal material and 5–10 parts solvent (for example, ethanol or wine). Tinctures can be prepared by extracting herbal materials usually with ethanol of a suitable concentration. The ratio of water to alcohol should be recorded.

Contd...

- ***Macerate***: Macerate is a liquid preparation prepared by soaking the herbal material(s), reduced to a suitable size, in water at room temperature for a defined period of time, usually for 30 minutes, when not otherwise specified.

2. **Soft extract:** Soft extract is a semi-solid preparation obtained by total or partial evaporation of the solvent from a liquid extract.
3 **Oleoresin:** Oleoresin is a semi-solid material composed of a resin in solution in an essential and/or fatty oil obtained by evaporation of the excess solvent.
4 **Dry extract:** Dry extract is a solid preparation obtained by evaporation of the solvent from a liquid/fluid extract. Dry extract can also be prepared by spray-drying with or without the use of an adsorbent (such as methyl cellulose), or by drying and milling to produce a powder. This may be further processed by compression or with use of a binding agent or granulation liquid to produce multiarticulate granules.

Factors influencing extraction of herbal materials: A number of factors influence the efficiency and reproducibility of the extraction process. Issues to consider include the solvent used to make an extract, particle size of the herbal material, the herb-to-solvent ratio, extraction process used (for example, percolation or maceration), extraction time, temperature and other relevant conditions. All these factors should be optimized and set out in the SOP.

Selection of extraction methods governed by the nature (stability, solubility, structural complexity and other properties of the chemical constituents) and amount of material to be extracted. It should be fast, simple, economical, environment-friendly and reproducible.

Distillation

Water or steam distillation is a method of choice for extracting volatile ingredients from herbs. Volatile oils that may be decomposed during distillation can be obtained by expression (mechanical pressing), solvent extraction, supercritical carbon dioxide extraction or by the enfleurage process suitable for delicate flowers.

Fractionation

Fractionation to separate mixture into a number of smaller quantities (fractions) can be achieved by liquid–liquid partition and various forms of chromatography. The method can be applied to produce preparations enriched in active compounds, or to remove inactive and/or toxic constituents.

Concentration and drying

Removal of excess solvent as soon as possible after extraction by evaporation or vaporization to enrich extracts/fractions with active ingredients is main objective of concentration step. For complete drying, use vacuum freeze-dryers (lyophilizers), cabinet vacuum dryers, continuously operating drum or belt dryers, microwave ovens or atomizers. Free flowing dry extract powders are obtained by drying the extract onto an inert excipient (methyl cellulose, maltodextrin etc.) to facilitate processing into the final finished product. Choice of technique depend on chemical and thermal stability of chemical constituents of interest.

Fermentation

Fermentation can be either natural (mixing with the juice of sugar- cane, brown sugar or honey and the mixture in an airtight utensil for several weeks) or by introducing an appropriate microbial organism (for example, Lactobacillus bacteria or yeast). Use non-corrosive utensils. Follow optimized and controlled temperature and length of fermentation.

Advanced cutting and powdering

Advanced cutting and powdering (or grinding) of the crude drug to a desirable uniform particle size facilitates the process of extraction and the preparation of dosage forms such as capsules. Various types of grinding machines can be utilized depending on the hardness, size, heat stability, friability and structural features of the plant part and output characteristics.

Processing documentation

An SOP including all processing steps should be adopted and documented in the Master Record. Batch records should be kept and any deviations from the SOP should be fully recorded and investigated. Name(s) of all operators, and the dates and time at which each step or stage are carried out should be documented. Herbal preparations documentation includes, as a minimum, the following information:

- Botanical information as specified in section 2.5;
- Batch number, batch size, and any other identification code;
- Supplier;
- Dates of receipt of the herbal material, processing of the material, and completion of the process;
- Name of person in charge of the processing;
- Name of quality assurance manager; and person in charge of batch release;
- Previous processes that the herbal material has already undergone;
- Characteristics of the herbal preparation (such as type of preparation, ratio of the herbal material to the herbal preparation, organoleptic characters);
- Methods used for processing to produce herbal preparation;
- Details of the procedures (master formula), including quantity of herbal materials, extraction solvent, additive, descriptions of the steps of operation, operational conditions used during the process, and other relevant information;
- Weight or amount of the herbal preparation;
- Batch production: give details of deviations or modifications of the master formula;
- Quality control parameters (such as identification tests, tests on water content and impurities, residual solvents, microbial contamination tests, shelf life), acceptance limits of the tests and quantitative assay results of active ingredients, markers or chemical reference standard(s);
- Storage conditions and containers; and
- Shelf life and retest period.

Good Herbal Processing Practices for the Production of Herbal Dosage forms

General information

In contrast to synthetic pharmaceutical preparations, certain herbal materials and herbal preparations may undergo simpler good practice processes to become suitable dosage forms and final products for administration. However, these dosage forms should be produced under applicable GMP conditions. Starting materials for the preparation and production of various herbal dosage/final dosage forms should consist of good quality medicinal plants cultivated or collected as prescribed by GACP. They should have been subjected to post-harvest processing, followed by further processing into herbal materials or herbal preparations under GHPP as described previously. Examples of a number of herbal dosage forms are presented in the Japanese Pharmacopoeia. The following describes some common dosage forms of herbal medicines. National and regional regulations and GMP guidelines must be followed for the production of finished products.

Preparation of liquid herbal dosage forms

Type of Preparation	Preparation Method
Fluidextract	Fluidextracts are prepared by percolation of herbal material(s) using an aqueous alcoholic menstruum. After being thoroughly moistened, the mixture is packed firmly into a percolator and covered with additional menstruum. It is macerated for 24 hours, then percolated at a moderate rate, adding fresh menstruum as necessary to completion. The first 700–800 mL of the percolate should be reserved for use to dissolve the residue from the additional percolate that has been concentrated to a soft extract at a temperature not exceeding 60°C. The extract is adjusted with menstruum, if necessary, so that it satisfies the requirements for content of solvent (in a ratio of one part (1.0 mL) of liquid to one part (1.0 g) of the herbal material). They may be filtered, if necessary.
Decoctions	In many traditional medicine contexts, decoctions are prepared by boiling the herbal materials in water for a certain period of time, after which they are strained and taken directly by the patients. The amounts of water used and the length of boiling are generally specified by the practitioners on a case-by- case basis.
Infusions	Infusions are prepared by macerating the herbal materials for a short period of time with warm or boiling water.
Tinctures	Tinctures are usually prepared by either maceration or percolation, using ethanol, wine or a hydroalcoholic mixture to extract the herbal material, or by dissolving a soft or dry extract of the herbal material in ethanol of the required concentration. Tinctures are adjusted, if necessary, so that they satisfy the requirement for content of solvent (1 part of herbal material and 5–10 parts of solvent). They may be filtered if necessary.
Syrups	Syrups are usually prepared by adding sucrose (at least 45% m/m) to the herbal solution or decoction, and then heating and straining it. Other polyol sweetening agents may be used. Sufficient purified water is then added to yield a product of the desired weight or volume. Syrups should be made in quantities that can be consumed within a reasonable period of time. If necessary, syrups may contain approved preservatives to prevent bacterial and mound growth
Oral emulsions	Various techniques can be applied to uniformly disperse one liquid in another immiscible liquid in the form of small droplets throughout the other. When emulsions are prepared, energy must be expended to form an interface between the oily and aqueous phases. Emulsification equipment includes a wide variety of agitators, homogenizers, colloid mills and ultrasonic devices.
Aromatic waters	Usually, an essential oil (1 part) is shaken in recently distilled water (999 parts) and set aside for 12 hours or longer after mixing with 10 parts of talcum powder. The solution is filtered and made up to a certain volume with water. Aromatic waters will deteriorate over time due to volatilization, decomposition or mould growth. They should, therefore, be made in small quantities for immediate use and protected from intense light, excessive heat and stored in airtight, light- resistant containers, if necessary.

Preparation of solid herbal dosage forms

Solid dosage forms as described here are those that are most commonly found in herbal medicine, but they are not limited to the following categories.

Type of Preparation	Preparation Method
Herbal tea bags	Herbal materials (for example, dried roots, leaves or flowers) are put into paper or cloth bags. Herbal tea bags should be free of bleach, gluten and dioxin. Metallic pins, used for attaching a piece of thread to the tea bag, should be avoided as this may release unsafe cations into the solution. When used, boiling water is poured into the vessel or cup containing the bag.
Plant powders	In many traditional medicine systems, ground powders of herbal materials are taken directly by patients as a dosage form. Powders are ground into various coarse or fine particle sizes, excluding nano powder.
Dry extract powders (powdered extracts)	Dry extract powders are prepared by spray-drying or freeze-drying of a fluid extract with or without the use of an adsorbent (such as methyl cellulose), or by drying and milling to produce a powder. Excipients are often used for purposes such as improving taste or facilitating the packaging step.
Granules	In the typical manufacture of granules, the dried liquid extract is blended with diluents, binders or other suitable excipients, then wetted with an appropriate binding solution or solvent to promote agglomeration. The composition is dried and sized to yield the desired material properties.
Pills	Pills may be prepared by trituration of dried powdered herbs or dry extract powders with suitable powdered excipients in serial dilution to attain a uniform mixture. Liquid excipients that act to bind and provide plasticity are added to the dry materials, and kneaded to form a mass. Typically, pills are swallowed with warm water.
Capsules	Capsules are prepared by enclosing a plant powder, or homogeneous dry extract powder or granules with excipients in a suitable capsule base such as gelatin, of a particular shape and size. In the case of gel capsules, liquid extract or soft extract can also be encapsulated. The process is carried out using specialized equipment.
Tablets	Tablets are usually prepared by mixing the homogeneous dry extract powder, plant powder or granules with excipients such as diluents and binders, followed by compression into a defined shape and size. Tablets may be coated or uncoated.
Lozenges	In the typical preparation of lozenges, sucrose (or another excipient such as sorbitol) is cooked with the herbal extract and water. Flavoring and coloring agents are added and thoroughly mixed while cooling. Individual units of the desired shape are formed by filling the molten mass into moulds. Care should be taken to avoid excessive moisture during storage to prevent crystallization of the sugar base.

Preparation of other herbal dosage forms

Type of Preparation	Preparation Method
Ointments, creams and salves	Ointments and creams can be formulated with a herbal extract or powder and a variety of oils and emulsifying agents. Preparation usually involves heating, mixing and stirring the lipid and aqueous portions until the mixture has congealed. They usually require the addition of preservative unless they are intended to be used within a relatively short period of time.
Inhalations	Dry powder inhalers are prepared by pulverizing dry extracts into fine particles. When necessary, lactose or other suitable excipients are added to make a homogeneous mixture. Inhalation liquid preparations are usually prepared by mixing dry herbal extracts with a vehicle and suitable pH-adjusting agents to make a solution or suspension. Suitable preservatives may be added to prevent the growth of microorganisms.
Plasters and patches	A dry or soft extract of herbal preparation is spread uniformly on an appropriate support that is usually made of a rubber base of synthetic resin. Plasters are available in a range of sizes or cut to size to effectively provide prolonged contact with the site of application. They adhere firmly to the skin but can be peeled off without causing injury.
Medicated oils	A fine paste of powdered herb or herbal material(s) together with a given media (if any, such as water, milk or fresh juices or decoctions of herbal materials) is mixed in a prescribed quantity of oil and macerated or boiled slowly with continuous stirring until complete removal of water or moisture (as the case may be). The oil is then decanted or strained while warm through muslin cloth and allowed to cool.

Technical Issues Supporting Good Herbal Processing Practices

Processing facilities

The ideal design and construction of a "post-herbal processing" facility descriptions are presented in Appendix 3. Additionally, relevant descriptions of a facility for processing herbal preparations and herbal dosage forms are provided in Appendix 4.

Packaging and labelling

Processed herbal materials, herbal preparations and herbal dosage forms should be packaged as quickly as possible to preserve their quality in non-polluted, clean, dry and undamaged, and conforming to the quality requirements. An appropriate label affixed to the packaging should include name, date of processing, name of processor or manufacturer, storage batch number, expiry date etc. The label should also contain information indicating quality approval and compliance with national and/or regional labelling requirements. Finished herbal product labelling should comply with the national/ regional regulation/requirements. Records should be kept of batch packaging, and should include the product name, place of origin, batch number, weight, assignment number and date. The records should be retained for a period of three years or as required by national and/or regional authorities.

Storage and transportation

All processed herbal medicines should be properly stored, preserved and comply with the "first-in and first-out" principle for use. They must be protected from pests, physical damage, moisture, light, heat, insect and animal attack. Separate quarantined area should be designated to rejected samples, Toxic or controlled herbal materials or preparations should be checked, labelled and stored according to the government's regulations. All refrigerated spaces should be equipped with temperature measurement and recording devices.

Equipment

All equipment, including tools and utensils used in the herbal processing procedures should be made of non-toxic, non-absorbent; non-corrosive materials.

Quality assurance and quality control

In general, compliance with quality assurance measures should be verified through regular internal oversight personnel (quality assurance manager) and external auditing visits to processing facilities by expert representatives of buyers and other stakeholders, and through inspection by national and/or local regulatory authorities.

Documentation

The SOPs should be adopted and documented. All methods and procedures used in the herbal processing including post-processing transportation, storage, the dates on which they are carried out and inspection report should be documented.

Personnel

All personnel should receive proper training in post-harvest handling, herbal processing, potentially toxic or allergenic herbs, safety, materials handling, sanitation, protective clothing, and hygiene and should perform tasks in compliance with local, national and/or regional regulations. All new staff should pass a medical examination. Personnel known or suspected to be suffering from or to be a carrier of a disease or illness likely to be transmitted, should not be allowed to work until deemed medically appropriate. Smoking, drinking and eating should not be permitted in herbal processing areas. Visitors to processing and handling areas should wear appropriate protective clothing and adhere to all of the personal hygiene provisions mentioned above.

Other Relevant Issues

Ethical and legal considerations

All herbal processing must be carried out in accordance with applicable legal and environmental requirements and with the ethical codes or norms of the community and country in which the activities take place.

Research, research training and information sharing

Research to understand and gain knowledge on the mechanism and scientific basis of processing procedures, new and better processing techniques and procedures, chemical conversion mechanism due to processing, GHPP for individual herbs or herbal materials and to document each in a monograph are strongly encouraged. Technical information resulting from research on processing methods is useful for promoting technical advancement, and should be shared through publication, conferences or otherwise conveyed to interested stakeholders.

Adoption of good herbal processing practices

Member States or nations that have not adopted GHPP for herbal medicines are encouraged to establish or adopt such practices as part of quality assurance and control measures, as well as a part of their regulatory requirements for herbal medicines.

Intellectual property rights and benefits-sharing

Agreements on intellectual property rights and the return of benefits and compensation for the use of source herbal materials or herbal preparations concluded in writing by the sourcing contractor, shall be acknowledged.

Threatened and endangered species

The processor shall ascertain and obtain appropriate documentation of relevant permission from the sourcing contractor about such materials.

Safety management of toxic herbs

The toxic herbal materials and their preparations or dosage forms have narrow therapeutic windows between effective dose and lethal dose. Examples- Powdered Digitalis and Digitalis Capsules. Hence, special attention and safety management measures are required like processor must use such materials under supervision, must be trained for proper processing procedures for the purpose of neutralizing the toxicity or reducing the side-effects prior to use and immediate proper medical treatment if poisoning and/or accidents occur.

Further Reading

1. WHO guidelines on good agricultural and collection practices (GACP) for medicinal plants. Geneva: World Health Organization; 2003.
2. WHO guidelines on assessing quality of herbal medicines with reference to contaminants and residues. Geneva: World Health Organization; 2007.
3. WHO guidelines for selecting marker substances of herbal origin for quality control of herbal medicines. In: WHO Expert Committee on Specification for Pharmaceutical Preparations: fifty-first report. Geneva: World Health Organization; 2017: Annex 1 (WHO Technical Report Series, No. 1003).
4. WHO good manufacturing practices (GMP): supplementary guidelines for the manufacture of herbal medicines. In: WHO Expert Committee on Specifications for Pharmaceutical Preparations: fortieth report. Geneva: World Health Organization; 2006: Annex 3 (WHO Technical Report Series, No. 937).
5. WHO guidelines on good manufacturing practices (GMP) for herbal medicines. Geneva: World Health Organization; 2007.

6. WHO good manufacturing practices (GMP): supplementary guidelines for the manufacture of herbal medicines. In: WHO Expert Committee on Specifications for Pharmaceutical Preparations: fifty-second report. Geneva: World Health Organization; 2018: Annex 2 (WHO Technical Report Series, No. 1010).
7. Quality control methods for herbal materials. Geneva: World Health Organization; 2011.
8. Good manufacturing practices for pharmaceutical products: main principles In: WHO Expert Committee on Specifications for Pharmaceutical Preparations: forty-eighth report. Geneva: World Health Organization; 2014: Annex 2 (WHO Technical Report Series, No. 986).
9. Safety issues in the preparation of homeopathic medicines. Geneva: World Health Organization; 2009.
10. The International Pharmacopoeia, seventh edition. Geneva: World Health Organization; 2017.
11. WHO monographs on selected medicinal plants, volume 1. Geneva: World Health Organization; 1999.
12. WHO monographs on selected medicinal plants, volume 2. Geneva: World Health Organization; 2002.
13. WHO monographs on selected medicinal plants, volume 3. Geneva: World Health Organization; 2007.
14. WHO monographs on selected medicinal plants, volume 4. Geneva: World Health Organization; 2009.
15. WHO monographs on selected medicinal plants commonly used in the Newly Independent States (NIS). Geneva: World Health Organization; 2010.
16. General guidelines for methodologies on research and evaluation of traditional medicine Geneva: World Health Organization; 2000 (WHO/EDM/TRM/2000.1)
17. European Medicines Agency 2006a. Guideline on Quality of Herbal Medicinal Products/Traditional Herbal Medicinal Products (CPMP/QWP/2819/00 Rev)
18. European Medicines Agency 2006b. Guideline on Specifications: Test Procedures and Acceptance Criteria for Herbal Substances, Herbal Preparations and Herbal Medicinal Products/Traditional Herbal Medicinal Products (CPMP/QWP/2820/00 Rev)
19. European Medicines Agency 2008. Reflection Paper on Markers used for Quantitative and Qualitative Analysis of Herbal Medicinal Products and Traditional Herbal Medicinal Products (EMEA/HMPC/253629/2007).
20. WHO guidelines on good herbal processing practices for herbal medicines. WHO Technical Report Series, No. 1010, 20

Scan QR code to view the website/guidelines

- WHO guidelines on good herbal processing practices for herbal medicines-

trs1010-annex1-herbal-processing.pdf (who.int)

CHAPTER 13

WHO Good Storage and Distribution Practices 2019

Introduction

Storage and distribution are important activities in the supply chain management of medical products. Various people and entities are generally responsible for handling, storage and distribution. Products may be subjected to various risks at different stages in the supply chain, i.e. during purchasing, storage, distribution, transportation, repackaging, and relabelling. Every activity in the storage and distribution of medical products should be carried out according to the principles of Good Manufacturing Practices (GMP), Good Storage Practice (GSP) and Good Distribution Practice (GDP) as applicable. This guideline does not deal with dispensing to patients as this is addressed in the World Health Organization (WHO) Good Pharmacy Practice (GPP) guide (xx). These guidelines should also be read in conjunction with other WHO guidelines (xx).

Scope

This document lays down guidelines for the storage and distribution of medical products for human and for veterinary use. The guidelines thus cover products for which a prescription is required by the patient, products which may be provided to a patient without a prescription, biologicals, vaccines and medical devices. The document does not specifically cover GMP aspects of finished products in bulk, distribution of labels or packaging as these aspects are considered to be covered by other guidelines. The principles for the distribution of starting materials (active pharmaceutical ingredients (APIs) and excipients) are also not covered here. These are laid down in the WHO guidance "Good Trade and Distribution Practices for Pharmaceutical Starting Materials".

Glossary

The various definitions provided in this guidelines apply to the words and phrases used in this guideline.

General Principles

The principles of GSP and GDP should be included in national legislation and guidelines for the storage and distribution of medical products, in a country or region as applicable, as a means of establishing minimum standards. The principles of GSP and GDP are applicable to:

- Working document
- Products moving forward in the distribution chain from the manufacturer;
- Products which are moving backwards in the chain, for example, as a result of the return or recall thereof; and
- Donations of products.

Quality Management

Entities involved in the storage and distribution of medical products must have an authorized, written quality policy describing the overall intentions and requirements regarding quality. This may be reflected in a quality manual. There should be an appropriate organizational structure. This should be presented in an authorized organizational chart. The responsibility, authority, interrelationships, duties and responsibilities of all personnel should be clearly indicated. The quality system should include appropriate procedures, processes and resources.

Quality Risk Management

There should be a system to assess, control, communicate and review risks identified at all stages in the supply chain based on scientific knowledge and experience with the process and ultimately linked to the protection of the patient.

Management Review

There should be a record-based system for periodic management review involving senior management, quality system and its effectiveness by using quality metrics and key performance indicators, continual improvement, and follow-up on recommendations from previous management review meetings.

Complaints

There should be a written procedure for the handling of complaints separately about a product or its packaging and distribution. All complaints should be recorded, risk assessed, informed to concerns including national regulatory authority if required and appropriately investigated.

Returned Goods

Returned medical products should be placed in quarantine upon receiving and handled in accordance with authorized procedures. A risk-based process should be followed when deciding on the fate of the returned goods. Destruction of products should be done in accordance with international, national and local requirements regarding disposal of such products and with due consideration to the protection of the environment. Records of all returned, rejected and destroyed medical products should be kept for a defined period.

Recalls

There should be a written procedure for the handling of recall medical products under well-defined responsibility. All recall products should be recorded, risk assessed, informed to concerns including national regulatory authority if required, appropriately transported, stored in secure, segregated conditions and clearly labelled.

Self-inspection

Self-inspections for implementation and compliance with the principles of regulations, GSP, GDP and other appropriate guidelines by non-biased individual members with appropriate knowledge and experience are integral part of quality system. The results containing all observations of all self-inspections should be recorded.

Premises

General

Premises should be suitably located, designed, constructed and maintained to ensure appropriate operations such as receiving, storage, picking, packing and dispatch of medical products. There should be sufficient space, lighting, ventilation, cleanliness, security, sufficient protection from weather conditions and pests. There should be appropriate controls for segregation, handling or storage of radio-active or other hazardous substances. Each incoming delivery should be checked and documented for purchase order, each container, label description, batch number, product and quantity. There should be appropriate designated space for returned, rejected and destroyed medical products.

Storage areas

Storage areas should be appropriately designed, constructed, maintained or adapted for various categories of materials like starting and packaging materials, intermediates, finished products, products in quarantine, and released, rejected, returned or recalled products. It should have sufficient safety measures, cleaning facilities, hazardous material control, temperature control, relative humidity control strategies depending upon products. The "first expired/first out" (FEFO) principle should be followed.

Storage conditions

The storage conditions for materials and medical products should be in compliance with the labelling, which is based on the results of stability testing. Heating, ventilation and air conditioning systems (HVAC) should be appropriately designed, installed, qualified, monitored at regular intervals and maintained to ensure that the required storage conditions are maintained. Data should be recorded and the records should be reviewed. All records pertaining to mapping and monitoring should be kept for a suitable period of time and as required by national legislation.

Stock Control and Rotation

Periodic stock reconciliation should be performed at defined intervals by comparing the actual and recorded stocks to identify discrepancies and inform to person responsible for quality.6666

Equipment

Equipment, including computerized systems should be appropriately designed, located, installed, qualified, maintained and suitable for their intended use. Procedures should be followed, and records maintained for the back-up and restoration of data.

Qualification and Validation

The scope and extent of qualification and validation should be determined using a documented risk assessment approach. Premises, utilities, equipment and instruments, processes and procedures should be considered and deviations should be investigated.

Personnel

There should be an adequate number of personnel with appropriate educational qualification, experience and training relative to the safety, health, personal hygiene and all job-related activities undertaken.

Documentation

Documentation means all procedures and records, either in paper or electronic form, should be prepared and maintained in accordance with the national legislation and principles of good documentation practices. Documents should be appropriately designed, completed, signed, dated, reviewed, authorized, distributed, accurate, legible, traceable, attributable, readily available and kept as required.

Activities and Operations

All activities and operations relating to procurement, storage and distribution of medical products should be conducted by authorized persons in accordance with documented procedures and national legislation, GSP, GDP and associated guidelines.

Repackaging and re-labelling

Repackaging and re-labelling of materials and products are not recommended. If allowed then should only be performed by authorized entities in compliance with the applicable national, regional and international requirements, and in accordance with GMP. Original packaging should be disposed to prevent re-use. Where feasible, consideration should be given to adding technology, such as global positioning system (GPS) electronic tracking devices and engine-kill buttons to vehicles, which would enhance the security and traceability of vehicles with products. Where possible, mechanisms should be available to allow for the segregation during transit of rejected, recalled and returned products as well as those suspected as falsified.

Outsourced Activities

Any activity relating to the storage and distribution of a medical product which is delegated to another person or entity should be performed by authorized parties, in accordance with national legislation, and the terms of a written contract.

Substandard and Falsified Products

The quality system should include procedures to assist in identifying, handling, storing and avoiding re-enter in market for materials that are suspected to be substandard and or falsified. Where these materials and products are identified, the holder of the marketing authorization, the manufacturer and the appropriate national and/or international regulatory bodies, as well as other relevant competent authorities, should be informed. Records should be maintained reflecting the investigations and action taken, such as disposal of the material or products.

Inspection of Storage and Distribution Facilities

Storage and distribution facilities should be inspected by authorized inspectors having appropriate educational qualifications, knowledge and experience in terms of compliance with national legislation, GSP, GDP and related guidelines (GxP) as appropriate. An inspection report should be prepared and provided to the inspected entity within 30 days from the last day of the inspection. Observations may be categorized based on risk assessment. Inspections should be closed with a conclusion after the review of the CAPAs.

Further Reading

1. World Health Organization. Good Storage and Distribution Practices. May 2019. https://www.who.int/medicines/ areas/ quality_safety/quality_assurance/qas19_793_ good_storage_and_ distribution_ practices_may_2019.pdf?ua=1

2. Guidelines on Good Distribution Practices For Pharmaceutical Products. Central Drugs Standard Control Organization Directorate General of Health Services, Ministry of Health and Family Welfare, Government of India, FDA Bhawan, ITO, Kotla Road, New Delhi -110002.
3. Good storage and Distribution for Drug Products, General Information-Good Storage and Distribution Practices USP-36. Available at:https://pharmacy.ks.gov/docs/default-source/defaultdocument-library/ups-36-good-storage-and-shipping-practices.pdf
4. Competition issues in the distribution of pharmaceutical- Russian Federation Available at: www.oecd.org/official document/public displaydocumentspdf/?col
5. WHO Technical Report Series No 961- Temperature mapping of storage areas Available at: www.who.int/..../areas/...TS-mapping – storage-area-final-sigh-off-a-pdf
6. HPRA- Guide to control and monitoring of storage and Transportation Temperature conditions for Medicinal products and active substances. Available at: https://www.hpra.ie/.../ia-g0011- guide-to-control-and-monitoring-of-storage-and-tran.
7. WHO 1991. Guidelines for the Assessment of Herbal Medicines. World Health Organization,
8. WHO 1995. Guidelines for Good Clinical Practice (GCP) for Trials on Pharmaceutical Products. World Health Organization, WHO Technical Series, No. 850, 1995, Annex 3. WHO 1999. WHO Expert Committee on Specifications for Pharmaceutical Preparations - WHO Technical Report Series, No. 885 – 35th Report. World Health Organization WHO 2009. Joint FAO/WHO Expert Committe on Food Additives: Evaluation of Certain Food Additives - WHO Technical Report Series, No. 952 - 69th Report. World Health Organization,
9. World Health Organization Research Office for the Western Pacific 1993. Research Guidelines for Evaluating the Safety and Efficacy of Herbal Medicines.

Scan QR code to view the website/guidelines

- WHO Good storage and distribution Practices- https://www.who.int/medicines/areas/quality_safety/quality_assurance/qas19_793_good_storage_and_distribution_practices_may_2019.pdf?ua=1

CHAPTER 14

Herbal Monograph, Pharmacopoeias, Markers

Herbal Monograph

Introduction

The following concepts are important in the development and setting of specifications and should be provided for each herbal monograph. The monograph should include: Title, Definition, Limits of active ingredients, Marker compounds, Description, Category, Identification, Chemical Tests, Assay of the marker constituents, Contaminants, Specific Tests, and Additional Requirements if any.

Monograph Title

For monographs intended for inclusion in pharmacopoeias, the title of the monograph should include the Latin binomial nomenclature or Synonym or Common Name whichever is appropriate and is followed by the name of plant part(s) or plant product (e.g., resin, gum-resin), and where applicable the processed form.

Definition

Some or all of the following are usually included in the definition: the state of the drug: whole, fragmented, peeled, cut, fresh or dried; the complete scientific name of the plant (genus, species, subspecies, variety, author); commonly used synonyms may be mentioned the part or parts of the plant used where appropriate, the stage in the growth cycle when harvesting takes place, or other necessary information wherever possible, the minimum content of quantifiable constituents (either responsible for the biological activity of the herb (bio-marker) or a chemical compound known to be present in the herb even if not responsible for biological activity (chemical/ analytical marker). Herbal drugs very often contain a mixture of related substances, in which case the total content of quantifiable constituents is determined and expressed as one of the constituents, usually the major constituent; separate limits may be given for different forms of the drug (whole/cut)

Characters: This section contains a brief description of the organoleptic characters of the drug such as colour, odour, taste etc.

Category: It includes the therapeutic/prophylactic category of the drug.

Identification: The purpose of the Identification in a monograph is to ensure that the article under examination is in agreement with what is stated in the Definition of the article. All the identifications mentioned below are not necessarily included: some may be absent when they are not feasible or are not significant for the purpose of identification. Macroscopic and microscopic requirements of an herbal monograph should be provided in detail with colour photographs.

Macroscopic: The important macroscopic botanical characters of the drug are specified to permit a clear identification. When two species/subspecies of the same plant are included in the definition, the individual differences between them are indicated.

Microscopic: It involves gross microscopic examination of the drug and it can be used to identify the organized/ unorganized drugs by their known histological characters. It is mostly used for qualitative evaluation of organized crude drugs in entire and powder forms with help of microscope. It involves using microscope for detecting various cellular tissues and their arrangements such as trichomes, stomata, starch granules and calcium oxalate crystals etc. Crude drug can also be identified microscopically by cutting the thin TS (transverse section)/ LS (Longitudinal section) especially in case of wood. Quantitative aspects of microscopy include study of stomatal number and index, palisade ratio, vein-islet number, size of starch grains and length of fibers etc.

Fingerprinting: Chromatographic or spectroscopic patterns, sometimes referred to as "fingerprints", may be used as standards for identification. These fingerprints can be obtained by HPLC, UHPLC, capillary electrophoresis, GC, TLC/HPTLC, IR, and Mass Spectroscopy.

The fingerprints must be able to distinguish these materials from other materials with potential for species substitution and suspected adulteration. The acceptance criteria for identification tests using chromatographic methods such as HPLC, UHPLC, capillary electrophoresis or GC methodology must contain a description of the critical features of the fingerprint chromatograms such as the presence of specified peaks, retention time, their order of elution, and where possible, their relative abundance. For methods of TLC/HPTLC, description must include colour and position of the characteristic bands. A colour image of a typical TLC/HPTLC chromatogram should be provided. A critical aspect of the identification of herbal materials by separation techniques is the use of reference standards for comparison.

In addition to the Sample solution, a Standard solution containing the reference standard is chromatographed concomitantly. The reference material used in the Standard solution may be an Authenticated Botanical Reference Substances (BRS), a reference standard extract, a single chemical entity, or a standardized mixture of substances.

Tests

- ***Physicochemical Evaluation:*** It is an important parameter in detecting adulteration or improper handling of drugs. It can serve as a valuable source of information and provide appropriate standard to establish the quality of herbs. These are:
- ***Extractable matter:*** It is considered useful to determine extractable matter only in herbal drugs where no constituent suitable for an assay is known or where the material is used to produce a preparation with a dry residue.
- ***Total ash:*** This test is always included unless otherwise justified. It is to be carried out on the powder drug.
- ***Acid- insoluble ash***: This test may be carried out depending on the nature of the particular herbal drug and is used to detect unacceptable quantities of certain minerals.
- ***Loss on Drying***: Herbal drugs are dried for preservation purposes. If they are insufficiently dried, growth of yeasts or moulds may occur. It is the loss of weight expressed as percentage w/w resulting from water and volatile matter of any kind that can be driven off under specified conditions. The limit is specified on the basis of the results obtained on a reasonable number of varied samples of acceptable quality.
- ***Swelling Index:*** Applicable to certain hydrocolloid-containing herbal drugs.
- ***Bitterness values:*** Applicable to herbal drugs containing bitter principles.

Contaminants- General

- ***Foreign Organic Matter***. It is the material consisting of any or all of the following:
- Parts of the organs from which the drug is derived other than the parts named in the definition and description or for the limit are prescribed in the individual monograph. Any part of organs other than those named in the definition and description. Matter not coming from the source plant and Moulds, insects or other animal contamination.
- Generally a limit of 2% of foreign matter is imposed, unless otherwise prescribed in a specific monograph. Where a limit for foreign matter greater than 2% is to be prescribed, it is stated in the specific monograph with an indication of the type of foreign matter. Where necessary, the monograph should indicate how the foreign matter is identified.
- ***Heavy Metals:*** The test is prescribed where there is the potential for contamination by heavy metals. The limit of heavy metals is indicated in the individual monograph in terms of ppm.
- ***Microbial contamination***: The Pharmacopoeial monographs should specify the total count of aerobic microorganisms, the total count of yeasts and molds, and the absence of specific pathogenic bacteria (e.g., *Staphylococcus aureus*, *Escherichia coli*, *Pseudomonas aeruginosa*, *Shigella* and *Salmonella* species)
- ***Contaminants- Specific:*** An individual herbal monograph may require certain specifications that are peculiar to that monograph, especially when safety is an issue. Limits may be set in certain specific monographs for the characters that are undesirable or have negative botanic characteristics. When one desires a limit for harmful substances that are present either naturally in the substance or formed as a result of postharvest processing practices, such submissions must be accompanied by toxicity data.

Assay

Wherever possible, an assay is included. Assay is carried out using suitable instruments such as UV-Visible spectrophotometer, LC, GC or by HPTLC system etc.

Additional Information

- ***Storage***: Storage conditions are applicable unless otherwise specified: store protected from light. Where applicable, additional specific conditions are given in the individual monograph.
- ***Labelling***: Labelling of herbal products includes the label both upon the immediate container and other associated labeling and written, printed or graphic materials. The label states the Latin binomial followed by the authorized name; the plant part(s), plant product, or processed form contained in the container or from which the article was derived. Content in percentage of active principles or marker compounds should be stated. Labelling should be in accordance with the applicable drug laws.

Pharmacopoeias

Introduction

Pharmacopoeia: the word derives from the ancient Greek φαρμακοποιΐα (pharmakopoiia), from φαρμακο- (pharmako-) "drug", followed by the verb-stem ποι- (poi-) "make" and finally the abstract noun ending -ια (-ia). These three elements together can be rendered as "drug-mak-ing" or "to make a drug". A pharmacopoeia, pharmacopeia, or pharmacopoea, in its modern sense, is a legally binding collection, prepared by a national or regional authority, of standards and quality specifications for medicines used in that country or region.

A quality specification is composed of a set of appropriate tests that will confirm the identity and purity of the product, ascertain the strength (or amount) of the active substance and, when needed, its performance characteristics. Reference substances, i.e. highly-characterized, physical specimens, are used in testing to help ensure the quality, such as identity, strength and purity, of medicines. The texts cover pharmaceutical starting materials, excipients, intermediates and finished pharmaceutical products (FPPs). General requirements may also be given in the pharmacopoeia on important subjects related to medicines quality, such as analytical methods, microbiological purity, dissolution testing, stability, etc. The role of a modern pharmacopoeia is to furnish quality specifications for active pharmaceutical ingredients (APIs), FPPs and general requirements, e.g. for dosage forms. The existence of such specifications and requirements is necessary for the proper functioning or regulatory control of medicines.

Some popular herbal pharmacopoeias of world are American Herbal Pharmacopoeia (AHP), British Herbal Pharmacopoeia (BHP), Korean Herbal Pharmacopoeia (KHP), etc. The AHP develops qualitative and therapeutic monographs on botanicals, including many of the Ayurvedic, Chinese, and Western herbs most frequently used in the United States. These monographs represent the most comprehensive and critically reviewed body of information on herbal medicines in the English language, and serve as a primary reference for academicians, health care providers, manufacturers, and regulators. Monographs of the BHP provide quality standards for 169 herbal raw materials. Subsequent work by the European Pharmacopoeia Commission (Council of Europe) has led to the introduction of many more herbal monographs in the European Pharmacopoeia. BHP is a very useful aid to quality assurance, particularly for herbs not featured in official pharmacopoeias. The third edition Korean Herbal Pharmacopoeia (KHP) contains total of 384 official monographs. The Indian Herbal Pharmacopoeia has 40 monographs published by Indian Drugs Manufacturers Association (IDMA) in collaboration with Regional Research Laboratory (RRL), Jammu. Most of the popular Indian Traditional systems of medicine has been developing pharmacopoeias for herbs used in it.

WHO and Pharmacopoeia

Pharmacopoeial requirements form a base for establishing quality requirements for individual pharmaceutical preparations in their final form. Index of pharmacopoeias published by World Health Association, Geneva has a comprehensive list of pharmacopoeias of different countries. According to the information available to the World Health Organization (WHO), 140 independent countries are at present employing some 30 national as well as the African, European and International Pharmacopoeias. Compared to national and regional pharmacopoeias, The International Pharmacopoeia (Ph. Int.) is issued by WHO as a recommendation with the aim to provide international standards – including less technically demanding alternatives where needed - for adoption by Member States and to help achieve a potentially global uniformity of quality specifications for selected pharmaceutical products, excipients and dosage forms.

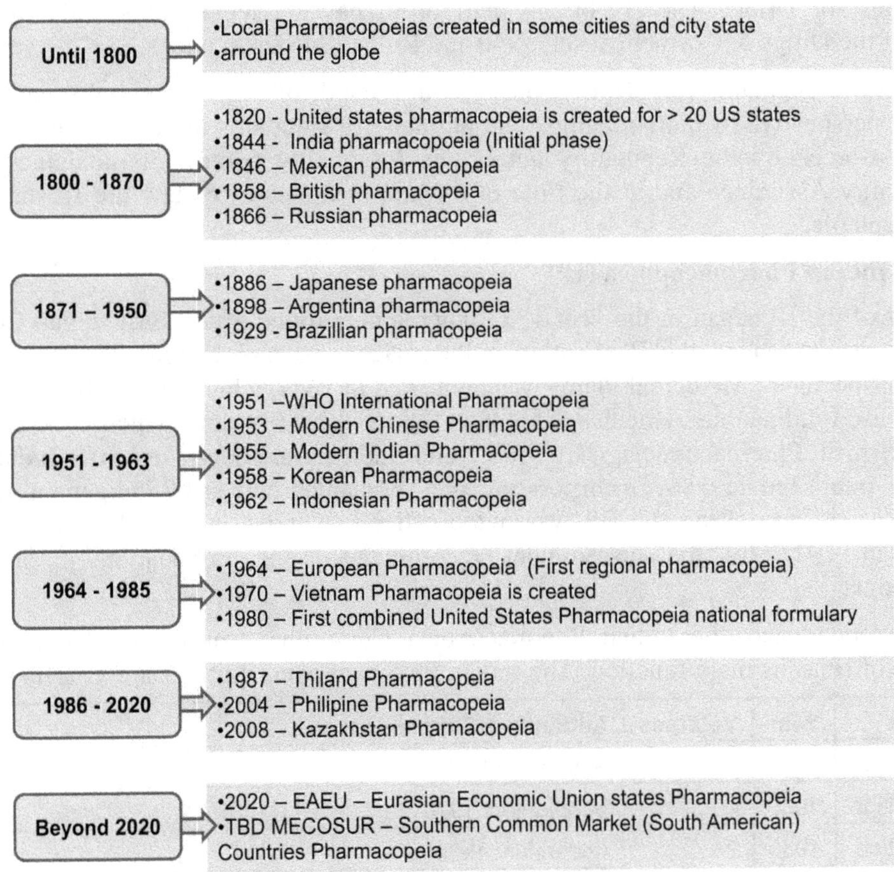

Figure 14.1 Timeline of Pharmacopeia development.

Indian Pharmacopoeia (IP)

In 1970, Pharmacopoeial Laboratory of Indian Medicine was formed to ensure standardization and testing of ASU drugs. Several others government recognized laboratories are also involved to lay down pharmacopoeial standards, preparation of monographs and Standard Operating Procedures (SOPs) for ASU drugs. Pharmacopoeial committees for ASU systems involve in the lay down of standards for quality, purity and strength of drugs and approve drug formularies. Pharmacopoeial Laboratories, Central Council for Research in Ayurveda and Siddha (CCRAS) laboratories, laboratories of Central Council for Research in Unani Medicine (CCRUM), Council for Scientific & Industrial Research (CSIR) laboratories and several other laboratories of private sector are involved in the mammoth job of controlling and maintaining of quality, formulation of standard for ensuring safety and quality of polyherbal/herbomineral preparations.

Indian Pharmacopoeia (IP) is an official document meant for overall Quality Control and Assurance of Pharmaceutical products marketed in India by way of contributing on their safety, efficacy and affordability. IP contains a collection of authoritative procedures of analysis and specifications for Drugs. The IP, or any part of it, has got legal status under the Second Schedule of the Drugs & Cosmetics Act, 1940 and Rules 1945 there under.

IP prescribes standards for identity, purity and strength of drugs essentially required from health care perspective of human beings and animals. IP standards are authoritative in nature. They are enforced by the Regulatory authorities for quality control of medicines in India. During Quality Assurance and at the time of dispute in the court of law the IP standards are legally acceptable.

History of Indian Pharmacopoeia (IP)

The history of the IP began in the year 1833 when a committee of the East Indian Company's Dispensary recommended the Publication a Pharmacopoeia and Bengal Pharmacopoeia and General Conspectus of Medicinal Plants was published in 1844, which mainly listed most of the commonly used indigenous remedies. This was followed by IP 1868, which covered both the drugs of British Pharmacopoeia (BP) 1867 and indigenous drugs used in India, with a supplement published in 1869 incorporating the vernacular names of indigenous drugs and plants. However, from 1885 the BP was made official in India. A drug Enquiry Committee appointed in 1927 by the government recommended the publication of a National Pharmacopoeia.

After independence, the Indian Pharmacopoeia Committee was constituted in 1948, for publication of IP as its main function. The Indian Pharmacopoeia editions are as follows: -

Edition	Year	Volumes	Addendum/Supplement
1st Edition	1955	-	Supplement 1960
2nd Edition	1966	-	Supplement 1975
3rd Edition	1985	2	Addendum 1989
			Addendum 1991
4th Edition	1996	2	Addendum 2000
			Vet Supplement 2000
			Addendum 2002
			Addendum 2005
5th Edition	2007	3	Addendum 2008
6th Edition	2010	3	Addendum 2012 and DVD of Indian Pharmacopoeia 2010
7th Edition	2014	4	Addendum 2015
			Addendum 2016
8th Edition	2018	4	Addendum 2019
			Addendum 2021

Addendum 2021 to IP 2018 contains a total of 66 new drug monographs [including 59 Chemical, 05 Herbs & Herbal Products, and 02 Blood & Blood-Related Products] and 04 new General Chapters. In addition, a total of 260 monograph amendments have also been included in the content of the IP Addendum 2021 that would further upgrade the quality of drug standards included in the IP.

Inclusion of monograph on herbal drug in Indian Pharmacopeia and formulation of Herbal Pharmacopeia are also a major step to achieve the goal. Along with pharmacopoeias and formularies other publications like 'Production of ISM Drugs with Current Good Manufacturing Practices', 'Quality Standards of Indian Medicinal Plants' could also be useful to maintain the standard and quality of ISM.

List of Monographs on Herbals in IP 2014

Raw Herbs			
1. Acacia	18. Birmi	35. Ivy Leaf	52. Punarnava
2. Ajwain	19. Brahmi	36. Kalmegh	53. Sahajana Leaf
3. Amalaki	20. Coleus	37. Kaunch	54. Sahajana Stick
4. Amaltas	21. Daruharidra Roots	38. Kundru	55. Shankhpushpi
5. Amra	22. Daruharidra Stems	39. Kutki	56. Sarpagandha
6. Anantmula	23. Draksha	40. Lasuna	57. Saunf
7. Arjuna	24. Ergot	41. Lavang	58. Senna Leaf
8. Artemisia	25. Garcinia	42. Lodhra	59. Senna Pods
9. Ashwagandha	26. Ginseng	43. Mandukaparni	60. Shatavari
10. Asthisamhrta	27. Gokhru	44. Manjistha	61. Shati
11. Bakuci	28. Gudmar	45. Maricha	62. Sunthi
12. Bala	29. Guduchi	46. Methi	63. Tulasi
13. Bassant	30. Guggul resin	47. Mirch	64. Valerian Root
14. Belladona Leaf	31. Haridra	48. Nagakesar	65. Vasaka
15. Bhibhitaki	32. Haritaki	49. Neem	66. Vidanga
16. Bhringraj	33. Hingu	50. Pippali Large	67. Vijayasara
17. Bhuiamla	34. Ispaghula Husk	51. Pippali Small	68. Yasti

Herbal extracts processed herbs/ Pharmaceutical aids/formulations	
1. Amla Juice Powder	16. Ivy Leaf Dry Extract
2. Arjuna Dry Extract	17. Kalmegh Dry Extract
3. Ashwagandha Dry Extract	18. Senna Dry Extract
4. Bassant Dry Extract	19. Sunthi Extract
5. Belladonna Dry Extract	20. Tulasi Dry Extract
6. Belladonna Soft Extract	21. Valerian Dry Extract
7. Bhibhitaki Aqueous extract	22. Vasaka Extarct
8. Brahmi Extract	23. Yasti Dry Extract
9. Coleus Dry Extract	24. Opium
10. Garcinia Aqueous extract	25. Bhuiamla Dry Extract
11. Ginseng Dry Extract	26. Gudmar Dry Extract
12. Gugulipid	27. Kunduru Dry Extract
13. Haridra Dry extract	28. Mandukaparani Dry Extract
14. Haritaki Aqueous extract	29. Malt Extract
15. Haritaki Extract	

Oil	
1. Arachis oil	21. Lemon Oil
2. Basil Oil	22. Lime Oil
3. Belladonna Tincture	23. Mentha Oil
4. Black pepper oil	24. Mentha Arvensis Oil
5. Caraway Oil	25. Nutmeg Oil
6. Cardamom Oil	26. Papain
7. Castor Oil	27. Peppermint Oil
8. Clove Bud Oil	28. Rosemary Oil
9. Clove Leaf Oil	29. Sarpagandha Powder
10. Clove Stem Oil	30. Sarpagandha Tablets
11. Coconut Oil	31. Shellac
12. Coriander Oil	32. Starch
13. Cumin Oil	33. Thyme Oil
14. Dill Seed Oil	34. Tolu Balsam
15. Prepared Ergot	35. Tragacanth
16. Eucalyptus oil	36. Opium powder
17. Guar Gum	37. Ipecac Tincture
18. Hydrogenated Castor Oil	38. Gugulipid Tablets
19. Lavender Oil	39. Senna Tablets
20. Lemon Grass Oil	

The United States Pharmacopeia (USP)

It is a pharmacopeia (compendium of drug information) for the United States published annually by the United States Pharmacopeial Convention (usually also called the USP), a nonprofit organization that owns the trademark and copyright. The USP is published in a combined volume with the National Formulary (a formulary) as the USP-NF. If a drug ingredient or drug product has an applicable USP quality standard (in the form of a USP-NF monograph), it must conform in order to use the designation "USP" or "NF." Drugs subject to USP standards include both human drugs (prescription, over-the-counter, or otherwise), as well as animal drugs. USP-NF standards also have a role in U.S. federal law; a drug or drug ingredient with a name recognized in USP-NF is deemed adulterated if it does not satisfy compendial standards for strength, quality or purity. USP also sets standards for dietary supplements, and food ingredients (as part of the Food Chemicals Codex). USP has no role in enforcing its standards; enforcement is the responsibility of FDA and other government authorities in the U.S. and elsewhere.

In the USP-NF

- Total Monographs: About 4,500
- Monographs for APIs: 1402
- Monographs for Finished Dosage Forms: 2454 in
- USP, 446 Excipients in NF
- Monographs for Biologicals: 153
- General Chapters: About 300
- Supplementary Texts: General Notices, Reagents,
- Indicators, and Solutions, Description and Solubility

The European Pharmacopoeia

(Pharmacopoeia Europaea, Ph. Eur. is a major regional pharmacopoeia which provides common quality standards throughout the pharmaceutical industry in Europe to control the quality of medicines, and the substances used to manufacture them. It is a published collection of monographs which describe both the individual and general quality standards for ingredients, dosage forms, and methods of analysis for medicines. These standards apply to medicines for both human and veterinary use. The 1st Edition of the European Pharmacopoeia was published in 1969, and comprised 120 texts. The 9th Edition, was published in July 2016 and is currently in force. It contains some 2,300 monographs, and more than 350 general chapters, illustrated with diagrams or chromatograms, and over 2,500 descriptions of reagents. With 121 new and 1,403 revised texts, over 50 percent of the 9th Edition's content is new compared to the 8th Edition. It consists of three initial volumes (9.0), and will culminate in a collection of eight non-cumulative supplements (9.1 to 9.8). A new edition is published every three years: in both English and French, by the Council of Europe.

Ayurveda, Siddha and Unani (ASU) Drug Pharmacopoeias and Formulary

ASU drug pharmacopoeias and formulary contains pharmacognostical, chemical and standards of the plant drugs. These pharmacopoeias and formularies contain information about the biological source, synonyms, description, TLC, important formulation, therapeutic indication, and details related to identity, purity, strength. Recently, chromatographic fingerprint profile as a supplementary to Ayurvedic Pharmacopoeia was also published. Identification and estimation of active therapeutic ingredients and marker compounds with reference to which drugs of Ayurveda, Siddha and Unani can be standardized are still developing and all these parameters are being added to pharmacopoeias.

Ayurvedic Pharmacopoeia of India (API) has monographs for 600 plant/animal/mineral derived drugs (Part I, Vol 1 to 8). Monographs for 152 compound Ayurvedic formulations are published in Ayurvedic Pharmacopoeia of India (Part II, Volume 1 to 3). Other than API, Siddha Pharmacopoeia of India (Volume 1 and 2), Homeopathic Pharmacopoeia of India (Volume 1 to 6) and Unani Pharmacopoeia of India (Volume 1 to 6) are the standards of books available for Indian herbs. The pioneering work Quality standards of Indian Medicinal plants by Indian Council of Medical Research (ICMR) is a non pharmacopoeial masterpiece for reference on standards of Indian herbs. Monographs on 449 plants (Volume 1 to 13) included in the book would help in improving monographs in API and other Pharmacopoeias of Indian origin. The Pharmacopoeia Commission for Indian Medicine (PCIM) under ministry of AYUSH is fully functional now to improve Pharmacopoeias for Indian Herbs

Ayurvedic Pharmacopoeia of India (Part I contain eight volumes and Part II contain three volume of compound formulation)

1. The Ayurvedic Pharmacopoeia of India Part I, Vol. I 2001
2. The Ayurvedic Pharmacopoeia of India Part I, Vol. II 2001
3. The Ayurvedic Pharmacopoeia of India Part I, Vol. III 2001
4. The Ayurvedic Pharmacopoeia of India Part I, Vol. IV 2004
5. The Ayurvedic Pharmacopoeia of India Part I, Vol. V 2006
6. The Ayurvedic Pharmacopoeia of India, Part II, Vol. I (Formulation) 2007

7. The Ayurvedic Pharmacopoeia of India Part I, Vol. VI 2008
8. The Ayurvedic Pharmacopoeia of India Part I, Vol. VII 2008
9. The Ayurvedic Pharmacopoeia of India, Part II, Vol. II (Formulation) 2009
10. The Ayurvedic Pharmacopoeia of India, Part II, Vol. III (Formulation) 2010
11. The Ayurvedic Pharmacopoeia of India Part I, Vol. VIII 2011
12. The Ayurvedic Pharmacopoeia of India, Part II, Vol. I (Hindi) 2011
13. The Ayurvedic Pharmacopoeia of India, Part II, Vol. II (Hindi) 2011

Ayurvedic Formulary of India

1. The Ayurvedic Formulary of India – Part I (2nd Revised Edition) 2003
2. The Ayurvedic Formulary of India – Part II 2000
3. The Ayurvedic Formulary of India – Part III 2012

Other official books

1. Thin layer Chromatographic Atlas of Ayurvedic Pharmacopoeial Drugs Part I, Vol. I 2009
2. Macroscopic & Microscopic Atlas of Pharmacopoeial Drugs Part I, Vol. V
3. Macroscopic & Microscopic Atlas of Pharmacopoeial Drugs Part I, Vol. I 2011

Unani Pharmacopoeia of India (Part I on signal drug contain six volume, Part II on formulation contain two volume), Unani Formulary of India (Part I–VI),

(a) National Formulary of Unani Medicine

1. National Formulary of Unani Medicine, Part-I (Size 107 MB)
2. National Formulary of Unani Medicine, Part-II (Size 0.5 MB)
3. National Formulary of Unani Medicine, Part-III (Size 21 MB)
4. National Formulary of Unani Medicine, Part-IV (Size 31 MB)
5. National Formulary of Unani Medicine, Part-V (Size 1.5 MB)
6. National Formulary of Unani Medicine, Part-VI (Size 1.3 MB)

(b) Unani Pharmacopoeia of India, Part-I (Single Drugs)

1. Unani Pharmacopoeia of India, Part-I, Vol.1 (Size 1 MB)
2. Unani Pharmacopoeia of India, Part-I, Vol.2 (Size 12.40 MB)
3. Unani Pharmacopoeia of India, Part-I, Vol.3 (Size 11.70 MB)
4. Unani Pharmacopoeia of India, Part-I, Vol.4 (Size 1 MB)
5. Unani Pharmacopoeia of India, Part-I, Vol.5 (Size 1.25 MB)
6. Unani Pharmacopoeia of India, Part-I, Vol.6 (Size 1.52 MB)

(c) Unani Pharmacopoeia of India, Part-II (Formulations)

1. Unani Pharmacopoeia of India, Part-II, Vol.1 (Size 1.35 MB)
2. Unani Pharmacopoeia of India, Part-II, Vol.2 (Size 1.44 MB)

(d) List of books proposed for incorporation in first schedule of drug and cosmetic act, 1940

Siddha Pharmacopoeia of India (volume I and II), Siddha Formulary of India (Part I & II) are playing a significant role in this area.

The Siddha Pharmacopoeia of India, Part I, Vol. I 2008

Markers in Standardization of Herbal Products

Insufficient information is available about the chemical constituents of most medicinal plants for guaranteeing their quality, safety, and efficacy. Therefore, it is necessary to establish comprehensive standards for assessing the quality of herbal drugs. Due to the complexity of phytomedicines, only a small group of compounds is chosen for quality purposes. Chemical and pharmacological studies represent useful tools for the selection of chemical markers for addressing the quality evaluation of medicinal plants. Phytochemical standardization encompasses all possible information generated with regard to the chemical constituents present in an herbal drug. Hence, the phytochemical evaluation for standardization purpose includes the following:

1. Preliminary testing for the presence of different chemical groups.
2. Quantification of chemical groups of interest (Example- total alkaloids, total phenolics, total triterpenic acids, total tannins).
3. Establishment of fingerprint profiles.
4. Multiple marker-based fingerprint profiles.
5. Quantification of important chemical constituents

Markers are chemically defined constituents of a herbal material utilized for control purposes. They may or may not contribute to the clinical efficacy. When they contribute to the clinical efficacy, however, evidence that they are solely responsible for the clinical efficacy may or may not be available. Markers are generally employed when constituents of known therapeutic activity are not known or are not clearly identified, and may be used to identify the herbal material or preparation or calculate their quantity in the finished product.

Types of Marker Compounds:

1. **Active Chemical Constituents as Marker:** One or a few of the compounds specific to the drug that are proved to be responsible for the claimed activity of the respective herbal drug like, vasicine and vasicinone from *Adhatoda vasica*, bacosoids from *Bacopa monnieri*, tylophorine from *Tylophora indica*, homoharringtonine from *Cephalo taxus*, camptothecin from *Camptotheca acuminate*, conessine from *Holarrhena antidysentrica*, morphine and codeine from *Papaver somniferum*, sarsasapogenin, asparanin A and asparanin B from *Asparagus adscendens*, shatavarin from *Asparagus racemosus*, atropine from *Atropa belladonna*, glycyrrhizin from *Glycyrrhiza glabra*, aloin from *Aloe vera*, protodioscin from *Tribulus terrestris*, sophoradin from *Sophora subprostrata*, quinine from *Cinchona* spp., trigonelline from *Trigonella foenum-graecum*, catechin from *Acacia catechu*, withanolides from *Withania somnifera*, tinosporic acid from *Tinospora*

cordifolia, cocaine from *Erythroxylum coca*, aegelin and marmelosin from *Aegle marmelos*, pristimerin from *Celastrus paniculata*, asiaticoside from *Centella asiatica*, emetine from *Cephaelis ipecacuanha*, psoralen from *Psoralea corylifolia*, glycyrrhizin from *G. glabra*, boeravinones from *Boerrhavia diffusa*, berberine from *Berberis aristata*, plumbagin from *Plumbago indica*, curcumin from *Curcuma longa*, podophyllin from *Podophyllum emodi*, jatamansone from *Nardostachys jatamansi*, quassinoids from *Ailanthus* spp., arjunolic acid from *Terminalia arjuna*, gingerols from *Zingiber officinale*, digoxin and digitoxin from *Digitalis lantana*, paclitaxel from *Taxus baccata* and *Taxus brevifolia,* allicin from *Allium sativum*, nimbidin from *Azadirachta indica*, forskolin from *Coleus forskohlii,* pilocarpine from *Pilocarpus jaborandi*, Dysobinin from *Dysoxylum binectariferum*, Diosgenin from *T. foenum-graecum* and plants of Dioscorea spp., vinblastine and vincristine from *Catharanthus rose*us and many more.

Medicinal Plants and their Chemical Markers mentioned in Indian Pharmacopeia 2014			
Sr. No.	**Plant Name**	**Markers Compound**	**Assay Used**
1.	Acacia	Quercetin, Rutin	HPTLC
2.	Aloe	Aloe emodin, Barbaloin	HPTLC
3.	Ashwagandha	Withanolide	HPLC
4.	Boswellia	α and β Amyrins and Boswellic acid	TLC
5.	Bramhi	Bacoside A	HPTLC
6.	Blue cherry	Procyanidine	TLC
7.	Clove	Caryophyllene, eugenol	GCMS
8.	Cardamom	γ- terpinene	HPTLC
9.	Cumin	p-cymine	TLC
10.	Cinnamon	d- α-phalandrene	TLC
11.	Dhatura	Dhaturametelin A and B	TLC
12.	Funnel	α -pinene, β-pinene	HPTLC
13.	Ginger	Gingerol, Shogaol	TLC
14.	Garlic	Allicin, Allyl Disulphide	TLC
15.	Gunja	Abraline	TLC
16.	Hingu	Piperine	TLC
17.	Haridra	Curcumin	TLC
18.	Kurchi	Conessine	TLC
19.	Liquorice root	Glycyrrhizine	TLC
20.	Marica	Chavicine, Piperdine	TLC
21.	Nutmeg	Myristicin	TLC
22.	Nux vomica	Brucine and Strychnine	TLC
23.	Katuka	Picrorhizine	TLC
24.	Piper root	Piperlongumine	TLC
25.	Senna	Senoside B	HPTLC
26.	Salmali	Saponins	TLC
27.	Yew	Taxine	TLC
28.	Vasaka	Vasicine and vasicinol	TLC
29.	Tulsi	β -Caryophyllene	TLC

2. **Chemical Markers:** Compounds reported from the respective drugs, although not specific to the drug, and activity specific to the drug has also not been proven (e.g., hederagenin, lapachol, cucurbitacins, rutin, quercetin). New classification suggests eight categories of chemical markers, namely (1) therapeutic components, (2) bioactive components, (3) synergistic components, (4) characteristic components, (5) main components, (6) correlative components, (7) toxic components, and (8) general components used with fingerprint spectrum.

Classification of chemical markers

1. Therapeutic components	Therapeutic components possess direct therapeutic effects of herbal medicine. They may be used as chemical markers for both qualitative and quantitative assessments. Example: Quinine in Cinchona
2. Bioactive components	Many structurally different bioactive components contribute to the therapeutic effects. Individual components may not have direct therapeutic effects. Hence, bioactive components may be used as chemical markers for qualitative and quantitative assessment. Example: Withanoloids from Ashwagandha
3. Synergistic components	Synergistic components do not contribute to the therapeutic effects or related bioactivities directly. However, they act synergistically to reinforce the bioactivities of other components, thereby modulating the therapeutic effects of the herbal medicine. Synergistic components may be used as chemical markers for qualitative and quantitative assessment. Example: Flavonoids from many plants
4. Characteristic components	While characteristic components may contribute to the therapeutic effects, they must be specific and/or unique ingredients of an herbal medicine. Example: Cordiofolioside from Giloy
5. Main components	Main components are the most abundant in an herbal medicine (or significantly more abundant than other components). They are not characteristic components and their bioactivities may not be known. Main components may be used for both qualitative and quantitative analysis of herbal medicines especially for differentiation and stability evaluation. Example: Gallic acid from many plants
6. Correlative components	Correlative components in herbal medicines have close relationship with one another. For example, these components may be the precursors, products or metabolites of a chemical or enzymatic reaction. Correlative components can be used as chemical markers to evaluate the quality of herbal medicines originated from different geographical regions and stored for different periods of time. Example: Tannins from many plants
7. Toxic components	Toxic chemical constituents present in plants may responsible for nephrotoxicity, heptotoxicity or other toxic effects can be used as marker. Example: Aconitine form Aconite rhizomes
8. General components used with fingerprint spectrum.	General components are common and specific components present in a particular species, genus or family. These components may be used with 'fingerprints' for quality control purposes. Example: Hyoscine and Hyocyamine from Solanaceae plants

3. **General Markers:** Compounds widely present in many plants (e.g. Quercetin, rutin, gallic acid, lupeol, stigmasterol, β-sitosterol) for which some activity may or may not be reported. For those plants for which active principles are known, their presence in the sample can be ascertained by co-chromatography and comparison of the Rf and absorption spectra with that of the standards of the marker compounds. Wherever active principles are not known, fingerprint profiles can include the general marker compounds. In addition, to have a complete picture of phytochemical profile, in the former case the fingerprint profiles should also include the other marker compounds.

Single or Multiple Marker-Based Evaluation

Single active or chemical marker based analysis is helpful in standardisation of raw material or extracts or single plant containing herbal formulations. But plants have complex mixtures of chemical compounds hence multiple-marker based analysis has recently been gaining importance. The multiple markers of a drug are usually a mixture of active principles and chemical markers. A few examples include quantification of four alkaloids of Cinchona officinalis stem bark.

Further Reading

1. The United States Pharmacopeia-National Formulary. USP 39-NF 34. Volume 1. Rockville: The United States Pharmacopeial Convention; 2016.
2. World Health Organization. The International Pharmacopoeia 9th ed. [Internet]. 2019; Available from: http://apps.who.int/phint/pdf/b/7.5.3.5.2-Uniformity-of-mass-for-single-dose-preparations.pdf.
3. British Pharmacopoeia Commission. British Pharmacopoeia 2016. Volume 5. London: The Stationery Office; 2015.
4. British Pharmacopoeia Commission. British Pharmacopoeia 2019. Volume 5. London: The Stationery Office; 2018.
5. Chan SSK, Li SL, Lin G. Pitfalls of the selection of chemical markers for the quality control of medicinal herbs. J Food Drug Anal. 2007;15:365–71.
6. Council of Europe. 2014. European pharmacopoeia. 8th ed. Strasbourg: Council of Europe.
7. Desai S, Tatke P. Phytochemical Markers: Classification, Applications and Isolation. Curr Pharm Des. 2019;25(22):2491-2498. doi: 10.2174/1381612825666190709203239. PMID: 31584364.
8. Dhamia N, Mishra AD. Phytochemical variation: How to resolve the quality controversies of herbal medicinal products? Journal of Herbal Medicine. 2015: 5; 118–127. Schwarz M, Klier B, Sievers H. Herbal reference standards. Planta Med. 2009 Jun;75(7):689-703.
9. European Medicines Agency 2006a. Guideline on Quality of Herbal Medicinal Products/Traditional Herbal Medicinal Products (CPMP/QWP/2819/00 Rev)
10. European Medicines Agency 2006b. Guideline on Specifications: Test Procedures and Acceptance Criteria for Herbal Substances, Herbal Preparations and Herbal Medicinal Products/Traditional Herbal Medicinal Products (CPMP/QWP/2820/00 Rev)

11. European Medicines Agency 2008. Reflection Paper on Markers used for Quantitative and Qualitative Analysis of Herbal Medicinal Products and Traditional Herbal Medicinal Products (EMEA/HMPC/253629/2007).
12. European Pharmacopoeia 8th ed. Volume 1. Strasbourg: Council of Europe; 2014.
13. European Pharmacopoeia 9th ed. Volume 1. Strasbourg: Council of Europe; 2017.
14. Hakamatsuka T. Standardization of Crude Drugs for the Japanese Pharmacopoeia. Yakugaku Zasshi. 2020;140(6):783-788. Japanese.
15. Helliwell K 2006. Herbal Reference Standards. Pharmeuropa 2: 235-238.
16. https://www.indianpharmacopoeia.in/index.php Accessed 20 Feb 2021
17. Jai Prakash Sushma Srivastava R.S. Ray Neha Singh Roshni Rajpali Gyanendra Nath Singh. Current Status of Herbal Drug Standards in the Indian Pharmacopoeia. Phytother Res. 2017 Dec;31(12):1817-1823
18. Joshi VK, Joshi A, Dhiman KS. The Ayurvedic Pharmacopoeia of India, development and perspectives. J Ethnopharmacol. 2017 Feb 2;197:32-38.
19. Leong F, Hua X, Wang M, Chen T, Song Y, Tu P, Chen XJ. Quality standard of traditional Chinese medicines: comparison between European Pharmacopoeia and Chinese Pharmacopoeia and recent advances. Chin Med. 2020 Jul 28;15:76.
20. Lu TL, Li JC, Yu JY, Cai BC, Mao CQ, Yin FZ. Application of traditional Chinese medicine reference standards in quality control of Chinese herbal pieces. Zhongguo Zhong Yao Za Zhi. 2014 Jan;39(1):149-52.
21. Montoro P, Sonia P, Cosimo P. 2012. Herbal medicines: development and validation of plant-derived medicines for human health. In: Quality issues of current herbal medicines. Boca Ratón (Florida): Taylor & Francis Group. Chapter 22; p. 413–438.
22. Rai N, Joshi SK, Sharma RK. Regulatory Requirements for Quality Control of Unani Medicines. J AOAC Int. 2020 Jun 1;103(3):634-648.
23. Roth L, Adler M, Jain T, Bempong D. Monographs for medicines on WHO's Model List of Essential Medicines. Bull World Health Organ. 2018 Jun 1;96(6):378-385. doi: 10.2471/BLT.17.205807. Epub 2018 Mar 28.
24. Ruparel P, Lockwood B 2011. The quality of commercially available herbal products. Nat Prod Commun 6: 733-744.
25. Sahoo N, Manchikanti P, Dey S 2010. Herbal drugs: Standards and regulation. Fitoterapia 81: 462-471
26. Sgamma T, Lockie-Williams C, Kreuzer M, Williams S, Scheyhing U, Koch E, Slater A, Howard C. DNA Barcoding for Industrial Quality Assurance. Planta Med. 2017 Oct;83(14-15):1117-1129.
27. Steinhoff B. Review: Quality of herbal medicinal products: State of the art of purity assessment. Phytomedicine. 2019 Jul;60:153003.
28. Suzuki H, Satake M. Determination of crude drugs in the pharmacopoeia. Eisei Shikenjo Hokoku. 1996;(114):145-6..
29. Tandon N, Yadav SS. Contributions of Indian Council of Medical Research (ICMR) in the area of Medicinal plants/Traditional medicine. J Ethnopharmacol. 2017 Feb 2;197:39-45.
30. Vivekanandan K, Prakash J, Muthusamy K, Singh GN. Quality Standards and Current Status of Ophthalmic Formulations in Indian Pharmacopoeia and National Formulary of India. Ther Innov Regul Sci. 2014 May;48(3):386-392. doi: 10.1177/2168479013513455.

31. World Health Organization [WHO]. 2000. General guidelines for methodologies on research and evaluation of traditional medicine. Geneva, Switzerland: WHO Press; p. 1–71.
32. World Health Organization [WHO]. 2011. Quality control methods for herbal materials. Geneva, Switzerland: WHO Press; p. 1–137.
33. World Health Organization. The International Pharmacopoeia 5th ed. [Internet]. 2015; Available from: http://apps.who.int/phint/pdf/b/2.7.The-International-Pharmacopoeia,-Fifth-Edition.pdf

Scan QR code to view the website/guidelines

- Herbal Monographs-
  Herbs and Herbal Products Monographs/General Chapters - Indian Pharmacopoeia Commission (ipc.gov.in)

- Good Pharmacopoeial Practices-
  TRS 1010 - Annex 7: WHO good pharmacopoeial practices: Chapter on herbal medicines

CHAPTER 15

WHO Guidelines for Selecting Marker Substances of Herbal Origin for Quality Control of Herbal Medicines 2017

Background

With the constant increase in the use of herbal medicines worldwide and the rapid expansion of the global market for them, the safety and quality of herbal materials and finished herbal products has become a major concern for health authorities, pharmaceutical industries and the public. The safety and efficacy of herbal medicines largely depend on their quality. Requirements and methods for quality control of finished herbal products, particularly for mixture herbal products, are far more complex than for chemical medicines. The quality of finished herbal products is also influenced by the quality of the raw materials used.

Objectives

The objectives of this document are to:

1. Provide selection criteria for marker substances of herbal origin for quality control of herbal medicines;
2. Identify methods and techniques for the identification and assay of these substances;
3. Provide examples of selected marker substances in selected herbal materials;
4. contribute to the technical guidance on methodologies for quality control of herbal materials, herbal preparations and finished herbal products, in order to meet the quality control requirements;
5. Promote the safety and efficacy of herbal medicines by contributing to consistent and reproducible quality.

Glossary and Terms

Medicinal plants are plants (wild or cultivated) used for medicinal purposes

Medicinal plant materials: See Herbal materials

Herbal medicines include herbs and/or herbal materials and/or herbal preparations and/or finished herbal products in a form suitable for administration to patients

Note: In some countries herbal medicines may contain, by tradition, natural organic or inorganic active ingredients that are not of plant origin (e.g. animal and mineral materials).

Herbs are crude plant material which may be entire, fragmented or powdered. Herbs include, e.g. the entire aerial part, leaves, flowers, fruits, seeds, roots, bark (stems) of trees, tubers, rhizomes or other plant parts.

Herbal materials include, in addition to herbs, other crude plant materials. Examples of these other plant materials include gums, resins, balsams and exudates.

Herbal preparations are produced from herbal materials by physical or biological processes. These processes may be extraction (with water, alcohol, supercritical carbon dioxide (CO^2)), fractionation, purification, concentration, fermentation and other processes. They also include processing herbal materials with a natural vehicle or steeping or heating them in alcoholic beverages and/or honey, or in other materials. The resulting herbal preparations include, among others, simply comminated (fragmented) or powdered herbal materials as well as extracts, tinctures, fatty (fixed) or essential oils, expressed plant juices, decoctions, cold and hot infusions.

Finished herbal products consist of one or more herbal preparations made from one or more herbs (i.e. from different herbal preparations made of the same plant as well as herbal preparations from different plants. Products containing different plant materials are called "mixture herbal products.

Finished herbal products and mixture herbal products may contain excipients in addition to the active ingredients. However, finished products or mixture herbal products to which chemically defined active substances have been added, including synthetic compounds and/or isolated constituents from herbal materials, are not considered to be "herbal

Substitute is a herbal material or herbal preparation that is replaced by another, appropriately labelled herbal material, or herbal preparation consistent with the national pharmacopoeia, or traditional (or complementary and alternative) medicine practice.

Adulterant is herbal material, an herbal constituent or other substance that is either deliberately or non-intentionally (through cross-contamination or contamination) added to a herbal material, herbal preparation, or finished herbal product.

Constituents are chemically defined substances or group(s) of substances found in a herbal material or herbal preparations.

Therapeutic activity refers to the successful prevention, diagnosis and treatment of physical and mental illnesses. Treatment includes beneficial alteration or regulation of the physical and mental status of the body and development of a sense of general well-being as well as improvement of symptoms.

Active ingredients refer to constituents with known therapeutic activity, when they have been identified. Where it is not possible to identify the active ingredients, the whole herbal medicine may be considered as one active ingredient.

Constituents with known therapeutic activity are substances or group(s) of substances which are chemically defined and known to contribute to the therapeutic activity of the herbal material or of a preparation.

Constituents with recognized pharmacological (biological) activities are characteristic constituents (substances or group(s) of substances) which are chemically defined and where the relevance of the pharmacological (biological) activities for the therapeutic or toxicological effects of the herbal material or herbal preparation has not yet been fully established.

Characteristic constituents are chemically defined substances or group(s) of substances that are specific for one medicinal plant or for certain plant species, families or genera.

Toxic constituents are substances or group(s) of substances that are chemically defined and their toxic property is predominant, although they may contribute to the therapeutic activities of the herbal material or herbal preparation.

Reference substances are chemically defined molecular entities (appropriate for intended uses in standardization or quality control of herbs and herbal materials).

Markers (marker substances) are reference substances that are chemically defined constituents of a herbal material. They may or may not contribute to the therapeutic activity. However, even when they contribute to the therapeutic activity, evidence that they are solely responsible for the clinical efficacy may not be available.

Primary chemical reference substances are substances that are widely acknowledged to have the appropriate qualities within a specified context, and whose assigned content when used as a (mostly as an assay) standard is accepted without requiring comparison to another chemical substance.

Secondary chemical reference substances (also called working standards) are substances whose characteristics are assigned and/or calibrated by comparison with a primary chemical reference substance. The extent of characterization and testing of a secondary chemical reference substance may be less than for a primary chemical reference substance

International Chemical Reference Substances (ICRS) are primary chemical reference substances established on the advice of the WHO Expert Committee on Specifications for Pharmaceutical Preparations. They are supplied primarily for use in physical and chemical tests and assays described in the specifications for quality control of medicines published in The International Pharmacopoeia or proposed in draft monographs. The ICRS may be used to calibrate secondary standards.

Certified reference substances are primary reference substances certified by regulatory bodies.

Pharmacopoeial reference substances (standards) are primary reference substances established and distributed by Pharmacopoeial authorities following the general principles of the ISO Guide 34.

Reference materials refer to materials other than substances appropriate for intended uses in standardization or quality control of herbs and herbal materials. Reference materials include, among others, herbarium samples, authentic specimens of herbal materials (such as extracts and their fractions), herbal reference preparations and authentic spectra or fingerprints.

Selection Criteria for Substances of Herbal Origin Relevant for Standardization and Quality Control of Herbal Medicines

General Considerations

Herbal materials, herbal preparations and finished herbal products are very complex. This can make the identification and quantification of herbal medicines very difficult and the detection of adulteration is very challenging. It should be emphasized that the identification of herbal medicines using markers, and quantification of marker substances in herbal medicines are not in themselves sufficient to guarantee the quality of herbal medicines. Quality control must cover all steps of their production and must be complemented by Good Agricultural and Collection Practices (GACP) and Good Manufacturing Practices (GMP),as appropriate.

Criteria for the selection of reference substances and quality control of herbal medicines should take into account that various ingredients may have different levels of influence on the final quality, safety and efficacy. For this reason, the order of selection of the substances for identification and quantification should follow the rules presented below.

1. If constituents with known therapeutic activity (activities) have been identified, they should be used as markers.
2. If 1 is not the case, but constituent(s) with recognized pharmacological activity (activities) is (are) known, they should be used as markers.
3. If the above cases are not applicable, the identity and quantity of herbal materials, preparations and medicines may be established by the production process and by analysing marker substance(s) containing other characteristic constituents(s).

Note that identification of herbal materials, and also to some extent herbal preparations and finished herbal products, may be be done or may be complemented by microscopic, macroscopic or DNA analytical methods using appropriate reference materials and descriptions.

Purpose and Expected Functions of Relevant Marker Substances

Markers used as chemical reference substances should be international chemical or pharmacopeial reference substances. If others are used, markers for quantitative determination should be of high purity as required by national regulations, determined by validated analytical methods, including physical and chemical ones. These analytical methods may be different from those employed for quantifying herbal materials. For markers used for identification, lower purity may be suitable. The general requirements for markers are:

- identity, specificity and selectivity using the specified analytical method(s);
- should be present in traceable quantity for identification or sufficient quantity for assay;
- should be easily obtained, stable under specified storage conditions;
- should be easily detected and quantified analytically.

Marker Substances of Constituents with known Therapeutic Activity

Purpose and Function: Markers of constituents with known therapeutic activity should serve their appropriate purpose (identification or quantification).

Selection criteria: The criteria for selection of a marker substance of constituents with known therapeutic activity are as follows:

- The marker must be readily available (for example, as an international or pharmacopoeia reference substance). New markers may only be selected if no such reference substance is available.
- In that case, detailed documentation should be provided on the identity and properties of the selected markers.
- It should be relatively easy to separate or distinguish the marker analytically from other structurally similar herbal constituents.

- Markers should be detectable and quantifiable with available analytical instrumental methods (such as thin-layer chromatography (TLC), high-performance thin-layer chromatography (HPTLC), gas chromatography(GC)or high-performance liquid chromatography(HPLC).
- Different marker substances may be selected for the same herbal medicines depending on the analytical instrumental methods available.
- Derivatives of the naturally occurring markers may be used where the latter are not easy to detect, are not stable or are not easily obtained.
- Different marker substances may be selected for the same herbal materials depending on the different forms of herbal preparations or finished herbal products.
- A group of markers may be selected if a single marker is not sufficient to identify and evaluate the herbal materials or finished herbal products.

Marker Substances of Constituents with Recognized Pharmacological Activities

***Purpose and Function*:** Markers of constituents with recognized pharmacological activities should serve as qualitative and quantitative measures in herbal medicines.

***Selection Criteria*:** The criteria for selection of a marker substance of constituents with recognized pharmacological activities are as follows:

- They occur naturally in sufficient quantities in herbal materials.
- Markers for quantification: should be representative of the main therapeutic or pharmacological profiles of the herbal materials and finished products.
- Markers for identification: should be specific for one plant or for certain plant species and genera. If not, other marker(s) should be selected for specific identification.
- They should be detectable and quantifiable by available instrumental analytical methods (such as TLC, HPTLC, HPLC, GC) or by another relevant analytical method.
- Different substances may be selected for the same herbal materials depending on the different forms of the herbal preparations (including different, e.g. aqueous and alcoholic extracts) or different therapeutic indications.
- A group of substances may be selected if a single one is not sufficient to evaluate the herbal material or finished herbal product.

Marker Substances of Characteristic Constituents

Purpose and Function: The main purpose of markers of characteristic constituents is identification and quantification of herbal materials in herbal preparations and finished herbal products.

Specific Requirements:

Markers for identification:

- The marker should be specific for one plant. If not, the marker should be specific for ascertain plant species, genus and family. *Note*: a plant family may contain many classes of biologically diverse species and chemically diverse ingredients, but the plants in the same genus are normally genetically close and contain structurally similar secondary metabolite constituents.
- If not specific for one plant, the marker should be specific at least for one herbal material or preparation in a mixture herbal preparation or herbal medicines.
- The marker should consist of one substance or group of substances, or characteristic pattern of substances. ***Note***: A pattern of substances characteristic for a specific herb may replace a single substance.

Markers for quantification:

- The marker for quantification should be available insufficient quantity for assay.

Selection criteria: The criteria for selection marker substances of characteristic constituents are as follows:

- They should occur naturally insufficient quantities in herbal materials.
- An authentic reference should be available.
- Spectral data on the substance should be recorded in an available library or database.
- TLC chromatogram pattern or other analytical identification should be illustrated in an available source.
- A simple identification and quantification test should be described for the substance or its chemical class.
- There should be adequate experimental evidence that the substance or group of substances is characteristic of the given herbal medicine.

Marker Substances for Toxic Constituents

Purposes and Function: Marker substances for toxic constituents are used to define maximum acceptable concentrations of toxic constituents in herbal materials, herbal preparations or finished herbal products.

Requirements: As a consequence of the composition of the herbal material or product, such a limit test is needed.

- There should be a defined upper tolerable limit for the mode of application and posology intended (e.g. oral, topical, inhalation, short-term, sub chronic or chronic application).
- A toxicological evaluation is required, but experience with traditional use should be taken into account.
- Genotoxicity, mutagenicity and carcinogenicity should also be considered when establishing toxicity criteria.

- An analytical detection procedure for the established tolerable limits should be available.
- These requirements should always be met by the finished herbal product destined for human use, since processing and conservation may alter toxicity.

Selection Criteria

- An appropriate reference substance should be available.
- For identity, specificity and selectivity are important characteristics.
- Limit of detection and limit of Quantitation values for the target herbal medicines should be specified.
- Highly sensitive instrumental analytical methods (such as TLC, HPTLC, GC, HPLC, GC/mass spectrometry (MS),liquid
- Chromatography (LC)/MS) should be available for detection of toxic substances.
- Simple identification tests for groups of toxic substances, such as alkaloids or terpenoids should be available.

Note: The criteria used for selecting marker substances for toxic constituents apply to detection of a toxic substance specific to a particular herbal material. To ensure its safety for human consumption, the toxic constituents of a herbal material, its herbal preparation or its finished herbal product should be identified accurately.

The toxicity may assess for control by the absence of a constituent or by establishing and testing allowable tolerable limit(s) for the toxic constituents using selected marker(s) and analytical methods. For example, the absence of thiamin as enzyme activity in horsetail (*Equisetum arvense*) as well as a method for the detection of kava lactone (a hepatotoxic agent) in kava kava (*Piper methysticum*) should be required.

- If it is not possible to exclude the toxic effect, e.g. because there is noappropriatemarkerconstituentorbecauseofthelackofananalyticalmethodor specific method of preparation, the herbal material or its herbal preparation should not be used in finished herbal products.

Use of Reference Materials

Various types of herbal reference materials are used as complements to analytical methods that were performed using markers and especially when no reference substances for the above-mentioned markers are available. They may also be used when markers are available, but are not adequate for identification of the herbal materials, preparations or finished products. For example, herbal medicines may contain a group of specified constituents or constituents with recognized pharmacological activities, such as flavonoids, alkaloids and saponins. There are also cases (e.g. well-identified extracts) when the reference material might be more stable than single ingredients with a high degree of purity (primary or secondary reference standards).

Purpose and Function: Identification and quantification of herbs, herbal materials and herbal medicines

Requirements

- Botanical reference materials and/or herbal preparations should be described by national pharmacopoeias or materia medica (e.g. those of China, Indonesia and Japan).
- Herbarium samples and authentic herbal material for microscopic and macroscopic comparison should be developed in cooperation with botanists for systematic authentication.
- If herbal preparations are used as the reference standard, full documentation on the preparation needs to be submitted to allow full traceability.
- Reference materials should be prepared following methods described in guidelines on validation.

Selection Criteria

- Herbal reference extracts should be prepared in accordance with standard operating procedures and the characteristic and/or active constituents should be well demonstrated on chromatograms (obtained by instrumental analytical methods such as TLC, high-performance thin-layer chromatography (HPTLC), HPLC, GC) and spectra (such as nuclear magnetic resonance (NMR) or MS) under specified conditions.
- The herbal reference extracts or herbal reference preparations and their main constituents should be stable and identifiable using available analytical instruments and analytical methods.
- There should be predetermined in-house criteria on how to use herbal reference preparations for identification of specified finished herbal products produced by manufacturers.

Analytical Methods for Substances of Herbal Origin in Herbal Medicines

This section describes testing methods employed for quality control.

General considerations regarding the test methods to be employed

Analytical methods used for quality control of herbal materials, herbal preparations and finished herbal products are generally based on:

(a) Chemical reactions;

(b) Chromatographic procedures (such as TLC, HPTLC, GC and HPLC), including fingerprinting;

(c) Spectroscopic and spectrometric methods;

(d) A combination of (b) and (c) and

(e) others.

Test methods should be specific and selective for the selected substances in the herbal materials, herbal preparations or finished herbal products. Test methods must be validated. It might be necessary to revalidate the method if the substance is tested at different stages of the production process (e.g., herbal preparations such as extracts and finished herbal products) because other substances, e.g. excipients may influence the analytical procedures.

Test methods, if applicable, should be able to detect substitutes or adulterants that are likely to be present in the sample.

Herbal materials, herbal preparations or finished herbal products with constituents with known therapeutic activity

The analytical methods used for quality control should be capable of detecting and quantifying the constituents with known therapeutic activity. The use of reference substances for the therapeutically important constituents in the analysis is recommended.

Herbal materials, herbal preparations or finished herbal products with characteristic constituents (whose pharmacologically or therapeutically active constituents are unknown)

When the pharmacological and the therapeutically active constituents are unknown, the identification and assay procedures should be based on characteristic constituents (markers) and fingerprint chromatograms, or on characteristic microscopic or macroscopic features of the herbal materials, herbal preparations or finished herbal products. Reference samples should be used in the analysis, where available.

Where the local laboratory has limited capacity, the use of dependable but simple basic technical and testing methods is recommended. However, the producer should not be discouraged from developing and applying more sophisticated methods for testing products intended for export.

Monographs

It is recommended that pharmacopeial monographs prepared by national or regional authorities should incorporate substances and constituents for quality control of herbal materials, herbal preparations or finished herbal products.

Further Reading

1. WHO Guidelines on good agricultural and collection practices (GACP) for medicinal plants. Geneva: World Health Organization; 2003.
2. WHO guidelines on assessing quality of herbal medicines with reference to contaminants and residues. Geneva: World Health Organization; 2007.
3. Good manufacturing practices: supplementary guidelines for the manufacture of herbal medicines. In: WHO Expert Committee on Specifications for Pharmaceutical Preparations: fortieth report. Geneva: World Health Organization; 2006: Annex 3 (WHO Technical Report Series, No. 937).
4. WHO guidelines on good manufacturing practices (GMP) for herbal medicines. Geneva: World Health Organization; 2007.
5. Quality control methods for medicinal plant materials. Geneva: World Health Organization; 1998.

6. Quality control methods for herbal materials. Geneva: World Health Organization; 2011.
7. General guidelines for the establishment, maintenance and distribution of chemical reference substances. In: WHO Expert Committee on Specifications for Pharmaceutical Preparations: forty first report. Geneva: World Health Organization; 2007: Annex 3 (WHO Technical Report Series, No. 943).
8. General requirements for the competence of reference material producers. ISO 17034:2016. Geneva: International Organization for Standardization; 2016.
9. Basic tests for drugs: pharmaceutical substances, medicinal plant materials and dosage forms. Geneva: World Health Organization; 1998.
10. General guidelines for methodologies on research and evaluation of traditional medicine. Geneva: World Health Organization; 2000 (WHO/EDM/TRM/2000.1).
11. Good manufacturing practices for pharmaceutical products: main principles. In: WHO Expert Committee on Specifications for Pharmaceutical Preparations: forty-eighth report. Geneva: World Health Organization; 2014: Annex 2 (WHO Technical Report Series, No. 986).
12. The International Pharmacopoeia, sixth edition. Geneva: World Health Organization; 2016.
13. National policy on traditional medicine and regulation of herbal medicines: Report of a WHO global survey. Geneva: World Health Organization; 2005.
14. Quality assurance of pharmaceuticals. WHO guidelines, good practices, related regulatory guidelines and GXP training materials. Geneva: World Health Organization; 2016.
15. Regulatory situation of herbal medicines: a worldwide review. Geneva: World Health Organization; 1998 (WHO/TRM/98.1).
16. WHO monographs on selected medicinal plants commonly used in the Newly Independent States (NIS). Geneva: World Health Organization; 2010.
17. WHO monographs on selected medicinal plants. Volume 1, Geneva: World Health Organization; 1999.
18. WHO monographs on selected medicinal plants. Volume 2, Geneva: World Health Organization; 2002.
19. WHO monographs on selected medicinal plants, Volume 3. Geneva: World Health Organization; 2007.
20. WHO monographs on selected medicinal plants, Volume 4. Geneva: World Health Organization; 2009.

Scan QR code to view the website/guidelines

- Herbal Marker-
trs1003-annex1-marker-substances-herbal-medicine-quality-control.pdf (who.int)

CHAPTER 16

WHO and ICH Guidelines for Quality Control of Herbal Materials

ICH Quality Control Guidelines

Introduction

There are no separate guidelines for herbal drugs or derived product recommended by ICH but whenever herbal medicines follows the criteria of drug then following ICH guidelines for synthetic drugs should be applicable to herb derived drugs and products. The International Council for Harmonisation of Technical Requirements for Pharmaceuticals for Human Use (ICH) is unique in bringing together the regulatory authorities and pharmaceutical industry to discuss scientific and technical aspects of drug registration. Since its inception in 1990, ICH has gradually evolved, to respond to the increasingly global face of drug development. ICH's mission is to achieve greater harmonisation worldwide to ensure that safe, effective, and high quality medicines are developed and registered in the most resource-efficient manner.

In November 2005, the ICH Steering Committee adopted a new codification system for ICH Guidelines. The purpose of this new codification is to ensure that the numbering / coding of ICH Guidelines is more logical, consistent and clear. Because the new system applies to existing as well as new ICH Guidelines a history box has been added to the beginning of all Guidelines to explain how the Guideline was developed and what is the latest version.

With the new codification revisions to an ICH Guideline are shown as (R1), (R2), (R3) depending on the number of revisions. Annexes or Addenda to Guidelines have now been incorporated into the core Guidelines and are indicated as revisions to the core Guideline (e.g., R1).

Categories and Codes of ICH Guidelines

The ICH topics are divided into four categories and ICH topic codes are assigned according to these categories.

Q-Quality Guidelines

Harmonisation achievements in the Quality area include pivotal milestones such as the conduct of stability studies, defining relevant thresholds for impurities testing and a more flexible approach to pharmaceutical quality based on Good Manufacturing Practice (GMP) risk management.

Q1A - Q1F Stability

Q2 Analytical Validation

Q3A - Q3D Impurities

Q4 - Q4B Pharmacopoeias

Q5A - Q5E Quality of Biotechnological Products

Q6A- Q6B Specifications

Q7 Good Manufacturing Practice

Q8 Pharmaceutical Development

Q9 Quality Risk Management

Q10 Pharmaceutical Quality System

Q11 Development and Manufacture of Drug Substances

Q12 Lifecycle Management

S-Safety Guidelines

ICH has produced a comprehensive set of safety Guidelines to uncover potential risks like carcinogenicity, genotoxicity and reprotoxicity. A recent breakthrough has been a non-clinical testing strategy for assessing the QT interval prolongation liability: the single most important cause of drug withdrawals in recent years.

S1A - S1C Carcinogenicity Studies

S2 Genotoxicity Studies

S3A - S3B Toxicokinetics and Pharmacokinetics

S4 Toxicity Testing

S5 Reproductive Toxicology

S6 Biotechnological Products

S7A - S7B Pharmacology Studies

S8 Immunotoxicology Studies

S9 Nonclinical Evaluation for Anticancer Pharmaceuticals

S10 Photosafety Evaluation

S11 Nonclinical Safety Testing

E- Efficacy Guidelines

The work carried out by ICH under the Efficacy heading is concerned with the design, conduct, safety and reporting of clinical trials. It also covers novel types of medicines derived from biotechnological processes and the use of pharmacogenetics/genomics techniques to produce better targeted medicines.

E1 Clinical Safety for Drugs used in Long-Term Treatment

E2A - E2F Pharmacovigilance

E3 Clinical Study Reports

E4 Dose-Response Studies

E5 Ethnic Factors

E6 Good Clinical Practice

E7 Clinical Trials in Geriatric Population

E8 General Considerations for Clinical Trials

E9 Statistical Principles for Clinical Trials

E10 Choice of Control Group in Clinical Trials

E11 Clinical Trials in Pediatric Population

E12 Clinical Evaluation by Therapeutic Category

E14 Clinical Evaluation of QT

E15 Definitions in Pharmacogenetics / Pharmacogenomics

E16 Qualification of Genomic Biomarkers

E17 Multi-Regional Clinical Trials

E18 Genomic Sampling

M-Multidisciplinary Guidelines

Those are the cross-cutting topics which do not fit uniquely into one of the Quality, Safety and Efficacy categories. It includes the ICH medical terminology (MedDRA), the Common Technical Document (CTD) and the development of Electronic Standards for the Transfer of Regulatory Information (ESTRI).

M1 MedDRA Terminology

M2 Electronic Standards

M3 Nonclinical Safety Studies

M4 Common Technical Document

M5 Data Elements and Standards for Drug Dictionaries

M6 Gene Therapy

M7 Genotoxic Impurities

M8 Electronic Common Technical Document (eCTD)

M9 Biopharmaceutics Classification System-based Biowaivers

M10 Bioanalytical Method Validation

WHO Quality Control Guidelines

Evaluation of Crude Drugs

Quality assurance of herbal medicinal products is the shared responsibility of manufacturers and regulatory bodies. National drug regulatory authorities have to establish guidelines on all elements of quality assurance, evaluate dossiers and data submitted by the producers, and check post-marketing compliance of products with the specifications set out by the producers as well as compliance with Good Manufacturing Practices (GMP). The manufacturers have to adhere to Good Agricultural and Collection Practices (GACP), GMP and Good Laboratory Practice (GLP) standards, establish appropriate specifications for their products, intermediates and starting materials and compile a well – structured, comprehensive documentation on pharmaceutical development and testing. The producers should make continued efforts to improve standards and adapt them to the present state of knowledge. A cooperative approach between different manufacturers, e.g. by establishing drug master-files for specifications and quality control, should be encouraged.

Evaluation of crude Drugs involves the process of identification of adulteration and determination of quality of crude drugs. Or Evaluation means "*confirmation of its identity and determination of its quality and purity.* This can be organoleptic or morphological, microscopic, biological, physical and chemical evaluation. Thus to determine impurities is also part of evaluation and one of the major reasons of impurity in crude drugs is d**rug adulteration. Adulteration** sub standardisation of drug with respect to therapeutic and chemical properties by replacing wholly or partially original drug. Types and terminologies related to adulteration are given in Table 20.1 and 20.2.

Table 16.1 Types of adulteration on the basis of reasons.

Unintentional	
Misidentification	**Due to confusion**: for herb Lakshmana different species are used *Arlia quinquefolia*, *Ipomea sepiaria* **Due to lack of knowledge of authentic plant**: All plants like *Cressa cretica, Selaginella bryopteris, Desmotrichum, fimbriatum, Malaxis acuminata (M. wallichii, Microstylis wallichii), Trichopus zeylanicus* and *Terminalia chebula* are consistently and repeatedly referred as Sanjeevani
Carelessness	Root of *Sida cordifolia* are replaced with the whole plant of *Sida cordifolia*
Geographical Unavaibility	For rasna, *Plucia lanceolata*is used in northern India while *Alpinia galanga* is in southern India.
Morphological similarity	*Cassia angustifolia* replaced with *Cassiaacutifolia* and *Euphorbia dracunculoides* Lam. (Euphorbiaceae) with*R. graveolens*
Intentional	
Adulteration with substandard commercial varieties	Rhubarb replaced with Chinese rhubarb or raphnotic rhubarb
Adulteration with superficially similar inferior drugs	Pimpalii *(Piper nigrum*) adulterated by papaya seeds
Adulteration with artificially manufactured substances	Artificial invert sugar are mixed with or replaced with pure Honey
Adulteration of exhausted drugs	Ginger is sold after extraction of its volatile oil
Adulteration with synthetic materials	Addition of synthetic Citral to oil of lime.
Adulteration with harmful substances	Pieces of limestone in asafoetida and of lead in opium.
Adulteration of the species belonging to same family	Mixing or replacement of*Datura metal*with*Datura stramonium*
Adulteration of different species	Mixing of*Tribulus terrestris*(zygophylaceae and *Pedalium murex* (Pedaliaceae)
Adulteration with totally different drugs	Bharangi (*Clerodendron indicum*) is totally replaced with Kantakari (*Solanum xanthocarpam*)
Adulteration with low cost drug	Kumkuma (saffron) being costly herb is substituted by Kusumbha (dried flowers of American saffron - *Carthamustinctorius*)

Table 16.2 Terminologies related to adulteration.

Inferiority	Impairment of quality with naturally substandard drug Example: The dried ripe seeds of *Strychnosnuxvomica* contain 1.15% of strychnine. Seeds containing less than 1.15% of strychnine, considered as inferior substandard drug.
Spoilage	Impairment of quality due to addition of Spoiled drug by the action of microorganism and thus renders the crude drug unfit for human consumption.
Deterioration	Impairment of the quality by destruction of any valuable constituent by extraction, moisture attack, heat treatment, microbial attack or by any other means. Example: Coffee that has largely lost its caffeine through over roasting is an example of deterioration.
Admixture	Impairment of the quality by addition of one product to another through accident, ignorance or carelessness. Example: *Senna* containing a few stems
Sophistication	Impairment of the quality by sophistication means the intentional addition of inferior material to any substance. Example: The addition of yellow soil to powdered turmeric powder
Substitution	Impairment of the quality by substitution means entirely different material is used instead of original drug. Example: Cotton seed oil is sold in the place of olive oil

Table 16.3 Adulterants of various crude drugs.

Crude drug name	**Adulterant**
Alexandrian senna (Cassia acutifolia)	Dog senna, Palthe senna, Bombay, Mecca or Arabian senna.
Aloes (Aloe barbadensis)	Natal aloes which contain natalion,homonatalion and resin with nataloresinotannol; Mochaaloes, black catechu, pieces of iron and stones.
Belladonna herb	Leaves of *Phytolacca americana* (Idioblast present), *Solanum nigrum*, and *Ailanthus glandulosa* (needle shaped crystals of calcium oxalate present).
Black pepper	*Piper attenuatum* , *Piper brachystachyum* , *Piper longum*
Cinchona	Cuprea bark (Remijia pedunculata, a coppery red coloured drug, contain quinine, quinidine and other alkaloid which resemble to those from cinchona bark. The bark contains numerous stone cells. Along with cinchona alkaloids, it also contains cupreine. False cupre bark (*R.purdiena*) contains alkaloids called cusconidine, traces of cinchonine, cinchonamine, but no quinine.
Cinnamon	Jungle cinnamom , Cinnamom chips, Saigol cinnamom, *Cinnamomum loureirii* (Lauraceae), Java cinnamom, *Cinaamomum burmanii* (Lauraceae).
Clove	Mother clove, Blown clove, Clove stalks
Digitalis	Leaves of *Verbascum thapsus* (Schophulariaceae) contain large woolly branched candelabra trichomes. The primrose leaves from *Primula vulgaris* (Primulaceae) contains uniseriate covering trichomes, which are 8 to 9 celled long. Comfrey leaves from *Symphytum officinale* (Boraginaceae) contains multicellular trichomes forming hook at the top.

Contd...

Crude drug name	Adulterant
Rauwolfia	*Reserpine containing*: African rauwolfia species(Rauwolfia vomitoria, caffra, R. cumminsfi, R.mombasiana, R. oreogiton, R. obscura, R. rosea and R. volkensii), R.tetraphylla and R. nitida, Alstonia venenata and A. constricta; *Ajmalicine containing*: Catharanthus roses; *Yohimbine containing*: Pausinystalia yohimba,
Rhubarb (Indian rhubarb)	Rhaphontic rhubarb obtained from rhizome of *R. rhaphonticum.* It lacks rhein , emodin or aloe-emodin butit contains rhaphonticin.
Saussurea	Vetiver oil.
Senega	Indian senega is *Polygala chinesis* Linn which does not contain Spurious Indian senega is *Glinus oppositifolia* family Molluginaceae. It contains a Saponins and starch. It shows several rings of vascular bundles. White senega is root of *Polygala alba* does not show keel
Shankhpushpi	*Canscora diffusa*

Standardization of Crude Drugs

Standardization of drug means technique which ensures quality, safety, efficacy and purity with respect to raw material, processing method, finished product and intended therapeutic effects. OR every product should have correct concentration of correct active principle and ingredient and it should induced intended therapeutic effect. The quality of herbal substances, herbal preparations and herbal medicinal products is determined by the quality of the starting plant material, develop-ment, in-process controls, GMP controls,and process validation, and by specifications applied to them throughout development and manufacture. Generally herbal extracts are categorized as:

- *Standardized extracts* have declared content of active constituents with therapeutic effects.
- *Quantified extracts* are defined range of constituents of known to contribute to therapeutic effects.
- *Other extracts* without known effective constituents are defined by their specifications i.e *Drug extract ratio (*DER) or *Genuine (Native) herbal preparation.*

Drug extract ratio (DER): Means the ratio between the quantity of herbal substance used in the manufacture of a herbal preparation and the quantity of herbal preparation obtained. The number (given as the actual range) written before the colon is the relative quantity of the herbal substance; the number written after the colon is the relative quantity of the herbal preparation obtained.

Genuine (Native) herbal preparation: Refers to the preparation without excipients, even if for technological reasons the genuine herbal preparation is not available. However, for soft and liquid herbal preparations the genuine herbal preparation may contain variable amounts of (extraction) solvent.

Ratio of herbal substance to genuine herbal preparation (DER genuine): Is the ratio of the mass of the herbal substance to the quantity of the resulting genuine herbal preparation. The number (given as the actual range) written before the colon is the relative quantity of the herbal substance; the number written after the colon is the relative quantity of the herbal preparation obtained.

Herbal medicinal products: Any medicinal product, exclusively containing as active substances one or more herbal substances or one or more herbal preparations, or one or more such herbal substances in combination with one or more such herbal preparations.

Herbal preparations: Are obtained by subjecting herbal substances to treatments such as extraction, distillation, expression, fractionation, purification, concentration or fermentation. These include comminuted or powdered herbal substances, tinctures, extracts, essential oils, expressed juices and processed exudates.

Herbal substances: All mainly whole, fragmented or cut plants, plant parts, algae, fungi, lichen in an unprocessed, usually dried form but sometimes fresh. Certain exudates that have not been subjected to a specific treatment are also considered to be herbal substances. Herbal substances are precisely defined by the plant part used and the botanical name according to the binomial system (genus, species, variety and author).

Herbal teas: Consist exclusively of one or more herbal substance(s) intended for oral aqueous preparations by means of decoction, infusion or maceration. The preparation is prepared immediately before use. Herbal teas are usually supplied in bulk form or in sachets.

Markers: Are chemically defined consti-tuents or groups of constituents of a herbal substance, a herbal preparation or a herbal medicinal product which are of interest for control purposes independent of whether they have any therapeutic or pharma-cological activity. Markers serve to calculate the quantity of herbal substance(s) or herbal preparation(s) in the Herbal Medicinal Product if the marker has been quantitatively determined in the herbal substance or herbal preparation.

There are two categories of markers:

Active markers are constituents or groups of constituents which are generally accepted to contribute to the therapeutic activity. Analytical markers are constituents or groups of constituents that serve for analytical purposes.

Need of Standardization

A major lacuna in natural drugs is the lack of drug standardization, information and quality control. Guidelines are necessary because:

- Biochemical and Geographical variation
- Deterioration during treatment & storage
- Substitution & adulteration,
- Export of quality natural drugs.
- Popularity of natural drugs for primary care in developing countries,
- Herbal medicines, however are not necessary always safe simply because they are natural. Some have given rise to serious adverse reactions & some contain chemicals that may produce long term side effects such as carcinogenicity & hepatotoxicity.

- Also herbal medicine will only benefit the health of human beings when they are of good quality
- Furthermore with the increased use of both herbal medicines & modern western pharmaceutical drugs, there is a need to monitor interactions.

WHO Guidelines

Herbal medicine is being used by about 80% of the world population for primary health care. They have faith, cultural acceptability and being natural believed to have better compatibility with the human body. Over time it is proved to have lesser side effects with good efficacy. Major Goals & objectives of the WHO guidelines are to promote the appropriate, safe and effective use of herbal medicines and to encourage the integration of herbal medicines into the mainstream medical systems. A WHO guideline involves policies on Quality, Safety and efficacy assessment of Crude plant materials and Stability of Finished products. It is also giving a lot emphasis on documentation of traditional use or and activity, determination (animal, human) and safety based on experience or/and toxicology studies.

Table 16.4 WHO parameters for standardization of herbal raw material, extracts and their products.

Preliminary evaluation	Sampling Foreign matter determination, Determination of total fiber
Morphological evaluation	Qualitative evaluation of color, odor and taste, size, shape, extra features etc
Microscopical evaluation	Qualitative histological evaluation of types and arrangements of tissues; quantitative assessment of palisade ratio, vein-islet, vein termination, stomatal index, stomatal number and Lycopodium method
Physical Qualitative evaluation	Solubility, refractive index, optical rotation, melting point, boiling point, density, viscosity, Chromatographic and spectroscopic evaluation
Physical quantitative or Physicochemical evaluation	Ash value, Extractive value, Moisture content, Volatile oil determination
Chemical evaluation	Qualitative evaluation to detect different classes of phytochemicals, quantitative determination of phytochemicals, assay etc
Biological evaluation	
Pharmacological evaluation	Animal activity, Animal organ or tissue activity
WHO Biological evaluation	Swelling index Foam index Hemolytic index Bitterness value Total tannin value
Toxicological evaluation	Microbial load determination Aflatoxin detection

Contd...

	Pesticide residue determination Radioactive contamination Heavy metal detection
Advanced Analytical evaluation	Chromatographic (TLC, Paper, HPTLC, HPLC and GC data) and spectroscopic evaluation
Along with above parameters there is need to evaluate herbal formulation for specific pharmaceutical parameters Such as: tablet: weight variation, friability, disintegration, and dissolution.	

Preliminary Evaluation

- ***Sampling:*** it is very crucial step in standardisation because of fact that whole quality control results are based on selected representative sample. So while selecting sample from raw material or finished product observes its packaging and labeling details carefully. It should not be poorly packaged or stored. Then take sufficient quantity of sample compared to total material quantity from top, bottom and middle region. Observe it for deterioration, adulteration, moisture, presence of any foreign matter etc. After satisfactory results use pooled sample for following evaluation parameters.
- **Foreign matter determination**: Anything other than biological source of crude drug is considered as foreign matter including dust, debris, sand, animal excreta, metals, minerals, insects etc. If leaves of Cassia angustifolia is authenticate source for anthraquinone glycosides then stems or roots of same plant are also considered as foreign matter. For determination of total foreign matter, spread the weighed quantity of sample on clean white paper or sheet, then observe through magnifying glasses and collect foreign matter. Weigh it and calculate percentage of total foreign matter. One can collect foreign matter according to different category (e.g. sand, other parts etc) and determine its percentage separately as well as in combine form.
- **Total Fiber Determination**: The crude fiber consists of the material other than ash which can't be dissolved in water and can't be digested by boiling with sulfuric acid or with sodium hydroxide solution. Thus it represents the most or less resistant part of the plant cell wall component like cellulose and pectin.Take about 2g of accurately weighed drug sample, extract with ether. Then extract with 200 ml of 1.25% sulfuric acid by boiling for the 30 min under reflux in a 500 ml flask. Then mixture is filtered through a hardened filter and the residue washed with boiling water until free from acid. The entire residue is rinsed back into the flask with 200ml of boiling 1.25% sodium hydroxide solution and again boiled under reflux for 30 min. The liquid is then quickly filtered through a tared filter and the residue on the filter is washed with boiling water until neutral, dried at 110^0C to constant weight and incinerated residue represents the weight of crude fiber. It is expressed as percentage of the original weight of the material.

Morphological Evaluation

Organoleptic evaluation or Preliminary examination can be considered as a first step towards establishment of identity and degree of purity. This is the evaluation by means of organs of senses to evaluate appearance of the drug, its odour and taste, occasionally the sound or snap of its fracture and feel of the drug to the touch. In the case of whole drugs the macroscopi-cally and sensory characters are usually sufficient to enable the drug to be identified. It provides simplest and quickest means of establish the identity and purity and thereby ensure quality of a particular sample. Judgment may vary from person to person and time to time based on individual's nature. Description of these features are very difficult so that often the characteristic like odour and taste can only described as "characteristic" and reference made to the analyst's memory. The organoleptic characterization is based on the shape, size, colour, surface characterrization, texture, fracture and appearance of the cut surface.

- **Color:** examined under an artificial light source or day light may be used. The color of the sample should be compared with that of a reference material.
- **Odour and taste**: slow and repeated inhalation of the material. where no distinct odour is perceptible, it is crushed using gentle pressure or if the material is known to be dangerous, by other suitable means such as pouring a small quantity of boiling water on to the crushed sample placed in a beaker. The strength of the odour like weak, distinct, strong is first determined and then the color sensation like musty, moldy, rancid, fruity, aromatic etc. are determined.
- **Size and shape:** The length, width and thickness of the crude materials are of great importance while evaluating a crude drug.
- **Extra features:** The texture is best examined by taking a small quantity of material and rubbing it between the thumb and forefinger, it is usually described as 'smooth', 'rough', 'gritty'. Touch of the material describes its softness or hardness. Bend and rupture caused to the sample, provides information of the brittleness and appearance of the fractured plane as fibrous, smooth, rough, granular, etc. all these characteristics are valuable in indicating the general type of material and the presence of more than one component.

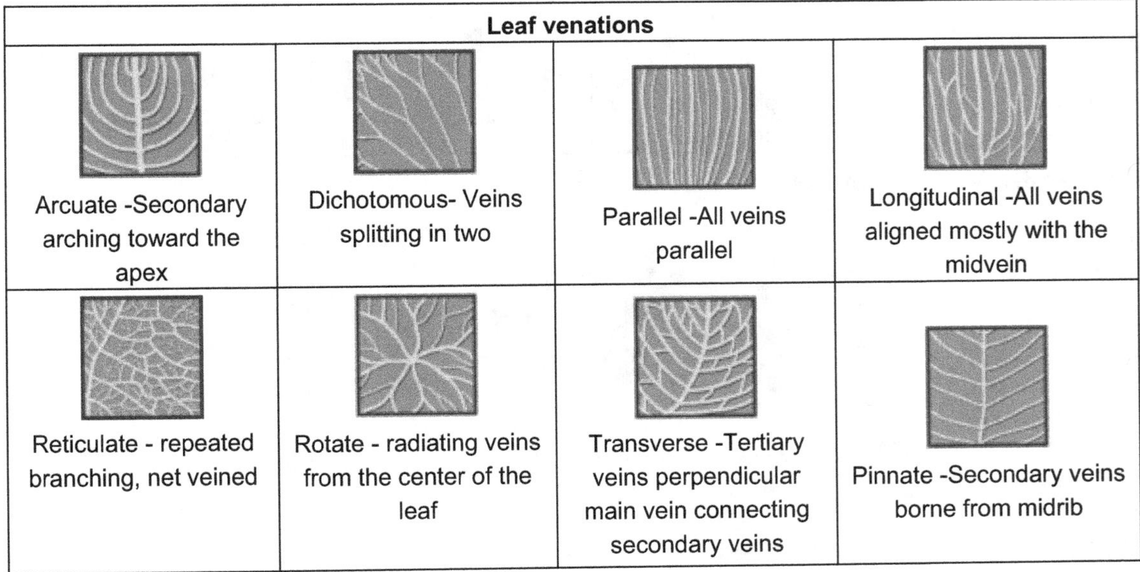

Leaf venations			
Arcuate -Secondary arching toward the apex	Dichotomous- Veins splitting in two	Parallel -All veins parallel	Longitudinal -All veins aligned mostly with the midvein
Reticulate - repeated branching, net veined	Rotate - radiating veins from the center of the leaf	Transverse -Tertiary veins perpendicular main vein connecting secondary veins	Pinnate -Secondary veins borne from midrib

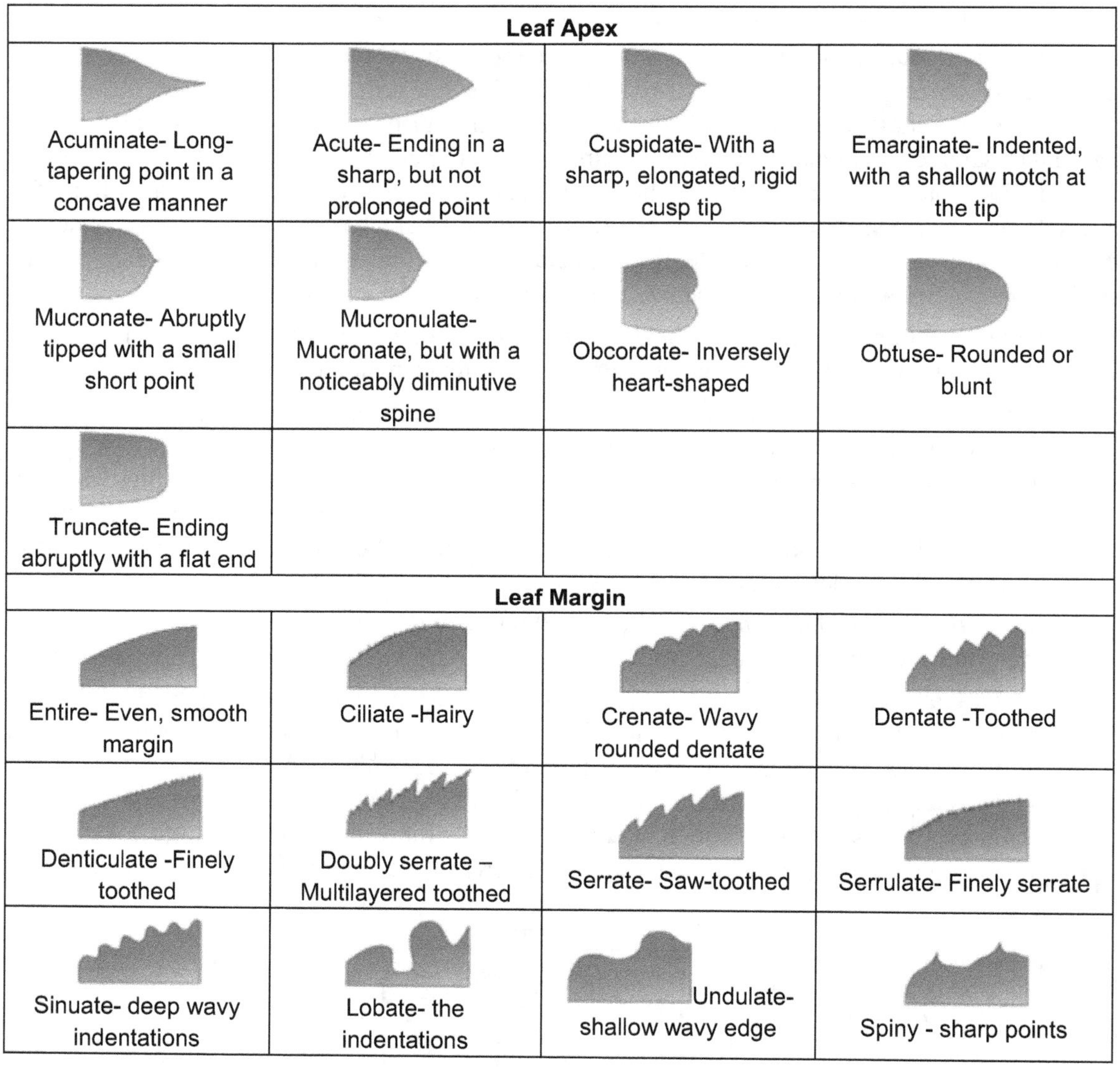

Leaf Apex
Acuminate- Long-tapering point in a concave manner
Acute- Ending in a sharp, but not prolonged point
Cuspidate- With a sharp, elongated, rigid cusp tip
Emarginate- Indented, with a shallow notch at the tip
Mucronate- Abruptly tipped with a small short point
Mucronulate- Mucronate, but with a noticeably diminutive spine
Obcordate- Inversely heart-shaped
Obtuse- Rounded or blunt
Truncate- Ending abruptly with a flat end
Leaf Margin
Entire- Even, smooth margin
Ciliate -Hairy
Crenate- Wavy rounded dentate
Dentate -Toothed
Denticulate -Finely toothed
Doubly serrate – Multilayered toothed
Serrate- Saw-toothed
Serrulate- Finely serrate
Sinuate- deep wavy indentations
Lobate- the indentations
Undulate- shallow wavy edge
Spiny - sharp points

Figure 16.1 Various features of leaf crude drugs.

Flat
Curved
Chanelled
Single quill
Double quill
Compound quill
Shapes of Barks

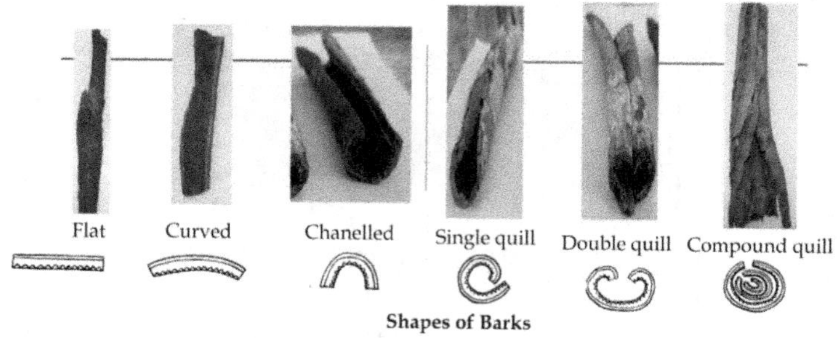

Figure 16.2 Various shapes of bark.

Microscopical Evaluation

Qualitative microscopical evaluation: It involves histological study of type and arrangement of tissues, presence of characteristic features such as stomata, starch grains, ca-oxalate crystals by using magnification power of microscopes. It utilizes stains to distinguish and identify different microscopical characters. E.g. iodine for starch, phloroglucinol and HCl for lignified fibers, sudan red –III for oil glands etc.

Clearing agents: Clearing agents used to remove interfering cell contents such as starch, protein, resin, lipids, chlorophyll etc so that to observe clear transparent images with maximum details. Material has to be either wash, mix or shake with these reagents. Chloral hydrate solution is actually mixture of Chloral hydrate and water in 5:2 proportions useful to remove common cell contents including chlorophyll. Cresol or acetophenol also removes many common cell contents. Dilute alkalis like Sodium hydroxide and potassium hydroxide solution useful to remove starch, proteins and cellulose tissues. Acids like Hydrochloric acid (20% v/v) removes starch by hydrolysis on boiling. Many organic solvents are also very useful to remove lipids, fats and pigments. Cedar wood and clove oils are especially useful to clear fatty oils.

Macerating / disintegrating agents: Macerating or Disintegrating reagents are very useful to remove cell wall contents like cellulose and or break the hard tissue such as stone cells, xylem vessels and fibers into isolated elements which further used for microscopical drawing, microscopical measurements, and quantitative microscopy and to study their other microscopical details. The disintegrated /macerated material gives a negative reaction for lignin. Following are most common Macerating / disintegrating agents.

- **Schult'z maceration fluid:** take50% v/v nitric acid solution in beaker, put it on water bath and add sufficient potassium chlorate until effervescence. Put small pieces of sample in this solution; again add potassium chlorate intermittently until starts separation of cells from tissue. Remove and Wash the material with water and make it free from acid.
- **Chromic acid-nitric acid solution:** It is solution of 10% of chromic anhydride in nitric acid (10%v/v). Take the pieces of material in beaker and addChromic acid-nitric acid in fuming cupboard. It attacks first cellulose later, lignin and finally after a long time, suberin.
- **Alkali solution:** take sample pieces in beaker containing either of dilute alkali [Sodium or potassium hydroxide solution (5%)] in water bath and boil until cell starts disintegrating.

Various Microscopical characters

Starch grains	Starch is composed of amylose and amylopectin, with the level of amylose ranging from 20% to 30% for most cereal starches. Starch grains are typically microscopically identified with either optical or electron microscopy. Starch grains can become clearer if they are stained a darker color with Iodine Stains. Logol's Iodine is one, used for staining starch because iodine reagents easily bind to starch but less easily to other materials. Features that allow identification of starch grains include: presence of hilum (core of the grain), lamellae (or growth layers), birefringence, and extinction cross (a cross shape, visible on grains under revolving polarized light) which are visible with a microscope and shape and size.

Contd...

Table 16.5 Structure and Amylose Content of Some Whole Granular Cereal Starches.

Source	Granule Shape	Granule Size (nm)	Amylose Content (%)
Wheat	Lenticular or round	20–25	22
Maize	Round or polyhedral	15	28
Waxy maize	Round	15 (5–15)	1
High-amylose	Round or irregular sausage-shaped	25	52
Barley	Round or elliptical	20–25	22
Rice	Polygonal	3–8	17–19[a] 21–23[b]
Oats	Polyhedral	3–10	23–24

a-Japonica, b-Indica

Adapted from Lineback (1984).

Calcium Crystals	There are two types' of calcium crystals forms due to excess carbonic acid or oxalic acid.

Calcium carbonate	Rare and generally associated with cell wall They are also called as cystoliths as they appear in the form of grapes in the tissues. Example: *Ficus elastica*
Cystolith	Cluster/Spheraphides; Prism; Raphides (Bundles of needle crystlas); Acicular/needle crystals; Rossette
Calcium oxalate	Very common and present in almost each part of plant. **Prisms/single crystals**: they are large, single or small groups and well developed. **Cluster crystals/ spheraphides**: they are group of numerous prisms/pyramids. The crystal are projecting, pointed, acute angled, and more or less spherical. **Rosette crystals**: they are large number of crystals in spherical mass (in the centre of which is an organic substance). Components of crystals radiate from the centre to the periphery and form a toothed circumference. **Acicular crystals/ raphids**: they re needle like, slender, long pointed at the ends. They may be single or in bundles. **Microcrystal/ crystal sand / micro sphenoid**: occur like an amorphous mass in cell. They are very minute and are present in large number in a single cell which is usually enlarged than other cells and is called idioblast.

Contd...

Table 16.6 Common crude drugs and their Calcium crystals.

Crude drugs	Type of calcium crystals
Asparagus, Aloe, Centella, Clove Flower Bud, Digitallis, Ephedra, Ginger, Isapgol, Nuxvomica	Absent
Azadircata, Senna, Clove, Rhubarb, Wild cherry bark, Tinosperma	Prism and cluster
Bacopa, Rauwolfia, Vasaka, Liquorice, Clove stalk, Senna, Kurchi, Cocca, Qaussia, Cascara	Prism
Cinchona	Microprism
Caraway	Rosette
Coriander, Dill, Fennel	Microrosette
Cassia, Cinnamon, Gentian	Acicular
Ipecac, Squill	Raphides
Cinnamon	Tubular
Datura	Spherophide crystals
Eucalyptus, Podophyllum	Clusters
Kurchi	Rhomboidal
Vinca	Microtubular, tactoid or needle shaped
Withania, Cinchona, Belladonna	Microsphenoid

Stomata

It is a pore, found in the upper epidermis of leaves, stems, and other organs, that controls the rate of gas exchange. The pore is bordered by a pair of specialized parenchyma cells known as guard cells that are responsible for regulating the size of the stomatal opening.There are different types of stomata and they are mainly classified based on their number and characteristics of the surrounding subsidiary cells. Listed below are the different types of stomata.

Types of stomatas present in Dicots:

- ***Paracytic (meaning parallel celled) or rubiaceous type:*** stomata have one or more subsidiary cells parallel to the opening between the guard cells. These subsidiary cells may reach beyond the guard cells or not. Examples families like Rubiaceae, Convolvulaceae and Fabaceae.
- ***Diacytic (meaning cross-celled) or caryophyllaceous type***: stomata have guard cells surrounded by two subsidiary cells, that each encircle one end of the opening and contact each other opposite to the middle of the opening. Examples families like Caryophyllaceae and Acanthaceae.
- ***Anomocytic (meaning irregular celled) or ranunculaceous type:*** stomata have guard cells that are surrounded by cells that have the same size, shape and arrangement as the rest of the epidermis cells. Examples families like Apocynaceae, Boraginaceae, Chenopodiaceae, and Cucurbitaceae.
- ***Anisocytic (meaning unequal celled) or cruciferous type:*** stomata have guard cells between two larger subsidiary cells and one distinctly smaller one. Examples families like Brassicaceae, Solanaceae, and Crassulaceae.
- ***Actinocytic (meaning star-celled)*** stomata have guard cells that are surrounded by at least five radiating cells forming a star-like circle. Examples families like Ebenaceae.
- ***Hemiparacytic stomata*** are bordered by just one subsidiary cell that differs from the surrounding epidermis cells, its length parallel to the stoma opening. Examples families like Molluginaceae and Aizoaceae.

Contd...

Types of stomatas present in Monocots:

- ***Gramineous (meaning grass-like) stomata*** have two guard cells surrounded by two lens-shaped subsidiary cells. The guard cells are narrower in the middle and bulbous on each end. This middle section is strongly thickened. The axis of the subsidiary cells are parallel stoma opening. Examples families like Poaceae and Cyperaceae.
- ***Hexacytic (meaning six-celled) stomata*** have six subsidiary cells around both guard cells, one at either end of the opening of the stoma, one adjoining each guard cell, and one between that last subsidiary cell and the standard epidermis cells.
- ***Tetracytic (meaning four-celled) stomata*** have four subsidiary cells, one on either end of the opening, and one next to each guard cell. This type occurs in many monocot families, but also can be found in some dicots. Examples families like Tilia and several Asclepiadaceae.

Types of stomatas present in ferns:

- ***Hypocytic stomata*** have two guard cells in one layer with only ordinary epidermis cells, but with two subsidiary cells on the outer surface of the epidermis, arranged parallel to the guard cells, with a pore between them, overlying the stoma opening.
- ***Pericytic stomata*** have two guard cells that are entirely encircled by one continuous subsidiary cell (like a donut).
- ***Desmocytic stomata*** have two guard cells that are entirely encircled by one subsidiary cell that has not merged its ends (like a sausage).
- ***Polocytic stomata*** have two guard cells that are largely encircled by one subsidiary cell, but also contact ordinary epidermis cells (like a U or horseshoe).

Table 16.7 Common crude drugs and their stomata.

Crude drugs	Type of Stomata
Senna, Coca	Paracytic (Rubiaceous)
Centella,Vasaka, mentha, peppermint, spearmint	Diacycytic (Caryophyllaceous)
Belladonna, stramonium, Datura, henbane, Vinca	Anisocytic(Cruciferous or unequal celled)
Digitallis, azadircata, bacopa, eucalyptus	Anomocyctic (Ranunculaceous)

Trichomes

Trichomes on plants areo epidermal outgrowths of various kinds.These are fine outgrowths or appendages on plants, algae, lichens, and certain protists. Trichomes can protect the plant from a large range of detriments, such as UV light, insects, transpiration, and freeze intolerance. Glandular trichomes found to store secondary metabolites like volatile oil, flavonoids etc.

Trichome type may assess the number of cells per trichome. A unicellular trichome consists of a single cell and is usually quite small. A multicellular trichome contains two or more cells. Multicellular trichomes can be either uniseriate, having a single vertical row of cells, or multiseriate, having more than one vertical row of cells. The number of cell layers in a trichome can also be diagnostic.

Many trichomes are diagnosed based on their general shape and morphology. Tapering trichomes are those ending in a sharp apex. Malpighian or dolabriform (also termed "two-armed" or "T-shaped") trichomes are those with two arms arising from a common base. (Malpighian is named after the family Malpighiaceae, where this trichome type is common.) Glandular trichomes are secretory or excretory trichomes, usually having an apical glandular cell. Glandular trichomes can be pilate-glandular, with a glandular cell atop an elongate basal stalk, or capitate-glandular, with a glandular cell having a very short or no basal stalk. Branched trichomes include two types: stellate, which are star-shaped trichomes having several arms arising from a common base (either stalked or sessile); and dendritic, which are treelike trichomes with multiple lateral branches. Peltate trichomes are those with a disk-shaped apical portion atop a peltately attached stalk.

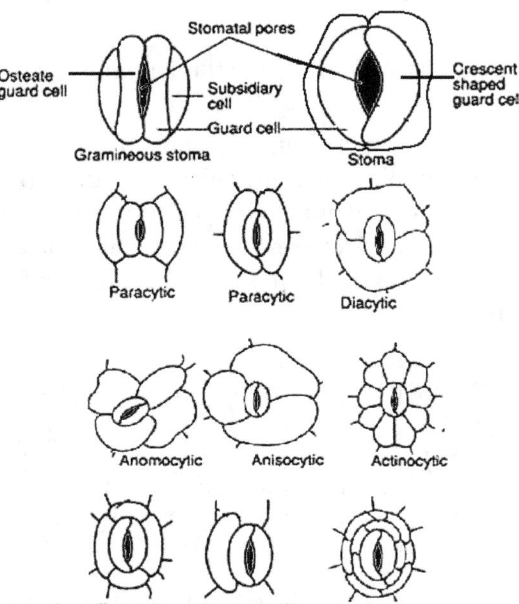

Figure 16.3 Various types of stomata.

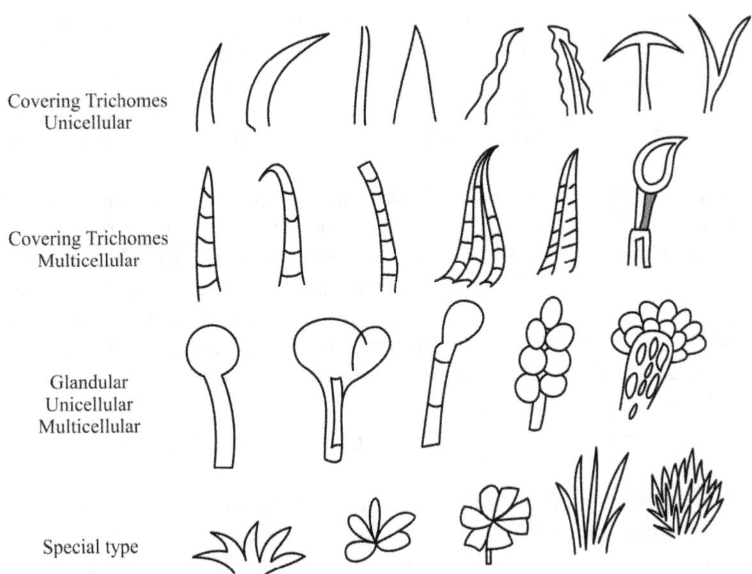

1. Unicelluar covering; 2. Feltate 3. Cylindrical 4. Conical 5. Wavy 6. T-shaped7. Forked 8. Ulticelluar 9. Unclinate 10. Multicellur 11. Multiseriate 12. Biseriate 13. Collapsed 14. Glandular inicellur both head and stalk 15. Glandular multicelluar head and unicellue stalk 16. Glandular muticelluar stalk and uncellue head17. Multicelluar head and unicelluar stalk 18. Multicelluar stalk 19. Stellate 20. Radiate 21. Peltate 22. Multiangualate 23. Echinoid

Figure 16.4 Various shapes of trichomes.

Quantitative microscopical evaluation: It involves determination of quantity of microscopical characters such as

- ***Leaf constant***: Palisade ratio, Vein islet number, Vein termination number, Stomatal number, Stomatal index
- ***Lycopodium spore method***: Newer technique which can be applied to determine percentage purity of any plant part crude drug unlike leaf constants which are applicable only to leaf crude drugs. Additional significance of this method is that it requires powder form of crude drugs unlike leaf constants which requires fresh or dry whole crude drug. Whole fresh or drug crude drugs cannot available throughout year while powder form of crude drug can be available and stored easily.

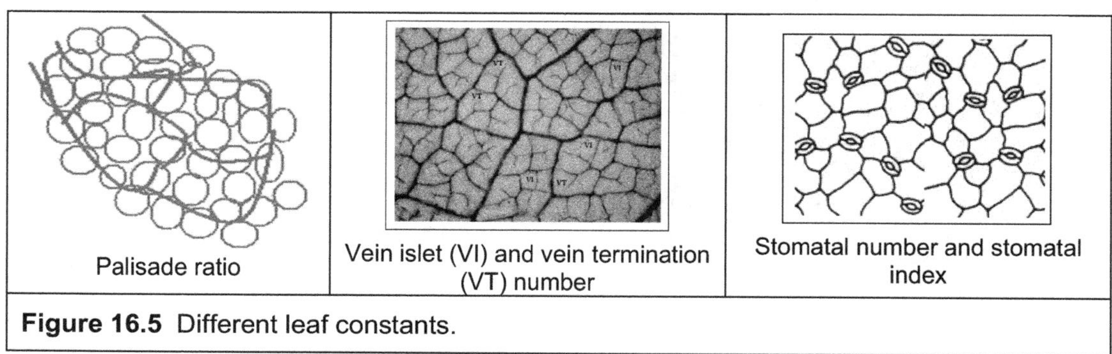

Figure 16.5 Different leaf constants.

Quantitative microscopical evaluation: It involves determination of quantity of microscopical characters such as Palisade ratio, Vein islet number, Vein termination number, Stomatal number, Stomatal index and newer technique Lycopodium spore method.

Palisade ratio:	This is average number of palisade cell beneath each epidermal cell. It can be also determined with powdered drugs. *Procedure:* Clear a piece of the leaf by boiling in choral hydrate solution for about thirty minutes. Arrange camera lucida and drawing board for making drawings to scale. Place stage micrometer on the microscope and using 16 mm objectives, draw a line equivalent to 1 mm as seen through the microscope. Construct a square on this line. Move the paper so that the square is seen in the eye piece, in the centre of the field. Place the slide with the cleared leaf (epidermis on the stage). Trace off at least four epidermal cells and draw palisade cells beneath each epidermal cell. Calculate average palisade cell beneath each epidermal cell.
Vein-islet number:	This is number of vein-islets per square mm of the leaf surface midway between midrib and margin. *Procedure:* Clear a piece of the leaf by boiling in choral hydrate solution for about thirty minutes. Arrange camera lucida and drawing board for making drawings to scale. Place stage micrometer on the microscope and using 16 mm objectives, draw a line equivalent to 1 mm as seen through the microscope. Construct a square on this line. Move the paper so that the square is seen in the eye piece, in the centre of the field. Place the slide with the cleared leaf (epidermis on the stage). Trace off the veins which are included within the square, completing the outlines of those islets which overlap two adjacent sides of the square. Count the number of vein islets in the square millimeter. Where the islets are intersected by the sides of the square, include

Contd...

those on two adjacent sides and exclude those islets on the other sides. (To obtain a critical result for a leaf, 4 sq mm should be used, preferably in one large area of 4 sq mm). Find the average number of vein islets from the four adjoining squares, to get the values for one sq mm.

Table 16.8 Vein-islet numbers of few medicinal plants.

Plant Name	Species	Range of vein-islet numbers	Average
Senna	Cassia senna	15–29.5	26
	Cassia angustifolia	19.5–22.5	21
Coca	Erythroxylum coca	8–12	11
	Erythroxylum truxillense	15–26	20
Digitalis	Digitalis purpurea	2–5.5	3.5
	Digitalis lanata	2–3.5	2.7
		3–8	4.4
	Digitalis lutea	1–1.5	1.2
	Digitalis thapsi	8.5–16	

Vein–termination number:

This is number of vein termination per square mm of the leaf surface midway between midrib and margin.

Procedure: Clear a piece of the leaf by boiling in choral hydrate solution for about thirty minutes. Arrange camera lucida and drawing board for making drawings to scale. Place stage micrometer on the microscope and using 16 mm objectives, draw a line equivalent to 1 mm as seen through the microscope. Construct a square on this line. Move the paper so that the square is seen in the eye piece, in the centre of the field. Place the slide with the cleared leaf (epidermis on the stage). Trace off the veins which are included within the square, completing the outlines of those islets which overlap two adjacent sides of the square. Count the number of veinlet terminations present within the square. Find the average number of veinlet termination number from the four adjoining squares, to get the values for one sq. mm.

Table 16.9 Vein-termination numbers of few medicinal plants.

Plant Name	Veinlet termination numbers
Atropa acuminata	1.4–3.5
Atropa belladonna	6.3–10.3
Cassia angustifolia	25.9–32.8
Cassia senna	32.7–40.2
Datura stramonium	12.6–20.1
Digitalis purpurea	2.5–4.2
Erythroxylum coca	16.8–21.0
Erythroxylum truxillense	23.1–32.3
Hyoscyamus niger	12.4–19.0

Stomatal number:

This is average number of stomata per square mm of epidermis of the leaf.

Procedure: Clear the piece of the leaf (middle part) by boiling with chloral hydrate solution or alternatively with chlorinated soda. Peel out upper and lower epidermis separately by means of forceps. Keep it on slide and mount in glycerin water. Arrange a camera lucida and drawing board for making the drawings to scale. Draw a square

Contd...

	of 1 mm by means of stage micrometer. Place the slide with cleared leaf (epidermis) on the stage. Trace the epidermis cell and stomata. Count the number of stomata present in the area of 1 sq. mm. Include the cell if at least half of its area lies within the square. Record the result for each of the ten fields and calculate the average number of stomata per sq mm.
Stomatal index:	This is percentage of the number of stomata forms to the total number of epidermal cells each stoma being counted as one cell. *Procedure:* Clear the piece of the leaf (middle part) by boiling with chloral hydrate solution or alternatively with chlorinated soda. Peel out upper and lower epidermis separately by means of forceps. Keep it on slide and mount in glycerin water. Arrange a camera lucida and drawing board for making the drawings to scale. Draw a square of 1 mm by means of stage micrometer. Place the slide with cleared leaf (epidermis) on the stage. Trace the epidermis cell and stomata. Count the number of stomata, also the number of epidermal cells in each field. Calculate the stomatal index using the above formula. Determine the values for upper and lower surface (epidermis) separately.

$$\text{Stomatal index} = \frac{\text{Stomatal number}}{\text{Total number of stomata} + \text{Total number of epidemal cells}} \times 100$$

Table 16.10 Vein-termination numbers of few medicinal plants.

Plant Name	Stomatal index	
	Upper surface	Lower surface
Atropa acuminata	1.7 to 4.8 to 12.2	16.2 to 17.5 to 1.83
Atropa belladonna	2.3 to 3.9 to 10.5	20.2 to 21.7 to 23.0
Cassia senna	11.4 to 12.4 to 13.3	10.8 to 11.8 to 12.6
Cassia angustifolia	17.1 to 19.0 to 20.7	17.0 to 18.3 to 19.3
Datura inermis	18.1 to 18.3 to 18.7	24.5 to 24.9 to 25.3
Datura metel	12.7 to 17.4 to 19.4	21.2 to 22.3 to 23.9
Datura stramonium	16.4 to 18.1 to 20.4	24.1 to 24.9 to 26.3
Datura tatula	15.6 to 20.2 to 22.3	28.3 to 29.8 to 31.0
Digitalis lanata	13.9 to 14.4 to 14.7	14.9 to 16.1 to 17.6
Digitalis lutea	2.5 to 5.5 to 8.4	21.6 to 22.9 to 25.2
Digitalis purpurea	1.6 to 2.7 to 4.0	17.9 to 19.2 to 19.5
Digitalis thapsi	5.9 to 7.0 to 7.8	11.9 to 12.4 to 13.5
Erythroxylum coca	Nil	12.2 to 13.2 to 14.0
Erythroxylum truxillense	Nil	8.9 to 10.1 to 10.7
Phytolacca acinosa	Nil	15.0
Phytolacca americana	2.9 to 4.2 to 5.7	13.0 to 13.2 to 13.4

Lycopodium spore method: Lycopodium is composed of the spores of *Lycopodium clavatum L.* each spore is tetrahedral in shape, the base is rounded and the three flat sides meet to form three well-marked covering ridges, which join one another at the apex. The whole surface of the spore is covered with minute reticulations and the interior is filled with fixed oil. The spores are exceptionally uniform in size (25μm), so that one can always know that a definite number of spores represent a particular weight of lycopodium.

The whole process can be simplified as 1 mg of spores contain averagely 94000 spores. By this figure one can calculate the weight of any number of spores under any condition under the microscope. If the lycopodium has been fixed with a definite proportion of another substance, one can find immediately how much of the second substance has been added, when examined microsopically. If it is admixed with any fine particles like pollen grains, starch etc. with characteristic countable particles it is possible to calculate the number of such characteristic particles per mg. in this way it is possible to have a standard figure that represents any such material. The number of characteristic particles per unit weight is often constant and is useful in assessing the quality of a sample. To use this method the number of particles in a good quality sample must either be known or first determined.

$$\%\text{Purity}: \frac{N \times W \times 940000}{S \times M \times P} \times 100$$

Where

N = Number of Characteristic particles of sample in 25 fields

W = weight of lycopodium spores taken in mg

S = number of lycopodium spores in 25 fields

M = weight of sample in mg

P = standard value of number of characteristic samples per mg in taken sample material (e.g. 1 mg ginger powder contains 2, 86, 000 starch grains)

Powder Microscopical Evaluation

Powder microscopical evaluation is done using powders of crude drugs unlike to histological studies where whole crude drug is used. Every time it is impossible to obtain fresh or to store whole dried crude drug so powder microscopy is most feasible. All microscopical characters can be observed in dispersed form without intact information like exact arrangement of cells, tissues.

***Procedure*:** Clear powder with clearing agents. Spread thin layer of powder on glass slide and observe under microscope. To differentiate cells (lignified and non-lignified, starch grains, oil glands) use staining reagents. Following characters can be observed according to plant parts:

Table 16.11 Common Powder characteristics of Various Plant parts.

Leaves	Epidermal cells, palisade cells, stomata, trichomes, calcium crystals, starch grains,
Roots/Rhizomes	Cork cell, parenchyma cells, phloem fibers, xylem, calcium crystals, starch grains, stone cells
Bark/wood	Cork cell, parenchyma cells, phloem fibers, xylem, calcium crystals, starch grains, stone cells, pericyclic fibers, sclerides, fibers
Flowers	Epidermal cells, anthers, pollen grains, oil globules, pigments,
Seeds	Endosperm, oil glands, aleurone grains, starch grains, pigment
Fruits	Epidermal cells, pericarp, mesocarp, oil glands (vittae), sclerenchymatous cells

Physical Qualitative Evaluation

Qualitative Physical Evaluation

This evaluation gives idea about quality of crude drug either pure or impure. This involves determination of following parameters:

- *Solubility*: Solubility is the property of a solid, liquid, or gaseous chemical substance called solute to dissolve in a solid, liquid, or gaseous solvent to form a homogeneous solution of the solute in the solvent.
  - Fats and oils: soluble in non polar solvents like petroleum, ether, benzene, and hexane
  - Carbohydrates, glycosides, tannins, flavonoids: soluble in different types of alcohols or water
  - Aglycone part of glycosides, bases of alkaloids: soluble in non-polar solvents

Table 16.12 Solubility chart.

Descriptive Term	Parts of Solvent for 1 part of solute
Very Soluble	Less than 1
Freely Soluble	From 1 to 10
Soluble	From 10 to 30
Sparingly Soluble	From 30 to 100
Slightly Soluble	From 100 to 1000
Very Slightly Soluble	From 1000 to 10,000
Practically Insoluble, or Insoluble	More than 10,000

- *Optical rotation* of a liquid is the angle through which the plane of polarization of light is rotated when the polarized light is passed through a sample of the liquid, rotation clockwise or anticlockwise. Clove oil 0 to -1.5 while eucalyptus oil having 0 to +10
- *Melting point*: All solid pure phytochemicals should be evaluated for its melting point. Difference in melting point indicates presence of impurities.
- *Boiling point*: This parameter is applicable to all liquid phytochemicals like essential oils or few alkaloids. Shift in boiling point range helps in determining purity of phytochemicals.
- *Refractive index (RI)*: The refractive index of a substance is the ratio between the velocity of light in air and the velocity in the substance under test. The refractive index of the material is given by the sine of the angle of incidence divided by the since of the angle of refraction. The RI varies with the temperature; Pharmacopoeial determinations are made at 20°C.
- *Viscosity*: Viscous natural drugs like gums, mucilages or pectin like compounds should be evaluated for its viscosity.
- *Density, specific gravity determination*: All liquid phytochemicals have to be evaluated for its density and specific gravity. This parameter is very essential for volatile oil standardization.

- *Spectroscopic evaluation:* λmax values in UV, wave number values in FTIR, delta values in NMR and m/e values in mass spectroscopy useful to identify impurities and thus to determine purity of samples. Spectroscopy is the study of the interaction between matter and radiation. It measures radiation intensity as a function of wavelength. Spectroscopic analyses are based on measuring the amount of radiation produced or absorbed by molecular or atomic species of interest. Spectroscopy is a common technique used in analytical chemistry for the identification of substances through the spectrum emitted from or absorbed by them. Spectroscopic methods can be classified according to the region of the electromagnetic spectrum involved in the measurement. The regions that have been used include gamma-ray, X-ray, Ultraviolet (UV), Visible, Infrared (IR), Microwave and Radio frequency (RF). Spectroscopic methods are mostly classified as atomic, molecular or ionic based on whether or not they apply to atoms, molecules or ions. The nature of their interactions can also be used to classify spectroscopic methods. These can be divided in three categories;
- *Absorption spectroscopy* which uses the range of the electromagnetic spectra in which substance absorbs photons. Example: Infrared, ultraviolet, visible and microwave spectroscopy are molecular techniques of absorption spectroscopy.
- *Emission spectroscopy* that uses the range of electromagnetic spectra in which photons are emitted by the substance. Example: Fluorescence spectroscopy, flame photometry
- *Scattering spectrometry* where the amount of light that a substance scatters depends on polarization angles and wavelength. Example: Raman spectroscopy.
- *Chromatographic evaluation*: Presence of extra band after development of chromatogram in paper or TLC, HPTLC indicates presence of impurities.Chromatography is based on the principle where molecules in mixture applied onto the surface or into the solid, and fluid stationary phase (stable phase) is separating from each other while moving with the aid of a mobile phase. The factors effective on this separation process include molecular characteristics related to adsorption (liquid-solid), partition (liquid-solid), and affinity or differences among their molecular weights. Because of these differences, some components of the mixture stay longer in the stationary phase, and they move slowly in the chromatography system, while others pass rapidly into mobile phase, and leave the system faster. Based on this approach three components form the basis of the chromatography technique.
- *Stationary phase:* This phase is always composed of a "solid" phase or "a layer of a liquid adsorbed on the surface a solid support".
- *Mobile phase:* This phase is always composed of "liquid" or a "gaseous component."
- Separated molecules

The type of interaction between stationary phase, mobile phase, and substances contained in the mixture is the basic component effective on separation of molecules from each other.

Chromatography methods based on partition are very effective on separation, and identification of small molecules as amino acids, carbohydrates, and fatty acids. However,

- Affinity chromatographies (ie. ion-exchange chromatography) are more effective in the separation of macromolecules as nucleic acids, and proteins.

- *Paper chromatography* is used in the separation of proteins, and in studies related to protein synthesis;
- *Gas-liquid chromatography* is utilized in the separation of alcohol, esther, lipid, and amino groups, and observation of enzymatic interactions,
- *Molecular-sieve chromatography* is employed especially for the determination of molecular weights of proteins.
- *Agarose-gel chromatography* is used for the purification of RNA, DNA particles, and viruses.

Types of chromatography

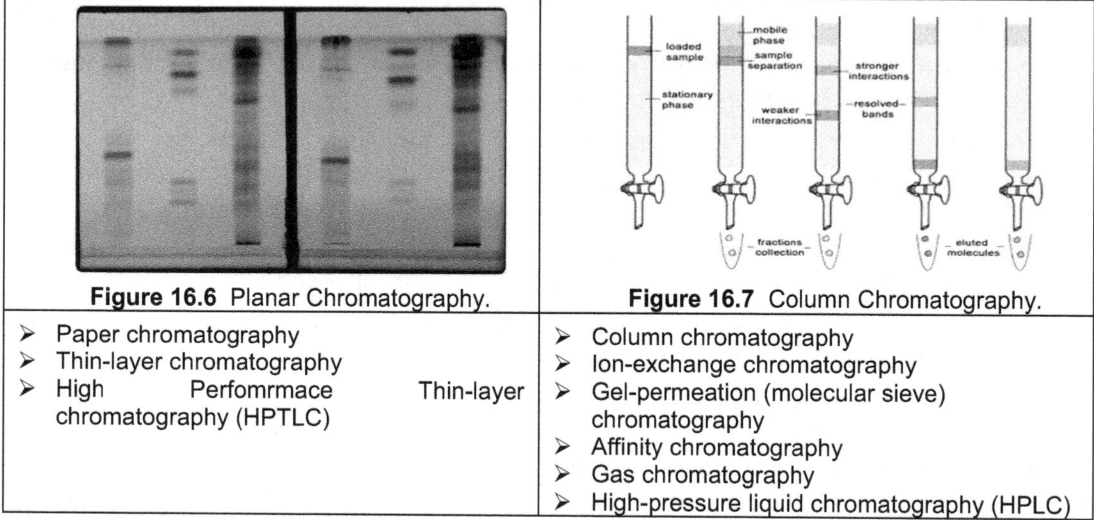

Figure 16.6 Planar Chromatography.	**Figure 16.7** Column Chromatography.
➢ Paper chromatography ➢ Thin-layer chromatography ➢ High Perfomrmace Thin-layer chromatography (HPTLC)	➢ Column chromatography ➢ Ion-exchange chromatography ➢ Gel-permeation (molecular sieve) chromatography ➢ Affinity chromatography ➢ Gas chromatography ➢ High-pressure liquid chromatography (HPLC)

Physical Quantitative Evaluation or Physicochemical Evaluation

Ash value determination

The residue remaining left after incineration of the crude drug is designated as ash. The residue obtained usually represents the inorganic salts naturally occurring in the drug and adhering to it. It varies with in definite limits according to the soils. It may also include inorganic matter deliberately added for the purpose of adulteration. Hence, an ash value determination furnishes the basis for judging the identity and cleanliness of any drug and gives information relative to its adulteration/contami-nation with inorganic matter, thus ash values are helpful in determining the quality and purity of drug.

Muffle furnace: Muffle furnace is an oven type instrument which can reach high temperatures. The furnace achieves the high-temperature on the basis of the insulating material which is fitted inside the chamber. The insulating material which is provided in the chambers acts as a muffle and stops the heat from escaping out of the chamber.

Crucible: There are a number of different types of crucible available for ashing crude drug samples, including quartz, pyrex, porcelain, steel and platinum. Selection of an appropriate crucible depends on the sample being analyzed and the furnace temperature used. The most widely used crucibles are made from porcelain because it is relatively inexpensive to purchase, can be used up to high temperatures (< 1200°C) and are easy to clean. Porcelain crucibles are resistent to acids but can be corroded by alkaline samples, and therefore different types of crucible should be used to analyze this type of sample. In addition, porcelain crucibles are prone to cracking if they experience rapid temperature changes.

Table 16.13 Ash values of few crude drugs.

Plant Name and Ash values	**Name of pharmacopeia and recommended Values**		
	Indian Pharmacopeia Vol-III, [2018]	**Ayurvedic Pharmacopeia Vol-I, [1986]**	**Indian Herbal Pharmacopeia [2002]**
Ashwagandha			
Ash value [NMT %]	7	4	7
Acid insoluble value [NMT %]	2	1	1.2
Turmeric			
Ash value [NMT %]	10	9	9
Acid insoluble value [NMT %]	2	1	1
Sarpagandha (Rauwolfia)			
Ash value [NMT %]	8	8	8
Acid insoluble value [NMT %]	2	1	2
Sunthi (Ginger)			
Ash value [NMT %]	8	6	6
Acid insoluble value [NMT %]	1.5	1.5	1.5

Types of ash values

***Total ash*:** The determination of ash is useful for detecting low grade products, exhausted drugs & excess of sandy and earthy material. Total ash is useful to exclude drugs which have been coated with chalk, lime or calcium sulphate to improve their appearance. Example: Ginger and Nutmeg. This test is designed to measure the amount of material remaining after ignition. Physiological ash is derived from the plant tissue. Nonphysiological ash is the residue after ignition of the extraneous matter (Example: sand and soil) adhering to the surface.

Procedure: Weigh accurately into previously ignited and tared crucible, usually platinum, silica about 2 to 3 g of the ground material. Spread the material in an even layer in the crucible. Ignite the material by gradually increasing the heat to 450 °C until free from carbon, cool in desiccator and weigh. If carbon-free ash can't be obtained in this manner, cool the crucible and moisten the residue with about 2 ml of water or a saturated solution of ammonium nitrate, dry on a water bath. Then on hot plate and ignite to constant weight without delay. Calculate the content of total ash in mg/g of air-dried material.

Acid-insoluble ash: Acid-insoluble ash is the residue obtained after boiling the ash with dilute Hcl and igniting the washed insoluble matter left on the filter. This determination measures the presence of silica especially sand and siliceous earth. Acid-insoluble ash is useful for detecting the presence of excessive earthy material.

Procedure: To the crucible containing the total ash, add 25 ml of Hcl(70 g/l) TS, cover with a watch-glass and boil gently for 5 mins. Rinse the watch-glass with 5 ml of hot water and add this liquid to the crucible. Collect the insoluble matter on an ash less filter paper and wash with hot water until the filtrate is neutral. Transfer the filter paper containing the insoluble matter to the original crucible, dry on hot plate and ignite to the constant weight. Allow the residue to cool in a suitable desiccator for 10 min and weigh without delay. Calculate the content of acid insoluble ash in mg/g of air dried material.

***Water-soluble ash**:* Water soluble ash is the calculated difference in wt between the total ash and the residue remaining after treatment of total ash with water. Water-soluble ash is useful to detect the presence of material exhausted by water. Ex: Tea leaves and Ginger. For the ginger the value of total ash is 2.5-6% and water-soluble ash is 1.9-3.0%. While for the exhausted ginger the value of total ash is 2-4% and water-soluble ash is 0.2-0.5%.

Procedure: To the crucible containing the total ash, add 25 ml of water and boil for 5 min. Collect the insoluble matter in a sintered glass crucible or on an ash less filter paper. Wash with hot water and ignite for 5 min at a temperature not exceeding 450 °C. Subtract the weight of this residue in mg obtained from the weight of total ash. Calculate the content of water soluble ash in mg/g of air dried material.

- ***Dry Ashing***: Dry ashing procedures use a high temperature muffle furnace capable of maintaining temperatures of between 500 and 600 °C. Water and other volatile materials are vaporized and organic substances are burned in the presence of the oxygen in air to CO_2, H_2O and N_2. Most minerals are converted to oxides, sulfates, phosphates, chlorides or silicates. Although most minerals have fairly low volatility at these high temperatures, some are volatile and may be partially lost. Example: iron, lead and mercury. If an analysis is being carried out to determine the concentration of one of these substances then it is advisable to use an alternative ashing method that uses lower temperatures. The food sample is weighed before and after ashing to determine the concentration of ash present. The ash content can be expressed on either a dry or wet basis:

$$\%\ \text{As(dry basis)} = \frac{M_{ASH}}{M_{DRY}} \times 100$$

$$\%\ \text{As(wet basis)} = \frac{M_{ASH}}{M_{DRY}} \times 100$$

where M_{ASH} refers to the mass of the ashed sample, and M_{DRY} and M_{ASH} refer to the original masses of the dried and wet samples.

A number of dry ashing methods have been officially recognized for the determination of the ash content of various foods (AOAC Official Methods of Analysis). Typically, a sample is held at 500-600°C for 24 hours.

Advantages: Safe, few reagents are required, many samples can be analyzed simultaneously, not labor intensive, and ash can be analyzed for specific mineral content.

Disadvantages: Long time required (12-24 hours), muffle furnaces are quite costly to run due to electrical costs, loss of volatile minerals at high temperatures, Example: Cu, Fe, Pb, Hg, Ni, Zn.

Recently, analytical instruments have been developed to dry ash samples based on microwave heating. These devices can be programmed to initially remove most of the moisture (using a relatively low heat) and then convert the sample to ash (using a relatively high heat). Microwave instruments greatly reduce the time required to carry out an ash analysis, with the analysis time often being less than an hour. The major disadvantage is that it is not possible to simultaneously analyze as many samples as in a muffle furnace.

- **Wet Ashing:** Wet ashing is primarily used in the preparation of samples for subsequent analysis of specific minerals (see later). It breaks down and removes the organic matrix surrounding the minerals so that they are left in an aqueous solution. A dried ground food sample is usually weighed into a flask containing strong acids and oxidizing agents (Example: nitric, perchloric and/or sulfuric acids) and then heated. Heating is continued until the organic matter is completely digested, leaving only the mineral oxides in solution. The temperature and time used depends on the type of acids and oxidizing agents used. Typically, a digestion takes from 10 minutes to a few hours at temperatures of about 350oC. The resulting solution can then be analyzed for specific minerals.

  Advantages: Little loss of volatile minerals occurs because of the lower temperatures used, more rapid than dry ashing.

  Disadvantages: Labor intensive, requires a special fume-cupboard if perchloric acid is used because of its hazardous nature, low sample throughput.

Extractive value determination:

Extractive value gives idea about soluble chemical constituents in particular solvents. According to IP, alcohol, Pet. Ether and water soluble extractive values should be determined.

Procedure: Weigh accurately quantity of crude drug and macerate it for 24 hr. With intermittent shaking for first 6 hr and allow to stand for further 18 hr. After 24 hr filter and evaporate filtrate. Residue remains after evaporation is value of extractive value of that particular solvent. While determining water extractive value, add 5% chloroform as a microbial growth inhibitor.

Table 16.14 Extractive values of few crude drugs.

Plant Name and Extractive values	Name of pharmacopeia		
	Indian Pharmacopeia Vol-III, [2018]	**Ayurvedic Pharmacopeia Vol-I, [1986]**	**Indian Herbal Pharmacopeia [2002]**
Ashwagandha			
Ethanol soluble extractive value [NLT %]	10	2	20
Water soluble extractive value [NLT %]	15	8	16
Turmeric			
Ethanol soluble extractive value [NLT %]	6	8	8
Water soluble extractive value [NLT %]	12	12	12
Sarpagandha (Rauwolfia)			
Ethanol soluble extractive value [NLT %]	2	4	9
Water soluble extractive value [NLT %]	5	10	8
Sunthi (Ginger)			
Ethanol soluble extractive value [NLT %]	2	3	2
Water soluble extractive value [NLT %]	10	10	10

Determination of Moisture Content: An excess of water in medicinal plant material will lead to deterioration through microbial growth or enzyme mediated hydrolysis in glycoside containing plants. Therefore limits for the amount of water should be set for every plant material. Methods of determination of moisture content include:

<table>
<tr>
<td>Loss on Drying: (Gravimetric method):</td>
<td>This test determines loss of both water and volatile matter by drying thermostabel substance at 100-105 °C in oven or thermo labile substances in a desiccators over phosphorus Pentoxide R under atmospheric or reduced pressure and temperature for a specified period of time. In an LOD test, the sample is weighed, dried, and weighed again. The difference in the two weights (Loss on Drying) is then compared with either the original weight
(Wet-base test) or final weight (Dry-base test) and the moisture content calculated. Tests can be manually conducted (weigh, oven dry, weigh) or automated (integrated weight and heating unit) with systems called Moisture Determination Balances. Depending on the balance and heating mechanism, a wide array of precision and accuracy is available. Today there are even micromoisture analyzers, using microbalances that can provide moisture measurement to the PPM level, consistent with the limits of KF testing. LOD Moisture Measurement can be done by:
▪ Forced air ovens.
▪ Convection ovens.
▪ Vacuum ovens.
▪ Infrared moisture balances.
▪ Microwave (drying) ovens.
Procedure: Take accurately weighed quantity of (about 2-5 g) of the material to be tested in silica crucible and dry the sample by one of the following techniques until constant weight is obtained. Calculate the loss of weight in mg/g of air dried material.
➢ Dry in an oven at 100-105 °C for 4 hr
➢ Dry in desiccator over phos-phorous pentaoxide R under</td>
</tr>
</table>

Contd...

<table>
<tr><td>Azeotropic Method (Toluene distillation method):
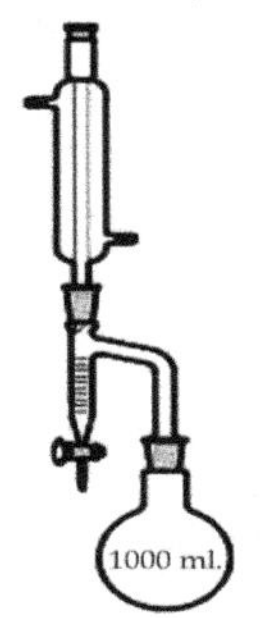

Figure 16.8
Water content determination - Dean Stark apparatus.</td><td>This method gives a direct measurement of the water present in the material being examined. When the sample is distilled together with an immiscible solvent, such as toluene R or xylene R. The water present in the sample is absorbed by the solvent, they are distilled together and separated in the receiving tube on cooling.
Procedure: Take accurately weighed quantity of the material expected to give about 2-3 ml of water into the flask. Heat the flask gently. When boiling begins, distill at a rate of 2 drops/sec until most of the water has distilled over, and then increase the rate of distillation to about 4 drops/sec. After complete distillation, rinse the inside of condenser tube with toluene R. Continue the distillation for 5 more min and again wash any droplets of water adhere to the walls of the receiving tube with toluene. Allow the water and toluene layers to separate and measure volume of the water. Calculate the content of water in % using the formula: % of Water = 100 (n'- n) / w
where
w = the weight in g of the material being examined.
n = the number of ml of water obtained in the first distillation
n'= the total number of ml of water obtained in both distillations.</td></tr>
<tr><td>Karl Fischer Method</td><td>In this method colored solution of Karl Fischer reagent (pyridine, sulfur dioxide, iodine, and anhydrous methanol) reacts quantitatively with water to form a colorless solution. This is coulometric or electrochemical titration method to determine water only unlike other methods of moisture content determination where volatile components are also estimated.
Principle: The working electrode is an iodine electrode, while the reference electrode is a platinum electrode. The reaction involves converting solid iodine into hydrogen iodide in the presence of sulfur dioxide and water. Pyridine, which is a base, is often used to counteract the formation of sulfuric acid. All reagents must be anhydrous for the analysis to be quantitative.
Procedure: The main compartment of the titration cell contains the anode solution plus the analyte. The anode solution consists of an alcohol (methanol or diethylene glycol monoethyl ether), a base Pyridine, Sulfur dioxide (SO_2) and iodine (I_2). The titration cell also consists of a smaller compartment with a cathode immersed in the anode solution of this main compartment. A dehydrating solvent suitable for the sample is placed in this flask. The sample is then added. Titration is carried out using a titrant. According to Faraday's laws, the iodine is produced in proportion to the quantity of electricity. This means that the water content can be determined immediately from the coulombs required for electrolytic oxidation.
1 mg of water = 10.71 Coulombs
Water reaction with Karl-Fischer reagent:
$H_2O + I_2 + SO_2 + 3\ C_5H_5N \rightarrow 2(C_5H_5N{+}H)\ I + C_5H_5N \cdot SO_3$
$C_5H_5N \cdot SO_3 + CH_3OH \rightarrow (C_5H_5N{+}H)\ O\text{-}O_2 \cdot OCH_3$</td></tr>
</table>

Contd...

<table>
<tr><td></td><td>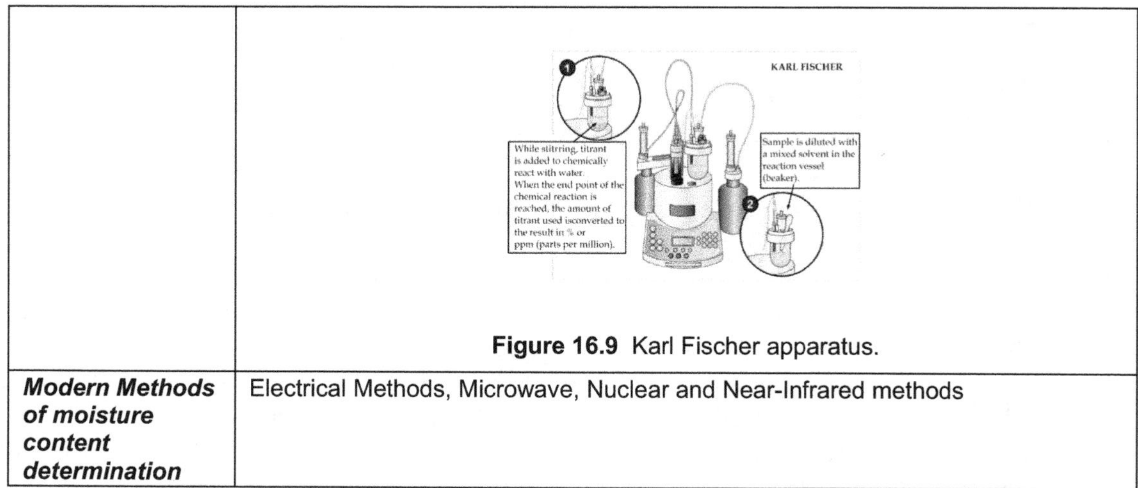

Figure 16.9 Karl Fischer apparatus.</td></tr>
<tr><td>Modern Methods of moisture content determination</td><td>Electrical Methods, Microwave, Nuclear and Near-Infrared methods</td></tr>
</table>

Determination of Volatile Oils

This determination is important standardization parameter for volatile oils containing plant materials. Initially in round bottom flask, add sufficient quantity of xylene R or the solvent given for the material, attach condenser and graduated collector tube. Heat the liquid in the flask until it begins to boil and adjust the distillation rate to 2-3 ml/min. Stop the heating after 30 min, turn off the heater and at least 10 min later, record the volume of solvent xylene collected in the graduated tube. Take the accurately weighed crude plant material and introduce into the flask and continue the distillation. After further 10 min, record the volume of the oil collected in the graduated tube and subtract the volume of the solvent (xylene) previously noted. The difference represents the volume of the volatile oil in the weight of plant material taken. Calculate the content in ml of oil per 100 g of plant material.

Chemical Evaluation

***Qualitative Chemical Evaluation*:** This involves various chemical tests to identify different phytochemicals. For example, Alkaloids can be detected by Mayer's reagent, Dragendroff's reagent, Wagner's reagent; cardiac glycosides by killer killani tests etc. Specific chemical tests can also be helpful in chemical evaluation. For example, Thalleoquin test for quinine.

***Quantitative Chemical Evaluation*:** Quantitative Chemical Assay procedure (Radio immuno assay, Enzyme-linked immunosorbent assay), values (Acid value, iodine value, saponification value for fats and oils while ester value, acetyl value, aldehyde content for volatile oil) and quantitative estimation of individual phytochemicals by using chromatography, spectroscopy etc. are parameters of quantitative chemical evaluation.

Biological or Pharmacological Evaluation

When potency of crude drug or its preparations is measured by its effect on microorganisms, organs or tissues of animal then it is known as biological evaluation and if on whole animals like rat, mice, monkey, guinea pig then it is known as pharmacological evaluation. When strength of drug in its preparation is to be evaluated then it is named as bioassays. This is preferred method when chemical or physical evaluation is not satisfactory for material.

<table>
<tr><td>In vivo methods</td><td>In vivo means "within the living. In this method drug effects are tested on whole, living organisms or cells, usually animals, including humans and plants. Animal testing and clinical trials are major elements of in vivo research.
Anti- inflammatory activity determination
<table>
<tr><td>Method/Model</td><td>:</td><td>Carrageenan rat paw edema model</td></tr>
<tr><td>Animal</td><td>:</td><td>Rats</td></tr>
<tr><td>Standard drug</td><td>:</td><td>Diclofenac</td></tr>
<tr><td>Disease inducing agent</td><td></td><td>Carrageenan</td></tr>
<tr><td>Duration</td><td>:</td><td>3 hr</td></tr>
<tr><td>Method of evaluation</td><td>:</td><td>Measurement of paw edema by using Plethysmometer or vernier caliper</td></tr>
<tr><td>Calculations</td><td>:</td><td>Percentage of inhibition of</td></tr>
</table></td></tr>
<tr><td>In vitro methods</td><td>In vitro studies are performed with microorganisms, cells, or biological molecules outside their normal biological context in labware such as test tubes, flasks, Petri dishes, and microtiter plates
In vitro anticancer activity on determination using animal cells or tissues: In metabolic assays in which, the cellular reduction of a colorless tetrazolium salt (MTT or XTT) yields a colored formazan in proportion to viable cell number. The formazans could be measured con-veniently in an automated colorimeter.
Procedure: Take cancer cells of 3 x 105 cells/well concentration in a 96 well plate except at least three wells without cells to serve as a control for the minimum absorbance. Incubate plate overnight at 37°C in a humidified incubator, 5% CO2 for the cancer cells to grow and adhere to the surface. Add Test compounds in to the plate. Include replicates for a range of concentrations. Include negative controls (including vehicle control) and a positive control. The final volume will be 100µl per well. Incubate plate for overnight (or for some other appropriate time) at 37°C in a humidified incubator, 5% CO_2. Then add 3-(4,5-dimethylthiazol-2-yl)-2,5-diphenyltetrazolium bromide (MTT) reagent (20µl/100µl per well of the 96 well plate). Incubate at 37°C for 3 hours then add 2.0 ml of 10% Trichloroacetic acid to stop further reaction and shake plate at room temperature for a minimum of 1 hour. After the 1 hour incubation, ensure the formazan precipitate is dissolved by pippeting each well up and down until no precipitate is visible. Read the plate on a plate reader using wavelength at 572 nm. Tabulate results and calculate the % viability.</td></tr>
<tr><td></td><td>Antimicrobial activity
Three methods can be useful to determine antimicrobial activity i.e. agar well method, turbidometric method and bioautographic method. In agar well method, select media specific to microorganisms and prepare plates of solid media Add microbial strains of optimum dilutions and then prepare well in plate by bore, add sample and standard solution in wells, incubate it for 24 hr for bacteria and 72 hr for Fungi. Measure zone of inhibition in mm by scale and compare with standard.
In turbidometric method, prepare tubes of liquid media; add strains and sample solutions, incubate it 24 hr for bacteria and 72 hr for Fungi.</td></tr>
</table>

Contd...

	Measure turbidity of liquid solutions by spectrophotometer and compare with standard. Bioautographic method involves use of TLC plates where media and microbial strain is applied over pre developed plates and allowed to incubate for 24 to 72 hr depending upon microorganism. Sepa-rated fractions on TLC having antimicro-bial activity would show zone of inhibition in visible light or after spraying with reagents like MTT which are able to differentiate between live or dead cells. **Figure 16.10** Zone of inhibition area indicates antimicrobial potency.
Ex vivo methods	Ex vivo refers to experimentation or measurements done in or on tissue from an organism in an external environment with minimal alteration of natural conditions. Ex vivo conditions allow experimentation on an organism's cells or tissues under more controlled conditions than is possible in in vivo experiments (in the intact organism), at the expense of altering the "natural" environment. Tissues may be removed in many ways, including in part, as whole organs, or as larger organ systems.
In silico methods	Experiments are performed on computer or via computer simulation. Virtual screening (VS) is a computational technique used in drug discovery to search libraries of small molecules in order to identify those structures which are most likely to bind to a drug target, typically a protein receptor or enzyme. There methods can be ligand-based, structure-based or hybrid techniques.

WHO Biological Evaluation

Determination of Swelling Index

This test is very useful for materials with swelling properties, especially gums and mucilage, pectin and hemicelluloses. “The swelling index is the volume in ml taken up by the swelling of 1g of plant material under specified conditions”. Introduce the quantity of the individual plant material, previously reduced to the required fitness and accurately weighed, into a 25 ml glass stoppered measuring cylinder of length of graduated portion of cylinder should be 125mm and internal diameter about 16 mm subdivided in 0.2 ml and marked from 0 to 25 ml in an upward direction. Add 25 ml of water unless otherwise indicated in the test procedure and shake the mixture thoroughly at intervals of every 10 min for 1 hr. Allow to stand for 3 hrs at room temperature or as otherwise given. Measure the volume in ml occupied by the plant material, including any sticky mucilage. Calculate the mean value of the individual determinations, related to 1g of plant material.

Determination of Foam Index

This test is to measure the foaming ability of an aqueous decoction of saponin containing medicinal plant materials which possesses property to form persistent foam when an aqueous decoction is shaken. Prepare aqueous decoction of about 1g of coarse powder plant material in 100 ml water by boiling for 30 min. Cool and filter into a 100 ml volumetric flask and add sufficient water to make up the volume to 100 ml. Now prepare 10 stoppered test tubes(ht-16cm, diameter-16 mm) in a series containing successive portions of above decoction 1,2,3, up to 10 ml and adjust the volume of the liquid in each tube with water to 10 ml. Stopper the tubes and shake them in a lengthwise motion for 15 sec , 2 frequencies per second. Allow to stand for 15 min and measure the height of the foam.

- If the height of the foam in every tube is less than 1 cm, the foaming index is less than 100.
- If in any tube a height of foam of 1cm is measured, the dilution of the plant material in this tube (a) is the index sought. if this tube is the first or second tube in a series, it is necessary to have an intermediate dilution prepared in a similar manner to obtain more precise results.
- If height of foam is more than 1cm in every test tube, the foaming index is over 1000.in this case the determination needs to be made on a new series of dilutions of the decoction in order to obtain results.
- Formula for foaming index: 1000/A where A= volume of decoction having exact 1 cm height

Determination of Haemolytic Activity

Saponins have ability to cause haemolysis where haemoglobin diffuses into the surrounding medium through a change in the erythrocytic membrane and makes blood a clear solution.

Requirement: Citrated ox blood (25% solution), phosphate buffer pH 7.4, 10 mg of saponin R in 100 ml phosphate buffer p^H 7.4,

Preliminary Test: Prepare a serial dilution of plant material or its extract with phosphate buffer pH 7.4 and blood suspension (25%) using 4 test tubes as given in following table 16.15. As soon as the tubes have been prepared, gently invert them to mix and avoid the formation of foam. Shake again after 30 min interval. Examine the tubes and record in which dilution total haemolysis has occurred indicated by a clear, resolution without any deposit of red cells and follow following observation steps for final results:

Table 16.15 Preliminary test dilutions of Haemolytic Activity.

Tube Number	1	2	3	4
Plant material extract (ml)	0.10	0.20	0.50	1.00
Phosphate buffer PH 7.4 (ml)	0.90	0.80	0.50	-
Blood suspension 2% (ml)	1.00	1.00	1.00	1.00

Table 16.16 Main test dilutions of Haemolytic Activity.

Tube Number	1	2	3	4	5	6	7	8	9	10	11	12	13
Drug extract	0.4	0.45	0.5	0.55	0.6	0.65	0.7	0.75	0.8	0.85	0.9	0.95	1.0
Phosphate buffer(ml)	0.6	0.55	0.5	0.45	0.4	0.35	0.3	0.25	0.2	0.15	0.1	0.05	0.0
Blood suspension	1.0	1.0	1.0	1.0	1.0	1.0	1.0	1.0	1.0	1.0	1.0	1.0	1.0

Observation steps:

- If total haemolysis is observed in tube no. 4, use the original plant material extract with phosphate buffer pH 7.4.
- If total haemolysis is observed in tubes tubes 3 and 4. Prepare a two fold dilution of original plant material extract with phosphate buffer pH 7.4.
- If total haemolysis is observed in tubes 2, 3 & 4 prepare 5-fold dilutions as described above.
- If after 6 hrs all test tubes contain a clear, red solution, prepare a tenfold dilution and carry out preliminary test as described above.
- If total haemolysis is not observed in any test-tube, repeat the preliminary test using a more concentration of plant material or its extract.

***Main Test*:** Prepare serial dilution of the plant material extract as per results of preliminary test with phosphate buffer pH 7.4 and blood suspension (2%) using 13 test-tubes as given in table.Carry out the evaluations as in the preliminary test but observe the results after 24 hrs. Calculate the amount of medicinal plant material in gm or of the preparation in gm or ml, which produce total haemolysis (b).

$$\text{Haemolytic activity} = 1000 * a/b$$

Where 1000 = the defined haemolytic activity of saponin R inrelation to OX blood, a= quantity of saponin R in gm, b = quantity of plant material in gm.

Determination of Bitterness Value

Medicinal plant materials which have a strong bitter taste are utilized mostly as appetizing agents. Bitter substance can be determined chemically. However since they are mostly composed of two or more than two constituents with various degrees of bitterness, it is first necessary to measure the total bitterness by using biological method .the bitter properties of plant material are determined by comparing the threshold bitter concentration of an extract of the material with that of a diluted solution of quinine hydrochloride R.This test should not be carried out until the identity of the plant material is confirmed.

Requirements: Stock solution of quinine HCL (sq) of 0.01mg/ml, well defined concentration of Sample solutions (St).

Method: Prepare dilutions as given in above tables. Rinse the mouth with safe drinking water. Then swirl 10 ml lowest concentration of the serial dilution in themouth mainly near thebase of tongue for

Table 16.17 Standard (Quinine) drug dilutions for bitterness value determination.

Tube No.	1	2	3	4	5	6	7	8	9
1.sq(ml)	4.2	4.4	4.6	4.8	5.0	5.2	5.4	5.6	5.8
2.safe DW	5.8	5.6	5.4	5.2	5.0	4.8	4.6	4.4	4.2
3.Quinine hcl	0.042	0.044	0.046	0.048	0.050	0.052	0.054	0.056	0.058

Table 16.18 Sample drug dilutions for bitterness value determination.

Tube no.	1	2	3	4	5	6	7	8	9	10
Sample	1.00	2.00	3.00	4.00	5.00	6.00	7.00	8.00	9.00	10.00 -
Safe drinking water (ml)	9	8	7	6	5	4	3	2	1	-

30 sec. If bitter sensation is no longer felt, withdraw the solution and wait for 1 min to ascertain that there is no delayed sensitivity. Then rinse with safe drinking water. The next highestconcentration of dilution should not be tasted until at least 10 min have passed. The threshold bitter concentration is the lowest concentration of dilution at which a material still provokes a bitter sensation.After first series of tests, rinse the mouth thoroughly with safe drinking water, until no bitter sensation remains and wait for at least 10 min before carrying out secondseries of tests. In order to save time, it is advisable to first ascertain whether the solution in tube no. 5 gives bitter sensation if noted, find the threshold bitterconcentration of the material by tasting the dilutions in tubes no 1-4. If tube no 5 does not give o bitter sensation, find the threshold bitter concentration in the dilutions of tube no 6-10.all solutions and the safe drinking water for mouth washing should be at 20-25^{0}C.

Calculation: 2000 * C / A * B = Bitterness Value in Units/gm

Where A = the quantity of material in mg/ml of standard, B = the volume of standard in ml/10ml of dilution threshold bitter conc., C = the quantity of quinine HCL R in mg/10ml of the dilution of threshold bitter conc.

Determination of Total Tannins Value

Tannins are substance capable of turning animal hides into leather by binding proteins to form water insoluble substances which are resistant to proteolytic enzymes. This process when applied to living tissue is known as an astringent action and is the reason for the therapeutic activity of tannins.

***Procedure*:** Take the powder plant material into conical flask, add 150 ml of water and heat over a boiling waterbath for 30 min, allow the solid material to settle and filter the liquid through a filter paper, discarding the first 50 ml of the filtrate. Determine the total amount of material extractable into water by evaporating 50 ml plant material extract to dryness and drying the residue in an oven at 105^{0}C for 4 hrsand weigh (T1).

Determine the amount of plant material not bound to the hide powder extractable into water by taking 80 ml of the plant extract, add 6 gm of hide powder R and shake well for 60 min. filter the evaporate 50 ml of the clear filtrate to dryness. Dry the residue in an oven at 1050C and weigh (T2).

Determine the solubility of hide powder by taking 6 gm of hide powder R. add 80 ml water and shake well for 60 min, filter and evaporate 50 ml of the clear filtrate to dryness. Dry the residue in an oven at 1050C and weigh (T0).

Calculation: Quantity of tannin in % = [T1 – (T2 – T0)] * 500 / W Where:W = the quantity of plant material in gm

Toxicological evaluation

Microbial Load Determination

Plant materials normally carry a great number of bacteria and moulds often originating in soil. Current practices of harvesting, handling and production may cause additional contamination and microbial growth.In addition the presence of aflatoxin in plant material can be hazardous to health if absorbed in very small amount.

(A) For contamination of crude plant material intended for further processing

- E. Coli - 10^4 per gram.
- Mould propagules - 10^5 per gram.

(B) For plant material that are used as topical dosage form.

- Aerobic bacteria max 10^7 per gram.
- Yeasts or mould max. 10^4 per gram.
- E. Coli max. 10^2 per gram.
- Other enterobacteria max 10^4 per gram.
- Salmonella - none.

(C) For plant material use for internal purposeAerobic bacteria 10^5per gram.

- Yeasts or mould max. 10^3 per gram.
- E. Coli max. 10 per gram.
- Other enterobacteria max 10^3per gram.
- Salmonella - none.

Table 16.19 Medias for various bacterias.

Bacteria	Media	Observation
Enterobacteriaceae and other Gram-negative bacteria	Violet red bile agar with glucose and lactose	Red or reddish in color
Escherichia coli	Maconkey broth	Reddish brown precipitation
Salmonella Species	Deoxycholate citrate agar	Well developed, colorless
Pseudomonas aeruginosa	Soyabean- casein digest medium	Green fluorescence
Pseudomonas aeruginosa	Baird-Parker agar	Black colonies

Prepare the selected media and transfer to petri plate, apply the herbal sample and allow incubating for 24-48hrs. Then observe and compare colonies.

Aflatoxin Determination

Aflatoxins produced by the growth of mold *Asperigillus flavus*, *A. Parasiticus* have carcinogenic properties because the toxin might be altered in a human body to a mutagenic compound. Aflatoxin B1, B2, G1 and G2 are highly dangerous contami-nation in any material of the plant origin.

***TLC Method*:** Initially follow the extraction procedure for aflatoxin isolation through non-polar solvents and then dissolve 0.2 ml extract in mixture of chloroform: acetonitrile (98:2). Take silica gel G as Stationary phase and chloroform: acetone: 2- propane (85:10:5) as mobile phase. Develop chromatogram, allow it to dry in air and examine chromatogram in a dark room under UV light 365 nm. Clear blue fluorescent spot are indicates presence of aflotoxins.

Table 16.20 Limits of Heavy Metals and Aflatoxins.

HM/Afla	IP	JP	EP	USP	AP	UP	WHO
Lead	NMT 20 ppm	NMT 20 ppm	5 ppm	NMT 5 ppm	NMT 10 ppm	10 ppm	10 ppm
Mercury	-	-	0.1 ppm	NMT 20 ppm	NMT 1 ppm	1 ppm	-
Bismuth	-	-	-	NMT 20 ppm	-		-
Arsenic	NMT 10 ppm	-	-	NMT 3 ppm	NMT 3 ppm	3 ppm	-
Antimony	-	-	-	NMT 20 ppm	-		-
Tin	-	-	-	NMT 20 ppm	-		-
Cadmium	-	-	0.5 ppm	NMT 20 ppm	NMT 0.3 ppm	0.3 ppm	0.3 ppm
Silver	-	-	-	NMT 20 ppm	-	-	-
Copper	-	-	-	NMT 20 ppm	-		-
Molybdenum	-	-	-	NMT 20 ppm	-		-
Vanadium	-	-	-	-	-		-
Palladium	-	-	-	-	-		-
Platinum	-	-	-	-	-		-
Gold	-	-	-	-	-		-

Contd...

HM/Afla	IP	JP	EP	USP	AP	UP	WHO
Ruthenium	-	-	-	-	-		-
Afla B1	-	10 µg/kg		NMT 5 ppb	0.5 ppm		
Afla G1	-	10 µg/kg		NMT 20 ppb	0.5 ppm		
Afla B2	-	10 µg/kg		NMT 20 ppb	0.1 ppm		
Afla G2	-	10 µg/kg		NMT 20 ppb	0.1 ppm		

HM- Heavy metal, Afla- aflatoxin, IP- Indian Pharmacopoeia, JP- Japanese Pharmacopoeia, EP- European Pharmacopoeia, USP-United states Pharmacopoeia, AP- the Ayurvedic Pharmacopoeia of India, UP- the Unani Pharmacopeia of India, WHO- World Health Organization, NMT- Not More Than, PPM-Parts Per Million and PPB- Parts Per Billion

Radioactive Contamination

A certain amount of exposure to ionizing radiation cannot be avoided since there are many sources, including radionuclide occurring naturally in the ground and the atmosphere. The WHO in collaboration with several other international organizations has developed guidelines for use in the event of widespread contamination by radionuclide resulting from a major nuclear accident. Even at a maximum observed levels of radioactive contamination with the more dangerous radionuclide, significant risk is associated only with consumption of quantities of over 20 kg of plant material per year so that a risk to health is most unlikely to be encountered given the amount of medicinal plant material that would need to be ingested. Additionally the level of contamination might be reduced during the manufacturing process. Therefore no limit radioactive contaminations are proposed. Detection of alpha, beta and gamma radiations: gas detector: Geiger Muller (GM) detector, solid detector: scintillation detector

Pesticide Residue Determination

The pesticides residues generally accumulate from agriculture practices of spraying, treating solids during cultivation and through the administration of fumigants during storage. Pollution is also increases amount of deposited pesticides. Thus it is necessary to limits the pesticides. Various methods like HPLC, LC, GC, along with MS are very useful and common methods of detection

Heavy Metal Determination

Trace elements and heavy metals analysis is used as a standardization tool of the plant material. As per WHO, limits for Lead is 10 mg/kg and for Cadmium is 0.3mg/kg.There are several laboratory methods that determine heavy metal concentrations with accuracy down to the ppm range or below: atomic absorption spectroscopy (AAS), colorimetry, inductively coupled plasma atomic emission spectroscopy (ICP-AES), polarography, selective ion electrodes, X-ray fluorescence, energy dispersive analysis via X-rays (EDAX), and electron microprobe analysis.

In ***AAS***, a light source emitting a narrow spectral line of the characteristic energy is used to excite the free atoms formed in the flame. The decrease in energy (absorption) is then measured. The absorption is proportional to the concentration of free atoms in the flame, given by lamberts-beer law.

Polarography is an electrochemical method of analysis based on the measurement of the current flow resulting from the electrolysis of a solution at a polarizable microelectrode as a function of applied voltage. Simple principle of polarography is the study of electro-reducible or electro-oxidsable solutions by means of electrolysis with two electrodes, one polarizable (Mercury Dropping Electrode) and another unpolarizable (large pool of mercury or a calomel half-cell). In polarography, the electric potential (i.e. voltage) of a dropping mercury drop in an electrolyte containing an electroactive species is varied as a function of time and the resulting current due to the electrochemical reaction is measured. Polarography is a specific type of measurement that falls into the general category of linear-sweep voltammetry where the electrode potential is altered in a linear fashion from the initial potential to the final potential.

***Procedure*:** The substance which is to be determined should be in solution form and a suitable portion added to the supporting electrolyte, gelatin is added and the resulting solution is transferred to the polarographic cell. Since oxygen reacts at the D.M.E. it is desirable to remove dissolved air from the solution by passing nitrogen through it before electrolysis. After shutting off the nitrogen the solution is electrolyzed by slowly applying an increasing voltage. The current is recorded at various values of the applied voltage and the results plotted. This gives the current-voltage curve known as a polarogram. It is then possible to determine the nature and concentration of the reacting substance from the polarogram.

Table 16.21 Limits of Residual Solvents.

Class-I toxic and carcinogenic		**Class-II less toxicity**		**Class-III low risk to human health**	
Solvent	**limit (PPM)**	**Solvent**	**Limit (PPM)**	**Solvent**	**Limit (PPM)**
Benzene	2	Acetonitrile	410	Acetic acid	5000 ppm
Carbon tetra chloride	4	Chloroform	60	Acetone	5000 ppm
1,2-dichloroethane	5	Cyclohexane	3880	1-Butanol	5000 ppm
1,1-dichloroethane	8	Hexane	290	Anisole	5000 ppm
1,1,1-trichloroethane	1500	Methanol	3000	2-Butanol	5000 ppm
-	-	Nitromethane	50	Dimethyl sulfoxide	5000 ppm
-	-	Pyridine	200	Ethanol	5000 ppm
-	-	Tetra hydro furan	720	Ethyl acetate	5000 ppm
-	-	Toluene	890	Ethyl ether	5000 ppm
-	-	Xylene	2170	Ethyl formate	5000 ppm
-	-	-	-	Formic acid	5000 ppm
-	-	-	-	Heptane	5000 ppm
-	-	-	-	Isobutyl acetate	5000 ppm

Contd...

Class-I toxic and carcinogenic		Class-II less toxicity		Class-III low risk to human health	
Solvent	limit (PPM)	Solvent	Limit (PPM)	Solvent	Limit (PPM)
-	-	-	-	Isopropyl acetate	5000 ppm
-	-	-	-	Methyl acetate	5000 ppm
-	-	-	-	Pentane	5000 ppm
-	-	-	-	1-Pentanol	5000 ppm
-	-	-	-	1-Propanol	5000 ppm
Ppm- parts per million					

Advanced Analytical Evaluation

Chromatography

Chromatography is the technique is used primarily for the separation of the components of a sample in which the components are distributed between two phases of which one is stationary (Solid/liquid) while other is mobile phase (liquid/gaseous). Chromatographic techni-que are generally classified on the basis of separation principle of it i.e. adsorption, partition, ion exchange or sieving These are as paper, column, TLC, HPTLC, HPLC, GLC, GSC, ion exchange chromatography, gel chromatography etc.All chromate-graphic techniques are useful for Qualitative as well as quantitative applications. Gradient and isocratic elution technique are generally preferred to separation on the basis of retention factor (Rf) or retention volume, area under curve, various chromatograms are evaluated. Pre and post derivitisation increases the sensitivity of detection.

Technique	Stationary phase/s	Mobile Phase	Detector/s	Application/s
Planar chromatographic techniques				
Paper	Whatman paper (Cellulose)	Organic solvents	UV-cabinet Or any non-corrosive derivitisation spraying agents	Identification Separation Purification Impurity detection **(Qualitative and preparative)**
TLC	Silica, alumina, calcium carbonate, starch,	Organic solvents	UV-cabinet Or any derivitisation spraying agents	Identification Separation Purification Impurity detection **(Qualitative and preparative)**

Contd...

HPTLC	Silica, alumina, calcium carbonate, starch,	Organic solvents	Densitometer based on UV-visible spectroscopy principle	**Qualitative and quantitative:** Identification Separation Purification Impurity detection **(Fingerprint)**
Column chromatographic techniques				
HPLC	Normal phase and reversed phase **Silica (C8, C18, Cyano, Diol)**	Organic solvents	UV-Detector, Photo-diode array detector, Refractive index detector	Identification Separation Purification Impurity detection
Gas	Polyethylene glycol, Polydimethyl siloxane, Poly (phynylmethyldimethylsiloxane) (10-50% phenyl)	Gases like nitrogen, helium, argon, air	Thermal Conductivity detector (TCD) Flame Ionization	Identification Separation Purification Impurity detection
	In gas liquid chromatography (GLC) generally non-volatile liquid is to be coated as a thin film on solid support like Diatomaceous earth)		detector (FID) Catalytic combustion detector (CCD) Electron capture detector (ECD) Mass spectrometer (MS) Infrared detector (IRD)	**(Gaseous and low molecular weight natural chemicals like volatile as well as non-volatile oils)**
Gel	Gelling materials like dextran, agarose	Organic solvents	UV-Detector	Identification Separation Purification Impurity detection **(High molecular weight phytochemicals like proteins, polymers, enzymes)**

Ultra-high performance liquid chromatography (UHPLC)

In recent years, UHPLC has been emerging as a feasible technique for the quality control of herbal products. UHPLC can withstand a pressure of at most 8000 psi and it brings liquid chromatographic analysis to another level by hardware modifications of the conventional HPLC machinery. UHPLC makes it possible to perform high-resolution separations superior to HPLC analysis by using solid phase particles of less than 2 μ m in diameter to achieve superior sensitivity and resolution. Smaller particle size leads to higher separation efficiency and shorter columns size leads to shorter analysis time with little solvent consumption. Within a period of last few years, UHPLC fingerprints of herbal products were developed instead of conventional HPLC approach. In comparison to HPLC, UHPLC analyses reported a decreased analysis time by a factor up to eight without loss of information. The results obtained not only showed decreased analysis time but also proved a great enhancement in selectivity compared to conventional HPLC analysis.

Hydrophilic interaction chromatography (HILIC)

HILIC has gained attention in herbal fingerprinting because of good separation quality of hydrophilic compounds. Many of polar compounds of herbal medicines are extracted by using aqueous solution, which might be better separated by means of HILIC. HILIC was introduced as an alternative for normal-phase liquid chromatography (NPLC); HILIC enables the separation of polar compounds on polar stationary phases with aqueous mobile phases. It is based on the principle of partitioning between a water-enriched layer in the hydrophilic stationary phase and a relatively hydrophobic mobile phase usually containing 5–40% water in organic solvent. This technique is more eco-friendly as compared to NPLC because of the use of water and polar organic solvents as mobile phase. In addition, the polar compounds are more soluble in the mobile phase of HILIC. As HILIC is a relatively recent technique, few papers analyzing herbal products have been published yet. Most papers usually describe a methodology exploiting the orthogonal character of the HILIC and reversed-phase liquid chromatography (RPLC) methods for quality control.

Chromatographic fingerprints of herbal medicines

In general, one could use the chromatographic techniques to obtain a relatively complete picture of an herbal, which is in common called chromatographic fingerprints of herbal medicines to represent the so-called phytoequivalence. Obtaining a good chromatographic fingerprint representing the phytoequivalence of an herb depends several factors, such as the extracting methods, measurement instruments, measurement conditions, etc. Furthermore, a chromatogram with good separation and a representative concentration profile of the bioactive components detected by a proper detector are also required. Thus, how to obtain a high quality chromatographic fingerprint of as more as possible information of the herbal medicines is an important task for chemists and pharmacologists. Some researchers have been done along with this direction. In order to understand bioactivities and possible side effects of active compounds of the herbal medicines and to enhance product quality control, it seems that one needs to determine most of the phytochemical constituents of herbal products so as to ensure the reliability and repeatability of pharmacological and clinical research. However, using the chemical fingerprints for the purpose of quality control of herbal medicines can only address to the problem of comparing the integrated sameness and/or difference and controlling their stability of the available herbal products. The complex relationship between the chromatographic fingerprints and efficacy of the herbal medicines is not taken into account yet, which seems to be the most important aspect for the quality control of herbal medicines. As it is well-known that the efficacy of traditional herbal medicines has a characteristic of a complex mixture of chemical compounds present in the herbs, thus how to evaluate reasonably their relationship is obviously not a trivial task.

Spectroscopy

Spectroscopy is defined as interaction between matter and electromagnetic radiation. Spectroscopy is the technique in which various electromagnetic radiations are studied. And spectrometer is the instrument which measure in electro-magnetic radiations. Spectroscopy can be absorption or emission spectroscopy. Various spectroscopy techniques are Absorption: UV-visible, IR, NMR, Mass and Emission: Flame, fluorescence spectroscopy.

Type of energy transfer	Region of electromagnetic spectrum	Spectroscopic technique	Quantic transition type
Absorption	γ-ray	Mossbauer spectroscopy	Nuclear
	X-ray	X-ray absorption spectroscopy	Inner electrons
	Ultraviolet/Visible	UV/Vis spectroscopy	Bounding electrons
		Atomic absorption spectroscopy	Bounding electrons
	Infrared	Infrared spectroscopy	Rotation/vibration of molecules
		Raman spectroscopy	Rotation/vibration of molecules
	Microwave	Microwave spectroscopy	Rotation of molecules
	Radio wave	Electron spin resonance spectroscopy	Spin of electrons in a magnetic field
		Nuclear magnetic resonance spectroscopy	Spin of nuclei in a magnetic field
Emission (thermal excitation)	Ultraviolet/Visible	Atomic emission spectroscopy	Bounding electrons
Photoluminescence	X-ray	X-ray fluorescence	Inner electrons
	Ultraviolet/Visible	Fluorescence spectroscopy	Bounding electrons
		Phosphorescence spectroscopy	Bounding electrons
		Atomic fluorescence spectroscopy	Bounding electrons
Chemiluminescence	Ultraviolet/Visible	Chemiluminescence spectroscopy	Bounding electrons

Applications of Spectroscopy

(i) ***UV-Visible Spectroscopy*:** To find out whether the system is conjugated (the coloured compounds such as β-carotene, crocetin are in system of extensively conjugated pi-electrons).

(ii) ***IR Spectroscopy*:** To identify the functional groups that are present in the compound.

(iii) ***Mass Spectroscopy*:** To determine the molecular structure and molecular weight of the compound and to identify the presence of isotopes patterns for Cl and Br.

(iv) ***NMR Spectroscopy*:** It gives idea about structural backbone of compound. 13C-NMR - To identify how many types of carbon atoms are present in the compound.1H-NMR -To find out how many types of hydrogen atoms are present in the compound and to find out how the hydrogen atoms are connected.

Further Reading

1. Denney RC, Barnes JD, Thomas MKJ, Vogel's Textbook of Quantitative Chemical Analysis, 6thedition, Pearson education, New Delhi, India, 2007, 29.
2. Skoog DA, Holler FJ, Crouch SR, Principles of Instrumental Analysis, 6thedition, Thomson brooks/cole, United states, 2007, 13
3. Willard HH, Merritt LL, Dean JA, Settle FA, Instrumental Methods of Analysis, 7thedition, CBS publishers and distributers Pvt Ltd, New Delhi, India, 1986, 7
4. Harborne JB, Phytochemical Methods: A Guide to Modern Techniques of Plant Analysis, 3rdedition, Thomson science, New York, London, 1998, 5-17, 32.
5. Chatwal GR, Anand SK, Instrumental Methods of Chemical Analysis, 5thedition, Himalaya Publising House, Mumbai, India, 2008,1.6.
6. Skoog DA, Holler FJ, Crouch SR, Principles of Instrumental Analysis, 6thedition, Thomson brooks/cole, United states, 2007, 157-377.
7. Siddhiqui MR, Alothman ZA, Rahman N, Analytical Techniques in Pharmaceutical Analysis: A Review, Arabian Journal of Chemistry, 2013, 1-46.
8. João Cajaiba Da Silva, Alex Queiroz, Alline Oliveira and Vinícius Kartnaller (January 25th 2017). Advances in the Application of Spectroscopic Techniques in the Biofuel Area over the Last Few Decades, Frontiers in Bioenergy and Biofuels, Eduardo Jacob-Lopes and Leila Queiroz Zepka, IntechOpen, DOI: 10.5772/65552. Available from: https://www.intechopen.com/books/frontiers-in-bioenergy-and-biofuels/advances-in-the-application-of-spectroscopic-techniques-in-the-biofuel-area-over-the-last-few-decade

Scan QR code to view the website/guidelines

- WHO Herbal Quality Control Methods-
Quality control methods for (who.int)

CHAPTER 17

Stability Testing and Shelf Life Determination of Herbal Medicines

Introduction

The term pharmaceutical stability encompasses several concepts. The first among them is the chemical stability of drug given as tablet, capsule, syrup or injection depends not only on drug content, but also on the hardness, friability, disintegration, dissolution, viscosity, etc. Nowadays, stability testing has become an integral part of formulation development. It generates information on which proposal for shelf life of drug or dosage form and their recommended storage conditions are based. It is also a part of dossier submission to regulatory agencies for licensing approval. Beside active ingredients, several excipients are used in modern herbal formulations to enhance the palatability, bio-absorption, and shelf-life of the formulations. These excipients vary based on the type of formulations. Solid dosage forms require diluents, binder or adhesives, lubricants, glidants, disintegrants, superdisintegrants, coloring agents, sweeteners, coating material, plasticizers. Similarly, liquid and semiliquid preparations require solvents, co-solvents, buffers, antimicrobial preservatives, thickening agents, wetting agents, humectants, emulsifying agents, sweetening agents, emollients, flavors. These excipients are basically of synthetic and natural origin. The nonclassical modern herbal formulations contain both types of excipients. In many cases, lack of compatibility studies pertaining to additives leads to instability of the formulations. Hence, compatibility and stability study of the additives in the formulation needs to be performed to ensure product quality.

Drug stability

The capability of a particular formulation(dosage form or drug product) in a specific container/ closure system to remain within it's physical, chemical, microbiological, therapeutics and toxicological specifications throughout it's shelf life. The term pharmaceutical stability encompasses several concepts. The first among them is chemical stability of the drug in the dosage form. But, the performance of a drug gives as tablet, capsule, syrup or injection depends not only on drug content, but also on the pharmaceutical properties of dosage form such as hardness, friability, disintegration, dissolution, viscosity etc. A study of the stability of pharmaceutical products and of stability testing techniques is essential for three main reasons.

1. It is important from the point of view of the safety of the patient.
2. It must be given to the relevant legal requirements concerned with identity, strength, purity and quality of the drug.
3. Finally such a study is important to prevent the economic repercussions of marketing an unstable product.

Factors affecting stability

Following factors affect the stability of dosage forms.

Storage time	The longer the storage time, the more the degradation of drug and the more the deterioration of dosage forms.
Storage conditions	Storage conditions such as storage temperature and percentage relative humidity at the storage place affect stability of dosage forms adversely.
Type of dosage form	The chemical stability of drug depends on the type of dosage forms. The liquid dosage forms such as solution exhibit more degradation than semisolid and solid dosage forms.

Contd..

Container and closure system	Container-closure systems adversely affect the stability of drug and dosage forms. The plastic containers and rubber closures are reported to absorb antioxidants and preservatives from the solutions in the contact with them leading to destabilization microbial attack.
Chemical degradation of products- Pharmaceutical products differ considerably in their composition, so naturally they are subject to different forms of chemical degradation (Hydrolysis, Oxidation, Autoxidation, Isomerization, Polymerization, Decarboxylation) and in addition they may be several simultaneous decomposition reaction occurring in a product. **Example-** the alkaloid ergometrine is susceptible to isomerization, oxidation and hydrolysis.	
Physical factors influencing chemical degradation	
Temperature	The rates of most chemical reactions increase with rise in temperature. It is, there fore important to be aware of this when formulating herbal products for use in tropical areas when a product has to heat sterilized before use. The observed variation of reaction rate with temperature is an important aspect of the collision theory of chemical reaction. According to this theory, a chemical reaction only takes place molecules collide. The thermal energy which is necessary to break chemical bonds and enable reaction to take place.
Moisture	Moisture absorbed on to the surface of a solid drug will often increase the rate of decomposition if it is susceptible to hydrolysis. **Example-** penicillin, streptomycin
Light	The instability of many products is when exposed to strong sunlight. In some instances, the instability of is due to the heat accompanying the sunrays, light is a form of energy that can initiate and accelerate decomposition. Many types of chemical reaction are induced by exposure to light of higher energy. There is often a relationship between the structure of the drug and sensitivity towards light. While the presence of a conjugated double bond system in the molecules, as in vitamin A and many unsaturated oils, can also induce photo ability. Autoxidation of volatile oil causes change in color like yellow-brown, while other fade. Phenolic substances such as phenol, thymol also tends to develop colours.

Stability Testing

Stability Testing is defined as "the test, which involves examining for and potency at suitable time intervals, is conducted for a period corresponding to the normal time that the product is likely to remain in stock or in use".

In recent years, the pharmaceutical dosage forms are becoming mire and more complex and diverse. Many novel dosage forms and drug targeting systems have been introduced. Hence, designing of stability testing protocol for a particular product has become much difficult. In addition, finding a right approach for estimating shelf life has become challenging. Traditionally, multi temperature accelerated studies and Arrhenius approach were used for determination of shelf life. But, this is not applicable in all the situations. It is applicable only in cases where the drug degradation is reasonable and temperature dependant and in cases where the rate and order of reaction can determine. Accelerating the decomposition process and extrapolating the result to normal storage conditions may make a prediction of the life of the product.

Types of changes occur on storage

1.Contents	➢ **Physical**- Viscosity, texture, colour, odour, pH, loss of volatile constituents, uptake of water, oxygen or carbon dioxide. ➢ **Chemical**- Degradation of active constituents, Interaction between constituents, Loss of constituents by sorption by container. ➢ **Microbiological** - Loss of antimicrobial preservative efficacy, Microbial spoilage.
2.Container	Leakage, Corrosion, Stress cracking.

Storage Conditions

Generally, for accelerated stability testing, the samples are store under isothermal conditions and for long term stability testing (real time testing), the containers are stored in open shelves in ventilated areas. But all the above mentioned guidelines suggest that both accelerated real time tests, the sample should be stored under controlled temperature and humidity conditions. Also, multi temperature accelerated testing according to Arrhenius approach has been replaced by single temperature accelerated testing. The guidelines describe storage conditions based on worldwide temperature and humidity (%Rh) conditions. Haynes's divided the countries of world in to four zones namely,

Zone-1 : Moderate

Zone-2 : Mediterranean

Zone-3 : Hot, dry

Zone-4 : Very hot, moist.

The mean kinetic temperatures and the yearly average %Rh of these zones are given in table

Table 17.1 Worldwide zones and temperature and humidity conditions.

Sr.no.	Zone	Mean kinetic temperature (MKT)	Yearly average humidity (%Rh)
1	Zone-I (moderate)	21°C	45
2	Zone-II (Mediterranean)	25°C	60
3	Zone-III (hot, dry)	30°C	35
4	Zone-IV (very hot, moist)	30°C	70

Table 17.2 Countries belonging to various stability zones.

Region	Zone I and II	Zone III and IV
Europe	All countries	
America	US, Canada, Mexico, Chile, peru.	Brazil, Columbia, Cuba, Guyana.
Asia	China, Iran, Japan, Nepal, Turkey.	India, Sri lanka, Taiwan< Malaysia, Pakistan.
Africa	Egypt, South Africa, Zimbabwe, Libya.	Kenya, Ghana, Angola.
Australian/ Oceanic	Australia, New Zealand	Fiji, Marshal Islands, Society Islands.

Table 17.3 Stability storage conditions for Zone-I and Zone-II countries.

Product	Type of study		
	Accelerated	Intermediate	Long-term
Solid oral dosage forms, solids for reconstitution, dry and lyophilized powders in glass vials.	40° C/75%RH	30° C/60%Rh	25° C/60%RH
Liquids in glass bottles, vials, glass ampoules.	40° C/ambient humidity	30° C/ ambient humidity	25° C/ ambient humidity
Drug products in semi permeable container.	40° C/15%RH	30° C/40%RH	25° C/40%RH
Drug products intended to be stored at refrigerator temperature	25° C/60%RH or 25° C/ ambient humidity for liquid products		5±3 °C with monitoring.
Drug products intended to be stored at freezer temperature	5±3 °C ambient humidity		-15±5 °C

Table 17.4 Stability storage conditions for Zone-III and Zone-IV countries.

Product	Type of study	
	Accelerated	Long-term
Solid oral dosage forms, solids for reconstitution, dry and lyophilized powders in glass vials.	40° C/75%RH	30° C and 35/70%RH (zone III/IV)
Liquids in glass bottles, vials, glass ampoules.	40° C/ambient humidity	30° C/ ambient humidity
Drug products in semi permeable container.	40° C/15%RH	30° C/40%RH
Drug products intended to be stored at refrigerator temperature	30° C and 35/70%RH (zone III/IV)	5±3 °C with monitoring.
Drug products intended to be stored at freezer temperature	5±3 °C ambient humidity	-15±5 °C

Table 17.5 Different test parameters for different dosage forms.

No.	Dosage form	Physical parameters
1	Solutions	A. Change of colour B. Change of odour C. Clarity D. Appearance(precipitation, cloudiness)

Contd..

No.	Dosage form	Physical parameters
2	Suspensions	A. Appearance B. P^H C. Colour, odour D. Redispersibility
3	Tablets	A. Appearance B. Friability C. Hardness D. Colour, odour E. Dissolution F. Moisture absorption
4	Hard gelatin capsules	A. Moisture B. Colour C. Appearance D. Brittleness E. Dissolution F. P^H
5	Soft gelatin capsules	A. Moisture B. Colour C. Appearance D. Brittleness E. Dissolution F. P^H G. Precipitation H. Cloudiness
6	Emulsions	A. Appearance B. Colour C. P^H D. Precipitation E. Cloudiness
7	Creams and ointments	A. Appearance B. Colour C. Homogeneity D. P^H

Prediction of the Shelf Life: "Shelf life of a pharmaceutical product can be defined as the time from the date of manufacture and packaging of the formulation until its chemical or biological activity is not less than a predetermined level or labeled potency and its physical characteristics have not changed appreciably or deleteriously".

Although there are exceptions, 90% of the labeled potency is generally recognized as the minimum acceptable level. Hence, expiry date "is the time in which the preparation will remain stable when stored under recommended conditions". After recording the data, the final step is the estimation of shelf life or expiry date. The guidelines suggest an approach, which is different from the conventional approach of stability testing. Conventionally, multi-temperature accelerated studies and Arrhenius approach were used for estimation of shelf life. But there are several inherent drawbacks in Arrhenius approach. They include

- Arrhenius approach is applicable only for cases where drug degradation is reasonable and reasonable and rate or order of reaction can be determined.
- In this approach, linear regression is applied even through the data is linear.
- Errors associated with determination of drug content are not included. Above critical temperature, degradation mechanism may change and in this case also, Arrhenius approach becomes invalid.

The ICH, CPMP and FDA guidelines suggest that instead of the accelerated stability testing, shelf life determination should be based on real time testing data through application of appropriate statistical techniques.

The shelf life determination from the data obtained is based on calculations of 95% one-side confidence limits. The calculations regarding calculation of one-sided confidence limit has been explained in detail by Carstensen.

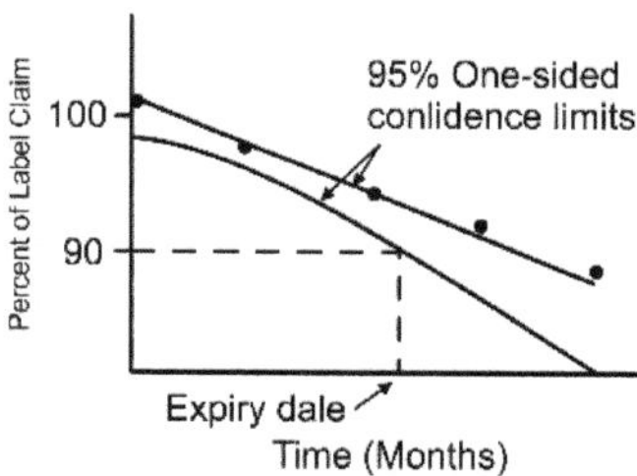

Figure 17.1 95% One way confidence limits.

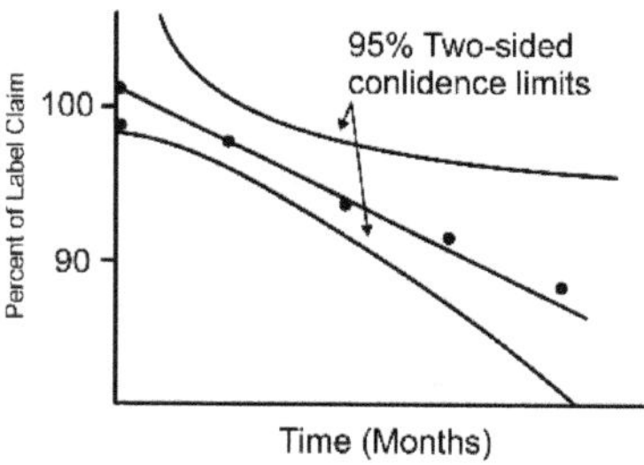

Figure 17.2 95% Two Way confidence limits.

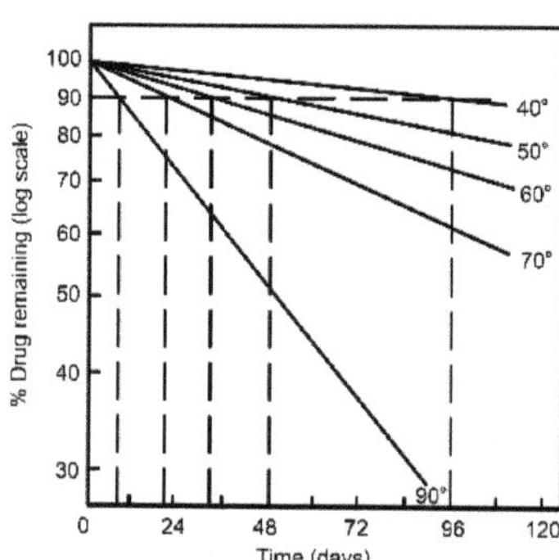

Figure 17.3 Time in days required for drug potency to fall to 90% of original value. These times, designated t90, are then plotted on a log scale in figure 17.6.

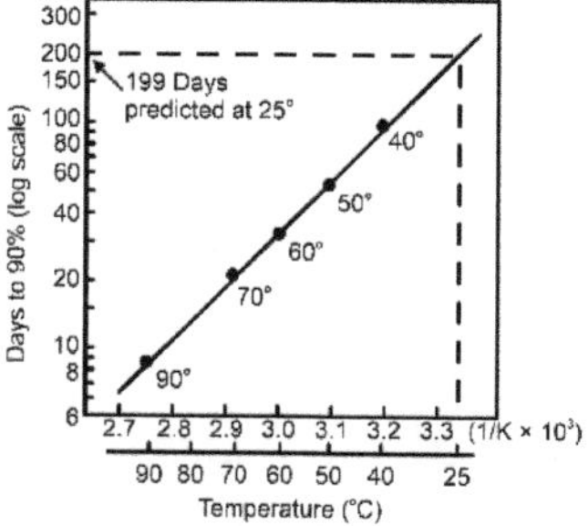

Figure 17.4 A log plot of t90 (i.e. time to 90% potency on the vertical axis against reciprocal temperature (both Kelvin and centigrade scales are shown on the horizontal axis.

Usually, 90% drug concentration is considered, as lowest specification limit, and the point on the X-axis at which the extension line cuts the 95% confidence limit line is considered as expiry date. If there is an increase in concentration of drug because of loss of vehicle, a 95% upper confidence limit should be defined.

A similar type of confidence limit analysis should be done for concentration-time data of degradation products. All the guidelines actually discourage the extrapolation of data beyond the range of storage times and permits only limited extrapolation. If the stability data shows very little change or no degradation, the guidelines suggest that no statistical treatment is necessary.

Global Scenario of Storage Stability Testing of Herbal Medicinal Products

Association of Southeast Asian Nations (ASEAN): Dosage form and testing parameters		
Sr. No	**Dosage forms**	**Testing parameter**
1	Oral powders	Organoleptic characteristics. Assay, Water content and Microbial contents
2	Hard capsules	Organoleptic characteristics. Assay, Water content, Microbial content, Dissolution, Disintegration,
3	Soft capsules	Organoleptic characteristics. Assay, Microbial content, Dissolution, Disintegration,
4	Tablets (Coated and uncoated)	Organoleptic characteristics. Assay, Hardness, Friability, Water content, Microbial content, Dissolution, Disintegration,
5	Pills and pellets (Coated and uncoated)	Organoleptic characteristics. Assay, Water content, Microbial content, Dissolution, Disintegration,
6	Suspensions	Organoleptic characteristics, Assay, Viscosity, pH, Microbial contents, Granules or Particle size variability, Resuspendability.
7	Emulsions	Organoleptic characteristics, Assay, Viscosity, pH, Microbial contents,
8	Semisolid preparations	Organoleptic characteristics, Assay, Viscosity, pH, Microbial contents,
9	Plasters	Organoleptic characteristics, Assay, Microbial contents, Adhesiveness.
10	Granules	Organoleptic characteristics, Assay, Water content, Microbial contents, Granules or particle size variation.
11	Herbal infusion bags	Organoleptic characteristics, Assay, Water content, Microbial contents,
12	Pastilles	Organoleptic characteristics, Assay, Water content, Microbial contents,

Contd..

Eurasian Economic Commission (EEC): Dosage form and testing parameters		
Sr. No	**Dosage forms**	**Testing parameter**
1	Pills	Dissolution*, Disintegration*, Water content, Resistance to abrasive for pills without a shell.
2	Hard gelatin capsules	Fragility, Dissolution*, Disintegration*, Water content, Microbiological purity.
3	Soft gelatin capsules	Dissolution*, Disintegration*, Microbiological purity., pH, Hermeticity, Adhesion.
4	Oral emulsion, suspension and solution	Sludge formation, pH, Viscosity, Extractable substances, Microbiological purity, Solution transparency.
5	Suspension	Dispersion, Rheological properties, Average particle size/ distribution, Polymorphic transformation*, Interconversion of polymorphs
6	Emulsion	Phase separation, Average size and distribution of globules.
7	Powders and granules (For oral solutions)	Water content and recovery.
8	Metered dose inhalers	Uniformity of dose content, Number of activation of container valve, Aerodynamic particle size distribution, Microscope evaluation, Water content, Hermeticity, Microbial contamination, Valve delivery or injection weight, Weight loss, Pump delivery, Foreign mechanical inclusion, Substances extracted and discharged from plastic and elastomeric components of the container, closure and pump.
9	Suspension aerosols	Microscopic analysis of valve and ingredients contents, Large inclusion, Particle's change in morphology, The agglomerates, Crystals, Foreign mechanical inclusion, Corrosion of the container
10	Suppositories	Degree of softening, Disintegration, Dissolution- at 37°C.
11	Nasal spray	Transparency for solutions, Microbial purity, pH, Mechanical inclusion, Uniformity of active ingredients
12	Topical dosage forms (eye, ear)	Transparency, Homogeneity, pH, Ability to resuspend for lotions, Thickness, Viscosity, Particle size distribution for suspension, Microbiological purity, Weight loss*, Sterility, Mechanical inclusion, Extractable volume.
13	Spray	Pressure weight loss, Total extractable weight, Speed of delivery, Microbiological purity, Spraying performance, Water content, Particle size distribution for suspension.
14	Parenteral medicinal products	Color, Transparency for solutions, Mechanical inclusions, pH, Sterility, Pyrogenicity, Endotoxin content, Volume.
15	Transdermal patches	Release rate in vitro, Hermeticity, Microbiological purity/sterility, Ungluing strength, Shear adhesion.

EMA: (European Medicines Agency): Dosage form and testing parameters		
Sr. No	**Dosage forms**	**Testing parameter**
1	Tablets (Coated, Uncoated) & Hard capsules	Dissolution, Disintegration, Hardness, Friability, Uniformity of mass, pH, Water content, Microbial limits.
2	Oral suspension	Uniformity of mass. pH, Microbial limits, Antimicrobial preservative contents, Antioxidant preservative content, extractable, Alcohol content, Particle size distribution, Redispersability, Rheological properties, Viscosity, Specific gravity, Reconstitution time, Water content. Dissolution- for oral suspension. Resuspension- for dry powders products.
3	Herbal teas	Loss on drying, Identification, Purity, Uniformity of mass of sachet, Assay, Particle size, Microbial limit.

ICH: (International Council of Harmonization): Dosage form and testing parameters		
Sr. No	**Dosage forms**	**Testing parameter**
1	Tablets (Coated & Uncoated) Hard capsules	Dissolution, Disintegration, Hardness, Friability, Uniformity, Water content, Microbial limit.
2	Oral liquids	Uniformity, pH, Preservative content, Extractables, Alcohol content, Dissolution, Partial distribution,Redisper- sibility, Rheology, Reconstitution time, Water content.
3	Parenteral drug products	Uniformity, pH, Sterility, Endotoxins, Pyrogen, Particulate matter, Water content, Microbial and antioxidant preservative content, Extractables, Functionality testing of delivery systems including prefilled syringes, Autoinjector cartridges or equivalent osmolarity, Particular size distribution for injectable suspensions, Redispersibility, Reconstitution time.

WHO: (World Health Organization): Dosage form and testing parameters		
Sr. No	**Dosage forms**	**Testing parameter**
1.	Liquid dosage forms (Fluid extract, Infusion, Tinctures, Syrups and oral solution) Oral suspension Oral emulsion Aromatic water, powders, granules for oral suspension	Precipitate formation, Clarity, pH, Viscosity, Extractable, Microbial contamination level, Precipitate formation, Clarity, pH, Viscosity, Extractable, Microbial contamination level, Dispersibility, Rheology, Mean size of distribution particle and polymorphism. Precipitate formation, Clarity, pH, Viscosity, Extractable, Microbial contamination level, Phase separation, Globule mean size or distribution, Water content and Reconstitution time.
2.	Solid dosage forms (Herbal tea bags, plant powders, Dry extract powder, Granule, Pills, Lozenges) Hard gelatin capsules Soft gelatin capsules, Tablets	Brittleness, Dissolution, Disintegration, Water content, Microbial contamination level, Dissolution, Disintegration, Microbial contamination level, pH, Leakage, Pellicle formation. Dissolution, Disintegration, Water content, Hardness, Friability.

Contd..

3.	Other dosage forms Ointments, Creams, salves	Clarity,, Homogeneity, pH, suspendability (For lotion), Consistency, Viscosity, Particle size distribution (For suspension), Microbial contamination level, Sterility, Weight loss, Ophthalmic & otic products. Sterility, Particulate matter, Extractable matter.

India: (AYUSH): Dosage form and testing parameters		
Sr. No	**Dosage forms**	**Testing parameter**
1	Tablets	Description, Identification, Uniformity of weight, Uniformity of diameter*, Disintegration test, Assay.
2	Capsules	Description, Identification, Uniformity of weight, Uniformity of diameter*, Disintegration test, Assay.
3	Parenteral preparation	Clarity, pH*, Identification, Volume in container, Sterility, Pyrogen test*, Toxicity test*, Assay.

Storage condition used for intermediate stability testing by various Global communities		
Global community	**Testing period (container type)**	**Storage condition (temperature/ relative humidity, RH)**
EEC	6 months (general container) 6 months (semipermeable container)	30°C ± 2°C/65% RH ± 5% RH 30°C ± 2°C/35% RH ± 5% RH
EMA	6 months (general container) 6 months (semipermeable container)	30°C ± 2°C/65% RH ± 5% RH 30°C ± 2°C/65% RH ± 5% RH
ICH	6 months (general container) 6 months (semipermeable container)	30°C ± 2°C/65% RH ± 5% RH 30°C ± 2°C/65% RH ± 5% RH
WHO	6 months (general case) 6 months (semipermeable case)	30°C ± 2°C/65% RH ± 5% RH 30°C ± 2°C/35% RH ± 5% RH
Australia	6 months (general container) 6 months (semipermeable container)	30°C ± 2°C/65% RH ± 5% RH 30°C ± 2°C/65% RH ± 5% RH
China	0, 1, 2, 3, and 6 months	30°C ± 2°C/65% RH ± 5% RH
Japan	6 months (general container) 6 months (semipermeable container)	30°C ± 2°C/65% RH ± 5% RH 30°C ± 2°C/65% RH ± 5% RH
Korea	More than 12 months (general container) More than 12 months (semipermeable container)	30°C ± 2°C/65% RH ± 5% RH 30°C ± 2°C/35% RH ± 5% RH

Contd...

Storage condition used for Long term Stability Testing by various Global communities				
Global community	Testing period (container type)			
		In ambient storage	In refrigerator	In freezer
ASEAN	0, 3, 6, 9, 12, 18, 24 months, and annually thereafter	30°C ± 2°C/75% RH ± 5% RH (moisturepermeable container1) 30°C ± 2°C (moisture-impermeable container2)	5°C ± 3°C	—
EEC	12 monthsa (general container) 6 or 12 monthsb (general container) 12 months (semipermeable container3)a 6 or 12 months (semipermeable container)b	25°C ± 2°C/60% RH ± 5% RH or 30°C ± 2°C/ 65% RH ± 5% RH or 30°C ± 2°C/75% RH ± 5% RH 25°C ± 2°C/40% RH ± 5% RH or 30°C ± 2°C/ 35% RH ± 5% RH	5°C ± 3°C —	-20°C ± 5°C —
EMA	6 or 12 months (general container) 6 or 12 months (semipermeable container)	30°C ± 2°C/60% RH ± 5% RH (6 months) 30°C ± 2°C/65% RH ± 5% RH (12 months) 25°C ± 2°C/40% RH ± 5% RH (6 months) 30°C ± 2°C/35% RH ± 5% RH (12 months)	5°C ± 3°C —	-20°C ± 5°C —
ICH	12 months (general container) 12 months (semipermeable container)	25°C ± 2°C/60% RH ± 5% RH or 30°C ± 2°C/ 65% RH ± 5% RH 25°C ± 2°C/40% RH ± 5% RH or 30°C ± 2°C/ 35% RH ± 5% RH	5°C ± 3°C —	- 20°C ± 5°C —
WHO	6 or 12 months (general case) 6 or 12 months (semipermeable case)	25°C ± 2°C/60% RH ± 5% RH or 30°C ± 2°C/ 65% RH ± 5% RH or 30°C ± 2°C/75% RH ± 5% RH 25°C ± 2°C/40% RH ± 5% RH or 30°C ± 2°C/ 35% RH ± 5% RH	5°C ± 3°C —	- 20°C ± 5°C —

Contd..

Storage condition used for Long term Stability Testing by various Global communities				
Global community	Testing period (container type)	In ambient storage	In refrigerator	In freezer
Australia	12 months (general container 12 months (semipermeable container)	25°C ± 2°C/60% RH ± 5% RH or 30°C ± 2°C/ 65% RH ± 5% RH 25°C ± 2°C/40% RH ± 5% RH or 30°C ± 2°C/ 35% RH ± 5% RH	5°C ± 3°C —	– 20°C ± 5°C —
Brazil	12 months (impermeable container) 12 months (semipermeable container)	30°C ± 2°C 30°C ± 2°C/75% RH ± 5% RH	5°C ± 3°C 5°C ± 3°C	– 20°C ± 5°C – 20°C ± 5°C
China	0, 3, 6, 9, 12, and 18 months (24 and 36 months, if necessary)	25°C ± 2°C/60% RH ± 10% RH or 30°C ± 2°C/65% RH ± 10% RH	6°C ± 2°C	—
Hong Kong	Every month for 3 consecutive months initially and then every 6 months	25°C ± 2°C/60% RH ± 5% RH	—	—
Japan	12 months (general container) 12 months (semipermeable container)	25°C ± 2°C/60% RH ± 5% RH or 30°C ± 2°C/ 65% RH ± 5% RH 25°C ± 2°C/40% RH ± 5% RH or 30°C ± 2°C/ 35% RH ± 5% RH	5°C ± 3°C —	– 20°C ± 5°C —
Kenya	12 months (general container) 12 months (semipermeable container)	25°C ± 2°C/60% RH ± 5% RH or 30°C ± 2°C/ 65% RH ± 5% RH 25°C ± 2°C/40% RH ± 5% RH or 30°C ± 2°C/ 35% RH ± 5% RH	5°C ± 3°C —	– 20°C ± 5°C —
Korea	0, 3, 6, 9, 12, 18, 24 months, and annually thereafter (general container) 0, 3, 6, 9, 12, 18, 24 months, and annually thereafter (semipermeable container4)	25°C ± 2°C/60% RH ± 5% RH or 30°C ± 2°C/ 65% RH ± 5% RH 25°C ± 2°C/40% RH ± 5% RH or 30°C ± 2°C/ 35% RH ± 5% RH	5°C ± 3°C —	– 20°C ± 5°C —

Contd...

Storage condition used for Long term Stability Testing by various Global communities				
Global community	Testing period (container type)			
		In ambient storage	In refrigerator	In freezer
Philippines	—	30°C ± 2°C/75% RH ± 5% RH	—	—
Zambia	3, 6, 9, 12, 18, 24, and 36 months	25°C ± 2°C/65% RH ± 5% RH	—	—
India	12 Months	30°C ± 2°C/60% RH ± 5%	—	—

Storage condition used for accelerated stability testing by various Global communities

Global community	Testing period (container type)			
		In ambient storage	In refrigerator	In freezer
ASEAN	0, 3, and 6 months (including the initial and final time points)	40°C ± 2°C/75% RH ± 5% RH	25°C ± 2°C/60% RH ± 5% RH	—
EEC	6 months (general container) 6 months (semipermeable container)	40°C ± 2°C/75% RH ± 5% RH 40°C ± 2°C/not more than 25% RH	25°C ± 2°C/60% RH ± 5% RH or 30°C ± 2°C/65% RH ± 5% RH or 30°C ± 2°C/75% RH ± 5% RH —	—
EMA	6 months (general container) 6 months (semipermeable container)	40°C ± 2°C/75% RH ± 5% RH 40°C ± 2°C/not more than 25% RH	25°C ± 2°C/60% RH ± 5% RH —	— —
ICH	6 months (general container) 6 months (semipermeable container)	40°C ± 2°C/75% RH ± 5% RH 40°C ± 2°C/not more than 25% RH	25°C ± 2°C/60% RH ± 5% RH —	—
Australia	6 months (general container) 6 months (semipermeable container)	40°C ± 2°C/75% RH ± 5% RH 40°C ± 2°C/not more than 25% RH	25°C ± 2°C/60% RH ± 5% RH —	—

Contd..

Global community	Testing period (container type)	In ambient storage	In refrigerator	In freezer
Brazil	6 months (impermeable container) 6 months (semipermeable container)	40°C ± 2°C 40°C ± 2°C/75% RH ± 5% RH	25°C ± 2°C 25°C ± 2°C/60% RH ± 5% RH	- 20°C ± 5°C - 20°C ± 5°C
China	0, 1, 2, 3, and 6 months (general container) 0, 1, 2, 3, and 6 month (semipermeable container)	40°C ± 2°C/75% RH ± 5% RH 40°C ± 2°C/20% RH ± 5% RH	25°C ± 2°C/60% RH ± 5% RH —	— —
Hong Kong	0, 1, 2, 3, and 6 months Every month for 3 consecutive months	30°C ± 2°C/65% RH ± 5% RH 37°C–40°C/75% RH ± 5% RH	— —	— —
Japan	6 months (general container) 6 months (semipermeable container)	40°C ± 2°C/75% RH ± 5% RH 40°C ± 2°C/not more than 25% RH	25°C ± 2°C/60% RH ± 5% RH —	— —
Korea	More than 6 months (general container) More than 6 months (semipermeable container)	40°C ± 2°C/75% RH ± 5% RH 40°C ± 2°C/not more than 25% RH	25°C ± 2°C/60% RH ± 5% RH —	— —
Philippines	—	40°C ± 2°C/75% RH ± 5% RH	—	—
Zambia	0, 1, 2, 3, and 6 months	40°C ± 2°C/75% RH	—	—
India	6 months	40°C ± 2°C/75% RH ± 5%	—	—

Further Reading

1. Kim JH, Lee K, Jerng UM, Choi G. Global Comparison of Stability Testing Parameters and Testing Methods for Finished Herbal Products. Evid Based Complement Alternat Med. 2019 Oct 20;2019:7348929.
2. Gupta PD, Daswani PG, Birdi TJ. Approaches in fostering quality parameters for medicinal botanicals in the Indian context. Indian J Pharmacol. 2014 Jul-Aug;46(4):363-71.
3. Bansal G, Suthar N, Kaur J, Jain A. Stability Testing of Herbal Drugs: Challenges, Regulatory Compliance and Perspectives. Phytother Res. 2016 Jul;30(7):1046-58.
4. Association of South East Asian Nations, ASEAN Guidelines on Stability Study and Shelf-Life of Traditional Medicines and Health Supplements, Association of South East Asian Nations, Jakarta, Indonesia, 2013.
5. The Eurasian Economic Commission Board, Quality Manual of Herbal Medicinal Preparation, The Eurasian Economic Commission Board, Moscow, Russia, 2018.
6. The Eurasian Economic Commission Board, Requirements to Stability Studies of Medicinal Products (Drugs) and Pharmaceutical Substances, The Eurasian Economic Commission Board, Moscow, Russia, 2018.
7. European Medicines Agency, Guideline on Specifications: Test Procedures and Acceptance Criteria for Herbal Substances, Herbal Preparations and Herbal Medicinal Products/traditional Herbal Medicinal Products, European Medicines Agency, Amsterdam, Netherlands, 2011.
8. European Medicines Agency, Guideline on Quality of Herbal Medicinal Products/traditional Herbal Medicinal Products, European Medicine Agency, Amsterdam, Netherlands, 2011.
9. The International Council for Harmonisation of Technical Requirements for Pharmaceuticals for Human Use, Specifications: Test Procedures and Acceptance Criteria for New Drugs Substances and New Drug Products: Chemical Substances, The International Council for Harmonisation of Technical Requirements for Pharmaceuticals for Human Use, Geneva, Switzerland, 1999.
10. Australian Government Department of Health Therapeutic Goods Administration, Technical Guidance on the Interpretation of the Manufacturing Standards: On-Going Stability Testing for Listed Complementary Medicines Version 1.1, Australian Government Department of Health Therapeutic Goods Administration, Canberra, Australia, 2013.
11. Australian Government Department of Health Therapeutic Goods Administration, Australian Regulatory Guidelines for Complementary Medicines (ARGCM) Version 7.2, Australian Government Department of Health Therapeutic Goods Administration, Canberra, Australia, 2018.
12. The Federative Republic of Brazil Agência Nacional de Vigilância Sanitária, Consolidado de normas da COFID (Versão IV), The Federative Republic of Brazil Agência Nacional de Vigilância Sanitária, Brasilia, Brazil, 2013.
13. The Federative Republic of Brazil Agência Nacional de Vigilância Sanitária, Determina a publicação da "Guia de orientação para registro de medicamentos fitoterápicos e registro e notificação de produtostradicionais fitoterápicos, The Federative Republic of Brazil Agência Nacional de Vigilância Sanitária, Brasilia, Brazil, 2014.
14. Government of Canada the Minister of Justice, Natural Health Products Regulations (SOR/2003-196), Government of Canada the Minister of Justice, Canada, 2003.

15. Health Canada, Quality of Natural Health Products Guide: Natural and Non-prescription Health Products Directorate, Health Canada, Ottawa, Canada, 2015.
16. China Food and Drug Administration, Notice of Technical Guiding Principles for the Study of Stability of Traditional Chinese Medicine and Natural Drugs, China Food and Drug Administration, Beijing, China, 2006.
17. Anhui Food and Drug Administration, Technical Guiding Principles for Pharmaceutical Research in Anhui Medical Institutions: 3. Technical Guiding Principles for Quality and Stability Research of Traditional Chinese Medicine Preparations, Anhui Food and Drug Administration, Hefei, China, 2009.
18. Egyptian Drug Authority, The Egyptian guidelines for registration of herbal medicines, Egyptian Drug Authority, Cairo, Egypt, 2017.
19. Legislative Council of the Hong Kong Special Administration Region of the People's Republic of China, Registration Of Proprietary Chinese Medicines, Legislative Council of the Hong Kong Special Administration Region of the People's Republic of China, Central, Hong Kong, 2011.
20. Legislative Council of the Hong Kong Special Administration Region of the People's Republic of China, Registration Of Proprietary Chinese Medicines. Product Quality Documents Technical Guidelines (Appendices), Legislative Council of the Hong Kong Special Administration Region of the People's Republic of China, Central, Hong Kong, 2004.
21. Department of Health, Ministry of Health and Family Welfare, Government of India, The Drugs and Cosmetic Rules. Notificaiton: No. F. 28-10/45-H (1), Department of Health, Ministry of Health and Family Welfare, Government of India, Bengaluru, Karnataka, 1945.
22. Ministry of Health, Labour and Welfare, "About partial revision of about the statement of application for prescription for over-the-counter products with approval criteria and the handling of attached materials," Drug Pharmacopoeia 0331, vol. 19, 2017.
23. Ministry of Health, Labour and Welfare, About revision of stability test guidelines, Medical Review, Article ID 0603001, 2003.
24. Republic of Kenya Pharmacy and Poisons Board, Registration Of Herbal and Complementary Products: Guidelines to Submission of Applications, Republic of Kenya Pharmacy and Poisons Board, Nairobi, Kenya, 2010.
25. Republic of Korea Ministry of Food and Drug Safety, Regulations on the approval and notification of Herb medication, Republic of Korea Ministry of Food and Drug Safety, 2016, no. 2016–112.
26. Republic of Korea Ministry of Food and Drug Safety, Stability Test Standards for Medicines, Republic of Korea Ministry of Food and Drug Safety, 2014, no. 2014–59.
27. Republic of the Philippines Department of Health, Guidelines On the Registration Of Herbal Medicines, Republic of the Philippines Department of Health, Manila, Philippines, 2004.
28. Republic of the Philippines Department of Health, Guidelines On the Registration Of Traditionally-Used Herbal Products, Republic of the Philippines Department of Health, 2004.
29. State of Qatar Ministry of Public Health, Registration Requirements: Herbal Products, Dietary Supplements and Medicated Cosmetics, State of Qatar Ministry of Public Health, Doha, Qatar, 2017.
30. Swiss Agency for Therapeutic Products, Requirements Of Quality Documentation for Asian Medicinal Products, Swiss Agency for Therapeutic Products, Bern, Switzerland, 2007.

31. United States Food and Drug Administration Center for Drug Evaluation and Research, Botanical Drug Development Guidance for Industry, United States Food and Drug Administration Center for Drug Evaluation and Research, 2016.
32. United States Food and Drug Administration Center for Drug Evaluation and Research, Guidance for Industry Botanical Drug Products, United States Food and Drug Administration Center for Drug Evaluation and Research, Silver Spring, MD, USA, 2004.
33. The Republic of Zambia Pharmaceutical Regulatory Authority, Guidelines On Application for Registration of Herbal Medicines, The Republic of Zambia Pharmaceutical Regulatory Authority, 2008.
34. European Medicines Agency, Guideline on Stability Testing: Stability Testing of Existing Active Substances and Related Finished Products, European Medicines Agency, Amsterdam, Netherlands, 2003.
35. The International Council for Harmonisation of Technical Requirements for Pharmaceuticals for Human Use, Stability Testing of New Drug Substances and Products Q1A (R2), The International Council for Harmonisation of Technical Requirements for Pharmaceuticals for Human Use, Geneva, Switzerland, 2003.
36. The Federative Republic of Brazil Agência Nacional de Vigilância Sanitária, Consolidado de normas da COFID, (Versão V), The Federative Republic of Brazil Agência Nacional de Vigilância Sanitária, The Federative Republic of Brazil, Brasilia, Brazil, 2015.
37. R. Enayatifard, H. Asgarirad, and B. Kazemi Sani, "Microbial quality of some herbal solid dosage forms," African Journal of Biotechnology, vol. 9, no. 11, pp. 1701–1705, 2010.
38. R. Guimarães, J. C. M. Barreira, L. Barros, A. M. Carvalho, and I. C. F. R. Ferreira, "Effects of oral dosage form and storage period on the antioxidant properties of four species used in traditional herbal medicine," Phytotherapy Research, vol. 25, no. 4, pp. 484–492, 2011.
39. H. J. Kim, H. N. Jang, J. Y. Bae, and S. N. Park, "A study on the stability of the cream containing Glycyrrhiza uralensis extract," Journal of the Society of Cosmetic Scientists of Korea, vol. 39, no. 2, pp. 117–125, 2013.

Scan QR code to view the website/guidelines

- Stability and shelf life of herbal medicines-

ASEAN Guidelines on Stability Study and Shelf-Life of Traditional Medicines and Health Supplements

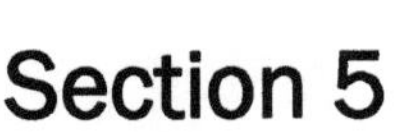

Section 5

Pre-clinical and Toxicity Regulations for Herbal Products

CHAPTER 18

CPCSEA and OECD Guidelines for Animal Experimentation

CPCSEA Standard Operating Procedures (SOP) for IAEC

Objective: The motto of Prevention of Cruelty to Animals (PCA) Act 1960 as amended in 1982, is to prevent infliction of unnecessary pain or suffering on animals. The Central Government has constituted a Committee for the Purpose of Control and Supervision of Experiments on Animals (CPCSEA) which is duty bound to take all such measuresas may be necessary to ensure that animals are not subjected to unnecessary pain or suffering before, during or after the performance of experiments on them. For this purpose, the Government has made "Breeding of and Experiments on Animals (Control and Supervision) Rules, 1998" as amended during 2001 and 2006, to regulate the experimentation on animals. The objective of this SOP is to contribute to the effective functioning of the Institutional Animal Ethics Committee (IAEC) so that a quality and consistent ethical review mechanism for research on animals is put in place for all proposals dealt bythe Committee as prescribed by the CPCSEA under PCA Act 1960 and Breeding and Experimentation Rules 1998.

IAEC objectives:

(a) experiments shall be performed in every case by or under the supervision of a person duly qualified in that behalf, that is, Degree or Diploma holders in Veterinary Science or Medicine or Laboratory Animal Science of a University or an Institution recognized by the Government for the purpose and under the responsibility of the person performing the experiment;

(b) that experiments are performed with due care and humanity and that as far as possible experiments involving operations are performed under the influence of some anesthetic of sufficient power to prevent the animals feeling pain;

(c) that animals which, in the course of experiments under the influence of anesthetics, are so injured that their recovery would involve serious suffering, are ordinarily destroyed while still insensible;

(d) that experiments on animals are avoided wherever it is possible to do so; as for example; in medical schools, hospitals, colleges and the like, if other teaching devices such as books, models, films and the like, may equally suffice;

(e) that experiments on larger animals are avoided when it is possible to achieve the same results by experiments upon small laboratory animals like guinea-'pigs,rabbits, mice, rats etc;

(f) that, as far as possible, experiments are not performed merely for the purpose of acquiring manual skill;

(g) that animals intended for the performance of experiments are properly looked afterboth before and after experiments;

(h) that suitable records are maintained with respect to experiments performed on animals

Functions of IAEC

As defined in "Breeding of and Experiments on Animals (Control and Supervision) Rules, 1998", "Institutional Animals Ethics Committee" means a body comprising of a group of persons recognized and registered by the Committee for the purpose of control and supervision of experiments on animals performed in an establishment which is constituted and operated in accordance with procedures specified for the purpose by the Committee;

The primary duty of IAEC is to work for achievement of the objectives as mentioned above.

IAEC will review and approve all types of research proposals involving small animal experimentation before the start of the study. For experimentation on large animals, the case is required to be forwarded to CPCSEA in prescribed manner with recommendation of IAEC. IAEC is required to monitor the research throughout the study and after completion of study through periodic reports and visit to animal house and laboratory where the experiments are conducted. The committee has to ensure compliance with all regulatory requirements, applicable rules, guidelines and laws.

Composition of IAEC

Institutional Animals Ethics committee shall include eight members as follows.

1. A biological scientist,
2. Two scientists from different biological disciplines,
3. A veterinarian involved in the care of animal,
4. Scientist in charge of animal's facility of the establishment concerned,
5. A scientist from, outside the institute,
6. A non-scientific socially aware member and
7. A nominee of CPCSEA

- Specialist may be co-opted while reviewing special project using hazardous agents such as radio-active substance and deadly microorganisms. The Chairperson of the Committee and Member Secretary would be nominated by the Institution from amongst the eight members. Members againstSerial number 5,6 and 7 will be nominated by CPCSEA, with a provision of a Link nominee for CPCSEA nominee. The duration of appointment is for a period of 3 years (coterminous with registration). IAEC is required to formulate a SOP for its working requirements and follow it in all the meetings. Socially aware member's presence is compulsory in cases referred to CPCSEA and at least in one meeting in a calendar year. The Member Secretary is responsible for organizing the meetings, maintaining the records and communicating with all concerned. A copy of minutes is required to be sent to Member Secretary CPCSEA within 15 days of the meeting, otherwise, the meeting will not be considered valid.

Application Procedures:

- All proposals should be submitted in the prescribed application form with
- Relevant documents as per checklist duly signed by the Principal Investigator (PI) and Co-investigators / Collaborators should be submitted to IAEC.

Guidelines on the Regulation of Scientific Experiments on Animals by Ministry of Environment & Forests (Animal Welfare Division), Government of India, June 2007

The use of animals in scientific research has been an area of concern in India, given the sharp polarization of views between animal welfare activists and the scientific community of the country regarding use of animals. This led to proliferation of litigation, which impeded the pace of research. In order to eliminate the potential for conflict, it was considered necessary to examine the international norms regarding the use of animals in scientific experiments, update regulations, streamline and simplify procedures, while ensuring ethical use of animals and reducing infliction of pain and stress on animals, during experimentation. The aim of these Guidelines is to ensure humane and ethical treatment of animals, while facilitating legitimate scientific research involving experiments on animals.

Persons engaged in conducting scientific experiments on animals must act in conformity with the provisions of the prevention of Cruelty to Animals Act, 1960, andthe Breeding of and Experiments on Animals (Control and Supervision) Rules, 1998, as amended. These provisions are enforced by the independent Committee for the Purpose of Control and supervision of Experimentation on animals (CPCSEA), a statutory body under the Prevention of Cruelty to Animals Act, 1960, in the Ministry of Environmentand Forests.

Compliance is also required with CPCSEA Guidelines for Laboratory animal facility.

Every establishment constituted and operated in accordance with the procedures specified by CPCSEA is required to constitute an Institutional Animals Ethics Committee (IAEC).

In terms of Rule 13 of the Breeding of and Experiments on Animals (Control and Supervision) Rules 1998, as amended, every IAEC shall include a biological scientist, two scientists from different biological disciplines, a veterinarian involved in the care of animals, the scientist in charge of the animal facility of the establishment concerned, a scientist from outside the institute, a non-scientific socially aware member and a representative or nominee of the CPCSEA. A specialist may be co-opted while reviewing special projects using hazardous agents such as radioactive substances and deadly microorganisms.

Experimental animals which are subject to regulation the relative sentience of different species of animals are as follows:

Invertebrates (e.g., cockroaches) <Birds <Rodents <Canines/Felines <Bovine/ Equines <Primates (e.g., Rhesus Macaque) <More evolved Primates(e.g., chimpanzee)

Anything higher than invertebrates in terms of level of sentience requires regulation. Thus rats, mice, birds, and farm animals are also subject to regulation.

Ethical principles adopted by CPCSEA for use of animals in scientific experiments

Principle 1: "Experiments on animals" (including experiments involving operations on animals) may be carried out for the purposes of advancement by new discovery of physiological knowledge; or of knowledge which is expected to be useful for saving or prolonging human life or alleviating suffering; or for significant gains in the wellbeing for the people of the country; or for combating any disease, whether of human being, animals or plants.

Principle 2: Animals lowest on the phylogenetic scale (i.e., with the least degree of sentience), which may give scientifically valid results, should be used for any Experimental procedure. Experiments should be designed with the minimum number of animals to give statistically valid results at 95% level of confidence. Alternatives not involving animal testing should be given due and full consideration and sound justification provided, if alternative, when available, are not used.

Principle 3: Proper use of animals in experiments and avoidance or minimization (when avoidanceis not possible) of pain and suffering inflicted on experimental animals should be an issue of priority for research personnel, and unless the contrary is scientifically established, investigators should process on the basis that procedures that cause painor suffering in human beings will also cause similar pain or suffering in animals. All scientific procedures adopted with animals that may cause more than momentary or slight pain and/or suffering should be performed with appropriate sedation, analgesia or anesthesia.

Principle 4: Persons engaged in animal experimentation have a moral responsibility for the welfare of the animals after their use in experiments. Investigators are responsible for the aftercare and/or rehabilitation of animals after experimentation, and may be permitted to euthanize Animals only in the following situations:

- When the animal is paralyzed and is not able to perform its natural functions; it becomes incapable of independent locomotion; and/or can no longer perceive the environment in an intelligible manner.
- During the course of experimental procedure, the animal has been left with a severe recurring pain and the animal exhibits obvious signs of long-term extreme pain and suffering.
- In situations where non-termination of the animal experimented upon would be life threatening to human beings or other animals.
- Costs of aftercare and/or rehabilitation of animal's post-experimentation are to be part of research costs and should be scaled per animal in positive correlation with the level of sentience of the animals.

Principle 5: The living conditions of animals should be appropriate for their species and contributeto their health and comfort. The housing, feeding, and care of all Animals used for biomedical purposes must be directed by a veterinarian or other scientist in a relevant discipline who is trained and experienced in the proper care, handling, and use of the species being maintained or studied. In all circumstances, veterinary care shall be provided as necessary.

CPCSEA Guidelines on specific aspects regarding the use of animals in scientific experiments

- Need to avoid/minimize pain and suffering inflicted on experimental animals with appropriate sedation, analgesia or anesthesia.
- Proper care, handling and use of experimental animals as directed by a veterinarian or other scientist in a relevant discipline
- The conventional regulatory framework may not be applied regarding use of experimental animals in agricultural production research..

- **Institutional Animals Ethics Committee (IAEC)** is not empowered to clear research project proposals that involve experiments on animals higher on the phylogenetic scale than rodents.
- Both announced and unannounced visits by duly authorized personnel (only) to inspect the animal house facilities of institutes may be carried out.

CPCSEA Guidelines for Laboratory Animal Facility – 2005

Goal

Good Laboratory Practices (GLP) for animal facilities is intended to assure quality maintenance and welfare of animals used in laboratory studies while conducting biomedical and behavioral research and testing of products. The goal of these Guidelines is to promote the humane care of animals used in biomedical and behavioral research and testing with the basic objective of providing specifications that will enhance animal wellbeing, quality in the pursuit of advancement of biological knowledge that is relevant to humans and animals.

Veterinary Care

Adequate veterinary care must be provided and is the responsibility of aveterinarian or a person who has training or experience in laboratory animal sciences and medicine. Daily observation of animals can be accomplished by someone other than a veterinarian; however, a mechanism of direct and frequent communication should be adopted so that timely and accurate information on problems in animal health, behavior, and well-being is conveyed to the attending veterinarian. The veterinarian can also contribute to the establishment of appropriate policies and procedures for ancillary aspects of veterinary care, such as reviewing protocols and proposals, animal husbandry and animal welfare; monitoring not and / or order closure. Occupational health hazards containment, and zoonosis control programs; and supervising animal nutrition and sanitation. Institutional requirements will determine the need for full-time or part-time or consultative veterinary services.

- Animals should be fed with palatable, non-contaminated, and nutritionally adequate food daily unless the experimental protocol requires otherwise. Diet should be free from heavy metals (e.g., Lead, Arsenic, Cadmium, Nickel, Mercury), naturally occurring toxins and other contaminants.
- Bedding should be absorbent, free from toxic chemicals or other substances that cause irritation, injure animals or personnel, and of a type not readily eaten by animals. Bedding should be used in amounts sufficient to keep animals dry between cage changes without coming into contact with watering tubes.
- Animals should have continuous access to fresh, potable, uncontaminateddrinking water, according to their requirements. Periodic monitoring of microbial contamination in water is necessary. Watering devices, such as drinking nozzles and automatic waterers should be examined routinely to ensure their proper operation.
- Sanitation is an essential activity in an animal facility. Animal rooms, corridors, storage spaces, and other areas should be properly cleaned with appropriate detergents and

disinfectants as often as necessary to keep them free of dirt, debris, andharmful agents of contamination. Cleaning utensils, such as mops, pails, and brooms, should not be transported between animal rooms.

- Adaptation of Programs designed to prevent, control, or eliminate the presence of or infestations by pests are essential in an animal home environment.

Animal Procurement

All animals must be acquired lawfully as a health surveillance program for screening incoming animals should be carried out to assess animal quality. Methods of transportation should also be taken into account (Annexure - 4).

Each consignment of animals should be inspected for compliance with procurement specifications, and the animals should be quarantined and stabilized according to procedures appropriate for the species and circumstances.

Physical Facilities

The physical condition and design of animal facility determine, to a great extent, the efficiency and economy of this operation. The design and size of an animal facility depend on the scope of institutional research activities, animals to be housed, physical relationship to the rest of the institution, and geographic location. A well planned, properly maintained facility is an important element in good animalcare.

Quarantine, Stabilization and Separation Surveillance, Diagnosis, Treatment and Control of Disease Animal Care and Technical Personnel

Animal care programs require technical and husbandry support. Institutions should employ people trained in laboratory animal science or provide for both formal and on-the-job training to ensure effective implementation of the program (Annexure4)

Personal Hygiene

Animal Experimentation Involving Hazardous Agents

Multiple Surgical Procedures on Single Animal

Durations of Experiments

Physical Restraint

Location of Animal Facilities to Laboratories:

Functional Areas

The size and nature of a facility will determine whether areas for separate servicefunctions are possible or necessary. Sufficient animal area required to:

- Ensure separation of species or isolation of individual projects when necessary;
- Receive, quarantine, and isolate animals; and
- Provide for animal housing.

- In facilities that are small, maintain few animals or maintain animals under special conditions (e.g., facilities exclusively used for housing germfree colonies or animalsin runs and pens) some functional areas listed below could be unnecessary or includedin a multipurpose area. Professional judgement must be exercised when developing a practical system for animal care.
- Specialized laboratories or
- Individual areas contiguous with or near animal housing areas for such activities as surgery, intensive care, necropsy, radiography, preparation of special diets, experimental manipulation, treatment, and diagnostic laboratory procedures containment facilities or
- Equipment, if hazardous biological, physical, or chemical agents are to be used
- Receiving and storage areas for food, bedding
- Pharmaceuticals and biologics, and supplies
- Space for administration, supervision, and direction of the facility
- Showers, sinks, lockers and toilets for personnel
- An area for washing and sterilization equipment and supplies,
- An autoclave for equipment
- Food, and bedding; and separate areas
- For holding soiled and cleaned equipment
- An area for repairing cages and equipment
- An area to store wastes prior to incineration or removal

Other Physical Facilities

Storage Areas

Facilities for Sanitizing Equipment and Supplies

Experimental Area

Environment

Animal Husbandry Caging or Housing System:

Sheltered or Outdoor Housing

Social Environment

Standard Operating Procedures (SOPs) / Guidelines

Personnel and Training

Transport of Laboratory Animals

Anaesthesia and Euthanasia

Laboratory Animal Ethics

Transgenic Animals

Breeding and Genetics

Maintenance and Disposal

Record Keeping

It is essential that animal House should maintain following records:

- Animal House plans, which includes typical floor plan, all fixtures etc.
- Animal House staff record - both technical and non - technical
- Health record of staff and animals
- All SOPs relevant to experiments, care, breeding and management of animals
- Breeding, stock, purchase and sales records
- Minutes of institutional Animals Ethics Committee Meetings
- Records of experiments conducted with the number of animals used (copy ofForm D)
- Mortality, Postmortem Record
- Clinical record of sick animals
- Training record of staff involved in animal activities
- Water, feed and bedding materials analysis report
- Health monitoring Records
- Rehabilitation Records

Annexure

Annexure – 1 Haematological Data of Common Laboratory Animals

Annexure – 2 Biochemical Data of Common Laboratory Animals

Annexure – 3A Minimum floor area recommended for laboratory animals (based on their weight/size and behavioral activity)

Annexure – 3B Example for calculating the number of Mice to be kept per cage, based on floor area recommended for animal according to their weight (size) and size of the cage

Annexure – 3C Example for calculating the number of rats to be kept per cage, based on floor area recommended per animal according to their weight (size) and size of the cage

Annexure – 3D Example for calculating the number of Hamster/ Gerbils/ Mastomys/Cotton rats to be kept per cage, based on floor area recommended per animal according to their weight (size) and size of the cage

Annexure - 3E Minimum floor area and height recommended for monkeys (rhesus and bonnet) based on their weight (size) and behavioral activity (for langurs, the recommended space is in the foot note below)

Annexure - 3F Recommended Space for Cats, Dogs and Birds

Annexure - 3G Recommended Space for Commonly Used Farm Animals

Annexure – 4 Specifications for Transport of Laboratory Animals By Road, Rail And Air

Annexure – 5 Commonly Used Anaesthetic Agents for Laboratory Animals

Annexure – 6 Euthanasia of Laboratory Animals

Annexure - 7 Qualifications & Knowledge Required for Laboratory Attendant

Annexure – 8 Institutional Biosafety Committee (IBSC)

OECD Guidelines for Testing Chemicals

Introduction

The OECD Guidelines for the Testing of Chemicals are a unique tool for assessing the potential effects of chemicals on human health and the environment. Accepted internationally as standard methods for safety testing, the Guidelines are used by professionals in industry, academia and government involved in the testing and assessment of chemicals (industrial chemicals, pesticides, personal care products, etc.). These Guidelines are continuously expanded and updated to ensure they reflect the state-of-the-art science and techniques to meet member countries regulatory needs. The Guidelines are elaborated with the assistance of experts from regulatory agencies, academia, industry, environmental and animal welfare organisations.

OECD Test Guidelines are covered by the OECD Mutual Acceptance of Data (MAD) system. Under this system, laboratory test results related to the safety of chemicals that are generated in accordance with OECD Test Guidelines and OECD Principles of Good Laboratory Practices are accepted in all OECD countries and adherent countries for the purpose of safety assessment and other uses relating to the protection of human health and the environment. The OECD Guidelines for the Testing of Chemicals are split into following five sections:

Section 1- Physical-Chemical properties

Section 2- Effects on Biotic Systems

Section 3- Environmental fate and behavior

Section 4 - Health Effects

Section 5 - Other Test Guidelines

Acute Oral Toxicity – Up-and-Down Procedure

Introduction

OECD guidelines for the Testing of Chemicals are periodically reviewed in the light of scientific progress or changing assessment practices. The concept of the up-and-down testing approach was first described by Dixon and Mood.

Principle of the Limit Test

The Limit Test is a sequential test that uses a maximum of 5 animals. A test dose of 2000, or exceptionally 5000 mg/kg, may be used. The procedures for testing at 2000 and 5000 mg/kg are slightly different. The selection of a sequential test plan increases the statistical power and also has been made to intentionally bias the procedure towards rejection of the limit test for compounds with LD50s near the limit dose; i.e., to err on the side of safety.

Principle of the Main Test

- The main test consists of a single ordered dose progression in which animals are dosed, one at a time, at a minimum of 48-hour intervals. The first animal receives a dose a step below the level of the best estimate of the LD50. If the animal survives, the dose for the next animal is increased by [a factor of] 3.2 times the original dose; if it dies, the dose for the next animal is decreased by a similar dose progression. (Note: 3.2 is the default factor corresponding to a dose progression of one half log unit).
- Each animal should be observed carefully for up to 48 hours before making a decision on whether and how much to dose the next animal. That decision is based on the 48-hour survival pattern of all the animals up to that time.
- A combination of stopping criteria is used to keep the number of animals low while adjusting the dosing pattern to reduce the effect of a poor starting value or low slope. Dosing is stopped when one of these criteria is satisfied, at which time an estimate of the LD50 and a confidence interval are calculated for the test based on the status of all the animals at termination. For most applications, testing will be completed with only 4 animals after initial reversal in animal outcome.

Data and Reporting

Individual animal data should be provided. Additionally, all data should be summarised in tabular form, showing for each test dose the number of animals used, the number of animals displaying signs of toxicity, the number of animals found dead during the test or killed for humane reasons, time of death of individual animals, a description and the time course of toxic effects and reversibility, and necropsy findings. A rationale for the starting dose and the dose progression and any data used to support this choice should be provided.

Calculation of LD50 for the main test

The LD50 is calculated using the maximum likelihood method. The following statistical details may be helpful in implementing the maximum likelihood calculations suggested (with an assumed *sigma*). All deaths, whether immediate or delayed or humane kills, are incorporated for the purpose of the maximum likelihood analysis. The likelihood function is written as follows:

$$L = L1\ L2\ \ldots.Ln,$$

Where

L is the likelihood of the experimental outcome, given *mu* and *sigma*, and n the total number of animals tested.

$$Li = 1 - F(Zi) \text{ if the } i^{st} \text{ animal survived, or}$$
$$Li = F(Zi) \text{ if the } i^{st} \text{ animal died,}$$

where

F = cumulative standard normal distribution,

$Zi = [\log(di) - mu] / sigma$

di = dose given to the i^{st} animal, and

sigma = standard deviation in log units of dose (which is not the log standard deviation).

An estimate of the true LD50 is given by the value of *mu* that maximizes the likelihood L. An estimate of *sigma* of 0.5 is used unless a better generic or case-specific value is available. Under some circumstances, statistical computation will not be possible or will likely give erroneous results. Special means to determine/report an estimated LD50 are available for these circumstances as follows:

(a) If testing stopped based on criterion (a) in paragraph 29 (i.e., a boundary dose was tested repeatedly), or if the upper bound dose ended testing, then the LD50 is reported to be above the upper bound.

(b) If all the dead animals have higher doses than all the live animals (or if all live animals have higher doses than all the dead animals, although this is practically unlikely), then the LD50 is between the doses for the live and the dead animals.

(c) If the live and dead animals have only one dose in common and all the other dead animals have higher doses and all the other live animals lower doses, or vice versa, then the LD50 equals their common dose. If a closely related substance is tested, testing should proceed with a smaller dose progression. If none of the above situations occurs, then the LD50 is calculated using the maximum likelihood method.

Further Reading

1. Alternatives, animal welfare and curriculum, workshop held on August 19, 2004. Bangalore Veterinary University, Bangalore, Karnataka, India.
2. Anon. Breeding of and Experiments on Animals (Control and Supervision) rules 1998. Gazette of India, Number 809, December 15th 1998.
3. Archna Mudgal. Pharmacy Council of India. Education (Amendment) regulations 2014. Gazette of India, Extraordinary, 10-1/2012 PCI, August 25, 2014.
4. Badyal DK, Desai C. Animal use in pharmacology education and research: The changing scenario. Indian J Pharmacol 2014;46:257-65
5. Committee for the Purpose of Control and Supervision on Experiments on Animals (2003) CPCSEA Guidelines for laboratory animal facility. Indian Journal of Pharmacology 35: 257–274.
6. Control of animal Experiments through Alternative Approaches, workshop held on March 25, 2000 at Defence Food Research Laboratory, Mysore, Karnataka, India.
7. Goyal RK et al, Practical Anatomy, Physiology and Biochemistry, 1985, BS Shah Prakashan, Ahmadabad.
8. Guidelines for care and use of Animals in Scientific Research, Indian National Science Academy, 200.
9. Guidelines for care and use of animals in scientific research. Indian National science academy. First edition, 1992 revised edition, 2000.
10. Guidelines for use of laboratory animals in medical colleges. Indian council of medical research, New Delhi, 2001.
11. International conference on alternatives to the use of animals in research and education held on February 18-20, 2003, New Delhi, India.
12. Liebsch M, Grune B, Seiler A, Butzke D, Oelgeschla¨ger M, Pirow R, et al. Alternatives to animal testing: current status and future perspectives. Arch Toxicol 2011;85:841-58

13. Mahesh NM. Different approaches to control animal experiments. Indian J. Pharm. Educ.2002; 36(2): 78-83.
14. Ministry of social justice and empowerment notification, New Delhi, 1998. The Breeding of and Experiments on Animals (Control and Supervision) Rules.
15. NV Giridharan, Vijay Kumar and Vasantha Muthuswamy. Use of animals in scientific research. A report from Indian Council of Medical Research, Ministry of Health and Family Welfare, New Delhi, May 2000: 1-25.
16. Pereira, S, Veeraraghavan, P, Ghosh, S. (2004) Animal experimentation and ethics in India: the CPCSEA makes a difference. Alternatives to Laboratory Animals 32 (Suppl. 1B): 411–415.
17. Prevention of Cruelty to Animals Act (PCA Act, 1960) as amended in 1982.
18. S Pereira and M. Tettamanti. Ahimsa and alternatives-the concept of the 4th R. The CPCSEA in India. Altex 2005; 22 (1/05): 3-6.
19. SK Kulkarni. Hand book of experimental pharmacology, 1999, Vallabh Prakashan, Delhi.
20. Solanki D. Unnecessary and cruel use of animals for medical undergraduate training in India. J Pharmacol Pharmacother 2010; 1(1): 59.
21. Zutphen, LFMv, Baumans, V, Beynen, AC (2001) Principles of laboratory animal science: a contribution to the humane use and care of animals and to the quality of experimental results. Amsterdam: Elsevier.
22. Alternatives, animal welfare and curriculum, workshop held on August 19, 2004. Bangalore Veterinary University, Bangalore, Karnataka, India.
23. Anon. Breeding of and Experiments on Animals (Control and Supervision) rules 1998. Gazette of India, Number 809, December 15th 1998.
24. Archna Mudgal. Pharmacy Council of India. Education (Amendment) regulations 2014. Gazette of India, Extraordinary, 10-1/2012 PCI, August 25, 2014.
25. Badyal DK, Desai C. Animal use in pharmacology education and research: The changing scenario. Indian J Pharmacol 2014;46:257-65
26. Baker, M (2013) Neuroscience. Through the eyes of a mouse. Nature 502: 156–158.
27. Balcombe, JP, Barnard, ND, Sandusky, C (2004) Laboratory routines cause animal stress. Contemporary Topics in Laboratory Animal Science 43: 42–51.
28. Committee for the Purpose of Control and Supervision on Experiments on Animals (2003) CPCSEA Guidelines for laboratory animal facility. Indian Journal of Pharmacology 35: 257–274.
29. Control of animal Experiments through Alternative Approaches, workshop held on March 25, 2000 at Defence Food Research Laboratory, Mysore, Karnataka, India.
30. Goyal RK et al, Practical Anatomy, physiology and biochemistry, 1985, BS Shah Prakashan, Ahmedabad.
31. Guidelines for care and use of animals in scientific research. Indian National science academy. First edition, 1992 revised edition, 2000.
32. Guidelines for use of laboratory animals in medical colleges. Indian council of medical research, New Delhi, 2001.
33. International conference on alternatives to the use of animals in research and education held on February 18-20, 2003, New Delhi, India.
34. Liebsch M, Grune B, Seiler A, Butzke D, Oelgeschla¨ger M, Pirow R, et al. Alternatives to animal testing: current status and future perspectives. Arch Toxicol 2011;85:841-58
35. Mahesh NM. Different approaches to control animal experiments. Indian J. Pharm. Educ.2002; 36(2): 78-83.

36. Ministry of social justice and empowerment notification, New Delhi, 1998. The Breeding of and Experiments on Animals (Control and Supervision) Rules.
37. NV Giridharan, Vijay Kumar and Vasantha Muthuswamy. Use of animals in scientific research. A report from Indian Council of Medical Research, Ministry of Health and Family Welfare, New Delhi, May 2000: 1-25.
38. Pereira, S, Veeraraghavan, P, Ghosh, S. (2004) Animal experimentation and ethics in India: the CPCSEA makes a difference. Alternatives to Laboratory Animals 32 (Suppl. 1B): 411–415.
39. Pratap, K, Singh, VP (2016) A training course on laboratory animal science: An initiative to implement the Three Rs of animal research in India. Alternative to Laboratory Animals 44: 21–41.
40. Prevention of Cruelty to Animals Act (PCA Act, 1960) as amended in 1982.
41. S Pereira and M. Tettamanti. Ahimsa and alternatives-the concept of the 4th R. The CPCSEA in India. ALTEX 2005; 22 (1/05): 3-6.
42. Sandercock, P, Roberts, I (2002) Systematic reviews of animal experiments. Lancet 360: 586.
43. SK Kulkarni. Hand book of experimental pharmacology, 1999, VallabhPrakashan, Delhi.
44. Solanki D. Unnecessary and cruel use of animals for medical undergraduate training in India. J Pharmacol Pharmacother 2010; 1(1): 59.
45. Van Luijk, J, Bakker, B, Rovers, MM. (2014) Systematic reviews of animal studies; missing link in translational research? PLoS One 9: e89981.
46. Zutphen, LFMv, Baumans, V, Beynen, AC (2001) Principles of laboratory animal science: a contribution to the humane use and care of animals and to the quality of experimental results. Amsterdam: Elsevier.
47. Buschmann J. The OECD guidelines for the testing of chemicals and pesticides. Methods Mol Biol. 2013;947:37-56.
48. Rao KS, Dong J. Nonclinical reproductive toxicity testing requirements for drugs, pesticides, and industrial chemicals in India and China. Methods Mol Biol. 2013;947:13-30.
49. Buschmann J. Critical aspects in reproductive and developmental toxicity testing of environmental chemicals. Reprod Toxicol. 2006;22(2):157-63.
50. Gelbke HP, Fleig H, Meder M; German Chemical Industry Association. SIDS reprotoxicity screening test update: testing strategies and use. Regul Toxicol Pharmacol. 2004;39(2):81-6.
51. Kühnel D, Nickel C. The OECD expert meeting on ecotoxicology and environmental fate--towards the development of improved OECD guidelines for the testing of nanomaterials. Sci Total Environ. 2014;472:347-53.
52. Dekant W, Melching-Kollmuss S, Kalberlah F. Toxicity assessment strategies, data requirements, and risk assessment approaches to derive health based guidance values for non-relevant metabolites of plant protection products. Regul Toxicol Pharmacol. 2010;56(2):135-42.
53. OECD Guideline for the Testing of Chemicals No. 407. Repeated Dose 28-day Oral Toxicity Study in Rodents, adopted on 3rd October, 2008.
54. OECD Guideline for the Testing of Chemicals No. 408. Repeated Dose 90-day Oral Toxicity Study in Rodents, adopted on 21st September, 1998.
55. OECD Guideline for the Testing of Chemicals No. 425. Acute Oral Toxicity - Up-and Down Procedure (UDP), adopted on 3rd October, 2008.

56. OECD Guideline for the Testing of Chemicals No. 420. Acute Oral Toxicity - Fixed Dose Procedure, adopted on 17th December, 2001.
57. OECD Guideline for the Testing of Chemicals No. 423. Acute Oral Toxicity - Acute Toxic Class Method, adopted on 17th December, 2001.
58. OECD Guideline for the Testing of Chemicals No. 414. Prenatal Development Toxicity Study, adopted on 22nd January, 2001.
59. OECD Guideline for the Testing of Chemicals No. 415. One-Generation Reproduction Toxicity Study, adopted on 26th May, 1983.
60. OECD Guideline for the Testing of Chemicals No. 416. Two-Generation Reproduction Toxicity, adopted on 22nd January, 2001.
61. https://www.oecd.org/chemicalsafety/testing/oecdguidelinesforthetestingofchemicals.htm accessed Dec. 2020

Scan QR code to view the website/guidelines

- CPCSEA Guidelines-

ACTS, RULES AND GUIDELINES: Committee for the Purpose of Control And Supervision of Experiments on Animals (ccsea.gov.in)

CHAPTER 19

Human Dose Calculation Guidelines

Introduction

This guidance outlines a process (algorithm) and vocabulary for deriving the maximum recommended starting dose (MRSD) for *first-in-human* clinical trials of new molecular entities in adult healthy volunteers, and recommends a standardized process by which the MRSD can be selected. The purpose of this process is to ensure the safety of the human volunteers. The goals of this guidance are to: (1) establish a consistent terminology for discussing the starting dose; (2) provide common conversion factors for deriving a human equivalent dose (HED); and (3) delineate a strategy for selecting the MRSD for adult healthy volunteers, regardless of the projected clinical use. This process is depicted in a flow chart that presents the decisions and calculations used to generate the MRSD from animal data (see Appendix E).

Background

- The process identified in this guidance pertains to determining the MRSD for adult healthy subjects when beginning a clinical investigation of any new drug or biological therapeutic that has been studied in animals. This guidance is not pertinent to endogenous hormones and proteins (e.g., recombinant clotting factors) used at physiologic concentrations or prophylactic vaccines. The process outlined in this guidance pertains primarily to drug products for which systemic exposure is intended; it does not address dose escalation or maximum allowable doses in clinical trials.
- Although the process outlined in this guidance uses administered doses, observed toxicities, and an algorithmic approach to calculate the MRSD, an alternative approach could be proposed that places primary emphasis on animal pharmacokinetics and modeling rather than dose. In a limited number of cases, animal pharmacokinetic data can be useful in determining initial clinical doses. However, in the majority of investigational new drug applications (INDs), animal data are not available in sufficient detail to construct a scientifically valid, pharmacokinetic model whose aim is to accurately project an MRSD.
- Toxicity should be avoided at the initial clinical dose. However, doses should be chosen that allow reasonably rapid attainment of the phase 1 trial objectives (e.g., assessment of the therapeutic's tolerability, pharmacodynamic or pharmacokinetic profile). All of the relevant preclinical data, including information on the pharmacologically active dose, the full toxicologic profile of the compound, and the pharmacokinetics (absorption, distribution, metabolism, and excretion) of the therapeutic, should be considered when determining the MRSD. Starting with doses lower than the MRSD is always an option and can be particularly appropriate to meet some clinical trial objectives.
- The remainder of this guidance focuses on the recommended algorithmic process for starting dose extrapolation from animals to humans based on administered doses, since this method will likely be useful for the majority of INDs seeking to investigate new drugs in healthy volunteers. Some classes of drugs (e.g., many cytotoxic or biological agents) are commonly introduced into initial clinical trials in patient volunteers rather

than healthy volunteers. Typically, patients are used instead of healthy volunteers when a drug is suspected or known to be unavoidably toxic. This guidance does not address starting doses in patients. However, many principles and some approaches recommended here may be applicable to designing such trials.

Overview of the Algorithm

The recommended process for selecting the MRSD is presented in Appendix E and described in this section. The major elements (i.e., the determination of the no observed adverse effect levels (NOAELs) in the tested animal species, conversion of NOAELs to HED, selection of the most appropriate animal species, and application of a safety factor) are all discussed in greater detail in subsequent sections. Situations are also discussed in which the algorithm should be modified. The algorithm is intended to be used for systemically administered therapeutics. Topical, intranasal, intratissue, and compartmental administration routes and depot formulations can have additional considerations, but similar principles should apply.

The process of calculating the MRSD should begin after the toxicity data have been analyzed. Although only the NOAEL should be used directly in the algorithm for calculating an MRSD, other data (exposure/toxicity relationships, pharmacologic data, or prior clinical experience with related drugs) can affect the choice of most appropriate species, scaling, and safety factors.

The NOAEL for each species tested should be identified, and then converted to the HED using appropriate scaling factors. For most systemically administered therapeutics, this conversion should be based on the normalization of doses to body surface area. Although body surface area conversion is the standard way to approximate equivalent exposure if no further information is available, in some cases extrapolating doses based on other parameters may be more appropriate. This decision should be based on the data available for the individual case. The body surface area normalization and the extrapolation of the animal dose to human dose should be done in one step by dividing the NOAEL in each of the animal species studied by the appropriate body surface area conversion factor (BSA-CF). This conversion factor is a unitless number that converts mg/kg dose for each animal species to the mg/kg dose in humans, which is equivalent to the animal's NOAEL on a mg/m^2 basis. The resulting figure is called a human equivalent dose (HED). The species that generates the lowest HED is called the most sensitive species.

When information indicates that a particular species is more relevant for assessing human risk (and deemed the *most appropriate species*), the HED for that species may be used in subsequent calculations, regardless of whether this species is the most sensitive. This situation is more applicable to biologic therapies, many of which have high selectivity for binding to human target proteins and limited reactivity in species commonly used for toxicity testing.

In such cases, in vitro binding and functional studies should be conducted to select an appropriate, relevant species before toxicity studies are designed (refer to ICH guidance for industry *S6 Preclinical Safety Evaluation of Biotechnology-Derived Pharmaceuticals* for more details). (However, if serious toxicities are observed in an animal species considered less relevant, those toxicities should be taken into consideration in determining the species to be used to calculate an HED. For example, in one particular case, dog was selected as the animal species used for calculation of an HED because of unmonitorable cardiac lesions, even though the rat was considered the most relevant species based on pharmacological activity data.)

Additionally, a species might be considered an inappropriate toxicity model for a given drug if the dose-limiting toxicity in that species was concluded to be of limited value for human risk assessment, based on historical comparisons of toxicities in the animal species to those in humans across a therapeutic class (i.e., the dose-limiting toxicity is species-specific). In this case, data from that species should not be used to derive the HED. Without any additional information to guide the choice of the most appropriate species for assessing human risk, the most sensitive species is designated the *most appropriate*, because using the lowest HED would generate the most conservative starting dose.

A safety factor should then be applied to the HED to increase assurance that the first dose in humans will not cause adverse effects. The use of the safety factor should be based on the possibility that humans may be more sensitive to the toxic effects of a therapeutic agent than predicted by the animal models, that bioavailability may vary across species, and that the models tested do not evaluate all possible human toxicities. For example, ocular disturbances or pain (e.g., severe headaches) in humans can be significant dose-limiting toxicities that may go undetected in animal studies.

In general, one should consider using a safety factor of at least 10. The MRSD should be obtained by dividing the HED by the safety factor. Safety concerns or design shortcomings noted in animal studies may increase the safety factor, and thus reduce the MRSD further.

Alternatively, information about the pharmacologic class (well-characterized classes of therapeutics with extensive human clinical and preclinical experience) may allay concerns and form the basis for reducing the magnitude of the default safety factor and increasing the MRSD. Although a dose lower than the MRSD can be used as the actual starting dose, the process described in this guidance will derive the maximum recommended starting dose. This algorithm generates an MRSD in units of mg/kg, a common method of dosing used in phase 1 trials, but the equations and conversion factors provided in this guidance (Table 1, second column) can be used to generate final dosing units in the mg/m^2 form if desired.

As previously stated, for purposes of initial clinical trials in adult healthy volunteers, the HED should ordinarily be calculated from the animal NOAEL. If the HED is based on an alternative index of effect, such as the pharmacologically active dose (PAD), this exception should be prominently stipulated in descriptions of starting dose calculations.

The remainder of this guidance provides a description of the individual steps in the recommended process and the reasoning behind each step.

Step 1: No Observed Adverse Effect Level (NOAEL) Determination

The first step in determining the MRSD is to review and evaluate the available animal data so that a NOAEL can be determined for each study. Several definitions of NOAEL exist, but for selecting a starting dose, the following is used: the highest dose level that does not produce a significant increase in adverse effects in comparison to the control group. In this context, adverse effects that are biologically significant (even if they are not statistically significant) should be considered in the determination of the NOAEL. The NOAEL is a generally accepted benchmark for safety when derived from appropriate animal studies and can serve as the starting point for determining a reasonably safe starting dose of a new therapeutic in healthy (or asymptomatic) human volunteers.

The NOAEL is not the same as the *no observed effect level(NOEL)*, which refers to any effect, not just an adverse one, although in some cases the two might be identical. The definition of the NOAEL, in contrast to that of the NOEL, reflects the view that some effects observed in the animal may be acceptable pharmacodynamic actions of the therapeutic and may not raise a safety concern. The NOAEL should also not be confused with *lowest observed adverse effect level(LOAEL)* or *maximum tolerated dose(MTD)*. Both of the latter concepts are based on findings of adverse effects and are not generally used as benchmarks for establishing safe starting doses in adult healthy volunteers. (The term *level* refers to dose or dosage, generally expressed as mg/kg or mg/kg/day.)

Initial IND submissions for first-in-human studies by definition lack in vivo human data or formal allometric comparison of pharmacokinetics. Measurements of systemic levels or exposure (i.e., AUC or C_{max}) cannot be employed for setting a safe starting dose in humans, and it is critical to rely on dose and observed toxic response data from adequate and well-conducted toxicology studies. However, there are cases where nonclinical data on bioavailability, metabolite profile, and plasma drug levels associated with toxicity may influence the choice of the NOAEL. One such case is when saturation of drug absorption occurs at a dose that produces no toxicity. In this instance, the lowest saturating dose, not the highest (nontoxic) dose, should be used for calculating the HED.

There are essentially three types of findings in nonclinical toxicology studies that can be used to determine the NOAEL: (1) overt toxicity (e.g., clinical signs, macro- and microscopic lesions); (2) surrogate markers of toxicity (e.g., serum liver enzyme levels); and (3) exaggerated pharmacodynamic effects. Although the nature and extent of adverse effects can vary greatly with different types of therapeutics, and it is anticipated that in many instances, experts will disagree on the characterization of effects as being adverse or not, the use of NOAEL as a benchmark for dose-setting in healthy volunteers should be acceptable to all responsible investigators. As a general rule, an adverse effect observed in nonclinical toxicology studies used to define a NOAEL for the purpose of dose-setting should be based on an effect that would be unacceptable if produced by the initial dose of a therapeutic in a phase 1 clinical trial conducted in adult healthy volunteers.

Step 2: Human Equivalent Dose (HEDs) Calculation

A. Conversion Based on Body Surface Area

After the NOAELs in the relevant animal studies have been determined, they are converted to HEDs. A decision should be made regarding the most appropriate method for extrapolating the animal dose to the equivalent human dose. Toxic endpoints for therapeutics administered systemically to animals, such as the MTD, are usually assumed to scale well between species when doses are normalized to body surface area (i.e., mg/m^2) (EPA 1992; Lowe and Davis 1998). The basis for this assumption lies primarily with the work of Freireich et al. (1966) and Schein et al. (1970). These investigators reported that, for antineoplastic drugs, doses lethal to 10 percent of rodents (LD_{10}s) and MTDs in nonrodents both correlated with the human MTD when the doses were normalized to the same administration schedule and expressed as mg/m^2. Despite the subsequent analyses showing that the MTDs for this set of drugs scale best between species when doses are normalized to $W^{0.75}$ rather than $W^{0.67}$ (inherent in body surface area normalization) (Travis and White 1988; Watanabe et al. 1992), normalization to body surface area has remained a widespread practice for estimating an HED based on an animal dose.

An analysis of the affect of the allometric exponent on the conversion of an animal dose to the HED was conducted (see Appendix A). Based on this analysis and on the fact that correcting for body surface area increases clinical trial safety by resulting in a more conservative starting dose estimate, it was concluded that the approach of converting NOAEL doses to an HED based on body surface area correction factors (i.e., $W^{0.67}$) should be maintained for selecting starting doses for initial studies in adult healthy volunteers. Nonetheless, use of a different dose normalization approach, such as directly equating the human dose to the NOAEL in mg/kg, may be appropriate in some circumstances. Deviations from the body surface area approach, when describing the conversion of animal dose to HED, should be justified. The basis for justifying direct mg/kg conversion and examples in which other normalization methods are appropriate are described in the following subsection.

Although normalization to body surface area is an appropriate method for extrapolating doses between species, consistent factors for converting doses from mg/kg to mg/m^2 have not always been used. Given that body surface area normalization provides a reasonable approach for estimating an HED, the factors used for converting doses for each species should be standardized. Since body surface area varies with $W^{0.67}$, the conversion factors are dependent on the weight of the animals in the studies. However, analyses conducted to address the effect of body weight on the actual BSA-CF demonstrated that a standard factor provides a reasonable estimate of the HED over a broad range of human and animal weights (see Appendix B). The conversion factors and divisors shown in Table 19.1 are therefore recommended as the standard values to be used for interspecies dose conversions for NOAELs. (These factors may also be applied when comparing safety margins for other toxicity endpoints (e.g., reproductive toxicity and carcinogenicity) when other data for comparison (i.e., AUCs) are unavailable or are otherwise inappropriate for comparison.)

Table 19.1 Conversion of Animal Doses to Human Equivalent Doses Based on Body Surface Area.

Species	To Convert Animal Dose in mg/kg to Dose in mg/m², Multiply by k_m	To Convert Animal Dose in mg/kg to HED[a] in mg/kg, Either:	
		Divide Animal Dose By	Multiply Animal Dose By
Human	37	---	---
Child (20 kg)[b]	25	---	---
Mouse	3	12.3	0.08
Hamster	5	7.4	0.13
Rat	6	6.2	0.16
Ferret	7	5.3	0.19
Guinea pig	8	4.6	0.22
Rabbit	12	3.1	0.32
Dog	20	1.8	0.54
Primates: Monkeys[c]	12	3.1	0.32
Marmoset	6	6.2	0.16
Squirrel monkey	7	5.3	0.19
Baboon	20	1.8	0.54
Micro-pig	27	1.4	0.73
Mini-pig	35	1.1	0.95

[a] Assumes 60 kg human. For species not listed or for weights outside the standard ranges,
[b] HED can be calculated from the following formula:$^{0.33}$. HED = animal dose in mg/kg x (animal weight in kg/human weight in kg)
[c] This k_m value is provided for reference only since healthy children will rarely be volunteers for phase 1 trials.
[d] For example, cynomolgus, rhesus, and stumptail.

B. Basis for Using mg/kg Conversions

The factors in Table 1 for scaling animal NOAEL to HEDs are based on the assumption that doses scale 1:1 between species when normalized to body surface area. However, there are occasions for which scaling based on body weight (i.e., setting the HED (mg/kg) = NOAEL (mg/kg)) may be more appropriate. To consider mg/kg scaling for a therapeutic, the available data should show that the NOAEL occurs at a similar mg/kg dose across species. The following circumstances should exist before extrapolating to the HED on a mg/kg basis rather than using the mg/m^2 approach. Note that mg/kg scaling will give a twelve-, six-, and twofold higher HED than the default mg/m^2 approach for mice, rats, and dogs, respectively. If these circumstances do not exist, the mg/m^2 scaling approach for determining the HED should be followed as it will lead to a safer MRSD.

1. NOAELs occur at a similar mg/kg dose across test species (for the studies with a given dosing regimen relevant to the proposed initial clinical trial). (However, it should be noted that similar NOAELs on a mg/kg basis can be obtained across species because of differences in bioavailability alone.)
2. If only two NOAELs from toxicology studies in separate species are available, one of the following should also be true:

- The therapeutic is administered orally and the dose is limited by local toxicities. Gastrointestinal (GI) compartment weight scales by $W^{0.94}$ (Mordenti 1986). GI volume determines the concentration of the therapeutic in the GI tract. It is then reasonable that the toxicity of the therapeutic would scale by mg/kg ($W^{1.0}$).
- The toxicity in humans (for a particular class) is dependent on an exposure parameter that is highly correlated across species with dose on a mg/kg basis. For example, complement activation by systemically administered antisense oligonucleotides in humans is believed to be dependent upon C_{max} mg/kg dose and in such instances mg/kg scaling would be justified.
- Other pharmacologic and toxicologic endpoints also scale between species by mg/kg for the therapeutic. Examples of such endpoints include the MTD, lowest lethal dose, and the pharmacologically active dose.
- There is a robust correlation between plasma drug levels (C_{max} and AUC) and dose in mg/kg.

C. Other Exceptions to mg/m^2 Scaling Between Species

Scaling between species based on mg/m^2 is not recommended for the following categories of therapeutics:

1. Therapeutics administered by alternative routes (e.g., topical, intranasal, subcutaneous, intramuscular) for which the dose is limited by local toxicities. Such therapeutics should be normalized to concentration (e.g., mg/area of application) or amount of drug (mg) at the application site.
2. Therapeutics administered into anatomical compartments that have little subsequent distribution outside of the compartment. Examples are intrathecal, intravesical, intraocular, or intrapleural administration. Such therapeutics should be normalized between species according to the compartmental volumes and concentrations of the therapeutic.
3. Proteins administered intravascularly with M_r> 100,000 daltons. Such therapeutics should be normalized to mg/kg.

Step 3: Most Appropriate Species Selection

After the HEDs have been determined from the NOAELs from all toxicology studies relevant to the proposed human trial, the next step is to pick one HED for subsequent derivation of the MRSD. This HED should be chosen from the most appropriate species. In the absence of data on species relevance, a default position is that the most appropriate species for deriving the

MRSD for a trial in adult healthy volunteers is the most sensitive species (i.e., the species in which the lowest HED can be identified).

Factors that could influence the choice of the most appropriate species rather than the default to the most sensitive species include: (1) differences in the absorption, distribution, metabolism, and excretion (ADME) of the therapeutic between the species, and (2) class experience that may indicate a particular animal model is more predictive of human toxicity. Selection of the most appropriate species for certain biological products (e.g., human proteins) involves consideration of various factors unique to these products. Factors such as whether an animal species expresses relevant receptors or epitopes may affect species selection (refer to ICH guidance for industry *S6 Preclinical Safety Evaluation of Biotechnology-Derived Pharmaceuticals* for more details).

When determining the MRSD for the first dose of a new therapeutic in humans, absorption, distribution, and elimination parameters will not be known for humans. Comparative metabolism data, however, might be available based on in vitro studies. These data are particularly relevant when there are marked differences in both the in vivo metabolite profiles and HEDs in animals. Class experience implies that previous studies have demonstrated that a particular animal model is more appropriate for the assessment of safety for a particular class of therapeutics. For example, in the nonclinical safety assessment of the phosphorothioate antisense drugs, the monkey is considered the most appropriate species because monkeys experience the same dose limiting toxicity as humans (e.g., complement activation) whereas rodents do not. For this class of therapeutics, the MRSD would usually be based on the HED for the NOAEL in monkeys regardless of whether it was lower than that in rodents, unless unique dose limiting toxicities were observed with the new antisense compound in the rodent species.

Step 4: Application of Safety Factor

Once the HED of the NOAEL in the most appropriate species has been determined, a safety factor should then be applied to provide a margin of safety for protection of human subjects receiving the initial clinical dose. This safety factor allows for variability in extrapolating from animal toxicity studies to studies in humans resulting from: (1) uncertainties due to enhanced sensitivity to pharmacologic activity in humans versus animals; (2) difficulties in detecting certain toxicities in animals (e.g., headache, myalgias, mental disturbances); (3) differences in receptor densities or affinities; (4) unexpected toxicities; and (5) interspecies differences in ADME of the therapeutic. These differences can be accommodated by lowering the human starting dose from the HED of the selected species NOAEL.

In practice, the MRSD for the clinical trial should be determined by dividing the HED derived from the animal NOAEL by the safety factor. The default safety factor that should normally be used is 10. This is a historically accepted value, but, as described below, should be evaluated based on available information.

A safety factor of 10 may not be appropriate for all cases. The safety factor should be raised when there is reason for increased concern, and lowered when concern is reduced because of available data that provide added assurance of safety. This can be visualized as a sliding scale, balancing findings that mitigate the concern for harm to healthy volunteers with those that suggest greater concern is warranted. The extent of the increase or decrease is largely a matter of judgment, using the available information. It is incumbent on the evaluator to clearly explain the reasoning behind the applied safety factor when it differs from the default value of 10, particularly if it is less than 10.

A. Increasing the Safety Factor

The following considerations indicate a safety concern that might warrant increasing the safety factor. In these circumstances, the MRSD would be calculated by dividing the HED by a safety factor that is greater than 10. If any of the following concerns are defined in review of the nonclinical safety database, an increase in the safety factor may be called for. If multiple concerns are identified, the safety factor should be increased accordingly.

- **Steep dose response curve:** A steep dose response curve for significant toxicities in the most appropriate species or in multiple species may indicate a greater risk to humans.
- **Severe toxicities:** Qualitatively severe toxicities or damage to an organ system (e.g., central nervous system (CNS)) indicate increased risk to humans.
- **Nonmonitorable toxicity:** Non-monitorable toxicities may include histopathologic changes in animals that are not readily monitored by clinical pathology markers.
- **Toxicities without premonitory signs:** If the onset of significant toxicities is not reliably associated with premonitory signs in animals, it may be difficult to know when toxic doses are approached in human trials.
- **Variable bioavailability:** Widely divergent or poor bioavailability in the several animal species, or poor bioavailability in the test species used to derive the HED, suggest a greater possibility for underestimating the toxicity in humans.
- **Irreversible toxicity:** Irreversible toxicities in animals suggest the possibility of permanent injury in human trial participants.
- **Unexplained mortality:** Mortality that is not predicted by other parameters raises the level of concern.
- **Large variability in doses or plasma drug levels eliciting effect:** When doses or exposure levels that produce a toxic effect differ greatly across species or among individual animals of a species, the ability to predict a toxic dose in humans is reduced and a greater safety factor may be needed.
- **Nonlinear pharmacokinetics:** When plasma drug levels do not increase in a dose related manner, the ability to predict toxicity in humans in relation to dose is reduced and a greater safety factor may be needed.
- **Inadequate dose-response data:** Poor study design (e.g., few dose levels, wide dosing intervals) or large differences in responses among animals within dosing groups may make it difficult to characterize the dose-response curve.

- **Novel therapeutic targets:** therapeutic targets that have not been previously clinically evaluated may increase the uncertainty of relying on the nonclinical data to support a safe starting dose in humans.
- **Animal models with limited utility:** Some classes of therapeutic biologics may have very limited interspecies cross-reactivity or pronounced immunogenicity, or may work by mechanisms that are not known to be conserved between (nonhuman) animals and humans; in these cases, safety data from any animal studies may be very limited in scope and interpretability.

B. Decreasing the Safety Factor

Safety factors of less than 10 may be appropriate under some conditions. The toxicologic testing in these cases should be of the highest caliber in both conduct and design. Most of the time, candidate therapeutics for this approach would be members of a well-characterized class. Within the class, the therapeutics should be administered by the same route, schedule, and duration of administration; should have a similar metabolic profile and bioavailability; and should have similar toxicity profiles across all the species tested including humans. A smaller safety factor might also be used when toxicities produced by the therapeutic are easily monitored, reversible, predictable, and exhibit a moderate-to-shallow dose-response relationship with toxicities that are consistent across the tested species (both qualitatively and with respect to appropriately scaled dose and exposure).

A safety factor smaller than 10 could be justified when the NOAEL was determined based on toxicity studies of longer duration compared to the proposed clinical schedule in healthy volunteers. In this case, a greater margin of safety should be built into the NOAEL, as it was associated with a longer duration of exposure than that proposed in the clinical setting. This assumes that toxicities are cumulative, are not associated with acute peaks in therapeutic concentration (e.g., hypotension), and did not occur early in the repeat dose study.

Step 5: Consideration of the Pharmacologically Active Dose

Selection of a PAD depends upon many factors and differs markedly among pharmacological drug classes and clinical indications; therefore, selection of a PAD is beyond the scope of this guidance. However, once the MRSD has been determined, it may be of value to compare it to the PAD derived from appropriate pharmacodynamic models. If the PAD is from an in vivo study, an HED can be derived from a PAD estimate by using a BSA-CF. This HED value should be compared directly to the MRSD.

If this *pharmacologic* HED is lower than the MRSD, it may be appropriate to decrease the clinical starting dose for pragmatic or scientific reasons. Additionally, for certain classes of drugs or biologics (e.g., vasodilators, anticoagulants, monoclonal antibodies, or growth factors), toxicity may arise from *exaggerated pharmacologic* effects. The PAD in these cases may be a more sensitive indicator of potential toxicity than the NOAEL and might therefore warrant lowering the MRSD.

Summary

A strategy has been proposed to determine the maximum recommended starting dose for clinical trials of new therapeutics in adult healthy volunteers. In summary, usually NOAELs from the relevant animal studies should be converted to the HEDs using the standard factors presented in Table 1. Using sound scientific judgment, a safety factor should be applied to the HED from the most appropriate species to arrive at the MRSD. This process is meant to define the upper limit of recommended starting doses and, in general, lower starting doses can be appropriate. The process described in this guidance should foster consistency among sponsors and Agency reviewers.

Glossary

- **Body surface area conversion factor (BSA-CF):** A factor that converts a dose (mg/kg) in an animal species to the equivalent dose in humans (also known as the *human equivalent dose*), based on differences in body surface area. A BSA-CF is the ratio of the body surface areas in the tested species to that of an average human.
- **Human equivalent dose (HED):** A dose in humans anticipated to provide the same degree of effect as that observed in animals at a given dose. In this guidance, as in many communications from sponsors, the term HED is usually used to refer to the human equivalent dose of the NOAEL. When reference is made to the human equivalent of a dose other than the NOAEL (e.g., the PAD), sponsors should explicitly and prominently note this usage.
- **K:** A dimensionless factor that adjusts for differences in the surface area to weight ratio of species because of their different body shapes.
- **k_m:** Factor for converting mg/kg dose to mg/m^2 dose
- **Lowest observed adverse effect level (LOAEL):** The lowest dose tested in an animal species with adverse effects.
- **Maximum recommended starting dose (MRSD):** The highest dose recommended as the initial dose in a clinical trial. In clinical trials of adult healthy volunteers, the MRSD is predicted to cause no adverse reactions. The units of the dose (e.g., mg/kg or mg/m^2) may vary depending on practices employed in the area being investigated.
- **Maximum tolerated dose (MTD):** In a toxicity study, the highest dose that does not produce unacceptable toxicity.
- **No observed adverse effect level (NOAEL):** The highest dose tested in an animal species that does not produce a significant increase in adverse effects in comparison to the control group. Adverse effects that are biologically significant, even if not statistically significant, should be considered in determining an NOAEL.
- **No observed effect level (NOEL):** the highest dose tested in an animal species with any detected effects.

- **Pharmacologically active dose (PAD):** The lowest dose tested in an animal species with the intended pharmacologic activity.
- **Safety factor (SF):** A number by which the HED is divided to introduce a margin of safety between the HED and the *maximum recommended starting dose.*
- **W:** Body weight in kg

APPENDIX A

Analysis of Allometric Exponent on HED Calculations

- An analysis was conducted to determine the effect of the allometric exponent on the conversion of an animal dose to the HED. One can derive the following equation (see Appendix C) for converting animal doses to the HED based on body weights and the allometric exponent (b):

  HED = animal NOAEL × (Wanimal/Whuman)(1-b)

- Conventionally, for a mg/m^2 normalization *b* would be 0.67, but a number of studies (including the original Freireich data) have shown that MTDs scale best across species when b = 0.75. The Interagency Pharmacokinetics Group has recommended that $W^{0.75}$ be used for interspecies extrapolation of doses in carcinogenicity studies (EPA 1992). There are no data, however, to indicate the optimal method for converting NOAELs to HEDs.
- Conversion factors were calculated over a range of animal and human weights using $(W_{animal}/W_{human})^{0.33}$ or $(W_{animal}/W_{human})^{0.25}$ to assess the effect on starting dose selection of using b = 0.75 instead of b = 0.67. The results are shown in Table 20.2. Using an allometric exponent of 0.75 had a big effect on the conversion factor for the smaller species mice and rats.
- Nonetheless, mice are not commonly used for toxicology studies to support the first-in-human clinical trials. In addition, there is evidence that the area under the plasma concentration versus time curves in rats and humans correlate reasonably well when doses are normalized to mg/m^2.
- We conclude that the approach of converting NOAEL doses to an HED based on body surface area correction factors (i.e., b = 0.67) should be maintained for selecting starting doses for initial studies in healthy volunteers since:
  1. mg/m^2 normalization is widely used throughout the toxicology and pharmacokinetic research communities;
  2. mg/m^2 normalization provides a more conservative conversion;
  3. there are no data to suggest a superior method for converting NOAELs; and
  4. CDER has significant experience in establishing safe starting doses based on mg/m^2, and it is readily calculated.

Table 19.2 Effect of Allometric Exponent on Conversion Factor[a].

Species	[b]Weight Range (kg)	Conversion Factors[c]	Ratio of 0.75 to 0.67		
		Standard	b = 0.67	b = 0.75	
Mouse	0.018-0.033	0.081	0.075	0.141	1.88
Rat	0.09-0.40	0.162	0.156	0.245	1.57
Rabbit	1.5-3	0.324	0.33	0.43	1.30
Monkey	1.5-4	0.324	0.37	0.47	1.27
Dog	6.5-13.0	0.541	0.53	0.62	1.17

[a]conversion factor = (Wanimal/Whuman)(1-b) [b]human weight range used was 50-80 kg (110-176 lb)
[c]mean conversion factor calculated across entire animal weight range and human weight range

The following summarizes the analysis of the effects of the allometric exponent on HED calculations:

- Changing the allometric exponent from 0.67 to 0.75 had a big effect on the conversion factor for the smaller rodent species; for mice the conversion factors differed by a factor of almost 2.
- Converting doses based on an exponent of 0.75 would lead to higher, more aggressive and potentially more toxic starting doses.
- The limited data available suggest that the most accurate allometric exponent for normalizing MTDs of antineoplastic agents for interspecies extrapolation is b = 0.75, but there are no data to indicate the optimal normalization method for interspecies extrapolation of NOAELs in a broad range of therapeutic classes. Using mg/m^2 is widely adopted throughout the drug development community.
- Unless evidence is provided to the contrary, HED calculations should be based on b =
- 0.67 (i.e., the standard conversions based on mg/m^2 relationships).
- There was no notable effect of body weight on calculation of the HED within the weight ranges examined.

APPENDIX B

Analysis of Body Weight Effects on HED Calculations

- Accurate conversion of a mg/kg dose to a mg/m^2 dose depends on the actual weight (and surface area) of the test species. A popular formula for converting doses is:

  mg/m^2 = k_m × mg/kg

  where km = 100/K × $W^{0.33}$ where K is a value unique to each species

  ork_m = 9.09 × $W^{0.35}$ where a K value unique to each species is not needed.

- The k_m value is not truly constant for any species, but increases within a species as body weight increases. The increase is not linear, but increases approximately proportional to $W^{2/3}$. For example, the k_m value in rats varies from 5.2 for a 100 g rat to 7.0 for a 250 g rat. Strictly speaking, the k_m value of 6 applies only to rats at the *reference weight* of 150 g.

- For standardization and practical purposes, a fixed k_m factor for each species is preferred. An analysis was undertaken to determine the effect of different body weights within a species on the conversion of an animal dose to the HED using k_m factors.

- The k_m factor was calculated for a range of body weights using k_m = 100/K × $W^{0.33}$. In Table 3, a working weight range is shown next to the reference body weight. This is the range within which the HED calculated by using the standard k_m value will not vary more than ±20 percent from that which would be calculated using a k_m value based on exact animal weight.

- This is a relativity small variance considering dose separation generally used in deriving the NOAEL, in toxicology studies, which are often twofold separations. For example, suppose a NOAEL in rats is 75 mg/kg and the average rat weight is 250 g. The k_m value for a 250 g rat is 7.0.

  HED = 75 × (7/37) = 14 mg/kg in humans.

  Using the standard k_m value of 6 for rats,

  HED = 75 × (6/37) = 12 mg/kg in humans.

- The HED calculated with the standard k_m value of 6 is within 15 percent of the value calculated using the actual k_m value of 7. As shown in Table 20.3, the body weights producing k_m factors for which the nominal, integer conversion factor was within 20 percent of the calculated factor covered a broad range. This working weight range encompassed the animal weights expected for the majority of studies used to support starting doses in humans.

Table 19.3 Conversion of Animal Doses to Human Equivalent Doses Based on Body Surface Area.

Species	Reference Body Weight (kg)	Working Weight Range[a] (kg)	Body Surface Area (m^2)	To Convert Dose in mg/kg to Dose in mg/m^2 Multiply by k_m	To Convert Animal Dose in mg/kg to HED[b] in mg/kg, Either	
					Divide Animal Dose By	Multiply Animal Dose By
Human	60	---	1.62	37	---	---
Child[c]	20	---	0.80	25	---	---
Mouse	0.020	0.011-0.034	0.007	3	12.3	0.081
Hamster	0.080	0.047-0.157	0.016	5	7.4	0.135
Rat	0.150	0.080-0.270	0.025	6	6.2	0.162
Ferret	0.300	0.160-0.540	0.043	7	5.3	0.189
Guinea pig	0.400	0.208-0.700	0.05	8	4.6	0.216
Rabbit	1.8	0.9-3.0	0.15	12	3.1	0.324
Dog	10	5-17	0.50	20	1.8	0.541
Primates: Monkeys[d]	3	1.4-4.9	0.25	12	3.1	0.324
Marmoset	0.350	0.140-0.720	0.06	6	6.2	0.162
Squirrel monkey	0.600	0.290-0.970	0.09	7	5.3	0.189
Baboon	12	7-23	0.60	20	1.8	0.541
Micro-pig	20	10-33	0.74	27	1.4	0.730
Mini-pig	40	25-64	1.14	35	1.1	0.946

[a]For animal weights within the specified ranges, the HED for a 60 kg human calculated using the standard k_m value will not vary more than ±20 percent from the HED calculated using a k_m value based on the exact animal weight.

[b]Assumes 60 kg human. For species not listed or for weights outside the standard ranges, human equivalent dose can be calculated from the formula: HED = animal dose in mg/kg x (animal weight in kg/human weight in kg)$^{0.33}$.

[c]The k_m value is provided for reference only since healthy children will rarely be volunteers for phase 1 trials.

[d]For example, cynomolgus, rhesus, and stumptail.

For the typical species used in nonclinical safety studies, Table 3 also shows the body surface area in m^2 for an animal at a particular *reference* weight. For example, a 400 g guinea pig has a body surface area of approximately 0.05 m^2. These values come from published sources with surface area determined experimentally by various methods. Compilations of this type of data can be found in published references.

For animal weights outside the working weight range in Table 3, or for species not included in the table, an alternative method is available for calculating the HED. In these cases the following formula can be used:

$$\text{HED} = \text{Animal dose (mg/kg)} \times [\text{animal weight (kg)} \div \text{human weight (kg)}]^{0.33}$$

For example, assume that a NOAEL of 25 mg/kg was determined in a study using rabbits weighing 4.0 kg. The 4.0 kg animals are outside the working range for rabbits of 0.9 to 3.0 kg indicated in Table 3.

$$\text{HED} = 25 \text{ mg/kg} \times (4.0 \div 60)^{0.33} = 25 \times (0.41) = 10 \text{ mg/kg}$$

Alternatively, if the standard conversion factor was used to calculate the HED

$$\text{HED} = 25 \text{ mg/kg} \div 3.1 = 8.1 \text{ mg/kg}$$

The value of 10 mg/kg for the HED is 25 percent greater than the value of 8.1 mg/kg that would be calculated using the standard conversion factor. For example, assume that a NOAEL of 25 mg/kg was determined in a study using rabbits weighing 4.0 kg. The 4.0 kg animals are outside the working range for rabbits of 0.9 to 3.0 kg indicated in Table 3.

$$\text{HED} = 25 \text{ mg/kg} \times (4.0 \div 60)^{0.33} = 25 \times (0.41) = 10 \text{ mg/kg}$$

Alternatively, if the standard conversion factor was used to calculate the HED

$$\text{HED} = 25 \text{ mg/kg} \div 3.1 = 8.1 \text{ mg/kg}$$

The value of 10 mg/kg for the HED is 25 percent greater than the value of 8.1 mg/kg that would be calculated using the standard conversion factor.

The k_m analysis addresses only half of the HED conversion process. The range of human sizes should also be considered to convert the mg/m^2 dose back to an HED dose in mg/kg. To examine the effect of both animal and human weights on the conversion factor, the principle of allometry was used. Interspecies biologic parameters are often related by the power function $Y = aW^b$ where W is body weight and b (allometric exponent) is the slope of the log-log plot, $\log y = b \times \log W + C$. Using algebraic manipulation (see Appendix C), one can derive an equation for converting an animal dose to the HED based on the body weights of the human and the animals for a given allometric exponent. For converting an animal NOAEL in mg/kg to the HED in mg/kg, the equation is:

$$\text{HED} = \text{animal NOAEL x } (W_{animal}/W_{human})^{(1-b)}$$

Since body surface area is believed to scale with an allometric exponent (b) of 0.67, one can explore how the animal and human body weights affect the conversion factor

(W-animal/W-human)/0.33.

The conversion factor was calculated over a range of animal weights and a range of human weights from 50-80 kg. The results are summarized in Table 4. Column B is the weight range of the animals used to calculate, in conjunction with the 50-80 kg range in humans, the conversion factor. The extremes of the conversion factors for the permutations chosen are shown in columns C and D.

The proposed standard conversion factors are shown in column E. The percentage difference of these extremes from the standard is shown in column F. Finally, the range of animal weights that produced a conversion factor for a 60 kg human within 20 percent of the standard factor is shown in column G. The ±10 percent and ±20 percent intervals across the entire range of weights are graphically illustrated for rats in Table 5.

Table 19.4 Effect of Body Weight on Human Equivalent Dose Conversions[a].

A	B	C	D	E	F	G
		Conversion Factor[c]				
Species	Animal Weight Range[b] (kg)	sm animal lg human	lg animal sm human	Standard[d]	% Difference of Extreme[e] from Standard	±20% Range[f] for 60 kg Human (kg)
Mouse	0.018-0.033	0.060	0.089	0.081	-22%	0.015-0.051
Rat	0.090-0.400	0.106	0.213	0.162	-35%	0.123-0.420
Rabbit	1.5-3.0	0.269	0.395	0.324	+22%	1.0-3.4
Monkey	1.5-4.0	0.319	0.435	0.324	+34%	1.0-3.4
Dog	6.5-13.0	0.437	0.641	0.541	-19%	4.7-16.2

[a]conversion factor = (W-animal/W-human)0.33
[b]human weight range used was 50-80 kg (110-176 lb)
[c]HED in mg/kg equals animal dose in mg/kg multiplied by this valued See Table 1 extreme from column C or D range of animal weights that produced a calculated conversion factor within 20 percent of the standard factor (column E) when human weight was set at 60 kg

Table 19.5 Human and Rat Body Weights Producing Body Surface Area Dose Conversion Factors Within 10 Percent and 20 Percent of the Standard Factor (0.162).

Effect of Body Weight on BSA-CF							
HED = animal NOAEL· (W_{animal}/W_{human})exp(1-b), b = 0.67 for mg/m² conversion							
Standard conversion to mg/kg = 0.162				± 10%	0.146-0.178		
				± 20%	0.130-0.194		
Rat Body Weight (kg)	Human Body Weight (kg)						
	50	55	60	65	70	75	80
0.090	0.124	0.120	0.117	0.114	0.111	0.109	0.106
0.100	0.129	0.125	0.121	0.118	0.115	0.113	0.110
0.110	0.133	0.129	0.125	0.122	0.119	0.116	0.114

Contd...

Effect of Body Weight on BSA-CF							
HED = animal NOAEL· (W_{animal}/W_{human})exp(1-b), b = 0.67 for mg/m² conversion							
Standard conversion to mg/kg = 0.162				± 10%		0.146-0.178	
				± 20%		0.130-0.194	
Rat Body Weight (kg)	Human Body Weight (kg)						
	50	55	60	65	70	75	80
0.120	0.137	0.132	0.129	0.125	0.122	0.119	0.117
0.130	0.140	0.136	0.132	0.129	0.126	0.123	0.120
0.140	0.144	0.139	0.135	0.132	0.129	0.126	0.123
0.150	0.147	0.142	0.138	0.135	0.132	0.129	0.126
0.160	0.150	0.146	0.141	0.138	0.134	0.131	0.129
0.170	0.153	0.149	0.144	0.141	0.137	0.134	0.131
0.180	0.156	0.151	0.147	0.143	0.140	0.137	0.134
0.190	0.159	0.154	0.150	0.146	0.142	0.139	0.136
0.200	0.162	0.157	0.152	0.148	0.145	0.141	0.138
0.210	0.164	0.159	0.155	0.151	0.147	0.144	0.141
0.220	0.167	0.162	0.157	0.153	0.149	0.146	0.143
0.230	0.169	0.164	0.159	0.155	0.152	0.148	0.145
0.240	0.172	0.166	0.162	0.157	0.154	0.150	0.147
0.250	0.174	0.169	0.164	0.160	0.156	0.152	0.149
0.260	0.176	0.171	0.166	0.162	0.158	0.154	0.151
0.270	0.179	0.173	0.168	0.164	0.160	0.156	0.153
0.280	0.181	0.175	0.170	0.166	0.162	0.158	0.155
0.290	0.183	0.177	0.172	0.168	0.164	0.160	0.157
0.300	0.185	0.179	0.174	0.179	0.165	0.162	0.158
0.310	0.187	0.181	0.176	0.171	0.167	0.163	0.160
0.320	0.189	0.183	0.178	0.173	0.169	0.165	0.162
0.330	0.191	0.185	0.180	0.175	0.171	0.167	0.163
0.340	0.193	0.187	0.181	0.177	0.172	0.169	0.165
0.350	0.194	0.188	0.183	0.178	0.174	0.170	0.167
0.360	0.196	0.190	0.185	0.180	0.176	0.172	0.168
0.370	0.198	0.192	0.187	0.182	0.177	0.173	0.170
0.380	0.200	0.194	0.188	0.183	0.179	0.175	0.171
0.390	0.202	0.195	0.190	0.185	0.180	0.176	0.173
0.400	0.203	0.197	0.191	0.186	0.182	0.178	0.174
0.410	0.205	0.199	0.193	0.188	0.183	0.179	0.175

Contd...

Effect of Body Weight on BSA-CF							
HED = animal NOAEL· (W_{animal}/W_{human})exp(1-b), b = 0.67 for mg/m² conversion							
Standard conversion to mg/kg = 0.162				**± 10%**		**0.146-0.178**	
				± 20%		**0.130-0.194**	
Rat Body Weight (kg)	**Human Body Weight (kg)**						
0.420	0.207	0.200	0.194	0.189	0.185	0.181	0.177
0.430	0.208	0.202	0.196	0.191	0.186	0.182	0.178
0.440	0.210	0.203	0.197	0.192	0.188	0.183	0.180
0.450	0.211	0.205	0.199	0.194	0.189	0.185	0.181
0.460	0.213	0.206	0.200	0.195	0.190	0.186	0.182

The following are conclusions from these analyses:

- The ±20 percent interval around the standard conversion factor includes a broad range of animal and human weights.
- Given that the human weights will vary broadly, it is not usually necessary to be concerned about the affect of the variation of animal weights within a species on the HED calculation.
- If an extreme animal weight is encountered in a toxicology study, one can calculate an accurate conversion factor using $(W_{animal}/W_{human})^{0.33}$.

APPENDIX C

Derivation of the Interspecies Scaling Factor $(W_a/W_h)^{(1-b)}$

Power equation (mg) = $aW^b \log(mg) = \log(a) + bC\log(W) = bC\log(W) + c$

Given the weights of animal and human, and animal dose in mg/kg, solve for HED in mg/kg:

Let

H = mg/kg dose in humans

A = mg/kg dose in animals

W_h = weight of human

W_a = weight of animal

for animal $\log(mg) = \log(a) + bC\log(W_a) = bC\log(W_a) + c$ replace mg $\log(ACW_a) = bC\log(W_a) + c$

solve for c $c = \log(ACW_a) - bC\log(W_a)$

$= \log(A) + \log(W_a) - bC\log(W_a)$

$= \log(A) + (1-b)\log(W_a)$

Like wise for human

$c = \log(H) + (1-b)\log(W_h)$

equate two equations $\log(A) + (1-b)\log(Wa) = \log(H) + (1\ b)\log(Wh)$

solve for log(H) $\log(H) = \log(A) + (1-b)\log(Wa) - (1\ b)\log(Wh)$

$= \log(A) + (1-b)[\log(W_a) - \log(W_h)]$

$= \log(A) + \log[(W_a/W_h)^{(1-b)}]\ \log(H)$

$= \log[AC(W_a/W_h)^{(1-b)}]$

solve for H $H = AC(W_a/W_h)^{(1-b)}$

For example, using mg/m^2 normalization (b = 0.67) the predicted human MTD in mg/kg based on a rat LD_{10} in mg/kg is $MTD = LD_{10}C(W_a/W_h)^{0.33}$.

Likewise the HED in mg/kg based on a surface area conversion given an animal NOAEL is $HED = NOAEL\ C(W_a/W_h)^{0.33}$.

APPENDIX D

Examples of Calculations for Converting Animal Doses to Human Equivalent Doses

This appendix provides examples of specific calculations to be taken in deriving an HED based on standardized factors. Tables 20.1 and 20.3 provide standardized conversion factors for changing animal or human doses expressed as mg/kg to doses expressed as mg/m^2. Tables 20.1 and 20.3 also have factors (and divisors) for converting animal doses in mg/kg to the human dose in mg/kg that is equivalent to the animal dose if both were expressed on a mg/m^2 basis. This human dose in mg/kg is referred to as the HED.

Example 1: Converting to mg/m^2 HED

To convert an animal or human dose from mg/kg to mg/m^2, the dose in mg/kg is multiplied by the conversion factor indicated as k_m (for mass constant). The k_m factor has units of kg/m^2; it is equal to the body weight in kg divided by the surface area in m^2.

Formula: mg/kg × km = mg/m2 to convert a dose of 30 mg/kg in a dog: 30 × 20 = 600 mg/m2 to convert a dose of 2.5 mg/kg in a human: 2.5 × 37 = 92.5 mg/m2

Example 2: Converting to mg/kg HED in two steps

To calculate the HED for a particular dose in animals, one can calculate the animal dose in mg/m^2 by ***multiplying*** the dose in mg/kg by the k_m factor for that species as described in Example 1. The dose can then be converted back to mg/kg in humans by ***dividing*** the dose in mg/m^2 by the k_m factor for humans.

Formula: animal mg/kg dose × animal k_m) ÷ human k_m = human mg/kg dose to calculate the HED for a 15 mg/kg dose in dogs: (15 × 20) ÷ 37 = 300 mg/m² ÷ 37 = 8 mg/kg

Example 3: Converting to mg/kg HED in one step

The calculation in Example 2 can be simplified by combining the two steps. The HED can be calculated directly from the animal dose by *dividing* the animal dose by the ratio of the human/animal k_m factor (third column in Table 20.1) or by *multiplying* by the ratio of the animal/human k_m factor (fourth column in Table 20.1).

Division method

NOAEL	calculation mg/kg ÷ [km human/km animal]	HED
15 mg/kg in dogs	15 mg/kg ÷ 1.8 =	8 mg/kg
50 mg/kg in rats	50 mg/kg ÷ 6.2 =	8 mg/kg
50 mg/kg in monkeys	50 mg/kg ÷ 3.1 =	16 mg/kg

Multiplication method

NOAEL	calculation mg/kg × [km animal/km human]	HED
15 mg/kg in dogs	15 mg/kg × 0.541 =	8 mg/kg
50 mg/kg in rats	50 mg/kg × 0.162 =	8 mg/kg
50 mg/kg in monkeys	50 mg/kg × 0.324 =	16 mg/kg

APPENDIX E

Selection of Maximum Recommended Starting Dose for Drugs Administered Systemically to Normal Volunteers

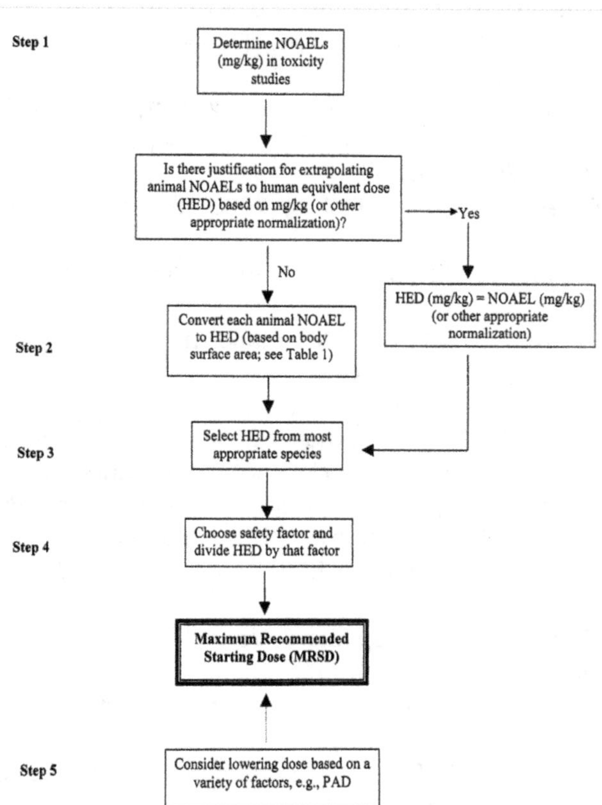

Further Reading

1. Boxenbaum, H and C DiLea, 1995, First-Time-in-Human Dose Selection: Allometric Thoughts and Perspectives, Journal of Clinical Pharmacology, 35:957-966.
2. Burtles, SS, DR Newell, REC Henrar, and TA Connors, 1995, Revisions of General Guidelines for the Preclinical Toxicology of New Cytotoxic Anticancer Agents in Europe, European Journal of Cancer, 31A:408-410.
3. Contrera, JF, AC Jacobs, RP Hullahalli, M Mehta, WJ Schmidt, and JA DeGeorge, 1995, Systemic Exposure — Based Alternative to the Maximum Tolerated Dose for Carcinogenicity Studies of Human Therapeutics, Journal of American College of Toxicology, 14:1-10.
4. EPA, 1992, A Cross-Species Scaling Factor for Carcinogen Risk Assessment Based on Equivalence of Mg/Kg$^{0.75}$/Day, Federal Register, 57:24152-24173.

5. Freireich, EJ, EA Gehan, DP Rall, LH Schmidt, and HE Skipper, 1966, Quantitative Comparison of Toxicity of Anticancer Agents in Mouse, Rat, Hamster, Dog, Monkey, and Man, Cancer Chemotherapy Reports, 50:219-244.
6. Geary, RS, JM Leeds, SP Henry, DK Monteith, and AA Levin, 1997, Antisense Oligonucleotide Inhibitors for the Treatment of Cancer: 1. QUESTION Pharmacokinetic Properties of PhosphorothioateOligodeoxynucleotides, Anti-Cancer Drug Design, 12:383-393.
7. Lowe, MC and RD Davis, 1998, The Current Toxicology Protocol of the National Cancer Institute, in K Hellman and SK Carter (eds.), Fundamentals of Cancer Chemotherapy, pp. 228235, New York: McGraw Hill.
8. Mahmood, I, MD Green, and JE Fisher, 2003, Selection of the First-Time Dose in Humans:
9. Comparison of Different Approaches Based on Interspecies Scaling of Clearance, 43(7):692-697.
10. Mordenti, J, 1986, Man Vs. Beast: Pharmacokinetic Scaling in Mammals, Journal of Pharmaceutical Sciences, 75:1028-1040.
11. Reigner, BG and KS Blesch, 2002, Estimating the Starting Dose for Entry into Humans: Principles and Practice, European Journal of Clinical Pharmacology, 57:835-845.
12. Schein, PS, RD Davis, S Carter, J Newman, DR Schein, and DP Rall, 1970, The Evaluation of Anticancer Drugs in Dogs and Monkeys for the Prediction of Qualitative Toxicities in Man, Clinical Pharmacology and Therapeutics, 11:3-40.
13. Spector, WS (ed.), 1956, Handbook of Biological Data, W.B. Saunders Co. Philadelphia. pp. 175.
14. Stahl, WR, 1967, Scaling of Respiratory Variables in Mammals, Journal of Applied Physiology, 22:453-460.
15. Travis, CC and RK White, 1988, Interspecies Scaling of Toxicity Data, Risk Analysis, 8:119125.
16. Watanabe, K, FY Bois, and L Zeise, 1992, Interspecies Extrapolation: A Reexamination of Acute Toxicity Data, Risk Analysis, 12:301-310.
17. International Conference on Harmonisation Guidances- ICH guidance for industry S6 Preclinical Safety Evaluation of Biotechnology-Derived Pharmaceuticals
18. ICH guidance for industry S3A Toxicokinetics: The Assessment of Systemic Exposure in Toxicity Studies
19. ICH guidance for industry M3 Nonclinical Safety Studies for the Conduct of Human Clinical Trials for Pharmaceuticals

Scan QR code to view the website/guidelines

- Human Dose Calculation- Guidance for Industry (fda.gov)

CHAPTER 20

WHO Guidelines for Assessment, Evaluation of Toxicity, Safety and Efficacy of Herbal Medicines 2000

WHO-Guidelines for the Assessment of Herbal Medicines 1991

Introduction

Herbal medicines means: Finished, labelled medicinal products that contain as active ingredients aerial or underground parts of plants, or other plant material, or combinations thereof, whether in the crude state or as plant preparations. Plant material includes juices, gums, fatty oils, essential oils, and any other substances of this nature. Herbal medicines may contain excipients in addition to the active ingredients. Medicines containing plant material combined with chemically defined active substances, including chemically defined, isolated constituents of plants, are not considered to be herbal medicines. Exceptionally, in some countries herbal medicines may also contain, by tradition, natural organic or inorganic active ingredients which are not of plant origin. The past decade has seen a significant increase in the use of herbal medicines.

The objective of these guidelines is to define basic criteria for the evaluation of quality, safety and efficacy of herbal medicines and thereby to assist national regulatory authorities, scientific organizations and manufacturers to undertake an assessment of the documentation/ submissions/dossiers in respect of such products. As a general rule in this assessment, traditional experience means that long-term use as well as the medical, historical and ethnological background of those products shall be taken into account. The definition of long-term use may vary according to the country but should be at least several decades. Therefore, the assessment should take into account a description in the medical/pharmaceutical literature or similar sources, or a documentation of knowledge on the application of a herbal medicine without a clearly defined time limitation. Marketing authorizations for similar products should be taken into account. Prolonged and apparently uneventful use of a substance usually offers testimony of its safety. In a few instances, however, investigation of the potential toxicity of naturally occurring substances widely used as ingredients in these preparations has revealed previously unsuspected potential for systematic toxicity, carcinogenicity and teratogenicity. Regulatory authorities need to be quickly and reliably informed of these findings. They should also have the authority to respond promptly to such alerts, either by withdrawing or varying the licences of registered products containing suspect substances, or by rescheduling the substances to limit their use to medical prescription.

Assessment of quality

- ***Pharmaceutical assessment:*** This should cover all important aspects of the quality assessment of herbal medicines. It should be sufficient to make reference to a pharmacopoeia monograph if one exists. If no such monograph is available, a monograph must be supplied and should be set out as in an official pharmacopoeia. All procedures should be in accordance with good manufacturing practices.
- ***Crude plant material:*** The botanical definition, including genus, species and authority, should be given to ensure correct identification of a plant. A definition and description of the part of the plant from which the medicine is made (e.g. leaf, flower, root) should be provided, together with an indication of whether fresh, dried or traditionally processed material is used. The active and characteristic constituents should be specified and, if possible, content limits should be defined. Foreign matter, impurities and microbial

content should be defined or limited. Voucher specimens, representing each lot of plant material processed, should be authenticated by a qualified botanist and should be stored for at least a 10-year period. A lot number should be assigned and this should appear on the product label.

- ***Plant preparations:*** Plant preparations include comminuted or powdered plant materials, extracts, tinctures, fatty or essential oils, expressed juices and preparations whose production involves fractionation, purification or concentration. The manufacturing procedure should be described in detail. If other substances are added during manufacture in order to adjust the plant preparation to a certain level of active or characteristic constituents or for any other purpose, the added substances should be mentioned in the manufacturing procedures. A method for identification and, where possible, assay of the plant preparation should be added. If identification of an active principle is not possible, it should be sufficient to identify a characteristic substance or mixture of substances (e.g. "chromatographic fingerprint") to ensure consistent quality of the preparation.
- ***Finished product:*** The manufacturing procedure and formula, including the amount of excipients, should be described in detail. A finished product specification should be defined. A method of identification and, where possible, quantification of the plant material in the finished product should be defined. If the identification of an active principle is not possible, it should be sufficient to identify a characteristic substance or mixture of substances (e.g. "chromatographic fingerprint") to ensure consistent quality of the product. The finished product should comply with general requirements for particular dosage forms.
- For imported finished products, confirmation of the regulatory status in the country of origin should be required. The WHO Certification Scheme on the Quality of Pharmaceutical Products Moving in International Commerce should be applied. General guidelines for methodologies on research and evaluation of traditional medicine
- ***Stability: The*** physical and chemical stability of the product in the container in which it is to be marketed should be tested under defined storage conditions and the shelflife should be established.

Assessment of safety

This should cover all relevant aspects of the safety assessment of a medicinal product. A guiding principle should be that, if the product has been traditionally used without demonstrated harm, no specific restrictive regulatory action should be undertaken unless new evidence demands a revised risk–benefit assessment. A review of the relevant literature should be provided with original articles or references to the original articles. If official monograph/review results exist, reference can be made to them. However, although long term use without any evidence of risk may indicate that a medicine is harmless, it is not always certain how far one can rely solely on long-term usage to provide assurance of innocuity in the light of concern expressed in recent years over the long-term hazards of some herbal medicines. Reported side-effects should be documented according to normal pharmacovigilance practices.

***Toxicological studies*:** Toxicological studies, if available, should be part of the assessment. Literature should be indicated as above.

Documentation of safety based on experience : As a basic rule, documentation of a long period of use should be taken into consideration when assessing safety. This means that, when there are no detailed toxicological studies, documented experience of long-term use without evidence of safety problems should form the basis of the risk assessment. However, even in cases of drugs used over a long period, chronic toxicological risks may have occurred but may not have been recognized. The period of use, the health disorders treated, the number of users and the countries with experience should be specified. If a toxicological risk is known, toxicity data must be submitted. The assessment of risk, whether independent of dose or related to dose, should be documented. In the latter case, the dosage specification must be an important part of the risk assessment. An explanation of the risks should be given, if possible. Potential for misuse, abuse or dependence must be documented. If long-term traditional use cannot be documented or there are doubts on safety, toxicity data should be submitted.

Assessment of efficacy

This should cover all important aspects of efficacy assessment. A review of the relevant literature should be carried out and copies provided of the original articles or proper references made to them. Research studies, if they exist, should be taken into account. The pharmacological and clinical effects of the active ingredients and, if known, their constituents with therapeutic activity should be specified or described. Evidence required to support indications The indication(s) for the use of the medicine should be specified. In the case of traditional medicines, the requirements for proof of efficacy should depend on the kind of indication. For treatment of minor disorders and for non-specific indications, some relaxation in requirements for proof of efficacy may be justified, taking into account the extent of traditional use. The same considerations may apply to prophylactic use. Individual experiences recorded in reports from physicians, traditional health practitioners or treated patients should be taken into account. Where traditional use has not been established, appropriate clinical evidence should be required.

Combination products: As many herbal remedies consist of a combination of several active ingredients, and as experience of the use of traditional remedies is often based on combination products, assessment should differentiate between old and new combination products. Identical requirements for the assessment of old and new combinations would result in inappropriate assessment of certain traditional medicines. In the case of traditionally used combination products, the documentation of traditional use (such as classical texts of Ayurveda, traditional Chinese medicine, Unani, Siddha) and experience may serve as evidence of efficacy. An explanation of a new combination of well-known substances, including effective dose ranges and compatibility, should be required in addition to the documentation of traditional knowledge of each single ingredient. Each active ingredient must contribute to the efficacy of the medicine. Clinical studies may be required to justify the efficacy of a new ingredient and its positive effect on the total combination.

Intended use Product information for the consumer

Product labels and package inserts should be understandable to the consumer or patient. The package information should include all necessary information on the proper use of the product. The following elements of information will usually suffice: ¨

- Name of the product ¨
- Quantitative list of active ingredient(s) ¨
- Dosage form ¨
- Indications ÿ dosage (if appropriate, specified for children and the elderly) general guidelines for methodologies on research and evaluation of traditional medicine
- Mode of administration
- Duration of use
- Major adverse effects, if any
- Overdosage information
- Contraindications, warnings, precautions and major drug interactions
- Use during pregnancy and lactation
- Expiry date
- Lot number
- Holder of the marketing authorization.

Identification of the active ingredient(s) by the Latin botanical name, in addition to the common name in the language of preference of the national regulatory authority, is recommended. Sometimes not all information that is ideally required may be available, so drug regulatory authorities should determine their minimal requirements. Promotion Advertisements and other promotional material directed to health personnel and the general public should be fully consistent with the approved package information.

Utilization of these guidelines

These guidelines for the assessment of herbal medicines are intended to facilitate the work of regulatory authorities, scientific bodies and industry in the development, assessment and registration of such products. The assessment should reflect the scientific knowledge gathered in that field. Such assessment could be the basis for future classification of herbal medicines in different parts of the world. Other types of traditional medicines in addition to herbal products may be assessed in a similar way. The effective regulation and control of herbal medicines moving in international commerce also requires close liaison between national institutions that are able to keep under regular review all aspects of production and use of herbal medicines, as well as to conduct or sponsor evaluative studies of their efficacy, toxicity, safety, acceptability, cost and relative value compared wit

WHO Research Guidelines for Evaluation the Safety and Efficacy of Herbal Medicines 1993

General Considerations in Herbal Medical Research

Governments should actively promote the rational use of herbal medicines that have been scientifically validated. Research on herbal medicines must be carried out in accordance with all relevant ethical guidelines.

Research Studies

Research on human subjects: When human subjects are involved, research must be conducted in accordance with four basic principles: justice, respect for persons, beneficence and non-malfeasance.

Research on animals: Research on animals must be carried out with respect for their welfare and consideration must be given to using in vitro laboratory methods that may reduce experimentation on intact animals

Respect for the environment: Proper consideration must be given to protection of the environment which supports the natural products that are the basis for herbal medicines and which may yield valuable medicinal products in the future

Traditional knowledge on herbal medicine

Herbal medicines have been used by the traditional system of medicine for a long time. Prolonged and apparently uneventful use of an herbal medicine may offer testimony of its safety and efficacy. The research approaches should differentiate between herbal medicines which have had documented experience from a long period of use with those whose traditional use has not been established.

Regulatory requirements

Regulatory requirements may be different in different countries. As a general rule, traditional experience which means that long- term use as well as the medical, historical and ethnological back- ground are well recorded, should be taken into account. In the design and conduct of researches on herbal medicine, the country's regulatory requirements must already be considered, particularly those required for registration of herbal medicine products.

Purposes of research

There are many reasons for carrying out research like to prove safety and efficacy of herbal medicines scientifically, to obtain purified or semi-purified compounds, to validate a new plant material or a new combination or even a new indication. a new dosage form or a new administrative route etc.

Selection of research projects

A thorough literature survey should be the starting point for every serious effort in herbal medicine research. Research projects should be selected with due consideration for several factors in addition to scientific interest Three of these are:

1. Potential value of the research results for improving the health of the community with due regard to the prevalence of disease and the feasibility of using alternative treatments
2. The medical value of indigenous plants
3. Technical and financial considerations.

Research approaches

Research on herbal medicines has generally been carried out by individual researchers or single multidisciplinary group to investigate pharmacodynamic studies to verify the traditional use, general pharmacological and toxicological tests to assure the safety of the medicinal product and clinical trial. Additional confirmatory clinical trials may be conducted if warranted. The clinical investigation of the therapeutic activity of such crude preparations maybe useful, because that activity may depend not only on a single substance but may be influenced by a large number of other components in the herbal medicine.

Non-clinical studies

The primary objectives of non-clinical studies are:

- To determine whether such studies support the clinical use of an herbal medicine;
- To characterize the range of pharmacological actions of herbal medicines; and
- To define the chemical characteristics of pharmacologically active natural products and to elucidate their mechanisms or actions

Pharmacodynamic investigations: Pharmacodynamic investigations are conducted in the light of the expected therapeutic effect of an herbal medicine using appropriate animal models or bioassays that closely relate to human disease as described by either traditional or modern medicine (see Guide- lines B, page 31).

General pharmacological investigations: General pharmacological investigations are conducted to elucidate various pharmacological activities other than the main pharmacodynamic action, such investigations usually cover the tests on nervous, cardiovascular and respiratory systems, and if necessary others, and should be performed on conscious or anaesthetised animals using adequate doses and proper routes of administration.

Toxicological investigations: Toxicological investigations are required to supplement human experience in defining possible toxicity from short-term use, but are particularly important in detecting toxicity that may occur either after prolonged exposure or years after the exposure has been discontinued. Generally, the longer the anticipated human use, the longer the test substance is administered to test animals. Animal and other toxicity studies are conducted according to generally accepted principles, referred to collectively as Good Laboratory Practice (GLP), which should be consulted in order to design appropriate studies (see Guidelines C, page 35).

(a) ***Systemic toxicity tests***: Systemic toxicity tests refer to alteration of either physiology, anatomy (gross or microscopic) or clinical chemistry (including haematology) that result from pathological changes in any organ distant from the site at which a herbal medicine is administered.

(i) ***Acute toxicity tests*** aim to deter- mine toxic manifestations of the test substance that occur when animals are exposed to one or more doses of the test substance within a single 24-hour period.

(ii) ***Long-term toxicity*** tests aim to determine toxic reactions when animals are exposed to the test drug for periods as long as their lifetime. In such tests, the animals are observed for behavioural changes as well as anatomical, physiological and biochemical manifestations of tissue damage. If pathological changes are detected during the period of drug administration, and the changes are not serious, it may be advisable to determine whether such changes are reversible after the drug is withdrawn. Thus, observations are made at intervals during continuous administration of the drug and then at intervals after the drug have been withdrawn to determine whether such pathology is reversible.

(b) ***Local toxicity tests*** are done to determine the local irritation and/or systemic absorption of an herbal medicine used for local applications (such as respiratory inhalants, drugs applied to skin or mucosa).

(c) ***Special toxicity test*** - regulatory requirements for special toxicity tests vary among Member States. For herbal medicines containing commonly used herbs which have been used clinically for a long period of time, some countries may not require special tests. Mutagenicity tests, however, are commonly required. If any deviation from traditional use is contemplated (such as new use, new preparation, new route of administration or more prolonged administration), additional toxicity tests such as carcinogenicity, teratogenicity and reproduction studies may be recommended

Clinical trials using herbal medicines

Clinical trials of herbal medicines may have two types of objectives. One is to validate the safety and efficacy that is claimed for a traditional herbal medicine. The other is to develop new herbal medicines or examine a purified or semi-purified compound derived from herbal medicines, a new indication for an existing herbal medicine or a change of dose formulation, or route of administration. Although special considerations may be required, the general principles of the clinical trials of herbal medicines are similar to those applied to synthetic drugs if clinical trial is regarded to be necessary.

Clinical trial protocol development

The development of a protocol should be the joint effort of representatives from several disciplines such as clinical pharmacologists, pharmacists, biostatisticians, physicians and other relevant health care workers, as well as experts in traditional medicine. Ordinarily, the protocol group is chaired by the chief investigator, who is a physician the protocol should include the following:

1. The title of the trial
2. A clear statement on the objectives of the study.
3. The justification of the proposed trial based on the available information on safety and efficacy, including a consideration of the non-clinical data as well as the drug utilization pattern and the disease spectrum for the country concerned
4. The rationale for the composition of the formula being studied and its relation to the principles of both herbal medicine and pharmacodynamic data.
5. The type of trial (such as controlled, open) and trial design (parallel groups, cross-over techniques), blind technique (double blind, single blind), randomization (methods and procedures).
6. Entry and exclusion criteria for study subjects (which may be based on diagnostic criteria of either modern or traditional medicine).
7. Number of trial subjects needed to achieve the trial objective, based on statistical considerations.
8. The therapeutic or clinical end points that are to be analysed at the conclusion of the trial (the unique nature of traditional medicine, which can relate to subjective wellness or quality of life, should also be considered when selecting the end points of the trial).
9. Control groups to be used (whether a therapeutic control group or a placebo group is used will depend on the disease being studied and the avail- ability of alternative modern drugs or herbal medicines of proven efficacy).

10. The subjective and objective clinical observations and laboratory tests which will be recorded during the course of the trial.
11. The treatment schedule for the duration of the trial, including dosage form and route of administration and the details of the product being used as a therapeutic control.
12. Criteria for other treatments that may or may not be given to subjects during the trial.
13. Procedures for the maintenance of subject identification code lists, treatment record, randomization list and/or Case Report Form (CRF).
14. Information on establishment of the trial code, where it will be kept and when, how and by whom it can be broken in the event of an emergency.
15. The qualifications and experience of the investigators.
16. The facilities and the sites where studies will be undertaken.
17. Methodology for the evaluation of results (such as statistical methods and reports on patients or participants who withdrew from the trial).
18. Information to be given to trial subjects.
19. Relevant communications with appropriate regulatory authorities.
20. Information given to the staff involved in the trial.
21. Medical care to be made available to patients after the trial.
22. List of literature referred to in the protocol.

When considering the above items, special attention must be given to designing a protocol that eliminates bias and reduces variance.

Ethics review board

The trial protocol should be considered by an ethics review board guided by the World Medical Association's Declaration of Helsinki under Good Clinical Practice (GCP). The board will generally be established at an institutional level but boards constituted of both medical and non-medical members existing at a regional or national level can also be used. The board will verify that the rights of the patients participating in the trial are protected and that the trial is justified in medical and social terms. The board will also consider the suitability of the trial protocol, patient selection and patient protection, and issues of informed consent of patients.

Responsibilities of investigators

The investigators who participate in the design of the protocol will also be responsible for preparing all necessary material for review by the ethics review board.

The investigators must be aware of such responsibilities as the following:

- The appropriate medical care of patients in the study;
- The ethical requirements for the trial (such as selection of patients. advice to patients);
- a knowledge of the product used in the trial;
- an appreciation of research methodology and the conduct of clinical trials (such as the recording and evaluation of results);
- An appreciation of the importance of careful monitoring of the trial and the need to take necessary action, to alter or terminate the trial if patients appear to be harmed by some aspect of the trial.

Responsibilities of the sponsor

If the product under investigation is supplied by a manufacturer, or if the trial is undertaken at the request of a manufacturer, the manufacturer (sponsor) has obligations to maintain the integrity of the investigators, the protocol group and the ethics review board and to prevent harm to a patient. The sponsor of a study can be an institution or an individual investigator as well as a manufacturer. The material supplied for the trial will be prepared according to Good Manufacturing Practices (GMP) to ensure the quality of the material used in the investigation. All data on the product will be made available to the investigator before the trial design is completed. The sponsor must meet all of the local requirements set by regulatory authorities and government agencies and should be aware of standards of good clinical practice.

Data management

The aim of record keeping and the handling of data is to gather information from the trial without error in a form that can later be analysed and reported. A Case Report Form (CRF) for each patient in the trial must be completed and signed by the investigator and the patient's files, CRFs and other sources of primary data must be kept for future reference. Patient data must be handled in a way that maintains confidentiality and yet ensures accuracy. All efforts should be made to maintain error-free records. When subjects are randomized to different groups, the randomization procedure used must be documented. In the case of a blinded trial, a code for the medicine actually administered must be kept under appropriate conditions.

Statistical Analysis

Bio statistical expertise is required when the trial is designed, and must continue to be available as data are collected, analysed and prepared for the final report on the trial. Statistical considerations will govern the number of patients needed to obtain a significant result from the trial, the number of patients needed depending on the anticipated difference in the result between the treatment groups of the trial. The plan for the statistical analyses to be used at the conclusion of the trial must be determined in advance and specified within the protocol. When results are finally analysed, they should be presented in a form that facilitates clinical interpretation.

Reporting

The Chief Investigator will be responsible for preparing a final report of the trial which should be provided to the sponsor, the ethics review board, and any other authorities determined by local legislation. The results of the trials conducted on a herbal medicine should be published in a timely fashion and must include all significant positive and negative results even studies which fail to demonstrate efficacy should be published, as selective publication, showing only results that are favourable, will only lead to s form of misconception known as publication bias.

Evaluation of herbal medicine research, technology transfer and education, herbal medical research, health care professions and public related aspects are also need to be considered while undergoing clinical trials of herbal medicines.

Using the Guidelines

These research guidelines for evaluating the safety and efficacy of herbal medicines are intended to facilitate the work of research scientists and clinicians in this field and to furnish some reference points for the governmental, industrial and non-profit organizations that provide financial support for their work.

A. Guidelines for quality specifications of plant materials and preparations

To ensure the reliability and repeatability of research on herbal medicines, the identity and quality (Information of plant materials, quality specifications like authenticity, purity, assay, packaging, labelling and storage, formula and composition of preparations) of the plant material and preparation (powders, granules, pills, extracts, tablets and injections), must be determined

B. Guidelines for pharmacodynamic and general pharmacological studies of herbal medicines

Herbal medicines have various pharmacological effects. The appropriate methods (animal species, disease model, route of administration, frequency of administration and control group) for evaluating the particular herbal medicine tested should be applied.

C. Guidelines for toxicity investigation of herbal medicines

These guidelines are intended to indicate the standard methods of non-clinical toxicological studies related to assessing the safety of herbal medicines Not a)l tests are necessarily required for each herbal medicine intended for human study.

Acute toxicity test, Long-term toxicity test

Commonly used ranges of administration periods	
Expected period of Clinical use	**Administration period for the toxicity study**
Single administration or repeated administration for less than one week	2 weeks to 1 month
Repeated administration, between one week to four weeks	4 weeks to 3 months
Repeated administration, between one to six months	3 to 6 months
Long term repeated administration for more than six months	9 to 12 months

Local toxicity test

Skin sensitization Test methods (in alphabetical order)

1. Adjuvant and patch test
2. Buehler test
3. Draize test
4. Freund's complete adjuvant test
5. Maximization test
6. Open epicutaneous test
7. Optimization test
8. Split adjuvant test

Other local toxicity tests: Other local toxicity tests may be conducted if the herbal medicine is intended for such use i.e. vaginal, rectal, respiratory, etc. irritations tests.

Special toxicity tests

Mutagenicity rest

I. Reverse mutation test in bacteria

II. Chromosomal aberration test with mammalian cells in culture

III. Micronucleus test with rodents

Carcinogenicity test

Reproductive and development toxicity test

Segment 1. Study on administration of the test substance prior to and in the early

Segment II. Study on administration of the test substance during the period of organogenesis.

Segment III. Study on administration of the test substance during the perinatal and lactation periods

Further Reading

1. WHO 1991. Guidelines for the Assessment of Herbal Medicines. World Health Organization,
2. WHO 1995. Guidelines for Good Clinical Practice (GCP) for Trials on Pharmaceutical Products. World Health Organization, WHO Technical Series, No. 850, 1995, Annex 3. WHO 1999. WHO Expert Committee on Specifications for Pharmaceutical Preparations - WHO Technical Report Series, No. 885 – 35th Report.
3. World Health Organization WHO 2009. Joint FAO/WHO Expert Committee on Food Additives: Evaluation of Certain Food Additives - WHO Technical Report Series, No. 952 - 69th Report. World Health Organization,
4. World Health Organization Research Office for the Western Pacific 1993. Research Guidelines for Evaluating the Safety and Efficacy of Herbal Medicines.
5. S. Thillaivanan, K. Samraj. Challenges, constraints and opportunities in herbal medicines – a review Int J Herb Med, 2 (2014), pp. 21-24
6. S.C. Mandal, M. Mandal. Quality, safety, and efficacy of herbal products through regulatory harmonization. Drug Info J, 45 (2011), pp. 45-53
7. S.K. Sharma, D.C. Katoch. Current Status & Infrastructure of Ayurveda (2006) Accessed from: http://herbalnet.healthrepository.org/bitstream/ 123456789/2075/6/3.%20Ayur53-65.pdf

Scan QR code to view the website/guidelines

- WHO safety and efficacy of herbal medicines guidelines-
Research guidelines for evaluating the safety and efficacy of herbal medicines (who.int)

CHAPTER 21

General Guidelines for Safety/Toxicity Evaluation of Ayurvedic Formulations 2018

Introduction

In spite of availability of several guidelines such as GCP guidelines for ASU drugs, ICMR guidelines for bio medical research for human participants, OECD guidelines, Schedule Y of Drug and Cosmetic Act, GCP guidelines for ASU Medicines, WHO guidelines for traditional medical research etc., there is need to evolve a comprehensive guideline to address system specific issues for conducting safety/toxicity studies of ASU drugs. The present document would certainly serve as a ready reference for researchers engaged in Research and Drug development in ASU systems.

Before conducting any toxicological testing in animals, the study should be approved by the Institute Animal Ethics Committee (IAEC) or the protocol should satisfy the guidelines of the local governing body. In India, the Committee for the Purpose of Control and Supervision of Experiments on Animals (CPCSEA) guidelines should be followed for the maintenance of experimental animals.

Safety/ toxicity studies of Ayurvedic drugs need fundamentally different approach and may only be conducted adopting similar Ayurvedic procedure like Anupana (Vehicle), Dose, Dosage, Age etc. which may play pivotal role in their therapeutic potential or processing such as Shodhna, Marana.

General Research Guidelines and Methodologies for Drug Development at a Glance

Table 21.1 Research criteria for evaluating the safety/ toxicity of ASU drugs.

S. No	Category	Ingredient(s)	Indication(s)	Requirement of Nonclinical Safety data	Requirement of Nonclinical Efficacy Data
(1)	(2)	(3)	(4)	(5)	(6)
Classical ASU	**Drugs as**	**Defined under**	**Section 3(a) of the**	**Drugs and**	**Cosmetics Act, 1940**
1.	1.1 Ayurvedic, Siddha and Unani drugs given in 158B as referred in Section 3(a) of Drugs and Cosmetics Act, 1940	As per text	As per text	Not Required	Not Required
	1.2 Any change in dosage form of ASU Drugs as described in Section 3(a) of Drugs and Cosmetics Act, 1940	As per text	As per text	Not Required	Not Required

Contd...

S. No	Category	Ingredient(s)	Indication(s)	Requirement of Nonclinical Safety data	Requirement of Nonclinical Efficacy Data
(1)	(2)	(3)	(4)	(5)	(6)
Classical ASU	**Drugs as**	**Defined under**	**Section 3(a) of the**	**Drugs and**	**Cosmetics Act, 1940**
	1.3 ASU Drugs referred in section 3(a) of Drugs and Cosmetics Act, 1940 to be used for new indication*	As per text	New	Not Required	Required
Patent or	**Proprietary Drugs**	**As defined under**	**Section 3(h) of the**	**Drugs and Cosmetics**	**Act, 1940**
2.	2.1 Patent or Proprietary Drugs as defined under section 3(h) of Drugs and Cosmetics Act, 1940 containing crude drugs /Aqueous Extract(s) / Hydro-Alcoholic Extracts).	As per text	Textual rationale	Not required	Not required
	2.2 Patent or Proprietary Drugs as defined under section 3(h) containing other than Aqueous and Hydro-alcoholic extract(s) / any other solvent based extract(s)*	As specified	As specified / claimed	Required: For Oral preparations*- 1. Single dose toxicity test (Acute toxicity) in mice and rats. 2. Repeated-dose Systemic Toxicity Studies (long term toxicity studies in rats. 3. Reproductive and Developmental Toxicity Studies 4. Genotoxicity 5. Carcinogenicity *metal associated toxicity in case of any metal/mineral as one of the	Required

Contd...

S. No	Category	Ingredient(s)	Indication(s)	Requirement of Nonclinical Safety data	Requirement of Nonclinical Efficacy Data
(1)	(2)	(3)	(4)	(5)	(6)
Classical ASU	Drugs as	Defined under	Section 3(a) of the	Drugs and	Cosmetics Act, 1940
				ingredients for topical preparations) Dermal toxicity study. b) Photo-allergy or dermal photo-toxicity. c) Allergenicity / Hypersensitivity in guinea pigs	
	2.4 Patent or Proprietary Drugs as defined under section 3(h) containing any of the ingredients of Schedule E (1) of the D&C Act, 194	As per text	Indication as claimed / specified	For oral preparations1. Single dose toxicity test (Acute toxicity) in mice and rats. 2. Repeated-dose Systemic Toxicity Studies (long term toxicity studies) in two species one rodent(rat) and one nonrodent Rabbit/dog. 3.Reproductive and Developmental Toxicity Studies 4. Genotoxicity 5. Carcinog-enicity *metal associated toxicity in case of any metal/mineral as one of the ingredients For Topical preparations) Dermal toxicity study. b) Photo-allergy or dermal photo-toxicity. c) Allergenicity / Hypersensitivity in guinea pigs	Required

Single-Dose Acute Toxicity Study (Acute Toxicity): Acute toxicity studies aim to determine toxic manifestations of the test substance that occur when animals are exposed to one or more doses within a 24-hour period.

Animal species: These studies should be carried out in two rodent species, mice and rats Sex: Both, males and females (nulliparous and non-pregnant) should be used

Number of animals: Each group should consist of at least six animals per sex.

Dose levels and route of administration: The limit of 2gm/kg or at least 10 times of the intended clinical therapeutic dose whichever is less, using the same route as recommended for human.

Frequency of administration: The test substance should be administered in one or more doses during a 24-hour period.

Study observations: Toxic signs and the severity, onset, progression and reversibility of the signs and mortality, if any, for 14 days after administration of test compound. Additional observations will be necessary if the animals continue to display signs of toxicity. Observations should include changes in skin and fur, eyes and mucous membranes, and also respiratory, circulatory, autonomic and central nervous systems, and somatoform activity and behaviour pattern. Attention should be directed to observations of tremors, convulsions, salivation, diarrhoea, lethargy, sleep and coma. Animals found in a moribund condition and animals showing severe pain or enduring signs of severe distress should be humanely killed. When animals are killed for humane reasons or found dead, the time of death should be recorded as precisely as possible. Autopsy of any animal which dies during study period has to be done. If necessary, a histopathological examination should be conducted on any organ/tissue showing macroscopic changes at autopsy.

Result: Body weight/body weight changes; Tabulation of response data and dose level for each animal (i.e., animals showing signs of toxicity including nature, severity, duration of effects, and mortality); Individual weights of animals at the day of dosing, in weekly intervals thereafter, and at the time of death or sacrifice; Time course of onset of signs of toxicity and whether these were reversible for each animal; Necropsy findings and any histopathological findings for each animal, if available; Maximum tolerated dose may be calculated. Statistical treatment of results (description of computer routine used and spreadsheet tabulation of calculations).

Repeated-Dose Oral Toxicity Study

Animal species: These studies should be carried out in two mammalian species of which one should be a non-rodent.

Sex: Males and females should be used.

Number of animals: In case of rodents, each group should consist of atleast ten males and ten females. In case of non-rodents, each group should consist of at least three males and three females.

Route of administration: It should be same as recommended for human.

Dose levels: The study is required to be done with three dose levels. High dose level should produce observable toxicity (to be selected on the basis of Maximum Tolerated dose calculated in Single-Dose Acute Toxicity Study)while low dose levels should not cause observable toxicity. Within this dose levels the addition of at least one more dose may enhance the possibility of observing a dose response relationship. In addition, vehicle control group should be included.

Period of exposure: The duration of exposure to study drug should be as per the intended therapeutic duration.

S. No.	Duration of proposed human administration	Period of exposure in toxicity study
1	Single dose	2 weeks
2	More than 2 weeks-less than 4 weeks	4 weeks
3	More than 4 weeks-less than 12 weeks	12 weeks
4	More than 12 weeks-less than 24 weeks	24 weeks
5	More than 24 weeks	Same as that of expected period of use of the trial drug

Recovery phase: In order to investigate the recovery phase from toxic changes, 50% of animals in each group are allowed to live for, atleast for 15 days or varying length of time after cessation period of administration of the test substance, should be examined.

Observations: General signs, Body weight, Food intake, Clinical Chemistry

Clinical Chemistry		
1	Urine qualitative	Appearance, Colour, Glucose, Bilirubin, Ketone, Specific Gravity, Blood, pH, Protein, Urobilinogen, Nitrites &Leucocytes
2	General parameters	Plasma Glucose, Serum Albumin/Globulin, Total Proteins
3	Liver function tests	Serum-Alkaline Phosphatase, Bilirubin, SGOT, SGPT, AST
4	Renal function tests	Blood Urea, Serum Creatinine
5	Lipid profile	Serum-Cholesterol, HDL, Triglyceride
6	Electrolytes	Serum-Na+, K+, Ca^.

Haematological examination: Blood samples should be taken from all groups of animals within 48 hours of last exposure to test material and before autopsy to monitor haemoglobin, complete blood picture, differential count etc. In addition, the below mentioned parameters must be estimated in post exposure (recovery) group of animals before termination of the experiment.

Clinical Haematology				
Haemoglobin (Hb/HGB)	**Total Red Blood Cell (RBC) count**	**Haematocrit (HCT)**	**Reticulocyte count**	**Total White Blood Cell (WBC) count**
Differential White Blood Cell (WBC) COUNT	Platelet Count (PLT)	Terminal bone marrow examination	ESR (Non-Rodents only)	General Blood picture: A special mention of abnormal and immature cells should be made

Other Function tests: If appropriate, ECG, visual, and auditory tests should be performed. For rodents, ophthalmological examination should be performed on a fixed number of animals from each group at least once during the administration period; for non-rodents, examination should be performed on all animals before the start of drug administration and at least once during the period of administration.

Necropsy and histopathological examination: A macroscopic examination of organs and tissues in all group animals within 48 hours of last exposure to test material should be performed. The organ weights must be measured wherever possible. The full histopathological examinations should be performed in an attempt to identify the severity or degree of the changes in all major and targeted organs. Similarly, in all post exposed group of animal's gross necropsy and histopathological examination should be conducted. Animals found dead during the examination should be autopsied as soon as possible in an attempt to identify the cause of death and the nature (severity or degree) of the toxic changes present.

Necropsy & histopathological examination			
Brain*: Cerebrum Cerebellum, and Midbrain	**(Spinal Cord)**	**Eye**	**(Middle Ear)**
Thyroid	(Parathyroid)	Spleen*	Thymus
Adrenal*	(Pancreas)	(Trachea)	Lung*
Heart*	Aorta	Oesophagus	Stomach
Duodenum	Jejunum	Terminal ileum	Colon
(Rectum)	Liver*	Kidney*	Urinary bladder
Epididymis	Testis* Uterus*	Ovary	Uterus*
Skin	Mammary gland	Mesenteric lymph node	Skeletal muscle

* Organs marked with an asterisk should be weighed. () Organs listed in parenthesis should be examined if indicated by the nature of the drug or observed effects.

Estimation of Metals: Heavy metal estimation will be carried out in blood and tissue homogenate in case the ASU drug contains any metal/mineral as one of the ingredients.

Reproduction and Developmental Toxicity Studies

Segment I.(Female Fertility Study):

Segment II(Teratogenicity Study):

Segment III.(Perinatal study):

Special Toxicity Tests

Test substance (described in ASU in 158-B as referred in Section 3(a), 3(h), and any of the ingredients of Schedule E (1) of Drugs and Cosmetics Rules, 1945 intended to be administered for chronic illnesses or otherwise over a long period of time (six months to one year) may be necessary to detect genotoxicity (early tumorigenic) effects and induce carcinogenicity.

Genotoxicity: Genotoxicity tests are conducted in-vitro and in-vivo to detect compounds which induce genetic damage directly or indirectly. These tests should enable hazard identification with respect to damage to DNA and its fixation. Genotoxicity data are not required before Phase I and II trials. But these studies should be completed before applying for Phase III trials. The following are the in-vitro and in vivo studies generally expected to be conducted:

(i) A test for gene mutation in bacteria.

(ii) An in-vitro test with cytogenetic evaluation of chromosomal damage with mammalian cells or an in vitro mouse lymphoma assay.

(iii) An in- vivo test for chromosomal damage using rodent hematopoietic cells.

Carcinogenicity Test: Carcinogenicity studies should be done in a rodent species (preferably rat). Mouse may be employed only with proper scientific justification. The selected strain of animals should not have a very high or very low incidence of spontaneous tumours. This test includes Preliminary and full-scale carcinogenicity study.

Local Toxicity Test for Topical preparations: Local Toxicity Investigations of the test substance are required for the following:

1. ASU drugs as referred to in the section 3(h) of the D&C Act containing crude drugs or Aqueous / Hydro-alcoholic extracts without textual rationale or not as per text;
2. ASU drugs containing other solvent based extracts;
3. ASU drugs containing ingredients of Schedule- E (1) of the D&C Rules, 1945. Application(s) of the test substance to an appropriate site (e.g., skin or vaginal mucous membrane) as topical/dermatological preparations are required for local toxicity investigations.

Dermal toxicity study:

Photo-allergy or dermal photo-toxicity:

Vaginal Toxicity Test:

Rectal Tolerance Test:

Other local toxicity tests:

Allergenicity/ Hypersensitivity:

Annexures

There are following annexure discussed in this guideline:

Guidelines for issue of license with respect to Ayurveda, Siddha or Unani drugs

Guidelines on the regulation of scientific experiments on animals

CPCSEA Guidelines for Laboratory Animal Facility-2005

Expert involved in development of Guidelines and consultative process

Further Reading

1. Drugs and Cosmetics Act, 1940 & Drugs & Cosmetics Rules 1945.
2. WHO guidelines for traditional system of medicine, 2000/ revised 2014.
3. WHO Research Guidelines for Evaluating the Safety and Efficacy of Herbal Medicines, 1993.
4. Handbook Non-Clinical Safety Testing - UNICEF/UNDP/World Bank/WHO Special Program for Research and Training in Tropical Diseases (TDR).
5. Operational guidance: Information needed to support clinical trials of herbal products UNICEF/UNDP/World Bank/WHO Special Program for Research and Training in Tropical Diseases (TDR).
6. US Food and Drug Administration's Guidance for Industry Botanical Drug Products Published on June 2004.
7. European Medicines Agency's CPMP (CPMP/SWP/1042/99 Rev 1) guideline on "Guideline on Repeated dose toxicity, adopted on 01st September 2010.
8. OECD Guideline for the Testing of Chemicals No. 407. Repeated Dose 28-day Oral Toxicity Study in Rodents, adopted on 3rd October, 2008.
9. OECD Guideline for the Testing of Chemicals No. 408. Repeated Dose 90-day Oral Toxicity Study in Rodents, adopted on 21st September, 1998.
10. OECD Guideline for the Testing of Chemicals No. 425. Acute Oral Toxicity - Up-and Down Procedure (UDP), adopted on 3rd October, 2008.
11. OECD Guideline for the Testing of Chemicals No. 420. Acute Oral Toxicity - Fixed Dose Procedure, adopted on 17th December, 2001.
12. OECD Guideline for the Testing of Chemicals No. 423. Acute Oral Toxicity - Acute Toxic Class Method, adopted on 17th December, 2001.
13. OECD Guideline for the Testing of Chemicals No. 414. Prenatal Development Toxicity Study, adopted on 22nd January, 2001.
14. OECD Guideline for the Testing of Chemicals No. 415. One-Generation Reproduction Toxicity Study, adopted on 26th May, 1983.
15. OECD Guideline for the Testing of Chemicals No. 416. Two-Generation Reproduction Toxicity, adopted on 22nd January, 2001.

Scan QR code to view the website/guidelines

- AYUSH Guidelines Safety and efficacy of Ayurvedic medicines-
CCRS_Guidline of Toxicity_Book-5_945-CD MATTER.pdf (ccras.nic.in)

Section 6

Pharmacovigilance and Clinical Trial Regulations for Herbal Products

CHAPTER 22

WHO Guidelines on Safety Monitoring of Herbal Medicines in Pharmacovigilance Systems 2004

Introduction

Safety is a fundamental principle in the provision of herbal medicines and herbal products for health care, and a critical component of quality control. These guidelines provide practical technical guidance for monitoring the safety of herbal medicines within pharmacovigilance systems. The safety monitoring of herbal medicines is compared and contrasted with that of other medicines currently undertaken in the context of the WHO International Drug Monitoring Programme. While there are regulatory and cultural differences in the preparation and use of different types of medicines, they are all equally important from a pharmacovigilance perspective.

The inclusion of herbal medicines in pharmacovigilance systems is becoming increasingly important given the growing use of herbal products and herbal medicines globally.

Herbal medicines are frequently used in conjunction with other medicines, and it is essential to understand the consequences of such combined use and monitor whether any adverse effects are arising. This can be achieved most readily within existing pharmacovigilance systems.

Among consumers, there is a widespread misconception that "natural" always means "safe", and a common belief that remedies from natural origin are harmless and carry no risk. However, some medicinal plants are inherently toxic.

Major causes of such events are adulteration of herbal products with undeclared other medicines and potent pharmaceutical substances, such as corticosteroids and non-steroidal antiinflammatory agents.

Adverse events may also arise from the mistaken use of the wrong species of medicinal plants, incorrect dosing, errors in the use of herbal medicines both by health-care providers and consumers, interactions with other medicines, and use of products contaminated with potentially hazardous substances, such as toxic metals, pathogenic microorganisms and agrochemical residues.

National pharmacovigilance systems should be closely linked to national drug regulatory systems. To function properly, a national safety monitoring programme for herbal medicines should be operated alongside an effective national drug regulatory system with the will and the potential to react to signals emanating from reports of adverse effects of herbal medicines and to take proper regulatory measures.

Objectives

The objectives of these guidelines are to:

- support Member States, in the context of the WHO International Drug Monitoring Programme, to strengthen national pharmacovigilance capacity in order to carry out effective safety monitoring of herbal medicines

- provide technical guidance on the principles of good pharmacovigilance and the inclusion of herbal medicines in existing national drug safety monitoring systems; and where these systems are not in place, to facilitate the establishment of an inclusive national drug safety monitoring system
- provide standard definitions of terms relating to pharmacovigilance, and safety monitoring of herbal medicines
- promote and strengthen internationally coordinated information exchange on pharmacovigilance, and safety monitoring of herbal medicines among Member States
- promote the safe and proper use of herbal medicines.

The regulation of herbal medicines and their place in national health-care systems differs from country to country, and these guidelines will therefore need to be adapted to meet the needs of the local situation.

Highlight

UMC suggests that the WHO-DD, the HATC classification and the checklist should prove useful tools for national pharmacovigilance centres to increase the clarity and accuracy of reports.

Challenges in Monitoring the Safety of Herbal Medicines

Regulation: National regulation and registration of herbal medicines vary from country to country. Where herbal medicines are regulated, they may be categorized as either prescription or non-prescription medicines. Herbal products may also be categorized other than as medicines. If trade in a particular herbal product is made between countries where different regulatory status is given, reclassification of the regulatory status in the importing country depends not on the nature or characteristics (medical or therapeutic value) of the product itself, but on the regulatory framework of the importing country. Further, herbal products categorized other than as medicines and foods are becoming increasingly popular, and there is potential for adverse reactions due to lack of regulation, weaker quality control systems and loose distribution channels (including mail order and Internet sales).

Quality assurance and control: Requirements and methods for quality control of finished herbal products, particularly for mixture herbal products, are far more complex than for other pharmaceuticals. The quality of such products is influenced by the quality of the raw material used. Good agricultural and good collection practices (GACP) for medicinal plants, including plant selection and cultivation, are therefore important measures. As with other medicines for human use, herbal medicines should be covered by a drug regulatory framework to ensure that they conform to required standards of safety, quality and efficacy.

Appropriate use: Due to lack of proper knowledge of herbal medicines, the education of health-care professionals, providers of herbal medicines and patients/consumers is vital for the prevention of potentially serious risks from misuse of herbal medicines.

Safety Monitoring of Herbal Medicines

Sources of reports	***Reports from health-care professionals*** ***Reports from consumers*** Reports from ***Manufacturers*** ***Reports from other sources*** ♦ **National poisons centres.** ♦ **Drug information centres** ♦ **Consumer organizations** ♦ **Clinical trials and studies**
Herbal products targeted for safety monitoring	– herbal medicines in the prescription medicines category – herbal medicines in the non-prescription medicines category – other herbal products intended for use in health care ♦ according to their registration/marketing status – herbal medicines undergoing the new drug development process: in clinical trials prior to national drug regulatory approval – herbal medicines undergoing the new drug development process: under post-marketing safety surveillance – herbal medicines undergoing re-evaluation under the current protocol: in clinical trials – herbal medicines undergoing re-evaluation under the current protocol: under post-marketing safety surveillance – herbal medicines on the market: under post-marketing safety surveillance – other herbal products marketed for health care, such as dietary supplements.
Reporting of suspected adverse reactions	***Who should report and to whom?*** • *Health professionals who are providers of herbal medicines*, including physicians, pharmacists and nurses, should report to the national pharmacovigilance centre. • *Patients/consumers* should normally report to their physicians or providers of herbal medicines. They may also report directly to the national pharmacovigilance centre, consumer organizations or manufacturers. • *Manufacturers* should report directly to the national pharmacovigilance centre or national regulatory authority. ***What information should be requested?*** • identification of the patient/consumer in order to avoid duplications and facilitate follow-up • age, sex and a brief medical history of the consumer/patient (when relevant); ethnicity • species name (Latin binomial name and common vernacular name of medicinal plant) and/or brand or ingredient name(s), including the part of medicinal plant used, preparation methods; manufacturer, country of origin, batch number, expiry date and provider • administration details: dose and quantity supplied, dosage form, route, start/stop dates • indication or reason for use • adverse reaction data: date of onset (or duration from first

Contd...

	administration to onset of event), description with symptoms and signs, severity and seriousness, results of clinical investigations and tests, course and outcome, and dechallenge/rechallenge with the same product, where appropriate • all other medicines used (including self-medication), with administration details • risk factors, e.g. age, impaired renal function, previous exposure to the herbal medicine(s) concerned, previous allergies, drug misuse or abuse, the social use of drugs • name and address of reporter (to be considered confidential and to be used only for data verification, completion and case follow-up). ***How to report*** A single standard printed or electronic reporting form covering all medicines, including herbal medicines, should be used. If possible, a sample of the herbal product and its packaging should be submitted with the report.
Recording and coding the identity of herbal medicines	• Use of a standardized classification and identification for transmitting reports • compatible Coding of adverse events/adverse reactions to herbal medicines with that for other medicines. • use of the WHO Drug Dictionary (WHO-DD) containing classified information on the names of herbal products and their ingredients in the same way as similar information on other medicines. • Use of herbal anatomical-therapeutic-chemical (HATC) classification, which is structurally equivalent to the anatomical-therapeutic-chemical (ATC) classification used for chemical substances in other medicines. • Use a system checklist for cross referencing of botanical and vernacular names used as names of ingredients. • Assistance in identification of multiple ingredients based on herbal product name • Local input by the reporter will help in correct documentation • establishment of a national inventory or catalogue should be encouraged. • Information from drug regulatory authority of the exporting country for imported herbs and or derived products will provide helpful information. • The precise Latin binomial botanical name together with a common vernacular name should be preferred. • National pharmacovigilance centres should collaborate with the pharmacognosy departments of universities and with botanists, zoologists and botanical garden staff regarding taxonomic (botanical and chemical) identification and botanical and vernacular nomenclature. • classification systems must cover additional products used in traditional medicine.
Other reporting issues	• The identity of both the patient and the reporter should remain confidential • Reporting on herbal medicines should be as accurate and complete as possible.

Assessment of Case Reports

Individual case reports

Assessment of reports on adverse reactions to herbal medicines should be undertaken by national pharmacovigilance centres in the same way as for other medicines. Each data element in the report should be considered and a causality assessment made using a standard approach. The assessment is usually based on:

- the association in time between administration of the herbal product and the event
- the outcome of dechallenge and rechallenge
- known pharmacology (including current knowledge of the nature and frequency of adverse reactions)
- medical or pharmacological plausibility (the sequence of symptoms, signs and laboratory tests and also pathological findings and knowledge of mechanisms)
- likelihood of other causes or their exclusion
- testing for adulterants or contaminants that could be the source of adverse events.
- inappropriate use.

The WHO causality categories are listed in Table 22.1.

Table 22.1 Causality categories.

The causality categories described by the Uppsala Monitoring Centre		
1	***Certain:***	a clinical event, including laboratory test abnormality, occurring in a plausible time relationship to drug administration, and which cannot be explained by concurrent disease or other drugs or chemicals. The response to withdrawal of the drugs (dechallenge) should be clinically plausible. The event must be definitive pharmacologically or phenomenologically, using a satisfactory rechallenge procedure if necessary.
2	***Probably/ Likely:***	a clinical event, including laboratory test abnormality, with a reasonable time sequence to administration of the drug, unlikely to be attributed to concurrent disease or other drugs or chemicals, and which follows a clinically reasonable response on withdrawal (dechallenge). Rechallenge information is not required to fulfil this definition.
3	***Possible:***	a clinical event, including laboratory test abnormality, with a reasonable time sequence to administrations of the drug, but which could also be explained by concurrent disease or other drugs or chemicals. Information on drug withdrawal may be lacking or unclear.
4	***Unlikely:***	a clinical event, including laboratory test abnormality, with a temporal relationship to drug administration which makes a causal relationship improbable, and in which other drugs, chemicals or underlying disease provide plausible explanations.

Contd...

5	***Conditional/ Unclassified:***	a clinical event, including laboratory test abnormality, reported as an adverse reaction, about which more data is essential for a proper assessment, or the additional data is under examination.
6	***Unassessable/ Unclassifiable:***	a report suggesting an adverse reaction which cannot be judged because information is insufficient or contradictory, and which cannot be supplemented or verified.
As a step towards harmonization in drug regulation in the countries of the European Union (EU), three causality categories were proposed by the EU pharmacovigilance working parties		
Category A:	"Reports including good reasons and sufficient documentation to assume a causal relationship, in the sense of plausible, conceivable, likely, but not necessarily highly probable".	
Category B:	"Reports containing sufficient information to accept the possibility of a causal relationship, in the sense of not impossible and not unlikely, although the connection is uncertain and may be even doubtful, e.g. because of missing data, insufficient evidence or the possibility of another explanation".	
Category C:	"Reports where causality is, for one or another reason, not assessable, e.g. because of missing or conflicting data".	

Feedback to reporters

The receipt of each report should be acknowledged and a new reporting form supplied to the reporter. The reporter will also appreciate receiving further information about the reaction concerned, for example, on experience held at the national pharmacolovigilance centre or that may be helpful in further use of the medicines, unless the provision of such information is in conflict with regulatory policy. Such feedback will motivate the reporter to send in further reports.

Detection of signals at national level

The national pharmacovigilance centre should, at regular intervals, analyse the case reports in its database by class of organ system and in smaller groups of clinically related events. This may reveal case series of similar events that could constitute a signal and/or indicate the need for further study or regulatory action. Such signals should be communicated to UMC. Weak signals may be strengthened by examination of reports from other countries held in the global WHO database.

Detection of signals at international level

The major aim of pharmacovigilance is the early detection of signals of previously unrecognized adverse reactions. Early signals may be strengthened by combining the experiences reported in various countries. Regional studies may be of particular value in the monitoring of herbal medicines. Data-mining techniques can be helpful in individual countries, but are most effective in the global WHO database managed by UMC.

Use of an advisory committee

Each national pharmacovigilance centre should have an advisory committee composed of experts to give advice on:

- maintaining quality standards in data collection and assessment procedures
- data interpretation
- publication of information
- follow-up action required.

The committee should be selected according to the expertise available but it should not be too large, so that it may not be possible to have all of the relevant disciplines represented. A committee might be selected from the following disciplines: general medicine, pharmacy, pharmaceutics, clinical pharmacology, clinical toxicology, pharmacogenetics, epidemiology, pharmacoepidemiology, pathology, drug regulation and quality assurance, drug information, information science, medical anthropology, communications, ethnopharmacology, pharmacognosy, phytochemistry, traditional medicine and/or complementary/alternative medicine.

Investigation and analysis of the cause of suspected adverse reactions

Some adverse reactions, particularly serious ones should be further investigated scientifically. The investigations may include the following:

- medical investigation of the adverse reactions: pathology, clinical pharmacology, clinical toxicology, pharmacogenetic studies
- pharmaceutical investigation of the adverse reactions: pharmacokinetics, pharmacodynamics and pharmaceutical, pharmacological and toxicological analysis
- pharmacognosical/phytochemical investigation (including authentification) of the herbal medicines
- physicochemical analysis to identify the constituents of the herbal medicines
- pharmacoepidemiology.

Technical expertise and basic equipment

Where possible, national pharmacovigilance centres should have the necessary technical expertise to handle herbal medicines. This might include:

- access to reliable information support on herbal medicines
- trained personnel in relevant technical areas (e.g. pharmacognosy, phytochemistry, ethnobotany, ethnopharmacology) and in the use and provision of herbal medicines
- access to facilities for analysis of potentially causative products about which there is often insufficient information.

Not all countries have access to suitable analytical laboratories. The establishment of regional laboratories specializing in the analysis of herbal products should be considered.

Data management

- Data quality. Strenuous efforts should be made to ensure that there are quality controls on data processing and that the data elements of reports are as complete and accurate as possible. Mechanisms to check for duplications should be instituted.

- Data storage. Computer databases should be managed to as high a standard as possible to facilitate access to and use of the data. Software should be selected with expert advice so that analytical needs can be met.
- Data analysis. Programmes should be developed to provide for regular analyses and data output appropriate for local needs.
- Analysis of the global WHO database. The global WHO database managed by UMC is being improved on the basis of the proposed "Database management and classification for coding of herbal medicines", of which the previously mentioned HATC is one part (Annex 6). Data-mining techniques that have proved effective on the very large numbers of reports for other medicines will be used for signal detection on reports for herbal medicines. The success of these techniques depends on the volume and quality of data submitted by national pharmacovigilance centres.
- Support on technical and data management is available from the WHO Collaborating Centre for International Drug Monitoring, UMC (http://www.who-umc.org/). Communication

General

The successful safety monitoring of herbal medicines depends on good communication (Annex 2). There are many barriers to be broken down if all the players in this field are to be involved. There is distrust between some and ignorance of the work and function of different groups. Transparent communication is essential to overcome these problems and ensure that all players collaborate to meet the goal of the safe and effective use of herbal medicines.

National pharmacovigilance centres should ensure that manufacturers receive timely information so that they can take appropriate action regarding their products. Effective communication of the results of monitoring is also essential so that pharmacovigilance activities can have a positive impact on the health of the people.

If there is no national pharmacovigilance centre, consideration should be given to designating other relevant organizations, such as the national regulatory authority, poisons centres, drug information centres and consumer complaints authorities as the focal point. Communication should be established at many different levels, for example between:

- the national pharmacovigilance centre and health professionals
- the national pharmacovigilance centre and providers of herbal medicines
- health professionals and providers of herbal medicines, and consumers and patients
- providers of herbal medicines and those for other medicines
- the national pharmacovigilance centre and consumers
- the national pharmacovigilance centre and the regulatory authority
- the national pharmacovigilance centre and such centres in other countries, within the region or in other regions
- the national pharmacovigilance centre and UMC
- the national pharmacovigilance centre and the mass media.

The development of effective communication needs to be adequately resourced. It is likely that this most important part of the safety monitoring programme for herbal medicines will require proportionately greater resources than is the case for other medicines.

Risk communication

Communication strategies should be established to effectively reach all relevant target audiences, such as providers of herbal medicines, other health professionals, manufacturers and patients/consumers. Communication of safety information is a shared responsibility between national pharmacovigilance centres, national regulatory agencies, manufacturers and health professionals. Different risk communication vehicles can be considered, including:

- adverse reaction bulletins or articles distributed in reputable journals
- public advisories or warnings
- "Dear Health Professional" letters.

Various methods of information dissemination can be considered, such as:

- internet posting
- direct mass mailing to providers of herbal medicines and health professionals
- briefings to the mass media
- briefings to patient/consumer associations
- education sessions at health professional society meetings.

In order to reach consumers and the wide range of providers of herbal medicines successfully, messages should be tailored to suit the recipients, including translation into local languages where appropriate.

Further Reading

1. Safety monitoring of medicinal products: guidelines for setting up and running a pharmacovigilance centre. Uppsala, Uppsala Monitoring Centre, 2000 (reproduced in Part II of this publication).
2. US report calls for tighter controls on complementary medicine. British Medical Journal, 2002, 324:870.
3. Three out of four Germans have used complementary or natural remedies. British Medical Journal, 2002, 325:990.
4. General guidelines for methodologies on research and evaluation of traditional medicine. Geneva, World Health Organization, 2000 (WHO/EDM/TRM/2000.1).
5. The importance of pharmacovigilance: safety monitoring of medicinal products. Geneva, World Health Organization, 2002.
6. Bowdler J. Effective communications in pharmacovigilance: the Erice report. Birmingham, W Lake, 1997.
7. WHO guidelines on good agricultural and collection practices (GACP) for medicinal plants. Geneva, World Health Organization, 2003.

8. Current challenges in pharmacovigilance: pragmatic approaches. Report of CIOMS Working Group V. Geneva, The Council for International Organizations of Medical Sciences, 2001.
9. Guidelines for good clinical practice (GCP) for trials on pharmaceutical products. In: The use of essential drugs. Sixth report of the WHO Expert Committee. Geneva, World Health Organization, 1995, Annex 3 (WHO Technical Report Series, No. 850).
10. WHO Drug Dictionary. Uppsala, Uppsala Monitoring Centre (electronic database, updated quarterly; information available at http//www.umcproducts.com/).
11. Bowdler J. Effective communications in pharmacovigilance: the Erice report. Birmingham, W Lake, 1997.
12. Current challenges in pharmacovigilance: pragmatic approaches. Report of CIOMS Working Group V. Geneva, The Council for International Organizations of Medical Sciences, 2001.
13. Edwards IR, Hugman B. The challenge of effectively communicating risk-benefit information. Drug Safety, 1999, 17:216–227.
14. Effective communications in pharmacovigilance. Uppsala, Uppsala Monitoring Centre, 1998. (Report of the International Conference on Developing Effective Communications in Pharmacovigilance, Erice, Sicily, 24–27 September 1997).
15. Elvin-Lewis M. Should we be concerned about herbal remedies? Journal of Ethnopharmacology, 2001, 75:141–164.
16. The importance of pharmacovigilance: safety monitoring of medicinal products. Geneva, World Health Organization, 2002. Viewpoint, watching for safer medicines, Part 1: issues, controversies and science in the search for safer and more rational use of medicines. Uppsala, The Uppsala Monitoring Centre, 2002.
17. Legal status of traditional medicines and complementary/alternative medicines: a worldwide review. Geneva, World Health Organization, 2001 (WHO/EDM/TRM/2001.2).
18. Regulatory situation of herbal medicines: a worldwide review. Geneva, World Health Organization, 1998 (WHO/TRM/98.1).
19. WHO global survey on national policy on traditional medicine and complementary/alternative medicine and regulation of herbal medicines. Geneva, World Health Organization (in preparation).
20. General guidelines for methodologies on research and evaluation of traditional medicines. Geneva, World Health Organization, 2000 (WHO/EDM/TRM/2000.1).
21. Guidelines for assessment of herbal medicines. In: WHO Expert Committee on Specifications for Pharmaceutical Preparations. Thirty-fourth report. Geneva, World Health Organization, 1996, Annex 11 (WHO Technical Report Series, No. 863). (These guidelines are also included in: Quality assurance of Pharmaceuticals: a compendium of guidelines and related materials, Vol. 1. Geneva, World Health Organization, 1997.)
22. Good Manufacturing Practices for pharmaceutical products: main principles. In: WHO Expert Committee on Specifications for Pharmaceutical Preparations. Thirty seventh report. Geneva, World Health Organization, 2003, Annex 4 (WHO Technical Report Series, No. 908).
23. Good Manufacturing Practices: supplementary guidelines for manufacture of herbal medicinal products. In: WHO Expert Committee on Specification for Pharmaceutical Preparations. Thirty-fourth report. Geneva, World Health Organization, 1996, Annex 8 (WHO Technical Report Series, No. 863). (These supplementary guidelines are

also included in Quality assurance of pharmaceuticals: a compendium of guidelines and related materials, Vol. 2. Good manufacturing practices and inspection. Geneva, World Health Organization, 1999. They are currently being updated).

24. Good trade and distribution practices (GTDP) for pharmaceutical starting materials. In: WHO Expert Committee on Specifications for Pharmaceutical Preparations. Thirty-seventh report. Geneva, World Health Organization, 2003, Annex 2 (WHO Technical Report Series, No. 908).
25. Guide to good storage practices for pharmaceuticals. In: WHO Expert Committee on Specifications for Pharmaceutical Preparations. Thirty-seventh report. Geneva, World Health Organization, 2003, Annex 9 (WHO Technical Report Series, No. 908).
26. Quality control methods for medicinal plant materials. Geneva, World Health Organization, 1998.
27. WHO guidelines for assessing safety and quality of herbal medicines with reference to contaminants and residues. Geneva, World Health Organization (in preparation).
28. WHO guidelines on good agricultural and collection practices (GACP) for medicinal plants. Geneva, World Health Organization, 2003.
29. WHO guidelines for developing consumer information on proper use of traditional medicines and complementary/alternative medicine. Geneva, World Health Organization, 2004.
30. WHO monographs on selected medicinal plants, Vol. 1. Geneva, World Health Organization, 1999.
31. WHO monographs on selected medicinal plants, Vol. 2. Geneva, World Health Organization, 2002.
32. WHO monographs on selected medicinal plants, Vol. 3. Geneva, World Health Organization

Scan QR code to view the website/guidelines

- Pharmacovigilance of herbal medicines-

WHO guidelines on safety monitoring of herbal medicines in pharmacovigilance systems

CHAPTER 23

Fundamentals of Clinical Trials and Phases of Trials

Introduction

- Experiments conducted on animals are essential to the development of new chemicals for the management of disease.
- Animal studies provide a general profile of the pharmacological actions, toxicity and pharmacokinetics of a new drug.
- Even with all this authentic information at hand, the safety and efficacy of new drugs however can be established only by adequate and well controlled studies on human subjects.
- Since findings in animals do not always accurately predict the human response to drugs, subjects who participate in clinical trials are put at some degree of risk.
- There are examples when drugs having passed the preclinical criteria for safety have shown serious side effects in humans.
- This may be due to the lack of correlation between toxicity data in animals and adverse effects in humans.
- However clinical evaluation of the candidate drug is important and necessary, as the drug is indicated for human use & this evaluation is nothing but performance of clinical trials.
- Purpose of this human evaluation is to determine whether the new drug is effective for its proposed therapeutic application (indication) in humans and to characterize its toxicity.

What is a Clinical Trial?

Definition: Clinical trial is a type of research study evaluating new drugs, medical devices, biologics or other interventions on human subjects in strictly scientifically controlled manner to assess the safety and effectiveness of new treatments in people.

- Clinical trial, clinical research or clinical studies are synonyms of each other.
- Carefully conducted clinical trials are the fastest and safest way to find treatments that work in people and ways to improve health.

Objectives of Clinical Trials

Trials may be assigned

1. To assess the safety & efficacy of an experimental therapy
2. To assess whether the new intervention is better than standard therapy.
3. To compare whether investigated agent is more effective than or equally as effective as other treatments already in the market.

Types of Clinical Trials

There are mainly **four** kinds of clinical trials.

1. **Treatment trials:** test experimental treatments, new combinations of drugs, or new approaches to surgery or radiation therapy.
2. **Prevention trials:** look for better ways to prevent disease in people who have never had the disease or to prevent a disease from returning. These approaches may include medicines, vitamins, vaccines, minerals, or lifestyle changes.
3. **Screening trials:** test the best way to detect or diagnose certain diseases or health conditions.
4. **Quality of Life trials (or Supportive Care trials):** explore ways to improve comfort and the quality of life for individuals with a chronic illness.

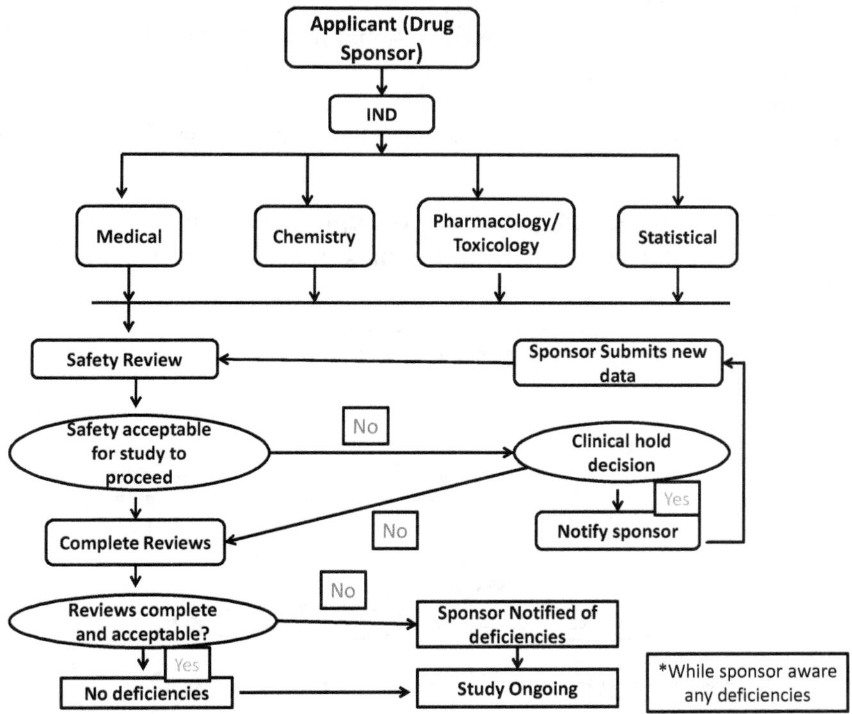

Figure 23.1 Investigational New Drug application (INDA) review process.

Performance of Clinical Trials

Before a pharmaceutical company can invite testing in humans, it must conduct extensive preclinical or laboratory research. This research typically involves years of experiments in animals, if this stage of testing is successful a pharmaceutical industry provides a data to the FDA, requesting approval to begin testing the drug in humans. This is called an Investigational

New Drug Development (IND). Once the approval of FDA [Figure 23.1] has been granted for performing clinical trials in humans, series of experiments started from phase 1 clinical testing.

Phases of Clinical Trials

Phase 0 (Zero)/Micro dosing : A Phase 0 clinical trial is a new idea from the US Food and Drug Administration and the Pharmaceutical Research and Manufacturers of America (PhRMA) that both organizations say they hope will streamline the process of drug development. With Phase 0 trials needing fewer preclinical studies than are usually required for a Phase I trial, researchers would give a few volunteers less than 1% of the therapeutic dose of an investigational drug, a microdose, thus necessitating manufacture of smaller batches. The trial would take no more than seven days, and the greatly reduced dose would ensure the absence of toxic effects. The official name of a Phase 0 trial is an exploratory investigational new drug (IND) study, and the goal is to quickly establish whether an agent will work as desired in humans. The theory is that such a trial should also quickly weed out ineffective drugs. These two factors are intended to give pharmaceutical companies faster answers about whether to move forward with regular clinical trials.

Phase 1 and 2 trials establish proof-of-concept, and phase 3 trials establish the efficacy and safety of the treatment in humans which is required for New Drug Application (NDA) approval.[Figure 23.2]

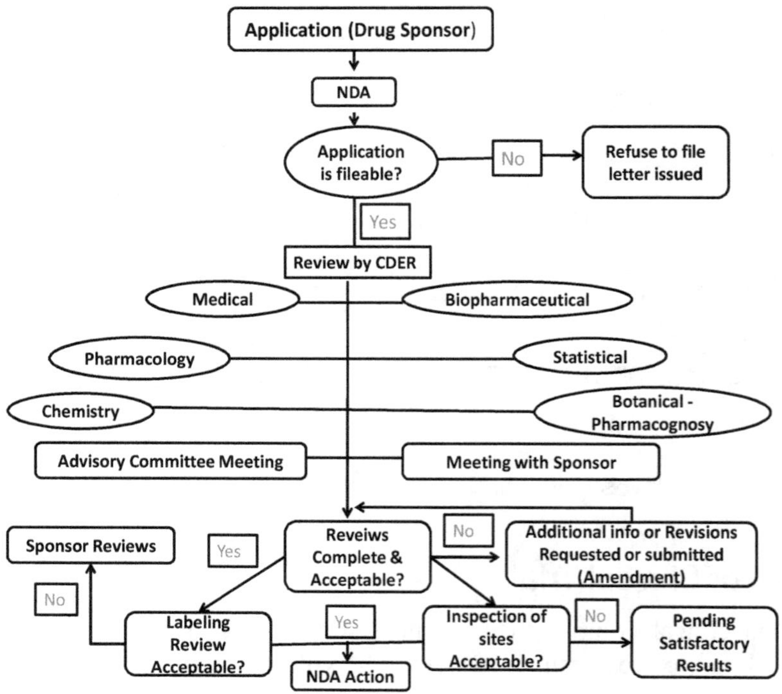

Figure 23.2 New Drug Application (NDA) Process.

Table 23.1 Different Phase Trials.

Phase	Primary goal	Dose	Patient monitor	Typical number of participants	Success rat	Notes
Preclinical	Testing of drug in non-human subjects to gather efficacy, toxicity and pharmacokinetic information	Unrestricted	Scientific researcher	No human subjects, in vitro and in vivo only		Includes testing in model organisms. Human immortalized cell lines and other human tissues may also be used.
Before beginning a phase I trial, the sponsor must submit an **Investigational New Drug application (INDA)** to the FDA detailing the preliminary data on the drug gathered from cellular models and animal studies.						
Phase I	Dose-ranging on healthy volunteers for safety	Often sub-therapeutic, but with ascending doses	Clinical researcher	20–100 normal healthy volunteers (or cancer patients for cancer drugs)	Approx. 70%	Determines whether drug is safe to check for efficacy.
Phase II	Testing of drug on participants to assess efficacy and side effects	Therapeutic dose	Clinical researcher	100–300 participants with a specific disease	Approx. 33%	Determines whether drug can have any efficacy; at this point, the drug is not presumed to have any therapeutic effect
Phase III	Testing of drug on participants to assess efficacy, effectiveness and safety	Therapeutic dose	Clinical researcher and personal physician	300–3,000 people with a specific disease	25–30%	Determines a drug's therapeutic effect; at this point, the drug is presumed to have some effect
Phase IV	Post marketing surveillance in public	Therapeutic dose	Personal physician	Anyone seeking treatment from a physician	N/A	Monitor long-term effects

Benefits and Risks of Participating in a Clinical Trial

Benefits: Clinical trials that are well-designed and well-executed are the best approach for eligible participants to:

- Play an active role in their own health care.
- Gain access to new research treatments before they are widely available.
- Obtain expert medical care at leading health care facilities during the trial.
- Help others by contributing to medical research.

Risks: There are risks to clinical trials.

- There may be unpleasant, serious or even life-threatening side effects to experimental treatment.
- The experimental treatment may not be effective for the participant.
- The protocol may require more of their time and attention than would a non-protocol treatment, including trips to the study site, more treatments, hospital stays or complex dosage requirements.

Ethics

What is scientifically desirable may not always be ethically acceptable. it is axiomatic that the comfort, health and safety of the participants take precedence over all other considerations, even if a promising clinical trial has to be abandoned or its design made less rigid, in order to secure them. Extreme diligence is needed to ensure that humanity does not leave the ward when science enters it. All the research involving human subjects should be conducted in accordance with applicable ethical principles.

Ethical Committee

As a consequence of unethical or questionably ethical practices committed in the past, most countries have established safeguards to protect the rights and welfare of persons who participate in clinical trials. The safeguard that has been established is the ethical committee also known as Institutional Review Board (IRB) or Human Subject's Protection Committee.

Protocol

Every well-designed clinical trial requires a protocol. The study protocol can be viewed as a written agreement between the investigator, the participant and the scientific committee. Clinical trial protocol is defined as a detailed documented plan that sets forth the objectives, study design, methodology, statistical considerations and organization of a clinical trial. A study protocol must be approved by an IRB before investigational drugs may be administered to humans.

Informed Consent

A document that describes the rights of the study participants, and includes details about the study, such as its purpose, duration, required procedures, and key contacts, risks and potential benefits is called as an informed consent. After reading it, you should be able to go over the information with the study doctors and ask questions about anything you do not understand. For example:

Volunteers

- Human volunteers who are involved in clinical trials called as participants, or research subjects or human subjects.
- All clinical trials have guidelines about who can participate. Using inclusion/exclusion criteria is an important principle of medical research that helps to produce reliable results.
- The factors that allow someone to participate in a clinical trial are called "inclusion criteria" and those that disallow someone from participating are called "exclusion criteria". These criteria are based on such factors as age, gender, the type and stage of a disease, previous treatment history, and other medical conditions. Before joining a clinical trial, a participant must qualify for the study.
- Some research studies seek participants with illnesses or conditions to be studied in the clinical trial, while others need healthy participants.
- It is important to note that inclusion and exclusion criteria are not used to reject people personally. Instead, the criteria are used to identify appropriate participants and keep them safe.

Investigator's Brochure

- The **Investigator's Brochure'** is a basic document which is required in a clinical trial, together with the clinical trial protocol.
- According to FDA regulations an Investigator's Brochure must contain a brief description of the drug substance and the formulation. At the moment when a new drug enters a Phase I clinical trial, preclinical information about the pharmacological and toxicological effects and the pharmacokinetics and biological disposition in animals must be available in the Investigator's Brochure.
- Once the drug candidate continues its way through Phase II and III clinical trials, information relating to safety and effectiveness in humans obtained from prior clinical studies must be included in the document. In addition possible risks and side effects to be anticipated on the basis of prior experience with the drug under investigation or with related drugs is to be included in the Investigator's Brochure.

Inclusion/Exclusion Criteria

- Establishing inclusion and exclusion criteria for study participants is a standard, required practice when designing high-quality research protocols. Inclusion criteria are defined as the key features of the target population that the investigators will use to answer their research question.
- Typical inclusion criteria include demographic, clinical, and geographic characteristics.
- In contrast, exclusion criteria are defined as features of the potential study participants who meet the inclusion criteria but present with additional characteristics that could interfere with the success of the study or increase their risk for an unfavorable outcome. Common exclusion criteria include characteristics of eligible individuals that make them highly likely to be lost to follow-up, miss scheduled appointments to collect data, provide inaccurate data, have comorbidities that could bias the results of the study, or increase their risk for adverse events (most relevant in studies testing interventions).
- It is very important that investigators not only define the appropriate inclusion and exclusion criteria when designing a study but also evaluate how those decisions will impact the external validity of the results of the study. Common errors regarding inclusion and exclusion criteria include the following: using the same variable to define both inclusion and exclusion criteria (for example, in a study including only men, listing being a female as an exclusion criterion); selecting variables as inclusion criteria that are not related to answering the research question; and not describing key variables in the inclusion criteria that are needed to make a statement about the external validity of the study results.
- Whether the benefits of enrolling in a study outweigh the potential risks is also a primary consideration for determining eligibility criteria.
- Older adults and patients with organ dysfunction or multiple chronic conditions may be excluded from clinical trials because of concerns about potential adverse impacts arising from co-morbidities and concomitant medications.
- Ethical considerations may lead to the exclusion of children, adolescents, and pregnant and lactating women in clinical trials. On the other hand, exclusion of such patients provides no information about a drug's benefits and risks in such patients, but they may use the drug if it is approved.
- Therefore, it is important to consider on a case by-case basis whether such exclusions are truly necessary.

Clinical Trial Design

There are a many ways to classify the many different types of experimental designs. In clinical trial, most commonly used designs are:

- **Parallel design** is one in which each patient receives only one of the treatments either test or control drug.

- **A change over/crossover design** is one in which each patient receives two or more of the treatments.

In any clinical trials, bias is one of the main concerns. Bias may be defined as systematic error or difference between the true value and that actually obtained due to all causes rather than sampling variability.

It can be occur at several places in a clinical trial from, the initial design through data analysis and interpretation. The general solution of the bias is to keep the participant and investigator blinded or masked to the identity of the assigned intervention.

Blinding

Definition: blinding (sometimes also called as masking) means using some procedures that prevents people involved in a clinical trials (patients, and/or investigators) from knowing which treatment each patient receives in a parallel study or the order of the treatments(in a changeover study).

Purpose of Blinding:

- The purpose of the blinding is to prevent bias, conscious or unconscious, from influencing the results or the interpretation of the results of a trial. The term bias is a very common on the part of both parties.
- In the case of investigators or their delegates, it can occur even in the reading and/or recording of readings of instruments and other so-called "objectives" devices.
- With patients, a knowledge of which drug has been taken often affects the disease condition, either objectively or in a patients opinion.

Types of trials based on blinding

According to blinding procedures, trials may be of two types

A. Open trials or unblinding trials

B. Blinding/Masked trials

1. Single blinding
2. Double blinding

A. Unblinding trials/open trials

- In an unblinding or open trial, both the participants and investigator know to which intervention the participants have been assigned.
- Some kinds of trials can only be conducted in this manner. Such studies include those involving most surgical procedures, comparisons of devices and medical treatments and changes in lifestyle (i.e. eating habits, exercise & cigarette smoking) or learning technique.

Advantages: An unblinding trial is appealing for two reasons:

1. All other things being equal, it is simpler to execute than other studies. The usual drug trial may be easier to design and carry out, and consequently less expensive, if blinding is not an issue.

2. Investigators are likely to be more comfortable making decision, such as whether or not to continue a participant on assigned medication, if they know the interventions identity.

Disadvantages:

1. Main drawback is the possibility of the bias. Participants reporting of symptoms and side effect and prescription of concomitant or compensatory treatment are all susceptible to bias.
2. Participants not on the new or experimental intervention may become dissatisfied and drop out of the trial in disproportionately large numbers. As more participants became aware of their medication's identity, the dropout rate increased. This was especially seen in the placebo group.

B. Blinding Masked trials

A clinical trial should ideally have a double-blind design to avoid potential problems of bias during data collection and assessment. In studies where such a design is impossible, a single blind approach and other measures to reduce potential bias are favored.

Methods of Blinding

In general blinding is accomplished simply by following these **two** methods.

1. Use of designations analogues to A, B, C & D that is specific letters or numbers invariably identified with each treatment.
   - With such a scheme if the code is broken for one of the patients, because of the occurrence of an adverse effect by accident, by guesswork, or for any other reason, that treatment is identified for all patients. If the trial has only two treatments, such an event destroys the blinding for the entire trial.
2. A satisfactory method widely used today, is the following: the doses are packaged with two-part labels of opaque paper. The visible part of each label is marked only with the patient number along with visit and dose numbers (if dose is to be repeated) and identification of the study and sponsor. The second part of the label cannot be seen until or unless it is torn off. This identifies the material, and is to be exposed only, if necessary, in an emergency. Furthermore, because there is no relationship between a patient, visit or dose number, and the nature of a treatment, any emergency exposure of the nature of a patient's treatment gives no information about those assigned to other patients. There is always check on the unauthorized opening of any label. Standard practice, which can be required by the FDA, is for the investigators to return both used and unused packages of drugs after the trial for continuing and examination.

1. Single Blind Trials

Definition: A study in which participant is unaware of what medication he/she is taking is called a single blind trial, also called single-masked study.

In this study, only the investigators are aware of which intervention each participant is receiving.

Advantages:

The advantages of this design are similar to those of an unblinded study:

(a) It is usually simpler to carry out than a double-blind design.

(b) Knowledge of the intervention may help the investigators exercise their best judgment when caring for the participants is main point. Indeed, certain investigators are reluctant to participate in studies in which they do not know the study group assignment. They recognize that bias is partially reduced by keeping the participants blinded but feel that the participants' health and safety are best served if they are not blinded.

Disadvantage:

1. The investigators avoid the problems of biased participant reporting, but they themselves can affect the administration of non-study therapy, data collection, and data assessment. Means when investigators already know the study therapy in some cases there may chance of partial adjustment during data collection & monitoring.

2. Double Blind Trials

Definition: A clinical trial design in which neither the participating individuals nor the study staff knows which participants are receiving the experimental drug and which are receiving a placebo (or another therapy) is called a double blind trial.

In this study neither the participants nor the investigators know the identity of the intervention assignment. Such designs are usually restricted to trials of drug efficacy.

Advantage:

- The main advantage of a truly double blind study is that the risk of bias is reduced. Because of investigators don't know which intervention a particular participant is receiving. Any effects of their actions theoretically would occur equally in intervention and control group.
- The possibility of bias may never be completely eliminated. However, a well-designed and properly run double-blind study can minimize bias.

Disadvantages:

1. Double-blind studies are usually more complex and therefore more difficult to carry out than other studies.
2. As the investigators remain blinded that any data that conceivably might endanger be kept from them during the study.
3. An effective data monitoring scheme must be set up, and emergency unblinding procedures must be established. These requirements pose their own problems and can increase the cost of a study.
4. In double blind trial certain functions, which in open or single blind studies could be accomplished by the investigators, must be taken over by others to maintain the blindness. Thus an outside body needs to monitor the data for toxicity and benefit especially in long-term trials.

(A) Cross-Over Designs

- The cross over design is a special case of randomized control trial and has some appeal to medical researchers.
- The cross-over design allows each participant to serve as his own control. In the simplest case, namely the two-period cross-over design, each participant will receive either intervention or control (A or B) in the first period and the alternative in the succeeding period.
- The order in which A and B are given to each participant is randomized. Thus approximately half of the participants receive the intervention in the sequence AB and the other half in the sequence BA.

Such cross-over study shall be carried out by **Latin square cross-over** design in which

- Each formulation is administered just once to each subject and once in each study period, and
- Unlike, parallel design all the subjects do not receive the same formulation at the same time; in a given study period, they are administered different formulations.

Such a randomized, balanced, cross-over study has several **advantages-**

- It minimizes the inter-subject variability in plasma drug levels.
- Minimizes the carry-over effects which could occur when a given dosage form influences the bioavailability of a subsequently administered product (intra-subject variability).
- Minimizes the variations due to time effect, and thus,
- Makes it possible to focus more on the formulation variables which is the key to the success for any bioequivalence study.

An example of Latin square design for a bioequivalence study in human volunteers is given here.

Latin Square Cross-Over Design for 6 Subjects To Compare Three Different Formulations, X, Y and Z.

	Drug formulation		
Subject number	**Study period 1**	**Study period 2**	**Study period 3**
1.7	X	Y	Z
2.8	Y	Z	X
3.9	Z	X	Y
4.10	X	Z	Y
5.11	Z	Y	X
6.12	Y	X	Z

A **drawback** of such a cross-over design is that

1. The study takes a long time since an appropriate washout period between two administrations is essential which may be very long if the drug has a longer $t_{1/2}$.
2. The study becomes more difficult and subject dropout rates are also high. This can be overcome by use of a balanced incomplete block design in which a subject receives no more than 2 formulations.

Randomization

Sound scientific clinical investigation almost demands that a control group be used against which the new intervention can be compared. Randomization is the preferred way of assigning participants to control and intervention groups.

- The randomized control clinical trial is the standard by which all trials are judged since other designs have certain undesirable features.

Definition: randomization is a process by which each participant has the same chance of being assigned to either intervention or control.

- An example would be the toss of coin, in which head indicates intervention group and tail indicates control group.
- Even in more complex randomization strategies, the element of chance underlies the allocation process. Of course, neither trial participant nor investigator should know what the assignment will be before the participant's decision to enter the study. Otherwise, the benefits of randomization can be lost.

Why randomization is necessary?

- Randomization tends to produce study groups comparable with respect to known and unknown risk factors, removes investigator bias in the allocation of participants, and guarantees that statistical tests will have valid significance levels.
- Randomization minimizes the differences among groups by equally distributing people with particular characteristics among all the trial arms. The researchers do not know which treatment is better. From what is known at the time, any one of the treatments chosen could be of benefit to the participant.

Methods of Randomization

Fixed allocation is the suitable method for the randomization phenomena. Fixed allocation procedures assign the intervention to participants with a pre-specified probability, usually equal, and that allocation probability is not altered as the study progresses. Several methods exist by which fixed allocation is achieved, but most popular and useful methods are:

(A) Simple randomization

(B) Blocked randomization

(A) Simple Randomization: The most elementary and simple form of randomization is the simple randomization. Methods by which simple randomization is achieved are described here.

1. One simple method is to toss an unbiased coin each time a participant is eligible to be randomized. For example, if the coin turns up heads, the participant is assigned to group A; if tails, to group B. using this procedure, approximately one half of the participants will be in group A and one half in group B.
2. For large studies, a more convenient method for producing a randomization schedule is to use a number-producing algorithm, available on most digital computer systems. A simple randomization procedure might assign participants to group A with probability p and participants to group B with probability 1-p.
    - One computerized process for simple randomization is to use a uniform random number algorithm to produce random numbers in the interval from 0.0 to 0.999.using a uniform random number generator, a random number can be produced for each participant. If the random number is between 0 and p, the participant would assigned to group A; otherwise to group B. for equal allocation, the probability cut point, p, is one half (i.e., p=0.50).
    - The **advantage** of the simple randomization procedure is that it is easy to implement.
    - The major **disadvantage** is that, although in the long run the number of the participants in each group will be in the proportion anticipated, at any point in the randomization, including the end, there could be a substantial imbalance.

(B) Blocked Randomization

- Blocked randomization, sometimes also called as permuted block randomization. It is used to avoid serious imbalance in the number of participants assigned to each group, an imbalance that could occur in the simple randomization procedure.
- Blocked randomization guarantees that at no time during randomization will the imbalance be large and that at certain points the number of participants in each group will be equal.
- If participants are randomly assigned with equal probability to groups A or B, then for each block of even size (e.g., 4, 6 or 8) one half of the participants will be assigned to A and the other half to B.
- The order in which the interventions are assigned in each block is randomized, and this process is repeated for consecutive blocks of participants until all participants are randomized.
- For example, the investigators may want to ensure that after every fourth randomized participant, the number of participants in each intervention group is equal. Then a block of size 4 would be used and the process would randomize the order in which two *A*'s and two *B*'s are assigned for every consecutive group of four participants entering the trial.
- One may write down all the ways of arranging the groups and then randomize the order in which these combinations are selected .in the case of block size 4, there are six possible combinations of these assignments: *AABB, ABAB, BAAB, BABA, BBAA* and *ABBA*. One of these arrangements is selected at random, and the four participants are assigned accordingly. This process is repeated as many times as needed.

Advantage: The main advantage of blocking is that balance between the numbers of participants in each group is guaranteed during the course of randomization.

Disadvantages:

1. Analysis of data is more complicated than simple randomization.
2. If blocking factor b is known by the study staff and the study is not double-blinded, the assignment for the last person entered in each block is known before randomization of that person. Example: if the blocking factor is 4 and the first three assignments are *ABB*, then the next assignment must be *A*. this could, of course, permit a bias in the selection of every fourth participant to be entered. This problem can be overcome by

(a) Using double blind study

(b) Size of a new block should be selected in a random fashion from few possibilities such as 2, 4, 6 and 8, instead of continuously repeating 4.

Placeboes-Controlled Study

A placebo is an inactive pill, liquid or powder that has no treatment value.

Definition: placebo controlled study is the method of investigation of drugs in which an inactive substance (the placebo) is given to one group of participants, while the drug being tested is given to another group.

- The results obtained in the two groups are then compared to see if the investigational treatment is more effective in treating the condition.
- Use of a placebo is acceptable if there is no known best therapy and in other special circumstances (e.g. the commonly used therapy is poorly tolerated).
- Of course, all participants must be told that there is a specified probability, for example, 50% of their receiving placebo. The use of a placebo also does not imply that control group participants will receive no treatment.

Placebo when administered for its therapeutic effects, the placebo preparation

- Must appear to be relevant to the illness.
- Must be harmless
- Should preferably conform to the patient's expectations.

In many trials, the objective is to see whether a new intervention plus standard care is better or worse than a placebo plus standard care. In all trials, there is the ethical obligation to allow the best standard care to be used.

In many single-blind and double-blind drug trials the control group is placed on a placebo.

Placebo-control trial is justified if two situations pertain.

1. If the investigator seeks to evaluate a new intervention without the participant receiving any other therapy for the condition being studied, there should be no standard intervention clearly superior to placebo. If a standard therapy is known to beneficial, the placebo and the intervention being assessed would be used in conjugation with the standard therapy.

2. The participants should fully understand that a placebo is being used and be aware of what their chances are of receiving either it or the alternative.

However, as noted, in many studies, the new intervention or placebo are added to the standard therapy and do not replace it.

Understanding Non-inferiority Trials

Non-inferiority clinical trials are being performed with an increasing frequency now-a-days, because it helps in finding a new treatment that have approximately the same efficacy, but may offer other benefits such as better safety profile. Non-inferiority clinical trials aim to demonstrate that the test product is no worse than the comparator by more than a pre-specified small amount. There are several fundamental differences between non-inferiority and superiority trials. Some practical issues concerning the non-inferiority trials are assay sensitivity, choice of the non-inferiority margin, sample size estimation, choice of active-control, and analysis of non-inferiority clinical trials. Noninferiority trials may be performed to demonstrate that a new treatment is better than an assumed placebo in situations where conducting a placebo control trial is unethical. US FDA guidelines state that non-inferiority design for a clinical trial is chosen when it would not be ethical to use a placebo, or a no treatment control, or a very low dose of an active drug, because there is an effective treatment that provides an important benefit (e.g., life-saving or preventing irreversible injury).

Details of Phases of Trials

1. **Phase 1 Trials:** Clinical pharmacology phase
   - A small number of generally healthy volunteers (approximately 20-80 people) are exposed to new drug closely, to assess compound's safety & also MTD (maximum tolerable dose) is determined & also pharmacokinetic profile of parent drug & all metabolites should be evaluated.
   - **Purpose**: Safety and dosage:
     - During Phase 1 studies, researchers test a new drug in normal volunteers (healthy people). In most cases, 20 to 80 healthy volunteers or people with the disease/condition participate in Phase 1. However, if a new drug is intended for use in cancer patients, researchers conduct Phase 1 studies in patients with that type of cancer.
     - Phase 1 studies are closely monitored and gather information about how a drug interacts with the human body. Researchers adjust dosing schemes based on animal data to find out how much of a drug the body can tolerate and what its acute side effects are.
     - As a Phase 1 trial continues, researchers answer research questions related to how it works in the body, the side effects associated with increased dosage, and early information about how effective it is to determine how best to administer the drug to

limit risks and maximize possible benefits. This is important to the design of Phase 2 studies.

- **Study Participants**: 20 to 100 healthy volunteers or people with the disease/condition.
- **Length of Study**: Several months
- **Approximately** 70% of drugs move to the next phase
- **Phase I trials can be further divided:**
- **Single ascending dose (Phase Ia):** In single ascending dose studies, small groups of subjects are given a single dose of the drug while they are observed and tested for a period of time to confirm safety. Typically, a small number of participants, usually three, are entered sequentially at a particular dose. If they do not exhibit any adverse side effects, and the pharmacokinetic data are roughly in line with predicted safe values, the dose is escalated, and a new group of subjects is then given a higher dose. If unacceptable toxicity is observed in any of the three participants, an additional number of participants, usually three, are treated at the same dose. This is continued until pre-calculated pharmacokinetic safety levels are reached, or intolerable side effects start showing up (at which point the drug is said to have reached the maximum tolerated dose (MTD). If an additional unacceptable toxicity is observed, then the dose escalation is terminated and that dose, or perhaps the previous dose, is declared to be the maximally tolerated dose. This particular design assumes that the maximally tolerated dose occurs when approximately one-third of the participants experience unacceptable toxicity. Variations of this design exist, but most are similar.
- **Multiple ascending dose (Phase Ib):** Multiple ascending dose studies investigate the pharmacokinetics and pharmacodynamics of multiple doses of the drug, looking at safety and tolerability. In these studies, a group of patients receives multiple low doses of the drug, while samples (of blood, and other fluids) are collected at various time points and analyzed to acquire information on how the drug is processed within the body. The dose is subsequently escalated for further groups, up to a predetermined level.
- **Food effect:** A short trial designed to investigate any differences in absorption of the drug by the body, caused by eating before the drug is given. These studies are usually run as a crossover study, with volunteers being given two identical doses of the drug while fasted, and after being fed.
- **Execution of Phase I trial:**

1. **Patient selection:** Generally, patients eligible for phase I studies have a confirmed disease. Each protocol specifies criteria for patient eligibility. Typically, these criteria involve patient organ function and the extent of prior therapy. Good organ function is usually required since pharmacologic mechanisms of metabolism and excretion are often unknown in these clinical trials. Patients with seriously impaired kidney, liver, or lung function may have less tolerance to the study agent, making it difficult to assess toxicity and increasing the risk of unacceptable toxicity in that patient.

2. **Informed consent:** Patients who enter phase I studies need to be fully informed that these studies usually represent the initial clinical experiments in humans. Expected side effects as noted in preclinical animal studies are presented, and the possibility that other, unpredictable side effects can occur must be stated.
3. **Treatment approach and endpoints:** Most phase I studies treat cohorts of patients (typically, three to six) at predefined dose levels. The studies start at very low doses that were minimally toxic in animals (e.g., 1/10 x LD10 in mice). If that dose is safe, a cohort of patients is treated at a higher dose, with escalation continuing until a maximum tolerated dose (MTD) is defined. Various escalation schemas with successively smaller increases in dose are used, with rapid escalation at lower, presumably more tolerable, doses and slower escalation as the dose increases. The toxicity defining the MTD is based on toxicity found in animal testing, with provisions for unexpected toxicities. A dose for phase II studies is decided based on the MTD; usually, the phase II dose is about 80% of the MTD. Phase I studies may also be designed to determine the toxicity of lengthening or shortening an infusion schedule or the interval between treatments, assess supportive care designed to reduce toxicity, and determine an optimum biologic dose (OBD, i.e., the dose associated with the maximum desired biologic response for which toxicity is still acceptable).

   The schedule of drug administration in phase I studies is determined from preclinical testing. Common schedules include administration once every two to four weeks, administration for five consecutive days every three to four weeks, or daily dosing. Schedules may also be based on maintaining a certain drug level in the blood. Scheduling may involve varying the length of intravenous infusion. Commonly, a study employs one schedule; however, some studies compare multiple schedules within the same study. Agents may be given intravenously, orally, intraperitoneally, intravascularly, or through other routes. Sometimes, investigators will randomize patients to multiple doses, schedules, or routes of administration to more quickly assess tolerance to various dosing routines and to rapidly follow up on the more promising one. Agents that are commonly used by one route or on an established schedule may return to phase I testing in order to determine a safe dose by another route or on a different schedule because an investigator has an important lead about how to improve the agent's effectiveness or reduce its toxicity. Also, phase I studies are employed to test the feasibility of combining drugs or different modalities of treatments.
4. **Required testing:** Because the purpose of phase I studies is to determine a tolerable dose and schedule, blood and other laboratory tests are performed at frequent intervals to monitor treatment effects on the function of major body systems. Additionally, blood levels of the agent are measured in order to establish the concentration and rate of disappearance of the agent from circulation and to correlate blood levels with side effects. This information helps researchers decide how to administer the agent in phase II studies and in patients with impaired organ function. For biological response modifiers, it is important to assess the effect on the immune function of the patient, For example anticancer drugs for which the antitumor effect appears to be mediated through alteration or stimulation of the immune system.

5. **Anticipated benefit:** While Phase I studies are primarily directed toward establishing a safe dose for further testing, there is always the possibility of therapeutic benefit in these studies.

2. **Phase II Trial: Clinical investigation of efficacy and safety**

➢ Phase-2 clinical testing shifts the focus of trials from safety to efficacy. In comparison to phase 1 Trials a large no. of people (100-300 patients) are enrolled in the trial and the majority of these participants suffer from the target illness. Side effect from new investigated product should also be monitored. Some Phase II trials are designed as case series, demonstrating a drug's safety and activity in a selected group of participants like cancer. Other Phase II trials are designed as randomized controlled trials, where some patients receive the drug/device and others receive placebo/standard treatment. Phase 2 trials are sometimes further divided into:

➢ **Phase 2a:** Phase 2a is focused specifically on dosing requirements. A small number of patients are administered the drug in different quantities to evaluate whether there is as a dose-response relationship, which is an increase in response that correlates with increasing increments of dose. In addition, the optimal frequency of dose is also explored.

➢ **Phase 2b:** Phase 2b trials are designed specifically to rigorously test the efficacy of the drug in terms of how successful it is in treating, preventing or diagnosing a disease.

➢ **Purpose**: Efficacy and side effects or efficacy vs side effects

- In Phase 2 studies, researchers administer the drug to a group of patients with the disease or condition for which the drug is being developed. Typically involving a few hundred patients, these studies aren't large enough to show whether the drug will be beneficial.
- Instead, Phase 2 studies provide researchers with additional safety data. Researchers use these data to refine research questions, develop research methods, and design new Phase 3 research protocols.

➢ **Study Participants**: Up to several hundred people with the disease/condition.

➢ **Length of Study**: Several months to 2 years

➢ **Approximately** 33% of drugs move to the next phase

➢ **Execution of Phase II trial:**

1. **Patient selection:** Patients enrolled on phase II studies are usually required to have measurable biopsy-proven disease, to have a good performance status, and to be free of serious intercurrent disease. Nearly normal renal, hepatic, cardiac, bone marrow, and pulmonary function are usually required. Often, patients treated with phase II agents must have failed treatment with other chemotherapy or surgery. A number of studies have demonstrated that patients who have received extensive prior therapy are unlikely to respond to phase II agents that are effective in minimally pretreated patients. Therefore, many phase II studies restrict the amount of prior therapy to one or two prior regimens.

2. **Informed consent:** Patients entering clinical trials must be counseled in detail about their prognosis and chances for being treated effectively with other investigational or standard therapies. The known side effects of new pharmaceutical agents must be conveyed to them. In addition, they must understand that unexpected side effects may occur.

3. **Treatment approach and endpoints:** Usually between 25 and 50 patients are treated for each dose and schedule selected from phase I testing. The decision on which cancers to treat may be based on preclinical efficacy against disease and from hints of activity in phase I studies. For example in phase II study of anticancer drugs most phase II studies require patients to have measurable or evaluable primary tumors or metastases. Measurable disease is serially measurable in two dimensions and includes the following: nodules on chest x-ray that are confined to the parenchyma, freely movable lymph nodes or masses, masses imaged on CT or MRI, and skin nodules. Examples of lesions that do not qualify as measurable are diffuse bony metastases on bone scan, pleural effusions, patchy pulmonary infiltrates, poorly defined subcutaneous masses, and ill-defined abdominal masses. Measurable disease is necessary to objectively define tumor response. A complete response means the disappearance of all known sites of disease without the development of any new disease for at least one month. Partial response is at least a 50% decrease in the sum of the products of the bidimensional measurement of all lesions with no new disease appearing for at least one month. Patients with ill-defined sites of disease cannot be accurately evaluated according to these criteria. Some studies will also allow enrollment of patients with evaluable disease. Evaluable disease may be measurable in one but not in two dimensions. Some studies consider any indicator of disease that can be followed serially as suitable for evaluability, including serum tumor markers and ascites.

    - The dose and schedule for phase II studies are taken from phase I studies. In the absence of unacceptable toxicity, some phase II protocols allow patients to continue treatment as long as their tumors respond or remain stable; other phase II protocols limit therapy to a specified number of treatments. Following treatment, patients are usually followed for outcome, i.e., for disease recurrence or progression, for survival, and for evidence of late toxicity.

    - An adequate number of patients needs to be treated to determine the level of drug activity. If no responses are seen in two trials, the agent is usually considered inactive. However, if the patients in these studies have received extensive prior therapy or failed to receive adequate doses of the new agent, negative results are less convincing. If responses are seen, the number of patients studied is increased to more precisely define the response rate. Some clinical trials combine phase I and phase II study designs within the same protocol, and patients treated at the recommended phase II dose during the phase I portion may be added to the statistical pool for the phase II portion.

    - Newer statistical approaches to phase II studies include randomization of patients to two or more treatment arms, each testing a new agent. The agent producing the highest response rate, even if the response rate is not significantly higher than that produced by other agents, is chosen for phase III testing.

4. **Required testing:** Since patients entered on phase II studies may be receiving a new agent, careful observation is mandatory and requires serial laboratory evaluations to monitor for organ damage. This requires a detailed history and physical examination, blood tests, x-rays, scans, and sometimes repeated surgical biopsies. Patients must be informed of the nature of the diagnostic monitoring required by the study as part of their informed consent.

5. **Anticipated benefit**

   - Phase II agents that demonstrate partial response rates of at least 15% may be considered for further testing, often combined with other agents of proven efficacy. New combinations are pilot tested in other phase II studies and may include only standard agents or both standard and new agents. A number of potentially effective agents are discarded after serious toxicity is noted in phase II studies. Ethical considerations require that investigators be willing to terminate phase II studies when severe toxicity without compelling efficacy is observed.

   - Once a new agent has demonstrated adequate efficacy and safety in phase II studies, it enters phase III testing where it can be compared to generally accepted therapies for efficacy and toxicity.

3. **Phase III Trials - later clinical development phase**

   Phase-3

   - Phase-3 trials are the longest, most comprehensive trials regarding efficacy and safety of new compounds. Significantly large numbers (1000-3000) of patients who are afflicted with the target illness are tested. In addition to monitoring the safety and efficacy, these trials also monitor adverse reactions and proper dosage regimen. Compounds that successfully complete phase-3 testing have a 95% chance of being approved by the FDA.

   - **Purpose**: Efficacy and monitoring of adverse reactions

     - Researchers design Phase 3 studies to demonstrate whether or not a product offers a treatment benefit to a specific population. Sometimes known as pivotal studies, these studies involve 300 to 3,000 participants.

     - Phase 3 studies provide most of the safety data. In previous studies, it is possible that less common side effects might have gone undetected. Because these studies are larger and longer in duration, the results are more likely to show long-term or rare side effects

   - **Study Participants**: 300 to 3,000 volunteers who have the disease or condition

   - **Length of Study:** 1 to 4 years

   - **Approximately** 25-30% of drugs move to the next phase

- **The New Drug Approval (NDA) Application:** Once the phase-3 trials have been completed, all preclinical & clinical data are compiled and submitted to the FDA for review. The NDA process is the last hurdle prior to approval and marketing. If NDA meets all the requirements of FDA, then approval granted to company for launching a new molecule to the market.

Execution of Phase III trial:

1. **Patient selection:** Generally, patients eligible for Phase III trials must have good performance status, be free of intercurrent disease, and have normal renal, hepatic, cardiac, bone marrow, and pulmonary function. Phase III studies may exclude patients who have received prior therapy for same disease, or they may enroll only patients who have had prior therapy. Studies that are designed to assess response rate require disease that is bidimensionally measurable or at least evaluable (capable of being objectively assessed for improvement or worsening over time).
2. **Informed consent:** Patients entering phase III studies must be counseled in detail about their prognosis and the expected benefits from participation in the study, as well as benefits that could be expected from treatment with other investigational or standard therapies. The known side effects of pharmaceutical agents must be conveyed, and they must understand that, despite prior phase I and II testing, unexpected side effects may occur. The expected length of the study and follow-up measures should also be made clear.
3. **Treatment approach and endpoints:** Patients are randomly allocated to the treatment options to help ensure unbiased comparison of the treatments. The numbers of patients who are treated with each regimen depends on the number of major events (usually recurrence or survival) predicted to occur during the course of accrual and follow-up. Anywhere from 100 to 1,000 or more patients may be required, and accrual may take 2-5 years or more. Studies must be designed to account for major prognostic categories by either entering large numbers of patients or by stratification on the basis of known prognostic factors. For example, a phase III study in breast cancer may randomize premenopausal and postmenopausal women separately. In spite of stratification and randomization, some studies will enroll more patients with good prognosis in one arm than in the others. In such cases, statistical techniques exist to retrospectively "balance" treatment arms for prognostic factors.

   The dose and schedule for the new arms are based on phase II studies. Dose and schedule for the standard arm are taken from published literature or prior phase III studies. In a few phase III studies, historical data are used instead of a standard arm and all patients are allocated only to investigational arms. There is considerable controversy about the validity of using historical data versus concurrently randomized controls in phase III studies.

   After completion or discontinuation of treatment, follow-up of patients typically lasts for life or until other treatment is initiated. The requirement for large enrollment and lengthy follow-up makes phase III studies expensive and difficult to run.

4. **Required testing:** Close observation of patients for both acute and chronic toxicity is necessary; unusual or chronic toxicities may be observed only in the large number of patients on phase III new regimen arms. Prognosis requires a detailed history and physical examination, blood tests, x-rays, scans, and sometimes repeated surgical biopsies. Patients must be informed of the nature of the diagnostic monitoring required by the study prior to their giving informed consent.

5. **Anticipated benefit:** Phase III studies offer the most up-to-date treatment for a given indication.

4. **Phase IV Trials or post marketing surveillance:** Sometimes adverse drug reactions only comes to light after the drug has been in the market for a while and has been used by very large no of patients. The medicine is made available to doctors, who start prescribing it. The effect can be monitored in thousands of patients to help identify any unforeseen side effects. Post-marketing surveillance is designed to detect any rare or long-term adverse effects over a much larger patient population and timescale than was possible during the initial clinical trials. Such adverse effects detected by Phase IV trials may result in the withdrawal or restriction of a drug - recent examples include cerivastatin (brand names Baycol and Lipobay), troglitazone (Rezulin) and rofecoxib (Vioxx).

Salient features of Phase IV trials:

- Many clinicians through out the approved marketing area.
- Update the clinical data relative to safety and efficacy.
- Elucidate the incidence of adverse reaction and explore a specific pharmacological effect or obtain more discrete information.
- Large scale, long term studies.
- Effect of drug on morbidity and mortality.

Need of Post Marketing Surveillance and Reporting of ADR

The information collected during the pre-marketing phase of drug development is inevitably incomplete with regard to possible ADRs. This is mainly because :

- Tests in animals are insufficient to predict human safety.
- Patients used in clinical trials are selected and limited in number, the conditions of use differ from those in clinical practice and the duration of trials is limited.
- By the time of licensing exposure of less than 5000 human subjects to a drug allows only the more common ADR to be detected.
- At least 30,000 people need to be treated with a drug to be sure that you do not miss at least one patient with an ADR which has an incidence of 1 in 10,000 exposed individuals.
- Information about rare but serious adverse reactions, chronic toxicity, use in special groups (such as children, the elderly or pregnant women) or drug interactions is often incomplete or not available,

Thus, post-marketing surveillance is important to permit detection of less common, but sometimes very serious ADRs. Therefore health professionals worldwide should report on ADRs as it can save lives of their patients and others.

- **Execution of Phase IV Trial:** FDA maintains a system of postmarketing surveillance and risk assessment programs to identify adverse events that did not appear during drug approval process.FDA monitors adverse events such as adverse reactions and poisoning. The agency may recommend this information to be updated in drug labeling, and in rare cases, to re-evaluate the approval and marketing decision.
    - The adverse drug reporting system (AERS) is a computerize information database designed to support the FDA's post marketing safety surveillance program for all approved drug and therapeutic biologic products.
    - The ultimate goal of AERS is to improve the public health by providing the best available tools for storing and analyzing the safety reports.
    - The reports in AERS are evaluated by multidisciplinary staff evaluators, epidemiologists and other scientists in the center of drug evaluation and research (CDER) office of drug safety to detect safety signals and to monitor drug safety.
    - As a result FDA may take regulatory actions to improve product safety and protect public health, such as updating a product's labeling information, sending out a "Dear health care Professional" letter or reevaluating an approval decision.
    - The **MEDWATCH** program is for health professionals and the public to voluntarily report serious reactions and problems with medical products, such as drugs and medical devices. It also ensures that new safety information is rapidly communicated to the medical community thereby improving patient care. All data contained in MEDWATCH form will be entered in the AERS database.

Methods of Post Marketing Surveillance

Four Methods of studies are generally used to identify drugs effects:

1. Controlled clinical trials,
2. Spontaneous or voluntary recording
3. Case control studies
4. Cohort studies

1. **Controlled Clinical Trials:** PMS studies conducted after the launch of a product is part of phase IV development of drug. Some of these studies may be retrospective case-control evaluation. These are done to evaluate rare suspected side effects.

   For example: when there was a suspicion that use of oral contraceptives may be associated with an increased incidence of thrombophlebitis (clotting of blood in the deep veins) and thromboembolism (blockage of smaller arteries due to detached blood clots) case- control studies were carried out.

   A group of cases of thromboembolism were compared with age matched controls that were similar to the cases as possible, but without the disease. • To minimize bias through such method as randomization and "double-blinding • Directly monitor patients for the duration of studies. • For evaluating a drug's efficacy and safety. • They are often costly.

2. **Spontaneous Reporting:** A communication from an individual (e.g: health care professional, consumer) to a company or regulatory authority. This describes a suspected adverse event. But the actual incidence of adverse drug reaction cannot be determined through spontaneous reporting. The spontaneous reporting system process 1. Data acquisition 2.data assessment 3.data interpretation

   - **Data acquisitio**n: which depends largely on the input of information derived from reports submitted by the health professionals who have encountered what they suspect is an ADR
   - **Data assessment**: which involves assessment of the individual case reports and assessment of pooled data obtained from various sources such as the international database of the WHO.
   - **Data interpretation based** on the available data and the assessments made, a signal related to the adverse reaction may be generated

   ➢ India – 'Suspected Adverse Drug Reaction Reporting Form'

   ➢ UK – 'Yellow Card', since 1964

   ➢ Australia – 'Blue Card', since 1964

   ➢ US – 'Med Watch'

3. **Case Control Studies or Individual Case Study Report (ICSR):** Case control studies identify patient with the adverse effects to be studied, and compare them with the sample drawn from the same cohort that gave rise to cases. A case control study involves two populations – cases and controls and has three distinct features: Both exposure and outcome have occurred before the start of the study. The study proceeds backwards from effect to cause. It uses a control or comparison group to support or refute an inference.

   Elements of a Case Control Study

   1. Selection of cases
   2. Selection of controls
   3. Information on exposure
   4. Analysis

   - **Selection of cases** -• All people in source population who develop the disease of interest -Sample of cases -Independent of the exposure under study • Clear definition of outcome studied • Prevalent vs. incident cases -Prevalent cases may be related more to survival with disease than to development of disease.
   - **Sources of cases-** • Hospital/clinic based -cases Easier to find -May represent severe cases • Population based (cancer registry) - not biased by factors drawing a patient to a particular hospital
   - **Selection of controls-**• Represent the distribution of exposure in the source population of cases -Selected from the same source population that gives rise to the cases • Selected independently of their exposure status

- SIGNAL- Reported information on a possible causal relationship which is being unknown or incompletely documented previously. -usually more than 1 report is required to generate a signal -before signals are published they are first clinically assessed by PV experts at UMC(Uppsala monitoring centre ,Sweden) There are 3types of signals 1.confirmed signals-causal relationship between the drug and adverse event 2.refuted(false) signals-no causal relationship 3.unconfirmed signals-require further investigation
- TRIAGE- Triage refers to the process of placing a potential adverse event report into one of three categories: 1) non-serious case 2) serious case or 3) no case (minimum criteria for an AE case are not fulfilled).
- WHOART- WHO -The WHO Adverse Reactions Terminology (WHOART) is a dictionary meant to serve as a basis for rational coding of adverse reaction terms. The system is maintained by the Uppsala Monitoring Centre (UMC), the World Health Organization Collaborating Centre for International Drug Monitoring.
- COSTART- Coding Symbols for a Thesaurus of Adverse Reaction Terms developed by USFDA . But recently COSTART was replaced by MedDRA.
- MedDRA- MedDRA or Medical Dictionary for Regulatory Activities is a clinically validated international medical terminology dictionary thesaurus
- HITECH act- Health Information Technology for Economic and Clinical Health act -by this data mining opportunities are maximized
- VIGI FLOW- web based ICSR(Individual Case Safety Report) system designed for national centres
- VIGIBASE- unique collection of international drug safety data. Vigibase is the name of the WHO ICSR data base
- VIGI SEARCH- a search service for accessing ICSRs stored in the vigibase , offered by UMC to national centres
- VIGIMED- Share point based conferencing facility, exclusive to member countries of the WHO. For fast communication of ADR
- VIGIMINE- statistical tool within vigisearch. It allows filtering of the results by age, gender , country.
- VIGILYZE- vigisearch & vigimine were replaced by this. It's a search and analysis tool that provide access to vigibase
- PVPI- Pharmacovigilance programme of India (23 November 2004)
- ▼ inverted black triangle symbol- medication is new to the market, or that an existing medicine (or vaccine) is being used for a new reason or by a new route of administration

4. **Cohort Studies:** Studies follow a defined group of patient for a period of time. Patient are not randomly assigned , & there is no blinding. Other names of cohort study are Longitudinal study, Incidence study and forward looking study.

Steps in Cohort Study

- Selection of study population
- Obtaining data exposure
- Selection of comparison group Follow-up
- Analysis

Features of cohort studies

- Cohorts are identified prior to appearance of disease under investigation
- The study groups are observed over a period of time to determine the frequency of disease among them
- The study proceeds from cause to effects

Indications for cohort study

- There is good evidence of an association between exposure and disease, from other studies.
- Exposure is rare.
- Attrition of study population can be minimized.
- Sufficient fund is available.

Consideration during selection of Cohort

- The cohort must be free from disease under study.
- Insofar as the knowledge permits, both the groups should be equally susceptible to disease under study.
- Both the groups must be comparable in respect of all variable which influence the occurrence of disease
- Diagnostic and eligibility criteria of the disease must be defined beforehand

Types of cohort study

• Prospective study • Retrospective cohort study • Ambi-directional cohort study

Advantage of Cohort Studies

- Temporality can be established
- Incidence can be calculated.
- Several possible outcome related to exposure can be studied simultaneously.
- Provide direct estimate of risk.
- Since comparison groups are formed before disease develops certain forms of bias can be minimized like misclassification bias.
- Allows the conclusion of cause effect relationship

Disadvantage of Cohort Studies

- Large population is needed

- Not suitable for rare diseases.
- It is time consuming and expensive
- Certain administrative problems like loss of staff, loss of funding and extensive record keeping are common.
- Problem of attrition of initial cohort is common
- Study itself may alter people's behavior

In a prospective study, investigators design the questions and data collection procedures carefully in order to obtain accurate information about exposures ***before*** disease develops in any of the subjects. In contrast, retrospective studies are conceived ***after*** some people have already developed the outcomes of interest. The investigators jump back in time to identify a cohort of individuals at a point in time before they have developed the outcomes of interest, and they try to establish their exposure status at that point in time. They then determine whether the subject subsequently developed the outcome of interest.

Retrospective cohort studies are very efficient for studying rare or unusual exposures, but there are many potential problems here. Sometimes exposure status is not clear when it is necessary to go back in time and use whatever data is available, especially because the data being used was not designed to answer a health question.

5. **Epidemiological Studies:** Epidemiology is the study of the distribution of diseases and other health-related conditions in populations, and the application of this study to control health problems. The purpose of epidemiology is to understand what risk factors are associated with a specific disease, and how disease can be prevented in groups of individuals; due to the observational nature of epidemiology, it cannot provide answers to what caused a disease to a specific individual. Epidemiologic studies can be used for many reasons, commonly to estimate the frequency of a disease and find associations suggesting potential causes of a disease. To achieve these goals, measures of disease (incidence) or death (mortality) are made within population groups. Epidemiology is fundamentally multidisciplinary and it uses knowledge from biology, sociology, statistics, and other fields.

   The four types of epidemiologic studies commonly used in radiation research are cluster, ecologic, case-control, and cohort studies. An additional approach for estimating risk in radiation research—although strictly not an epidemiologic study—is risk-projection models. These models are used to predict excess cancer risks by combining population dose estimates with existing risk coefficients to transfer risks across populations with different baseline rates.

6. **Observational Studies:** Cohort, cross sectional, and case-control studies are collectively referred to as observational studies. Often these studies are the only practicable method of studying various problems, for example, studies of aetiology, instances where a randomised controlled trial might be unethical, or if the condition to be studied is rare. Cohort studies are used to study incidence, causes, and prognosis. Because they measure events in chronological order they can be used to distinguish between cause and effect. Cross sectional studies are used to determine prevalence. They are relatively quick and easy but do not permit distinction between cause and effect. Case controlled studies compare groups

retrospectively. They seek to identify possible predictors of outcome and are useful for studying rare diseases or outcomes. They are often used to generate hypotheses that can then be studied via prospective cohort or other studies.

Meta-analysis

Meta-analysis is a quantitative, formal, epidemiological study design used to systematically assess previous research studies to derive conclusions about that body of research. Outcomes from a meta-analysis may include a more precise estimate of the effect of treatment or risk factor for disease, or other outcomes, than any individual study contributing to the pooled analysis. The examination of variability or heterogeneity in study results is also a critical outcome. The benefits of meta-analysis include a consolidated and quantitative review of a large, and often complex, sometimes apparently conflicting, body of literature. The specification of the outcome and hypotheses that are tested is critical to the conduct of meta-analyses, as is a sensitive literature search. A failure to identify the majority of existing studies can lead to erroneous conclusions; however, there are methods of examining data to identify the potential for studies to be missing; for example, by the use of funnel plots. Rigorously conducted meta-analyses are useful tools in evidence-based medicine. The need to integrate findings from many studies ensures that meta-analytic research is desirable and the large body of research now generated makes the conduct of this research feasible.

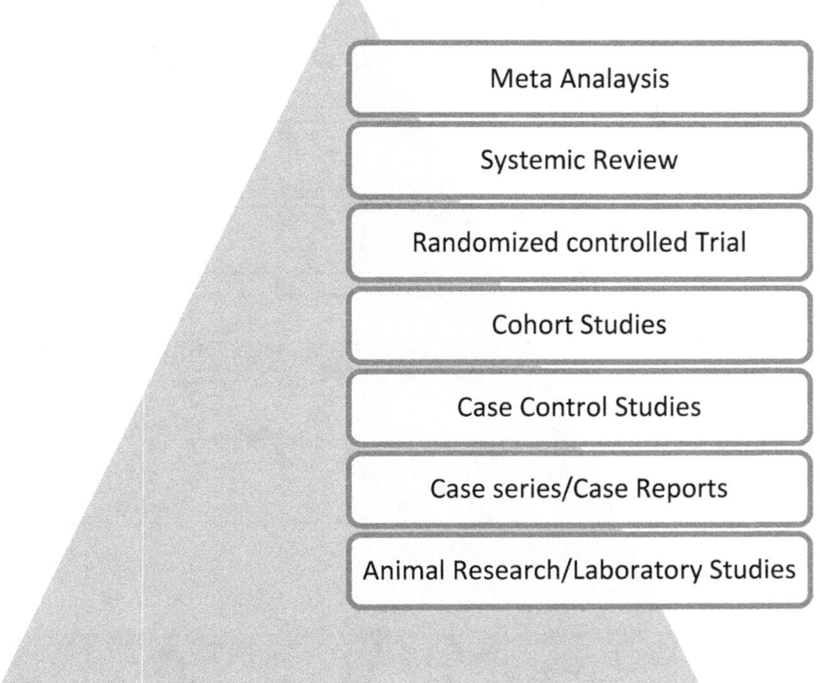

Figure 23.3 Hierarchy of Evidence programme of India.

SUSPECTED ADVERSE DRUG REACTION REPORTING FORM

For VOLUNTARY reporting of Adverse Drug Reactions by Healthcare Professionals

INDIAN PHARMACOPOEIA COMMISSION

(National Coordination Centre-Pharmacovigilance Programme of India)
Ministry of Health & Family Welfare, Government of India
Sector-23, Raj Nagar, Ghaziabad-201002
www.ipc.nic.in

FOR AMC/NCC USE ONLY

AMC Report No. :

Worldwide Unique No. :

A. PATIENT INFORMATION

1. Patient Initials	2. Age at time of Event or Date of Birth ________	3. M ☐ F ☐ Other ☐ 4. Weight________Kgs

12. Relevant tests/ laboratory data with dates

B. SUSPECTED ADVERSE REACTION

5. Date of reaction started (dd/mm/yyyy)

6. Date of recovery (dd/mm/yyyy)

7. Describe reaction or problem

13. Relevant medical/ medication history (e.g. allergies, race, pregnancy, smoking, alcohol use, hepatic/renal dysfunction etc.)

14. Seriousness of the reaction (Yes ☐ No ☐)

☐ Death (dd/mm/yyyy) ☐ Congenital-anomaly
☐ Life threatening ☐ Required intervention to Prevent permanent impairment/damage
☐ Hospitalization/Prolonged
☐ Disability ☐ Other (specify)

15. Outcomes

☐ Recovered ☐ Recovering ☐ Not recovered
☐ Fatal ☐ Recovered with sequelae ☐ Unknown

C. SUSPECTED MEDICATION(S)

S.No	8. Name (Brand/Generic)	Manufacturer (if known)	Batch No. / Lot No.	Exp. Date (if known)	Dose used	Route used	Frequency (OD, BD etc.)	Therapy dates		Indication
								Date started	Date stopped	
i										
ii										
iii										
iv										

S.No as per C	9. Action Taken						10. Reaction reappeared after reintroduction			
	Drug withdrawn	Dose increased	Dose reduced	Dose not changed	Not applicable	Unknown	Yes	No	Effect unknown	Dose (if reintroduced)
i										
ii										
iii										
iv										

11. Concomitant medical product including self medication and herbal remedies with therapy dates (Exclude those used to treat reaction)

D. REPORTER DETAILS

16. Name and Professional Address:______________________

Pin:__________E-mail______________________

Tel. No. (with STD code)______________________

Occupation:________________ Signature:______________

17. Causality Assessment:

18. Date of this report (dd/mm/yyyy):

Additional Information:

Confidentiality: The patient's identity is held in strict confidence and protected to the fullest extent. Programme staff is not expected to and will not disclose the reporter's identity in response to a request from the public. Submission of a report does not constitute an admission that medical personnel or manufacturer or the product caused or contributed to the reaction.

Form: Medicines side effect reporting form for consumers by Pharmacovigilance programme of India

Version 1.0

MEDICINES SIDE EFFECT REPORTING FORM (FOR CONSUMERS)

Indian Pharmacopoeia Commission, National Coordination Centre- Pharmacovigilance Programme of India, Ministry of Health & Family Welfare, Government of India.

IPC

1. Patient Details

Patient Initials: ☐☐ | Gender (√): Male ☐ Female ☐ Other ☐ | Age (Year or Month) :

2. Health Information

a. Reason(s) for taking medicine(s)(Disease/Symptoms):

b. Medicines Advised by (√): Doctor ☐ Pharmacist ☐ Friends/Relatives ☐ Self (Past disease experienced/No past disease experienced) ☐

3. Details of Person Reporting the Side Effect

Name (Optional):

Address:

Telephone No: | Email:

4. Details of Medicine Taking/Taken

Name of Medicines	Quantity of Medicines taken (e.g. 250 mg, Two times a day)	Expiry Date of Medicines	Date of Start of Medicines	Date of Stop of Medicines

Dosage form (√) : Tablet ☐ Capsule ☐ Injection ☐ Oral Liquids ☐ If Others (Please Specify..........................)

5. About the Side Effect

When did the side effect start? ☐ Side Effect is still Continuing (Yes/No): ☐

When did the side effect stop? ☐

6. How bad was the Side Effect? (Please √ the boxes that Apply)

☐ Did not affect daily activities ☐ Affect daily activities

☐ Admitted to hospital ☐ Death

☐ Others

7. Describe the Side Effect (What did you do to manage the side effect?)

This reporting is voluntary, has no legal implication and aims to improve patient safety. Your active participation is valuable. The information provided in this form will be forwarded to ADR Monitoring Centre for follow-up. You are requested to cooperate with the programme officials when they contact you for more details. Please do report even if you do not have all the information.

Please turn the page to read the instructions

Abbreviated New Drug Application (ANDA) Submission

An Abbreviated New Drug Application (ANDA) contains data that, when submitted to FDA's Center for Drug Evaluation and Research, Office of Generic Drugs, provides for the review and ultimate approval [Figure 25.4] of a generic drug product. Generic drug applications are called "abbreviated" because they are generally not required to include preclinical (animal) and clinical (human) data to establish safety and effectiveness. Instead, a generic applicant must scientifically demonstrate that its product is bioequivalent (i.e., performs in the same manner as the innovator drug). Once approved, an applicant may manufacture and market the generic drug product to provide a safe, effective, low cost alternative to the American public.

Generic drug applications are referred to Abbreviated New Drug Application.

- Pharmaceutical companies must admit ANDAs and receive FDA's approval before marketing new generic drugs according to 21CFR 314.105(d).
- Once ANDA is approved, an applicant can manufacture and market generic drug to provide safe, effective and low cost alternative of innovator drug product to the public. A generic drug is comparable to Innovator drug for dosage form, strength, route of administration, quality, performance and intended use.
- One of the ways to demonstrate bioequivalence is to measure the time taken by generic drug to reach bloodstream in 24-36 healthy volunteers. The time and amount of active ingredients in the bloodstream should be comparable to those of Innovator drug.
- Use of bioequivalence as base for approving generic drug products was established in 1984, also known as WAXMAN-HATCH ACT. It is because of this act that generic drugs are cheaper without conducting costly and duplicative clinical trials.

Code of Federal Regulations

- The following regulations apply to ANDA process:
- 21 CFR 314- Applications for FDA approval to market a New Drug or Antibiotic Drug
- 21 CFR 320- Bioavailability and Bioequivalence requirements
- 21 CFR 310- New Drugs.
- Office of Generic Drug(OGD) strongly encourages submission of bioequivalence, chemistry and labeling portions of the application in electronic format.

Format and Content of ANDA

- Copies of the Abbreviated application are required to be submitted; an archival copy, a review copy and a field copy. An Archival copy shall contain the following:
- Application form
- Table of Contents
- Basis for ANDA submission
- Conditions of use
- Active Ingredients
- Route of Administration

- Dosage form and Strength
- Bioequivalence and Bioavailability
- Labeling
- Chemistry, Manufacturing and Controls
- Samples
- Patent Certification
- Financial Certification or disclosure statement.
- Other Information.
    - Under Sec 314.94 (a) (12), the patent certification includes one of the following:
    - Paragraph I Certification- That the patent information has not been submitted to FDA.
    - Paragraph II Certification- That the patent has expired
    - Paragraph III Certification- That the patent will expire (on date of marketing)
    - Paragraph IV Certification- That the patent is invalid, unenforceable, or will not be infringed by manufacture, use or sale of generic drug.

Difference between submission of NDA and ANDA

ANDA requires submission of :	**NDA requires submission of:**
1. Detailed description of components. 2. Manufacturing, Controls, Packaging, data to assure bioequivalence and bioavailability and Labeling. Labeling should be prepared in accordance with DESI (Drug efficacy study implementation).	1. Well-controlled clinical studies to demonstrate effectiveness. 2. Preclinical and clinical data to show safety. 3. Details of Manufacturing and Packaging. 4. Proposed annotated Labeling

Exclusivity

Exclusivity is a statutory provision designed to promote a balance between an Innovator and Generic drug competitor. As long as a drug patent lasts, a reference listed drug company enjoys a period of market exclusivity or monopoly. Expiration of patent removes the monopoly of the patent holder.

Terms of Exclusivity

Orphan drugs---------- 7 years

New Chemical Entity----------5 years

Pediatric Exclusivity---------6 months additional

Patent Challenge----------180 days.

Hatch-waxman amendments and 180 days exclusivity

- Before Hatch Waxman Amendment, generic manufacturer could file ANDA only after innovator's patent expiry or cancellation. But under Sec 505(j)(5)(B) of Hatch Waxman amendment it permits preparation and filing of ANDA before patent expiration, so that the effective approval date of generic drug would be on expiration date of the patent of Innovator Original drug.

- The Act also establishes another procedure in which the generic company can challenge patent of the Innovator. For generic companies, the amendment provide an inventive 180-day exclusivity period in which no other ANDA for that drug can be approved. This 180-day period is to encourage generic companies to challenge validity of Orange book listed patents or to design around these patents to bring more quickly a generic drug to market.
- For Innovator company, filing of an ANDA is an act of patent infringement. So, if innovator company brings suit within 45 days, the approval of generic company's ANDA is delayed for upto 30 months.

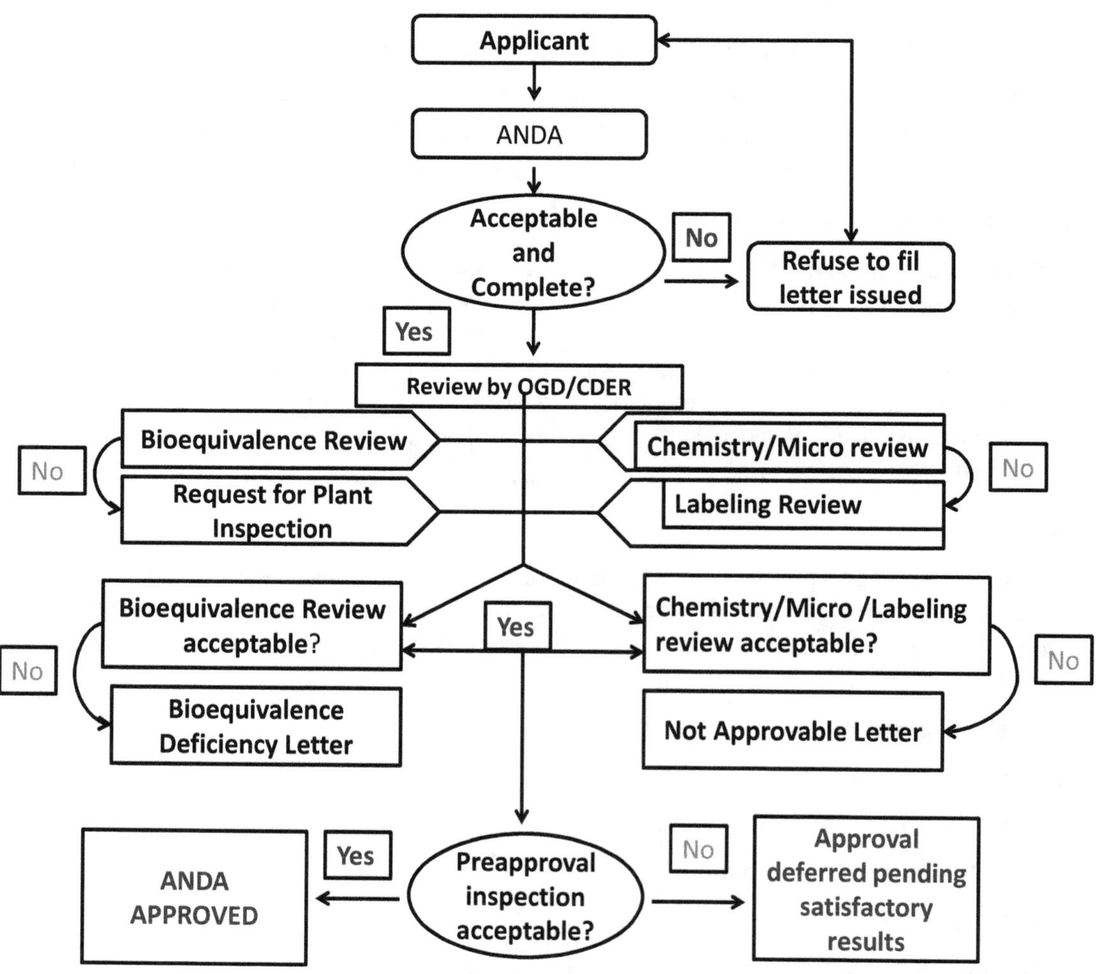

Figure 23.4 ANDA Review Process.

Further Reading

1. Ameh SJ, Obodozie OO, Abubakar MS, Garba M. Current phytotherapy – An inter-regional perspective on policy, research and development of herbal medicine. J Med Plants Res. 2010;4:1508–16.
2. Bansal D, Hota D, Chakrabarti A. Research methodological issues in evaluating herbal interventions. J Clin Trial. 2010;2:15–21.
3. Bian ZX, Li YP, Moher D, Dagenais S, Liu L, Wu TX, et al. Improving the quality of randomized controlled trials in Chinese herbal medicine, part I: Clinical trial design and methodology. Zhong Xi Yi Jie He Xue Bao. 2006;4:120–9.
4. Bower H. Double standards exist in judging traditional and alternative medicine. Br Med J. 1998;316:1694.
5. Brewin CR, Bradley C. Patient preferences and randomised clinical trials. BMJ. 1989;299:313–5.
6. Buchanan DR, White JD, O'Mara AM, Kelaghan JW, Smith WB, Minasian LM. Research-design issues in cancer-symptom-management trials using complementary and alternative medicine: Lessons from the National Cancer Institute Community Clinical Oncology Program experience. J Clin Oncol. 2005;23:6682–9.
7. Chadwick L, Fong H. Herb quality assurance and standardization in herb-drug interaction evaluation and documentation. In: Lam YW, Huang SM, Hall SD, editors. Herbal Supplement-Drug Interactions. Taylor and Francis: New York; 2006. pp. 191–203.
8. Critchley JA, Zhang Y, Suthisisang CC, Chan TY, Tomlinson B. Alternative therapies and medical science: Designing clinical trials of alternative/complementary medicines – Is evidence-based traditional Chinese medicine attainable? J Clin Pharmacol. 2000;40:462–7
9. De Smet PA. Herbal remedies. N Engl J Med. 2002;347:2046–56.
10. Drug and Cosmetic Act, 1940; Drugs and Cosmetics Rules 1945
11. Eisenberg DM, Kessler RC, Foster C, Norlock FE, Calkins DR, Delbanco TL. Unconventional medicine in the United States. Prevalence, costs, and patterns of use. N Engl J Med. 1993;328:246–52.
12. Ernst E, Siev-Ner I, Gamus D. Complementary medicine – A critical review. Isr J Med Sci. 1997;33:808–15.
13. Ethical Guidelines For Biomedical Research on Human Participants- ICMR 2006 (http://icmr.nic.in/ethical_guidelines.pdf)
14. Fong HH. Integration of herbal medicine into modern medical practices: Issues and prospects. Integr Cancer Ther. 2002;1:287–93.
15. General Guidelines for Methodologies on Research and Evaluation of Traditional Medicine, World Health Organization 2000 (http://whqlibdoc.who.int/hq/2000/WHO_EDM_TRM_2000.1.pdf)
16. Geneva, Switzerland: World Health Organization; 2005. Operational Guidance: Information Needed to Support Clinical Trials of Herbal Products.
17. Geneva: World Health Organization; 1993. World Health Organization. Research Guidelines for Evaluating the Safety and Efficacy of Herbal Medicines.

18. Geneva: World Health Organization; 1998. World Health Organization. Regulatory Situation of Herbal Medicines. A Worldwide Review.
19. Geneva: World Health Organization; 2000b. World Health Organization. General Guidelines for Methodologies on Research and Evaluation of Traditional Medicine. WHO/EDM/TRM/2000.
20. Geneva: World Health Organization; 2001. World Health Organization. Legal Status of Traditional Medicine and Complementary/Alternative Medicine: A Worldwide Review. WHO/EDM/TRM/2001.
21. Geneva: World Health Organization; 2003a. World Health Organization. WHO Guidelines on Good Agricultural and Collection Practices (GACP) for Medicinal Plants
22. Good Clinical Practices For Clinical Research In India, Central Drugs Standard Control Organization, Directorate General of Health Services, Ministry of Health and Family Welfare, Government of India, (http://cdsco.nic.in/html/GCP.htm)
23. Guideline For Good Clinical Practice, E6(R1), International Conference On Harmonisation Of Technical Requirements For Registration Of Pharmaceuticals For Human Use (http://www.ich.org/fileadmin/Public_Web_Site/ICH_Products/ Guidelines/ Efficacy/ E6_R1/Step4/E6_R1__Guideline.pdf)
24. Howard KI, Orlinsky DE, Perilstein J. Contribution of therapists to patients' experiences in psychotherapy: A components of variance model for analyzing process data. J Consult Clin Psychol. 1976;44:520–6.
25. Jonas WB, Linde K. Conducting and evaluating clinical research on complementary and alternative medicine. In: Gallin JI, editor. Principles and Practice of Clinical Research. San Diego, CA: Academic Press; 2002. pp. 401–26.
26. Kleinman A, Eisenberg L, Good B. Culture, illness, and care: Clinical lessons from anthropologic and cross-cultural research. Ann Intern Med. 1978;88:251–8.
27. Kumar K. USA: Howard University, USA in Collaboration with NIPRD, Abuja, Nigeria, and Xechem International Inc; 2005. Fundamentals of Clinical Trials; p. 178.
28. Lai SL. Ch 1. Guangdong: People's Publishing House; 2000. Clinical Trials of Traditional Chinese Materia Medica.
29. Leung PC. Textbook of Clinical Trials. In: Machin D, Day S, Green S, editors. 1st ed. John Wiley and Sons: Chichester; 2004. pp. 63–84.
30. Manila: World Health Organization, Western Pacific Region; 2000a. World Health Organization. Traditional and Modern Medicine, Harmonizing the Two Approaches.
31. Mason S, Tovey P, Long AF. Evaluating complementary medicine: Methodological challenges of randomised controlled trials. BMJ. 2002;325:832–4.
32. Mills S. Clinical Research in Complementary Therapies: Principles, Problems and Solutions. In: Lewith GT, Jonas WB, Walach H, editors. Elsevier Science: Churchill Livingstone; 2003. pp. 211–27.
33. New Delhi: Regional Office for South-East Asia; 2003b. World Health Organization. Guidelines for the regulation of herbal medicines in the South-East Asia Region.
34. Palevitch D, Earon G, Carasso R. Feverfew (Tanacetum parthenium) as a prophylactic treatment for migraine: A double-blind placebo-controlled study. Phytother Res. 1997;11:508–11.

35. Protocols Developed by Central Council for Research in Ayurvedic Sciences (http://www.ccras.nic.in/)

36. Richardson J. The use of randomized control trials in complementary therapies: Exploring the issues. J Adv Nurs. 2000;32:398–406.

37. Shetti S, Kumar CD, Sriwastava NK, Sharma IP. The growing use of herbal medicines: Issues relating to adverse reactions and challenges in monitoring safety. Front Pharmacol. 2014;4:177.

38. Skalli S, Soulaymani Bencheikh R. Safety monitoring of herb-drug interactions: A component of pharmacovigilance. Drug Saf. 2012;35:785–91.

39. US Food and Drug Administration. Guidance for Industry: Botanical drug products. 2004.

40. Walker LG, Anderson J. Testing complementary and alternative therapies within a research protocol. Eur J Cancer. 1999;35:1614–8.

41. WHO Guidelines on Safety Monitoring of Herbal Medicines in Pharmacovigilance Systems, World Health Organization, Geneva, 2004 (http://apps.who.int/ medicinedocs/ documents/ s7148e/s7148e.pdf)

Scan QR code to view the website/guidelines

- Clinical trial basics-

The Basics | National Institutes of Health (NIH)

CHAPTER 24

AYUSH Guidelines of Good Clinical Practices 2018

Introduction

Definitions

Traditional Medicine

Investigational ASU Drug/Patent or Proprietary Medicines

Pre-Clinical supporting data, Protocol and relevant components of Protocol, Ethical & Safety Considerations, Ethical Principles, Ethics Committee, Informed Consent Process, Responsibilities (Sponsor, Monitor, Investigator), Data safety management, Record Keeping and Data Handling, Quality Assurance, Statistics, Special Concerns,

Appendices

Appendix I: Guidelines for Evaluation of Ayurveda, Siddha and Unani Medicine

Appendix II: Ethical Issues (Ethical Guidelines for Biomedical Research Human Participants, Indian Council of Medical Research 2006

Appendix III: Investigator's Brochure (IB)

Appendix IV: Essential Documents

Further Reading

Introduction

The history of Good Clinical Practice (GCP) statute traces back to one of the oldest enduring traditions in the history of medicine. Ayurveda has emphasized much on ethical guidelines while treating a patient through medical/surgical interventions. Utmost priority has been accorded to ethical issues and prior consent of the patient was suggested in the Ayurvedic texts. Further it has been enlisted the qualities of a physician, drug, supporting para-medical staff and role and responsibilities of the patient to achieve success in managing a patient.

As the guiding ethical code it is primarily known for its edict to do no harm to the patient. However, the complexities of ASU medicine research necessitate a more elaborate set of guidelines that address a Physician's ethical and scientific responsibilities such as obtaining informed consent or disclosing risk while involved in ASU medicine research.

Good Clinical Practice is a set of guidelines which encompasses the design, conduct, termination, audit, analysis, reporting and documentation of the studies involving human subjects. The fundamental tenet of GCP is that in research on man, the interest of science and society should never take precedence over considerations related to the well being of the study subject. It aims to ensure that the studies are scientifically and ethically sound and that the clinical properties of the ASU medicine under investigation are properly documented. The guidelines seek to establish two cardinal principles: protection of the rights of human subjects and authenticity of ASU medicine clinical trial data generated.

These guidelines are formulated based on CDSCO Document on GCP Guidelines (2001) for Clinical Trials on Pharmaceutical Products. They should be followed for carrying out all ASU medicine research in India at all stages of drug development, whether prior or subsequent to product registration in India.

Definitions

Ayurveda Siddha Unani Drugs- Ayurvedic, Siddha or Unani drug includes all medicines intended for internal or external use for or in the diagnosis, treatment, mitigation or prevention of disease or disorder in human beings or animals, and manufactured exclusively in accordance with the formulae described in, the authoritative books of Ayurvedic, Siddha and Unani Tibb system of medicine, specified in the First Schedule;

Patent or Proprietary Medicine - In relation to Ayurvedic, Siddha or Unani Tibb systems of medicine of all formulations containing only such ingredients mentioned in the formulae described in the authoritative books of Ayurveda, Siddha or Unani Tibb system of medicine specified in the first Schedule, but does not include a medicine which is administered by parenteral route and also a formulation included in the authoritative books as specified in clause (a);

Phases of clinical trial for ASU drug / Patent or Proprietary Medicines

- **Human Pharmacology (Phase I)**
- **Therapeutic exploratory trials (Phase II)**
- **Therapeutic confirmatory trials (Phase III)**
- **Post Marketing Trials (Phase IV)**

Traditional Medicine

'Traditional Medicine' / Folk medicine is the sum total of the knowledge, skills and practices based on the theories, beliefs and experiences indigenous to different cultures, societies, communities, folklores in India, used for the maintenance of health, as well as in the prevention, diagnosis, improvement or treatment of physical and mental illnesses, and which may not find a mention in the list of authoritative texts listed under First Schedule of Drugs and Cosmetics Act 1940.

Investigational ASU Drug/Patent or Proprietary Medicines: Physical, chemical (wherever available), pharmaceutical properties and the formulation of the Investigational ASU drug / Patent or Proprietary Medicines must be documented to permit appropriate safety measures to be taken during the course of a study. Instructions for the storage and handling of the dosage form should be documented.

Pre-clinical supporting data	The available pre-clinical data and clinical information on the Investigational ASU drug / Patent or Proprietary Medicines should be adequate and convincing to support the proposed study as per guidelines.
Protocol	A well designed study relies predominantly on a thoroughly considered, well-structured and complete protocol.
	Relevant components of Protocol: Same as CDSCO Guidelines o **Study design**: Same as CDSCO Guidelines. Information on Anupan, Desh, Kala, Pratyatmniyata, or Paynaya/pathya, samprpti vighatan etc. and /other relevant scientific considerations of respective system of medicine if appropriate and required. o **Inclusion, Exclusion and Withdrawal of Subjects:** Same as CDSCO Guidelines. Questionnaire for Prakriti evaluation if applicable.
Ethical & Safety Considerations	Same as CDSCO Guidelines
Ethical Principles	Same as CDSCO Guidelines
Ethics Committee	**Same as CDSCO Guidelines** **Composition:** The composition may be as follows:- 1. Chairperson 2. 1-2 basic medical scientists (one pharmacologist and one preferably from Dravyaguna / Rasshastra / Bhaishajya Kalpana or Gunapadam or Ilm-ul advia /Taklis-Wa-Dawa-Sazi). 3. 2 clinicians from various Institutes, one out of which should be from respective system 4. One legal expert or retired judge 5. One social scientist / representative of non-governmental voluntary agency 6. One philosopher / ethicist / theologian 7. One lay person from the community 8. Member Secretary 9. One expert member of ASU

Contd...

Informed Consent Process	Same as CDSCO Guidelines Following topics are discussed in detail in these guidelines: • Informed Consent Form with Participant/ Patient Information Sheet. • Fresh or re-consent is taken in following conditions: • Waiver of consent • Obligations of investigators regarding informed consent • Essential information for prospective research participants: • Compensation for Participation • Conflict of Interest • Selection of Special Groups as Research Participants o *Pregnant or nursing women* o *Children* o *Vulnerable groups* • Essential Information on Confidentiality for Prospective Research Participants • Compensation for Accidental Injury • Post-Trial Access
Responsibilities	***Sponsor, Monitor, Investigator:*** **Same as CDSCO Guidelines** Qualifications of investigator should be qualified by education, training and experience to assume responsibility for the proper conduct of the study and should have qualifications prescribed by the Central Council of Indian Medicine (CCIM)/. Medical Council of India (MCI)/Dental council of India (DCI). However, if the clinical trial is conducted in allopathic hospital, one Investigator / Co-Investigator must be from respective ASU system. If investigational products of more than one system are used, then investigator from all respective systems should be included in the study as Co-investigator(s).
Data safety management	**Same as CDSCO Guidelines**
Record Keeping and Data Handling	**Same as CDSCO Guidelines**
Quality Assurance	**Same as CDSCO Guidelines**
Statistics	**Same as CDSCO Guidelines**
Special Concerns	**Same as CDSCO Guidelines** Panchakarma including Snehana, Swedana, Dhara, Pizhichil and para-surgical procedures like Ksharasutra, Leech therapy, Agni karma, Hajamat, Hammam, NutulDalk, Riazat, Prachhanna, Raktamokshana, Tarpana, Vidalaka, Varmam etc. are special strength areas of ASU systems of medicine. Proper documentation of end point, procedure, standardization of ASU drug / Patent or Proprietary Medicines used in the procedures, parameters of evaluation, statistical consideration should be given special attention while conducting clinical trials on them.

Contd...

***Appendix III:* Investigator's Brochure (IB)**	The Investigator's Brochure is a compilation of the clinical and non-clinical data on the Investigational Product(s) that are relevant to a study of the product(s). It provides the investigator(s) and others involved in the study with the information on the rationale to facilitate compliance with the key features of the protocol, such as the dose, dose frequency/interval, methods of administration and safety monitoring procedures. The IB also provides background material to support the clinical management of the study subjects. The information contained in the IB should be in a concise, simple, objective, balanced, and non-promotional form to enable an understanding unbiased risk-benefit assessment of the appropriateness of the proposed trial.
***APPENDIX IV:* Essential Documents (for the conduct of a Clinical Trial)**	The various Essential Documents needed for different stages of the study are classified under three groups: 1. before the clinical phase of the study commences, 2. during the clinical conduct of the study, and 3. after completion or termination of the study.

Further Reading

1. General Guidelines for Methodologies on Research and Evaluation of Traditional Medicine, World Health Organization 2000 (http://whqlibdoc.who.int/hq/2000/WHO_EDM_TRM_2000.1.pdf)
2. Ethical Guidelines for Biomedical Research on Human Participants- ICMR 2006 (http://icmr.nic.in/ethical_guidelines.pdf)
3. Good Clinical Practices for Clinical Research in India, Central Drugs Standard Control Organization, Directorate General of Health Services, Ministry of Health and Family Welfare, Government of India, (http://cdsco.nic.in/html/GCP.htm)
4. Guideline for Good Clinical Practice, E6(R1), International Conference on Harmonisation of Technical Requirements for Registration of Pharmaceuticals for Human Use (http://www.ich.org/fileadmin/Public_Web_Site/ICH_Products/ Guidelines/Efficacy/E6_R1/Step4/E6_R1__Guideline.pdf)
5. Drug and Cosmetic Act, 1940; Drugs and Cosmetics Rules 1945.
6. WHO Guidelines on Safety Monitoring of Herbal Medicines in Pharmacovigilance Systems, World Health Organization, Geneva, 2004(http://apps.who.int/ medicinedocs/documents/s7148e/s7148e.pdf)
7. Protocols Developed by Central Council for Research in Ayurvedic Sciences (http://www.ccras.nic.in/)

Scan QR code to view the website/guidelines

- AYUSH Guidelines Clinical evaluation-
CCRS_Clinical _BOOK-6_945-CD MATTER.pdf (ccras.nic.in)

CHAPTER 25

CDSCO Guidelines of Good Clinical Practices 2013

Introduction

The history of Good Clinical Practice (GCP) statute traces back to one of the oldest enduring traditions in the history of medicine: The Hippocratic Oath. As the guiding ethical code it is primarily known for its edict to do no harm to the patient. However, the complexities of modern medicine research necessitate a more elaborate set of guidelines that address a Physician's ethical and scientific responsibilities such as obtaining informed consent or disclosing risk while involved in biomedical research.

Following are Regulatory bodies in India involved in Drug regulations:	
Central Drugs Standard Control Organisation (CDSCO)	Regulates drugs in India under ministry of health and family welfare
Drugs Controller General India (DCGI)	Assess the quality, safety and efficacy of drugs
Indian council of medical research (ICMR)	Formulates, promotes and coordinates biomedical research
Drugs Consultative Committee (DCC)	Provides technical guidance to the CDSCO
Central Drugs Laboratory (CDL)	National statutory laboratory of the Indian government for quality control of drugs
Drugs Technical Advisory Board (DTAB)	Provides technical advice to the CDSCO.

Good Clinical Practice is a set of guidelines for biomedical studies which encompasses the design, conduct, termination, audit, analysis, reporting and documentation of the studies involving human subjects. The fundamental tenet of GCP is that in research on man, the interest of science and society should never take precedence over considerations related to the well being of the study subject. It aims to ensure that the studies are scientifically and ethically sound and that the clinical properties of the pharmaceutical substances under investigation are properly documented. The guidelines seek to establish two cardinal principles: protection of the rights of human subjects and authenticity of biomedical data generated.

Highlight

The clinical trials can be initiated only

- After permission from the Drugs Controller general India (DCGI)
- Approval from respective ethics committee and
- Mandatory registration on website www.ctri.in being maintained by ICMR before the enrolment of the first trial participant for the clinical trial

These guidelines have been evolved with consideration of WHO, ICH, USFDA and European GCP guidelines as well as the Ethical Guidelines for Biomedical research on Human Subjects issued by the Indian Council of Medical Research. They should be followed for carrying out all biomedical research in India at all stages of drug development, whether prior or subsequent to product registration in India.

Content of CDSCO Good Clinical Practice Guidelines is as follows:

Introduction

Pre-requisites for the study

- Investigational Pharmaceutical Product
- Pre-Clinical supporting data
- Protocol
- Relevant components of Protocol
  - General Information
  - Objectives and Justification
  - Ethical Considerations
  - Study design
  - Inclusion, Exclusion & Withdrawal of Subjects
  - Handling of the Product(s)
  - Assessment of Efficacy
  - Assessment of Safety
  - Statistics
  - Data handling and management
  - Quality control and quality assurance
  - Finance and Insurance
  - Publication policy
  - Evaluation

Ethical & Safety Considerations

- Ethical Principles
- Ethics Committee
  - Basic Responsibilities
  - Composition
  - Terms of Reference
  - Review Procedures
  - Submission of Application
  - Decision Making Process
  - Interim Review
  - Record Keeping
  - Special Considerations

Informed Consent Process

- Informed Consent of Subject
- Essential information for prospective research subjects
- Informed Consent in Non-Therapeutic Study
- Essential Information on Confidentiality for Prospective Research Subjects
- Compensation for Participation
- Selection of Special Groups As Research Subject:.Pregnant or nursing women, Children, Vulnerable groups
- Compensation for Accidental Injury

Responsibilities

Sponsor

- Investigator and Institution Selection
- Contract
- SOP
- Allocation of duties and responsibilities
- Study management, data handling and record keeping

Contd...

- Compensation for Participation
- Confirmation of review by the Ethics Committee
- Information on Investigational Products
- Supply, storage and handling of Pharmaceutical Products
- Safety Information
- Adverse Drug Reaction Reporting
- Study Reports
- Monitoring
- Audit
- Multicentre Studies
- Premature Termination or Suspension of a Study
- Role of Foreign Sponsor

Monitor

- Qualifications
- Responsibilities

Investigator

- Qualifications
- Medical Care of the Study Subjects
- Monitoring and Auditing of records
- Communication with Ethic Committee
- Compliance with the Protocol
- Investigational Product(s)
- Selection and recruitment of Study Subjects
- Records/Reports

Record Keeping and Data Handling

- Documentation
- Corrections
- Electronic Data Processing
- Validation of Electronic Data Processing Systems
- Language
- Responsibility of Investigator
- Responsibilities of Sponsor and Monitor

Quality Assurance

Statistics

- Role of Biostatistician
- Study design
- Randomisation and Blinding
- Statistical Analysis

Special Concerns

- Clinical Trials of Vaccines: Phases of Vaccine Trials, Guidelines
- Clinical Trials of contraceptives
- Clinical Trials with Surgical Procedures / Medical devices:Definitions, Guidelines
- Clinical Trials for Diagnostic agents – Use of radioactive materials and X-rays Guidelines
- Clinical Trials of Herbal Remedies and Medicinal Plants: Categories of Herbal Product, Guidelines

Appendices

Types of Clinical Trials

Observational Studies	Interventional Studies (Blinded or non-blinded trials)
1. Descriptive • Case report • Case series • Population	1. Randomised controlled trials • Placebo • No treatment control • Historical control • Active control
2. Analytical • Cohort: Prospective, retrospective, Time series • Case control • Cross sectional • Ecological	2. Adaptive trials 3. Non-randomised trials

GSR/notification with date	Amendment/gazette notification/regulation
SO 1468 (E); September 06, 2005	Devices such as cardiac stents, heart valves, intravenous cannulas, catheters, orthopedic implants, and internal prosthetic replacements specified as "drugs
GSR 53 (E); January 30, 2013	" Introduction of "compensation for clinical trial-related injury or death.
GSR 63 (E); February 01, 2013	Introduction of SAE analysis and timelines for reporting SAEs Requirement conditions for conduct of clinical trials
GSR 72 (E); February 08, 2013	Introduction of clinical trial inspections and actions in case of noncompliance Registration of ECs with DCGI made mandatory
File No GCT/20/SC/ClinJ2013 DCGI; November 19, 2013	Introduction of AV recording of informed consent process of clinical trials
File no 12-01/14-DC Pt 47; July 03, 2014	Clinical trial waiver for approval of new drugs already approved outside India specified
	under certain conditions-national emergency, extreme urgency, epidemic and orphan drugs and drugs indicated for diseases in which no therapy exists
File no. ECR/Misc/Indt.EC/007/2013; July 30, 2017	Independent ECs registered by CDSCO to oversee BA/BE studies only
GSR 889 (E); December 12, 2014	Clarification regarding compensation in case of trial-related injury
	Change in timelines for SAE reporting
GSR 611 (E); July 31, 2015	Modification and relaxation of AV consenting norms- for "vulnerable" populations only and where a "NCE" or "NME" is being studied
GSR 313 (E); March 6, 2016	A "new" drug undergoing a clinical trial for IIS no longer needs approval from the DCGI. Approval from the IEC would suffice
File 12-01/14-Pt 47; August 02, 2016	The only three trials per investigator norm revoked
Circular by CDSCO; August 02, 2016	The condition that trials could not be conducted at sites with<50 beds revoked Only IEC permission required for addition of new trial site or investigator (no DCGI approval)
CDSCO/IT/2015 (48); September 05, 2016	"SUGAM" portal for online applications for clinical trials

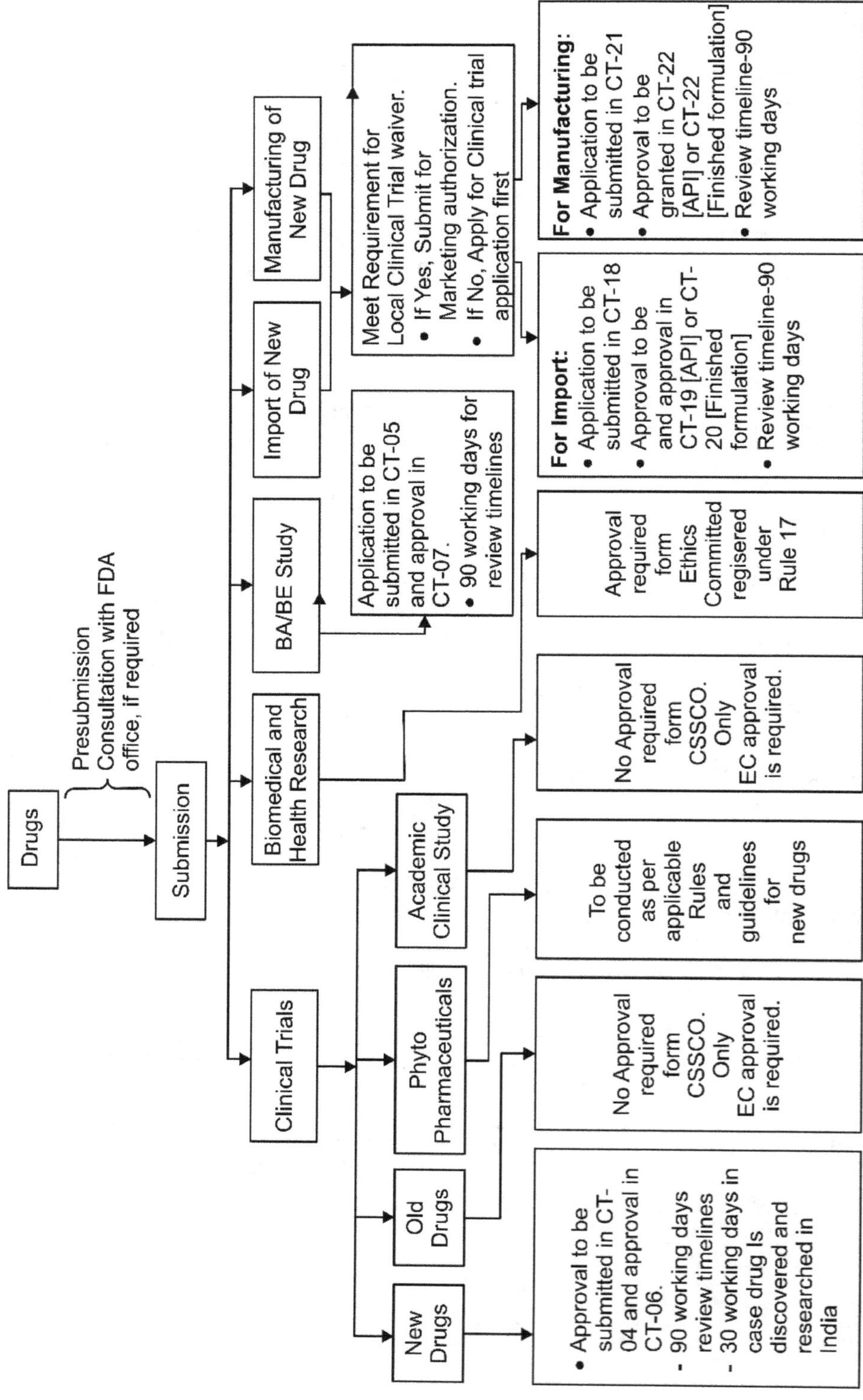
Drugs
Presubmission Consultation with FDA office, if required
Submission
Clinical Trials
Biomedical and Health Research
BA/BE Study
Import of New Drug
Manufacturing of New Drug
New Drugs
Old Drugs
Phyto Pharmaceuticals
Academic Clinical Study
• Approval to be submitted in CT-04 and approval in CT-06.
- 90 working days review timelines
- 30 working days in case drug Is discovered and researched in India
No Approval required form CSSCO. Only EC approval is required.
To be conducted as per applicable Rules and guidelines for new drugs
No Approval required form CSSCO. Only EC approval is required.
Approval required form Ethics Committed regisered under Rule 17
Application to be submitted in CT-05 and approval in CT-07.
• 90 working days for review timelines
Meet Requirement for Local Clinical Trial waiver.
• If Yes, Submit for Marketing authorization.
• If No, Apply for Clinical trial application first
For Import:
• Application to be submitted in CT-18
• Approval to be and approval in CT-19 [API] or CT-20 [Finished formulation]
• Review timeline-90 working days
For Manufacturing:
• Application to be submitted in CT-21
• Approval to be granted in CT-22 [API] or CT-22 [Finished formulation]
• Review timeline-90 working days

Table 3: Overall comparison of new rules with former rules.

Sl. No.	Key features	New Drugs and Clinical trials Rules, 2019	Former rules
1	Clarity of terms and definition	Terms like biomedical and health research, clinical trial site, efficacy, Good clinical practice guidelines, orphan drugs, post-trail access, A registered pharmacist, similar biologic and trial subjects are clearly defined.	Not clearly defined
2	Reorganisation of term New drug	The definition has been extended to for sustained or modified released formulation or a novel drug which has been approved earlier and shall be considered new for 4 years from the date of approval.	Sustained or modified released formulation or a novel drug was not regarded as a new drug for 4 years after approval
3	Significance of Central Licensing Authority (CLA)	CLA will be the drug controller nominated by the Central Government and who is not below the rank of Assistant Drug Controller (India). He can delegate his powers after obtaining the consent from central government to the officers of CDSCO who is not below the rank of assistant drug controller.	Delegation of powers was limited to signing the license and registration certificate and the powers can be given to any person who the licensing authority wishes for after obtaining approval from the central government.
4	Amendments in the constitution of ethics committee	Minimum of 50% members nominated must be outside the organization in which the ethics committee is constituted. It also mandates the requirement of at least one woman in the committee.	Not highlighted on this requirement
5	Responsibility of ethics committee	Rules highlights on the training that every member must undergo in order to be eligible for an ethics committee.	Rule compelled that the members of an ethics committee must be familiar with the schedules of clinical trials, he must follow good clinical practices and must follow the principles to protect human subjects.
6	Validity of approved licence	5 years, the renewal must be done 90 days prior to the expiry of license.	3 years
7	Timelines for reporting changes in the constitution of ethics committee	Reported within 30 working days to the central licensing authority	Timeline was not lucid
8	Maintenance of records and the documents required	5 years from the date of completion of trials. Documents submitted are Recommendation given by Ethics Committee for determination of compensation. Records relating to the serious adverse event, medical management of trial subjects and compensation paid	5 years from the date of completion of trials. No compulsion on the requirement of specific documents.
9	Responsibility of ethics committee in the aspect of conducting trials for biomedical and health research	Compelled to follow National Ethical Guidelines for Biomedical and Health Research Involving Human Participants. The ethics committee must register with authority as stated by central government in the Ministry of Health and Family Welfare, Department of Health Research.	Ethics committee must be registered with DCGI office under rule 122DD.
10	Application filed for conducting clinical trials	CT-04	Form 44
11	Consent granted in the form of application	CT-06	No specific application, permission is granted through an application letter

<table>
<tr><th colspan="2">New Rules, 2019</th></tr>
<tr><td>Revised Fees Structure</td><td>
<table>
<tr><th colspan="4">New and Old License applications Fees structure</th></tr>
<tr><th colspan="2">Types of applications</th><th>New Fee structure (2019)</th><th>Old Fees Structure</th></tr>
<tr><td>Clinical trials</td><td>Phase-I</td><td>3,00,000</td><td>50000</td></tr>
<tr><td></td><td>Phase-II & III</td><td>2,00,000</td><td>25000</td></tr>
<tr><td></td><td>Phase-IV</td><td>50,000</td><td>No Fees</td></tr>
<tr><td colspan="2">Bioavaibility-Bio equivalence (BA/BE) study</td><td>2,00,000</td><td>25000 (drugs approved within 1 year) 15,000 (Drugs b/w 1 to 4 years)</td></tr>
<tr><td colspan="2">Registration of bioavailability-bioequivalence study centre</td><td>5,00,000</td><td>No Fees</td></tr>
<tr><td rowspan="3">Reconsideration of</td><td>Clinical trial application</td><td>50,000</td><td>No Fees</td></tr>
<tr><td>BA/BE Study application</td><td>50,000</td><td>No Fees</td></tr>
<tr><td>BA/BE Centre study application</td><td>50,000</td><td>No Fees</td></tr>
</table>
</td></tr>
<tr><td>Ethics Committees (ECs)</td><td>As per new rules, ECs need to include at least one female member and 50% of membership must consist of those who are not affiliated with the institution or organization in which the committee is constituted. The new rules also mandate each EC member to undergo such training and development programs as may be specified from time-to-time by CLA. Further, any change in membership or constitution of registered E, is to be reported to CLA in writing within 30 working days. ECs will have to go through reconstitution (and subsequent re-registration) to comply with new rules before taking up any new CTs for review. ECs reviewing biomedical and health research proposals should register by using Form CT-01 with the authority designated by the Department of Health Research (and not with the CLA), within the Ministry of Health (MoH). Initially, provisional registration would be granted, with a validity of two years. Subsequently, based on scrutiny of the documents furnished, the designated authority may grant final registration using Form CT-03.</td></tr>
<tr><td>Academic Clinical Trials</td><td>• only for approved drug
• CT initiated by investigator, academic or research institute
• can be conducted for new indication, new route, new dose or dosage form
• results only for academic or research purpose and not for commercial purpose. Data cannot be used for seeking approval in any country
• EC can seek clarity from Central Licensing Authority (CLA) and CLA must respond in 30 days (or deemed that no approval is needed)
• medical management and compensation is applicable as per ICMR Guidelines for Biomedical Research on Human Participants</td></tr>
</table>

	• academic CTs are required to be conducted in accordance with the CT protocol approved by the EC and ethical principles specified in the ICMR *Guidelines for Biomedical Research on Human Participants*
Regulations on Biomedical and Health Research (BHR)	The study types include: • *In Vitro* Diagnostics (*IVDs*) performance testing for research • new surgical intervention • Assisted Reproductive Technology (ART) • public health survey • epidemiological health survey • observational and non-interventional study of old drug These types of studies would be approved by ethics committees constituted under Rule 16 and registered under Rule 17 with CDSCO office as the "Ethics Committee for Biomedical and Health Research." Apart from approving such studies, ethics committees also are responsible for medical management and compensation for injury or death in these types of studies. Rules applicable to biomedical and health research would be applicable from 15 September 2019. Twelve (12) new drug advisory committees (NDAC) and six (6) medical device advisory committees have been constituted. Fresh Applications of clinical trial proposals of new drug (INDs) are being evaluated by these committees. All IND applications are evaluated by IND Committees.
Presubmission Meeting	*New Rules, 2019* has included a provision for presubmission meetings with the CLA or any other officer authorized by the CLA for seeking guidance about the requirements of laws and procedures for obtaining license or permission of manufacturing processes, clinical trials and other requirements. The application for a presubmission meeting should be accompanied by documents referred to in the Second Schedule, as available with the applicant to support their proposal along with a fee specified in the Sixth Schedule. CLA, within a period of 30 days, will relate the facts to the applicant in writing and direct them to provide further information or documents as necessary.
Revising New Drug Definition	The definition of 'new drugs' has been revised to include following: • phytopharmaceutical drugs • novel drug delivery system of any drug • living modified organisms, monoclonal anti-body, stem cell-derived products and gene therapeutic products or xenografts, intended to be used as drug New drugs are classified into two categories. The first category would convert to an old drug after four years of its approval; the second category has always been considered 'new drugs,' irrespective of the period since they were first approved by the CLA. Class (i) is part of first category and Class (ii) and (iii) are part of second category. Sustained release and modified release dosage forms have been moved from the first category to the second. For products in the second category, CTs and marketing approvals undertaken with these products would legally come under the control of CLA. Even for generic products (after four years of innovator approval) companies first need to take approval from CLA, followed by State FDA, for local manufacturing. For sustained and modified release dosage forms, there would be additional timelines for generic product approval, as this would be first approved by CLA.

<table>
<tr><td>Phase IV and Postmarketing Studies (PMS)</td><td>Previously, there was ambiguity in the definition and requirements for Phase IV and PMS. New Rules, 2019 have differentiated the requirements for conducting Phase 4 CT and postmarketing surveillance studies for new drugs. In New Rules, 2019, Phase IV Study would include studies related to:
drug-drug interactions
dose-response or safety studies
trials designed to support use under the approved indications
In such trials, the ethical aspects for protection of rights, safety and well-being of the trial subjects will be followed as per the regulatory provisions, including that for compensation in case of clinical trial-related injury or death and good clinical practices guidelines. Study drugs should be provided to the trial subject free-of-cost in such studies, unless there is a specific concern or justification for not providing the drug free-of-cost after approval from CLA and the EC.</td></tr>
<tr><td>Postmarketing Surveillance Studies</td><td>Such studies are conducted with a new drug under approved conditions of its use and with a scientific objective approved by CLA. Inclusion or exclusion of subjects are decided as per recommended use in the prescribing information or approved package insert. In such studies, the study drugs included in the protocol are a part of the patient's treatment according to prescriber's directions. The regulatory provisions and guidelines applicable for clinical trial of a new drug are not applicable when a drug is already approved for marketing.</td></tr>
<tr><td>Difference Between Phase IV and Postmarketing Studies From Regulations Perspective</td><td>
<table>
<tr><th></th><th>Phase IV</th><th>PMS</th></tr>
<tr><td>Approval required from CLA</td><td colspan="2">Approval required in case of new drug and not in case of old drug*</td></tr>
<tr><td>Drugs to be provided</td><td>Study drug to be provided</td><td>Discretion of applicant</td></tr>
<tr><td>Design</td><td>As per study protocol design</td><td>As per prescribing information</td></tr>
<tr><td>Compensation</td><td>Applicable</td><td>Not applicable</td></tr>
<tr><td>Fees</td><td>INR 200,000 ($2,900)</td><td>Not applicable</td></tr>
<tr><td colspan="3">* Advised to check with CDSCO if truly old drug</td></tr>
</table>
There is an expectation that number of Phase IV studies being conducted in India will increase. This expectation is based on the assumption that with local clinical trial waiver, a Phase IV study might need to be conducted, except in special situations.</td></tr>
<tr><td>Orphan Drug Registration</td><td>• New Rules, 2019 define orphan drugs as a "drug intended to treat a condition which affects not more than five lakh (500,000) persons in India." To promote research in orphan drugs, there has been favorable provisions in New Rules, 2019 as follows:
provision for fast-track approval process and special status for orphan drugs, including a complete fee waiver for CT filing
• provision for expeditious review process. In situations where the evidence for clinical safety and efficacy have been established. Even if the drug has not completed all clinical trial phases, the sponsor or applicant may apply to the CLA for expedited review process. After accelerated approval, applicants could be required to conduct postmarketing trials for validating anticipated clinical benefits
• provision for waiver of local clinical study and Phase IV on satisfaction of CLA</td></tr>
</table>

These guidelines are also applicable to clinical Trials of Vaccines, surgical procedures/ medical devices and Diagnostic Agents - Use of Radio-active Materials and X- Raysunder special Concerns. All procedures for clinical trials are applicable**to Contraceptives**. Subjects should be clearly informed about the alternative available. In women where implant has been used as a contraceptive for trial, a proper follow up for removal of the implant should be done, whether the trial is over or the subject has withdrawn from the trial. Children borne due to failure of contraceptives under study should be followed up for any abnormalities if the woman does not opt for medical termination of pregnancy.

Clinical trials of Herbal Remedies and Medicinal Plants

For the herbal remedies and medicinal plants that are to be clinically evaluated for use in the Allopathic System and which may later be used in allopathic hospitals, the procedures laid down by the office of the DCG (I) for allopathic drugs should be followed. This does not pertain to guidelines issued for clinical evaluation of Ayurveda, Siddha or Unani drugs by experts in those systems of medicine which may be used later in their own hospitals and clinics. All the general principles of clinical trials described earlier pertain also to herbal remedies. However, when clinical trials of herbal drugs used in recognized Indian systems of Medicine and Homoeopathy are to be undertaken in Allopathic Hospitals, associations of physicians from the concerned system as co-investigators/ collaborators/ members of the expert group is desirable for designing and evaluating the Study.

Categories of Herbal Products: The herbal products can belong to any of the three categories given below:

(a) A lot is known about the use of a plant or its extract in the ancient Ayurveda, Siddha or Unani literature or the plant may actually be regularly used by physicians of the traditional systems of medicine for a number of years. The substance is being clinically evaluated for same indication for which it is being used or as has been described in the texts.

(b) When an extract of a plant or a compound isolated from the plant has to be clinically evaluated for a therapeutic effect not originally described in the texts of traditional systems or, the method of preparation is different, it has to be treated as a new substance or new chemical entity (NCE) and the same type of acute, subacute and chronic toxicity data will have to be generated as required by the regulatory authority before it is cleared for clinical evaluation.

(c) An extract or a compound isolated from a plant which has never been in use before and has not ever been mentioned in ancient literature, should be treated as a new drug, and therefore, should undergo all regulatory requirements before being evaluated clinically.

Guidelines

- It is important that plants and herbal remedies currently in use or mentioned in literature of recognized Traditional System of Medicine is prepared strictly in the same way as described in the literature while incorporating GMP norms for standardization. It may not be necessary to undertake phase I studies. However, it needs to be emphasized that since the substance to be tested is already in used in Indian Systems of Medicine or has been described in their texts, the need for testing its toxicity in animals has been considerably reduced. Neither would any toxicity study be needed for phase II trial unless there are reports suggesting toxicity or when the herbal preparation is to be used for more than 3 months. It should be necessary to undertake 4-6 weeks toxicity study in 2 species of animals in the circumstances pointed out in the preceding sentence or when a larger multicentric phase III trial is subsequently planned based on results of phase II study.

- Clinical trials with herbal preparations should be carried out only after these have been standardized and markers identified to ensure that the substances being evaluated are always the same. The recommendations made earlier regarding informed consent, subject, inducements for participation, information to be provided to the subject, withdrawal from study and research involving children or persons with diminished autonomy, all apply to trials on plant drugs also. These trials have also got to be approved by the appropriate scientific and ethical committees of the concerned Institutes. However, it is essential that such clinical trials be carried out only when a competent Ayurvedic, Siddha or Unani physician is a co-investigator in such a clinical trial. It would neither ethically acceptable nor morally justifiable, if an allopathic physician, based on references in ancient literature of above-mentioned traditional systems of Medicine, carries out clinical evaluation of the plant without any concept or training in these systems of medicine. Hence, it is necessary to associate a specialist from these systems and the clinical evaluation should be carried out jointly.
- When a Folklore medicine / Ethno-medicine is ready for commercialisation after it has been scientifically found to be effective, then the legitimate rights/ share of the Tribe or Community from whom the knowledge was gathered should be taken care of appropriately while applying for the Intellectual Property Rights and / Patents for the product.

Appendices

- Appendix I: Declaration of Helsinki [For details see chapter 28]
- Appendix II: Schedule Y [For details see chapter 29]
- Appendix III: Format for submission of Pre-clinical and clinical data for r-DNA based vaccines, diagnostics and other biologicals. [For details visit CDSCO Website]
- Appendix IV: Investigator's Brochure [For details visit CDSCO Website]
- Appendix V: Essential Documents [For details visit CDSCO Website]

Further Reading

1. Frequently Asked Questions (FAQs) on New Drugs and Clinical Trialfaqnd.pdf (cdsco.gov.in)Accessed in Dec 2020
2. European Medicines Agency. ICH Harmonised Tripartite Guideline E6: Note for Guidance on Good Clinical Practice (PMP/ICH/135/95) London: European Medicines Agency; 2002.

3. https://cdsco.gov.in/opencms/opencms/en/Clinical-Trial/clinical-trials/ Accessed in Dec 2020
4. https://database.ich.org/sites/default/files/E6_R2_Addendum.pdf Accessed in Dec 2020
5. Kumar M, Kher S. Regulatory Considerations for Conducting Clinical Trials in India. Regulatory Affairs Focus. 2007;12(3):26-31.
6. Kumar M, Tate K. Designing a Global Product Development strategy. Regulatory Affairs Focus. 2008;13(6):16-21.
7. Kumar M. Agencies Involved in Approving Clinical Trials in India. Regulatory Affairs Focus. 2007;12(8):34-9.
8. Office of Human Subjects Research. The Nuremberg Code [Web Page] 1949. Available at http://ohsr.od.nih.gov/guidelines/nuremberg.
9. Otte A, et al. Good Clinical Practice: Historical background and key aspects. 2005;26:563–74.
10. Schedule – Y, Amendment version 2005, Drugs and Cosmetics Rules, 1945 Available online https://rgcb.res.in/documents/Schedule-Y.pdf. Accessed Feb. 2021
11. The Doctors Trial (the Medical Case of the Subsequent Nuremberg Proceedings) [Web Page] Available at http://www.ushmm.org/research/doctors/Nuremberg_Code.htm.
12. The World Medical Association. Declaration of Helsinki [Web Page] 2004. Available at http://www.wma.net/e/policy/b3.htm.
13. Vadivale M. ICH-GCP Guidelines for Clinical Trials. Berita MMA. 1999;7(29)
14. Vijayananthan A, Nawawi O. The importance of Good Clinical Practice guidelines and its role in clinical trials. Biomed Imaging Interv J. 2008;4(1):e5. doi:10.2349/biij.4.1.e5
15. www.clinicaltrials.gov Accessed Feb. 2021
16. WHO 1995. Guidelines for Good Clinical Practice (GCP) for Trials on Pharmaceutical Products. World Health Organization, WHO Technical Series, No. 850, 1995, Annex 3

Scan QR code to view the website/guidelines

- Indian GCP Guidelines- cdsco.gov.in/opencms/opencms/system/modules/CDSCO.WEB/elements/download_file_division.jsp?num_id=MzM5NQ==

CHAPTER 26

Ethical Principles for Clinical Trials

Introduction

Ethics in clinical research focuses largely on identifying and implementing the acceptable conditions for exposure of some individuals to risks and burdens for the benefit of society at large. Ethical guidelines for clinical research were formulated only after discovery of inhumane behavior with participants during research experiments. World War II led the states to take more interest in science and research resulting in initiation of larger, systematic clinical investigations to gain knowledge for better treatment of patients, especially the soldiers. Most of the studies were carried out through defense efforts and used mainly the prisoners without concern of their consent and well being. The discovery of these experiments stunned the whole world which led to formulation of Nuremberg code in Germany. The Nuremberg Code was the first international code laying ethical principles for clinical research. With increasing research all over, World Health Organization formulated guidelines in the form of Declaration of Helsinki in 1964. In 1982, the Council for International Organizations of Medical Sciences (CIOMS) in association with World Health Organization (WHO) developed 'International Ethical Guidelines for Biomedical Research Involving Human Subjects'. The US laid down its guidelines for ethical principles in the Belmont Report after discovery of the Tuskegee's Syphilis study. The Indian Council of Medical Research has laid down the 'Ethical Guidelines for Biomedical Research on Human Subjects' in the year 2000 which were revised in 2006.

Nuremberg 10 Point Code

Four American judges presiding issued a ten point code that described basic principles of ethical behavior in the conduct of human experimentation. This ten-point code is known as the Nuremberg Code. The Code is an "ethical standard" and reflects the modern thinking that:

1. Informed consent should be obtained without coercion.
2. The experiment should be useful and necessary.
3. Human experiments should be based on previous experiments with animals.
4. Physical and mental suffering should be avoided.
5. Death and disability should not be expected outcomes of an experiment.
6. The degree of risk to be taken should not exceed the humanitarian importance of solving the problem.
7. Human subjects should be protected against even remote possibilities of harm.
8. Only qualified scientists should conduct medical research.
9. Human subjects should be free to end an experiment at any time.
10. The scientist in charge must be prepared to end an experiment at any stage.

Belmont Report

The Belmont Report is a report created by the National Commission for the Protection of Human Subjects of Biomedical and Behavioral Research. Its full title is the Belmont Report: Ethical Principles and Guidelines for the Protection of Human Subjects of Research, Report of the National Commission for the Protection of Human Subjects of Biomedical and Behavioral Research.

The report, prompted in part by problems arising from the Tuskegee Syphilis Study (1932–1972), was issued on 30 September 1978 and published in the Federal Register on 18 April 1979. The report took its name from the Belmont Conference Center where the document was drafted in part.

The Belmont Report summarizes ethical principles and guidelines for research involving human subjects. Three core principles are identified: respect for persons, beneficence, and justice. Three primary areas of application are also stated. They are informed consent, assessment of risks and benefits, and selection of subjects. According to Vollmer and Howard, the Belmont Report allows for a positive solution, which at times may be difficult to find, to future subjects who are not capable to make independent decisions.

The Belmont Report explains the unifying ethical principles that form the basis for the National Commission's topic-specific reports and the regulations that incorporate its recommendations. The three fundamental ethical principles for using any human subjects for research are:

1. **Respect for persons**: protecting the autonomy of all people and treating them with courtesy and respect and allowing for informed consent. Researchers must be truthful and conduct no deception;
2. **Beneficence**: the philosophy of "Do no harm" while maximizing benefits for the research project and minimizing risks to the research subjects; and
3. **Justice**: ensuring reasonable, non-exploitative, and well-considered procedures are administered fairly — the fair distribution of costs and benefits to potential research participants — and equally.

These principles remain the basis for the United States Department of Health and Human Services (HHS) human subject protection regulations.

Today, the Belmont Report continues as an essential reference for Institutional Review Boards (IRBs) that review HHS-conducted or -supported human subjects research proposals involving human subjects, in order to ensure that the research meets the ethical foundations of the regulations.

Applications of these principles to conduct research requires careful consideration of i) informed consent, ii) risks benefit assessment, and iii) selection of subjects of research.

Nurses, as primary caregivers for individuals participating in a study, must do to ensure the rights of the participant are met.

1. Ensure the study is approved by an IRB
2. Get informed consent from the patient
3. Ensure that the patient understands the full extent of the experiment, and if not, will contact the study coordinator
4. Ensure the patient wasn't coerced into doing the experiment by means of threatening or bullying

5. Be careful of other effects of the clinical trial that were not mentioned, and report it to the proper study coordinator
6. Support the privacy of the patient's identity, their motivation to join or refuse the experiment.
7. Ensure that all patients at least get the minimal care needed for their condition

Today, the Belmont Report serves as a historical document and provides the moral framework for understanding regulations in the United States on the use of humans in experimental methods.

World Medical Association Declaration of Helsinki

The World Medical Association has developed the Declaration of Helsinki as a statement of ethical principles to provide guidance to physicians and other participants in medical research involving human subjects. Medical research involving human subjects includes research on identifiable human material or identifiable data. The Declaration of Geneva of the World Medical Association binds the physician with the words, "The health of my patient will be my first consideration," and the International Code of Medical Ethics declares that, "A physician shall act only in the patient's interest when providing medical care which might have the effect of weakening the physical and mental condition of the patient." Medical research is subject to ethical standards that promote respect for all human beings and protect their health and rights. Some research populations are vulnerable and need special protection. The particular needs of the economically and medically disadvantaged must be recognised. Special attention is also required for those who cannot give or refuse consent for themselves, for those who may be subject to giving consent under duress, for those who will not benefit personally from the research and for those for whom the research is combined with care.

Basic Principles under Declaration of Helsinki for All Medical Research

1. It is the duty of the physician in medical research to protect the life, health, privacy, and dignity of the human subject.
2. Medical research involving human subjects must conform to generally accepted scientific principles, be based on a thorough knowledge of the scientific literature, other relevant sources of information, and on adequate laboratory and, where appropriate, animal experimentation.
3. Appropriate caution must be exercised in the conduct of research which may affect the environment, and the welfare of animals used for research must be respected.
4. The design and performance of each experimental procedure involving human subjects should be clearly formulated in an experimental protocol. This protocol should be submitted for consideration, comment, guidance, and where appropriate, approval to a specially appointed ethical review committee, which must be independent of the investigator, the sponsor or any other kind of undue influence. This independent committee should be in conformity with the laws and regulations of the country in which the research experiment is performed. The committee has the right to monitor ongoing trials. The researcher has the obligation to provide monitoring information to the

committee, especially any serious adverse events. The researcher should also submit to the committee, for review, information regarding funding, sponsors, institutional affiliations, other potential conflicts of interest and incentives for subjects.

5. The research protocol should always contain a statement of the ethical considerations involved and should indicate that there is compliance with the principles enunciated in this Declaration.
6. Medical research involving human subjects should be conducted only by scientifically qualified persons and under the supervision of a clinically competent medical person. The responsibility for the human subject must always rest with a medically qualified person and never rest on the subject of the research, even though the subject has given consent.
7. Every medical research project involving human subjects should be preceded by careful assessment of predictable risks and burdens in comparison with foreseeable benefits to the subject or to others. This does not preclude the participation of healthy volunteers in medical research. The design of all studies should be publicly available.
8. Physicians should abstain from engaging in research projects involving human subjects unless they are confident that the risks involved have been adequately assessed and can be satisfactorily managed. Physicians should cease any investigation if the risks are found to outweigh the potential benefits or if there is conclusive proof of positive and beneficial results.
9. Medical research involving human subjects should only be conducted if the importance of the objective outweighs the inherent risks and burdens to the subject. This is especially important when the human subjects are healthy volunteers.
10. Medical research is only justified if there is a reasonable likelihood that the populations in which the research is carried out stand to benefit from the results of the research.
11. The subjects must be volunteers and informed participants in the research project.
12. The right of research subjects to safeguard their integrity must always be respected. Every precaution should be taken to respect the privacy of the subject, the confidentiality of the patient's information and to minimize the impact of the study on the subject's physical and mental integrity and on the personality of the subject.
13. In any research on human beings, each potential subject must be adequately informed of the aims, methods, sources of funding, any possible conflicts of interest, institutional affiliations of the researcher, the anticipated benefits and potential risks of the study and the discomfort it may entail. The subject should be informed of the right to abstain from participation in the study or to withdraw consent to participate at any time without reprisal. After ensuring that the subject has understood the information, the physician should then obtain the subject's freely given informed consent, preferably in writing. If the consent cannot be obtained in writing, the non-written consent must be formally documented and witnessed.
14. When obtaining informed consent for the research project the physician should be particularly cautious if the subject is in a dependent relationship with the physician or may consent under duress. In that case the informed consent should be obtained by a

well-informed physician who is not engaged in the investigation and who is completely independent of this relationship.

15. For a research subject who is legally incompetent, physically or mentally incapable of giving consent or is a legally incompetent minor, the investigator must obtain informed consent from the legally authorised representative in accordance with applicable law. These groups should not be included in research unless the research is necessary to promote the health of the population represented and this research cannot instead be performed on legally competent persons.
16. When a subject deemed legally incompetent, such as a minor child, is able to give assent to decisions about participation in research, the investigator must obtain that assent in addition to the consent of the legally authorised representative.
17. Research on individuals from whom it is not possible to obtain consent, including proxy or advance consent, should be done only if the physical/mental condition that prevents obtaining informed consent is a necessary characteristic of the research population. The specific reasons for involving research subjects with a condition that renders them unable to give informed consent should be stated in the experimental protocol for consideration and approval of the review committee. The protocol should state that consent to remain in the research should be obtained as soon as possible from the individual or a legally authorised surrogate.
18. Both authors and publishers have ethical obligations. In publication of the results of research, the investigators are obliged to preserve the accuracy of the results. Negative as well as positive results should be published or otherwise publicly available. Sources of funding, institutional affiliations and any possible conflicts of interest should be declared in the publication. Reports of experimentation not in accordance with the principles laid down in this Declaration should not be accepted for publication.

Additional Principles for Medical Research Combined With Medical Care

19. The physician may combine medical research with medical care, only to the extent that the research is justified by its potential prophylactic, diagnostic or therapeutic value. When medical research is combined with medical care, additional standards apply to protect the patients who are research subjects.
20. The benefits, risks, burdens and effectiveness of a new method should be tested against those of the best current prophylactic, diagnostic, and therapeutic methods. This does not exclude the use of placebo, or no treatment, in studies where no proven prophylactic, diagnostic or therapeutic method exists.
21. At the conclusion of the study, every patient entered into the study should be assured of access to the best proven prophylactic, diagnostic and therapeutic methods identified by the study.
22. The physician should fully inform the patient which aspects of the care are related to the research. The refusal of a patient to participate in a study must never interfere with the patient-physician relationship.

In the treatment of a patient, where proven prophylactic, diagnostic and therapeutic methods do not exist or have been ineffective, the physician, with informed consent from the patient, must be free to use unproven or new prophylactic, diagnostic and therapeutic measures, if in the physician's judgement it offers hope of saving life, re-establishing health or alleviating suffering. Where possible, these measures should be made the object of research, designed to evaluate their safety and efficacy. In all cases, new information should be recorded and, where appropriate, published. The other relevant guidelines of this Declaration should be followed.

Indian Perspective

The Indian Council of Medical Research (ICMR), in February 1980, released a 'Policy Statement on Ethical Considerations involved in Research on Human Subjects'. This was the first policy statement giving official guidelines for establishment of ethics committees (ECs) in all medical colleges and research centres. But as with other nations of the world, these guidelines were not respected by many researchers and India was not free of controversial research works. In 1970s and 1980s researchers at the Institute for Cytology and Preventive Oncology in New Delhi, carried out a study on 1158 women patients of different stages of cervical dysplasia or precancerous lesions of the cervix.

These patients were left untreated to see how many lesions progressed to cancer and how many regressed. By the end of the study seventy one women had developed malignancies and lesions in nine of them had progressed to invasive cancer. Sixty-two women were treated only after they developed localised cancer. After the controversy about the study became public in 1997, the ICMR started developing 'Ethical Guidelines for Biomedical Research on Human Subjects' and finalised them in the year 2000.

These are a set of guidelines which every researcher in India should follow while conducting research on human subjects. Although not a law, these guidelines have been put into force through **Schedule Y.** With the changing scenario in the research field and development of modern techniques, the guidelines were revised in 2006. These guidelines have elaborated the three basic ethical principles: respect for person, beneficence and justice by inducting twelve general principles as follows:

1. **Principle of essentiality**: The research being carried out should be essential for the advancement of knowledge that benefits patients, doctors and all others in aspects of health care and also for the ecological and environmental well being of the planet.
2. **Principles of voluntariness, informed consent and community agreement**: The research participant should be aware of the nature of research and the probable consequences of the experiments and then should make a independent choice without the influence of the treating doctor, whether to take part in the research or not. When the research treats any community or group of persons as a research participant, these principles of voluntariness and informed consent should apply to the community as a whole and also to each individual member who is the participant of the research or experiment.

3. **Principle of non-exploitation**: Research participants should be remunerated for their involvement in the research or experiment. The participants should be made aware of all the risks involved irrespective of their social and economic condition or educational levels attained. Each research protocol should include provisions of compensation for the human participants either through insurance cover or any other appropriate means to cover all foreseeable and hidden risks.
4. **Principle of privacy and confidentiality**: All the data acquired for research purpose should be kept confidential to prevent disclosure of identity of the involved participant and should not be disclosed without valid legal and/or scientific reasons.
5. **Principle of precaution and risk minimisation**: Due care and caution should be taken at all stages of the research and experiment (from its beginning as a research idea, formulation of research design/ protocol, conduct of the research or experiment and its subsequent applicative use) to prevent research participant from any harm and adverse events. EC has to play an active role in risk minimization.
6. **Principle of professional competence**: Clinical research should be carried out only by competent and qualified persons in their respective fields.
7. **Principle of accountability and transparency**: The researcher should conduct experiments in fair, honest, impartial and transparent manner after full disclosure of his/her interests in research. They should also retain the research data, subject to the principles of privacy and confidentiality, for a minimum period of 5 years, to be scrutinized by the appropriate legal and administrative authority, if necessary.
8. **Principle of the maximisation of the public interest and of distributive justice**: The results of the research should be used for benefit of all humans, especially the research participants themselves and/or the community from which they are drawn and not only to those who are socially better off.
9. **Principle of institutional arrangements:** It is required that all institutional arrangements required to be made in respect of the research and its subsequent use or applications should be duly made in transparent manner.
10. **Principle of public domain**: The results of any research work done should be made public through publications or other means. Even before publication, the detailed information of clinical trials should be made public before starts of recruitment via clinical trial registry systems that allow free online access like: www.ctri.in/; www.actr.org.au/; www.clinicaltrials.gov/ or www.isrctn.org/.
11. **Principle of totality of responsibility:** All those directly or indirectly connected with the research should take the professional and moral responsibility, for the due observance of all the principles, guidelines or prescriptions laid down in respect of the research.
12. **Principle of compliance**: All those associated with the research work should comply by the guidelines pertaining to the specific area of the research. For research to be conducted ethically we need to follow these twelve general principles laid down by the ICMR. In order to follow these principles we should be aware about the informed consent process, vulnerable population, therapeutic misconception, post trial access and structure and role of ethics committees. These concepts hold special importance in developing countries

like ours, as most of the research participants are uneducated and economically backwards, hence we discuss them here.

Ethical Principles of ICH GCP

1. Clinical trials should be conducted in accordance with the ethical principles that have their origin in the Declaration of Helsinki, and that are consistent with GCP and the applicable regulatory requirement(s).
2. Before a trial is initiated, foreseeable risks and inconveniences should be weighed against the anticipated benefit for the individual trial subject and society. A trial should be initiated and continued only if the anticipated benefits justify the risks.
3. The rights, safety, and well-being of the trial subjects are the most important considerations and should prevail over interests of science and society.
4. The available nonclinical and clinical information on an investigational product should be adequate to support the proposed clinical trial.
5. Clinical trials should be scientifically sound, and described in a clear, detailed protocol.
6. A trial should be conducted in compliance with the protocol that has received prior Institutional Review Board (IRB)/Independent Ethics Committee (IEC) approval/favourable opinion.
7. The medical care given to, and medical decisions made on behalf of, subjects should always be the responsibility of a qualified physician or, when appropriate, of a qualified dentist.
8. Each individual involved in conducting a trial should be qualified by education, training, and experience to perform his or her respective task(s).
9. Freely given informed consent should be obtained from every subject prior to clinical trial participation.
10. All clinical trial information should be recorded, handled, and stored in a way that allows its accurate reporting, interpretation and verification.

Addendum

1. This principle applies to all records referenced in this guideline, irrespective of the type of media used.
2. The confidentiality of records that could identify subjects should be protected, respecting the privacy and confidentiality rules in accordance with the applicable regulatory requirement(s).
3. Investigational products should be manufactured, handled, and stored in accordance with applicable good manufacturing practice (GMP). They should be used in accordance with the approved protocol.
4. Systems with procedures that assure the quality of every aspect of the trial should be implemented.

Further Reading

1. Anderson JA. The ethics and science of placebo-controlled trials: assay sensitivity and the Duhem–Quine thesis. J Med Philos. 2006;31:65–81.
2. Appelbaum PS, Lidz CW. In: The Therapeutic Misconception The Oxford Textbook of Clinical Research Ethics. Emanuel EJ, et al., editors. Oxford: Oxford University Press; 2008. pp. 633–43.
3. Berg JW, et al. Informed Consent: Legal Theory and Clinical Practice 2nd edn. New York: Oxford University Press; 2001.
4. Deng C, et al. Challenges of clinical trial design when there is lack of clinical equipoise: use of a response conditional crossover design. J Neurol. 2012;259:348–52.
5. Edwards SJ, et al. Ethical issues in the design and conduct of randomised controlled trials. Health Technol Assess. 1998;2(15):1–132.
6. Englev E, Petersen KP. ICH-GCP Guideline: kvalitetssikring af kliniske laegemiddelforsøg. Status og perspektiver [ICH-GCP Guideline: quality assurance of clinical trials. Status and perspectives]. Ugeskr Laeger. 2003 Apr 14;165(16):1659-62..
7. Freedman B. Equipoise and the ethics of clinical research. N Engl J Med. 1987;317: 141–5.
8. Giordano S. The 2008 Declaration of Helsinki: some reflections. J Med Ethics. 2010;36:598–603.
9. Glantz LH, et al. Research in developing countries: taking "benefit" seriously. Hastings Cent Rep. 1998;28:38–42.
10. Good clinical practice research guidelines reviewed, emphasis given to responsibilities of investigators: second article in a series. J Oncol Pract. 2008;4(5):233-235.
11. Hellman S, Hellman DS. Of mice but not men: problems of the randomized clinical trial. N Engl J Med. 1991;324(22):1585–9.
12. Herz DA, Looman JE, Lewis SK. Informed consent: is it a myth? Neurosurgery. 1992;30(3):453–8.
13. Howick J. Questioning the methodologic superiority of 'placebo' over 'active' controlled trials. AJoB. 2009;9:34–48.
14. Lilford RJ. Ethics of clinical trials from a Bayesian and decision-analitic perspective: whose equipoise is it anyway? BMJ. 2003;326:980–81.
15. McCulloch P, et al. Randomised trials in surgery: problems and possible solutions. BMJ. 2002;324:1448–51.
16. Miller F, Brody H. A critique of clinical equipoise: therapeutic misconception in the ethics of clinical trials. Hastings Cent Rep. 2003;33:19–28.
17. Miller FG, Wertheimer A. Facing up to paternalism in research ethics. Hastings Cent Rep. 2007;37(3):24–34.
18. Nardini C. The ethics of clinical trials. *Ecancer medical science*. 2014;8:387. Published 2014 Jan 16.
19. National Commission for the Protection of Human Subjects of Biomedical and Behavioral Research. Bethesda, MD: ERIC Clearinghouse; 1978. The Belmont report: Ethical principles and guidelines for the protection of human subjects of research.
20. Palmer CR, Rosenberger WF. Ethics and practice: alternative designs for phase III randomized clinical trials. Control Clin Trials. 1999;20(2):172–86.
21. Riis P. Thirty years of bioethics: the Helsinki Declaration 1964–2003. New Rev Bioeth. 2003;1:15–25.

22. Sackett D. Why randomized controlled trials fail but needn't: 1. failure to gain "coal-face" commitment and to use the uncertainty principle. CMAJ. 2000;162:1311–14.
23. Shapiro H, Meslin E. Ethical issues in the design and conduct of clinical trials in developing countries. N Engl J Med. 2001;345:139–42.
24. Temple R, Ellenberg SS. Placebo-controlled trials and active-control trials in the evaluation of new treatments. Part 1: ethical and scientific issues. Ann Intern Med. 2000;133(6):455–63.
25. The Nuremberg Code. Trials of war criminals before the Nuremberg military tribunals under control council law. 1949. [14/10/13]. http://nuremberg.law.harvard.edu/php/docs_swi.php?%20DI=1&text=medical.
26. Wendler D, Miller F. Deception in the pursuit of science. Arch Intern Med. 2004;164:597–600.
27. World Medical Association. Declaration of Helsinki, 6th revision. 2008. [14/10/13]. http://www.wma.net/en/30publications/10policies/b3/
28. Worrall J. Evidence and ethics in medicine. Perspect Biol Med. 2008;51(3):418–31

Scan QR code to view the website/guidelines

- Ethics in Clinical Research-
Ethics in Clinical Research | Clinical Center Home Page (nih.gov)

CHAPTER 27

ICH Guidelines of Good Clinical Practices 2016

Introduction

Good Clinical Practice (GCP) is an international ethical and scientific quality standard for designing, conducting, recording and reporting trials that involve the participation of human subjects. Compliance with this standard provides public assurance that the rights, safety, and well-being of trial subjects are protected, consistent with the principles that have their origin in the Declaration of Helsinki, and that the clinical trial data are credible.

The objective of this ICH [International Council for Harmonisation of Technical Requirements for Pharmaceuticals for Human Use (ICH) (formerly the International Conference on Harmonisation of Technical Requirements for Registration of Pharmaceuticals for Human Use)] guidance is to provide a unified standard for to facilitate the mutual acceptance of clinical data by the regulatory authorities.

This guidance should be read in conjunction with other ICH guidance's relevant to the conduct of clinical trials (e.g., E2A (clinical safety data management), E3 (clinical study reporting), E7 (geriatric populations), E8 (general considerations for clinical trials), E9 (statistical principles), and E11 (paediatric populations)).

The Principles of ICH-GCP

1. Clinical trials should be conducted in accordance with the ethical principles that have their origin in the Declaration of Helsinki, and that are consistent with GCP and the applicable regulatory requirement(s).
2. Before a trial is initiated, foreseeable risks and inconveniences should be weighed against the anticipated benefit for the individual trial subject and society. A trial should be initiated and continued only if the anticipated benefits justify the risks.
3. The rights, safety, and well-being of the trial subjects are the most important considerations and should prevail over interests of science and society.
4. The available nonclinical and clinical information on an investigational product should be adequate to support the proposed clinical trial.
5. Clinical trials should be scientifically sound, and described in a clear, detailed protocol.
6. A trial should be conducted in compliance with the protocol that has received prior institutional review board (IRB)/independent ethics committee (IEC) approval/favourable opinion.
7. The medical care given to, and medical decisions made on behalf of, subjects should always be the responsibility of a qualified physician or, when appropriate, of a qualified dentist.
8. Each individual involved in conducting a trial should be qualified by education, training, and experience to perform his or her respective task(s).
9. Freely given informed consent should be obtained from every subject prior to clinical trial participation.
10. All clinical trial information should be recorded, handled, and stored in a way that allows its accurate reporting, interpretation, and verification.

11. The confidentiality of records that could identify subjects should be protected, respecting the privacy and confidentiality rules in accordance with the applicable regulatory requirement(s).
12. Investigational products should be manufactured, handled, and stored in accordance with applicable good manufacturing practice (GMP). They should be used in accordance with the approved protocol.
13. Systems with procedures that assure the quality of every aspect of the trial should be implemented.

Aspects of the trial that are essential to ensure human subject protection and reliability of trial results should be the focus of such systems.

Institutional Review Board/Independent Ethics Committee (IRB/IEC)

Responsibilities: An IRB/IEC should safeguard the rights, safety, and well-being of all trial subjects. Special attention should be paid to trials that may include vulnerable subjects. The IRB/IEC should obtain the following documents:

- Trial protocol(s)/amendment(s), written informed consent form(s) and consent form updates that the investigator proposes for use in the trial, subject recruitment procedures (e.g., advertisements), written information to be provided to subjects, Investigator's Brochure (IB), available safety information, information about payments and compensation available to subjects, the investigator's current curriculum vitae and/or other documentation evidencing qualifications, and any other documents that the IRB/IEC may need to fulfil its responsibilities.
- The IRB/IEC should review a proposed clinical trial within a reasonable time and document its views in writing, clearly identifying the trial, the documents reviewed and the dates for the following:
    - Approval/favourable opinion;
    - Modifications required prior to its approval/favourable opinion;
    - Disapproval/negative opinion; and
    - Termination/suspension of any prior approval/favourable opinion.
- The IRB/IEC should consider the qualifications of the investigator for the proposed trial, as documented by a current curriculum vitae and/or by any other relevant documentation the IRB/IEC requests.
- The IRB/IEC should conduct continuing review of each ongoing trial at intervals appropriate to the degree of risk to human subjects, but at least once per year.
- The IRB/IEC should ensure that information regarding payment to subjects, including the methods, amounts, and schedule of payment to trial subjects, is set forth in the written informed consent form and any other written information to be provided to subjects. The way payment will be prorated should be specified.

Composition, Functions, and Operations

The IRB/IEC should consist of a reasonable number of members, who collectively have the qualifications and experience to review and evaluate the science, medical aspects, and ethics of the proposed trial. The IRB/IEC should retain all relevant records (e.g., written procedures, membership lists, lists of occupations/affiliations of members, submitted documents, minutes of meetings, and correspondence) for a period of at least 3 years after completion of the trial and make them available upon request from the regulatory authority.

Investigator

Investigator's Qualifications and Agreements	The investigator(s) should be qualified by education, training, and experience to assume responsibility for the proper conduct of the trial, should meet all the qualifications specified by the applicable regulatory requirement(s), and should provide evidence of such qualifications. The investigator should be thoroughly familiar with the appropriate use of the investigational product(s), recruitment of subjects, GCP and the applicable regulatory requirements.
Adequate Resources	The investigator should be able to demonstrate (e.g., based on retrospective data) a potential for recruiting the required number of suitable subjects within the agreed recruitment period, have sufficient time to properly conduct and complete trial and have adequate number of qualified staff with well informed protocol, the investigational product(s), and their trial-related duties and functions and adequate facilities for the foreseen duration of the trial to conduct the trial properly and safely. The investigator is responsible for supervising any individual or party to whom the investigator delegates trial-related duties and functions conducted at the trial site.
Medical Care of Trial Subjects	A qualified physician (or dentist, when appropriate), who is an investigator or a sub investigator for the trial, should be responsible for all trial-related medical (or dental) decisions and adequate medical care. Although a subject is not obliged to give his/her reason(s) for withdrawing prematurely from a trial, the investigator should make a reasonable effort to ascertain the reason(s), while fully respecting the subject's rights.
Communication with IRB/IEC	Before initiating a trial, the investigator/institution should have written and dated approval/favourable opinion from the IRB/IEC for the trial protocol, written informed consent form, consent form updates, subject recruitment procedures (e.g., advertisements), and any other written information to be provided to subjects. During the trial the investigator/institution should provide updated Investigator's Brochure (if any) and all documents subject to review to the IRB/IEC.
Compliance with Protocol	The investigator/institution should conduct the trial in compliance with the protocol agreed to by the sponsor and, if required, by the regulatory authority, and which was given approval/favourable opinion by the IRB/IEC. The investigator should not implement any deviation from, or changes of, the protocol without agreement by the sponsor and prior review and documented approval/favourable opinion from

Contd...

	the IRB/IEC of an amendment, except where necessary to eliminate an immediate hazard(s) to trial subjects, or when the change(s) involves only logistical or administrative aspects of the trial (e.g., change in monitor(s), change of telephone number. Such changes should be informed to IRB/IEC for review and approval/favourable opinion, regulatory authority and sponsor for agreement.
Investigational Product	Responsibility for investigational product(s) accountability and use only in accordance with the approved protocol at the trial site(s) rests with the investigator/institution. Investigator/institution may/should assign some or all duties for investigational product(s) to an appropriate pharmacist or another appropriate individual who is under the supervision of them. They should maintain records of the product's delivery to the trial site, the inventory at the site, the use by each subject, and the return to the sponsor or alternative disposition of unused product(s). These records should include dates, quantities, batch/serial numbers, expiration dates (if applicable), and the unique code numbers assigned to the investigational product(s) and trial subjects.
Randomization Procedures and Unblinding	The investigator should follow the trial's randomization procedures, if any, and should ensure that the code is broken only in accordance with the protocol. If the trial is blinded, the investigator should promptly document and explain to the sponsor any premature unblinding (e.g., accidental unblinding, unblinding due to a serious adverse event) of the investigational product.
Informed Consent of Trial Subjects	In obtaining and documenting informed consent, the investigator should comply with the applicable regulatory requirement(s), and should adhere to GCP and to the ethical principles that have their origin in the Declaration of Helsinki. Prior to the beginning of the trial, the investigator should have the IRB/IEC's written approval/favorable opinion of the written informed consent form and any other written information to be provided to subjects. Any revised written informed consent form, and written information should receive the IRB/IEC's approval/favorable opinion in advance of use. Investigator or assigned staff should not unduly influence a subject to participate or to continue to participate in a trial and should provide ample time and opportunity to inquire about details of the trial and final decision. The language used in the oral and written information about the trial, including the written informed consent form, should be as non-technical as practical and should be understandable to the subject or the subject's legally acceptable representative and the impartial witness, where applicable. Before beginning a trial, the written informed consent form should be signed and personally dated by the subject or by the subject's legally acceptable representative, and by the person who conducted the informed consent discussion. The witness should sign, personally date the consent form if information is read to subjects to confirm that information is accurately explained to, and apparently understood by, the subject. Both the informed consent discussion and the written informed consent form and any other written information to be provided to subjects should include detail explanations of the following:

Contd...

	trial research details, purpose, trial treatment(s), random assignment, procedures, subject's responsibilities, experimental aspects, expected benefits, foreseeable risks or inconveniences, alternative procedure(s) or treatment with potential benefits and risks, compensation, anticipated prorated payment (if any), anticipated expenses (if any), expected duration of the subject's participation, approximate number of subjects involved in the trial. That the subject's participation in the trial is voluntary and that the subject may refuse to participate or withdraw from the trial, at any time, without penalty or loss of benefits to which the subject is otherwise entitled. That the monitor(s), the auditor(s), the IRB/IEC, and the regulatory authority will be granted direct access to the subject's original medical records for verification of clinical trial procedures and/or data, without violating the confidentiality of the subject, to the extent permitted by the applicable laws and regulations and that, by signing a written informed consent form, the subject or the subject's legally acceptable representative is authorizing such access. Nontherapeutic trials may be conducted in subjects with consent of a legally acceptable representative provided with some conditions.
Records and Reports	The investigator/institution should maintain adequate and accurate source documents and trial records that include all pertinent observations on each of the site's trial subjects. Source data should be attributable, legible, contemporaneous, original, accurate, and complete. Changes to source data should be traceable, should not obscure the original entry, and should be explained if necessary (e.g., via an audit trial). Essential documents should be retained until at least 2-years after the last approval of a marketing application in an ICH region and until there are no pending or contemplated marketing applications in an ICH region or at least 2 years have elapsed since the formal discontinuation of clinical development of the investigational product or should be retained for a longer period as per regulatory requirements or by an agreement with the sponsor. The financial aspects of the trial should be documented in an agreement between the sponsor and the investigator/institution.
Progress Reports	The investigator should promptly provide written reports and submit written summaries of the trial's status to the IRB/IEC annually, or more frequently, if requested by the IRB/IEC.
Safety Reporting	All SAEs should be reported immediately to the sponsor except for those SAEs that the protocol or other document (e.g., Investigator's Brochure) identifies as not needing immediate reporting. The immediate and follow-up reports should identify subjects by unique code numbers assigned to the trial subjects rather than any confidential information. For reported deaths, the investigator should supply the sponsor and the IRB/IEC with any additional requested information (e.g., autopsy reports and terminal medical reports).
Premature Termination or Suspension of	If the trial is prematurely terminated or suspended for any reason, the investigator/institution should promptly inform the trial subjects, should assure appropriate therapy and follow-up for the subjects, and, where required by the

Contd...

a Trial	applicable regulatory requirement(s), should inform the regulatory authority with a detailed written explanation of the termination or suspension.
Final Report(s) by Investigator	Upon completion of the trial, the investigator, where applicable, should inform the institution; the investigator/institution should provide the IRB/IEC with a summary of the trial's outcome, and the regulatory authority with any reports required.

Sponsors

Quality Management	The sponsor should implement a system to manage quality throughout all stages (clinical trial protocols, tools, and procedures) for data collection of the trial process to ensuring human subject protection and the reliability of trial results. The quality management system should use a risk-based approach: Critical Process and Data Identification, Risk Identification, Risk Evaluation and Risk Control
Quality Assurance and Quality Control	The sponsor is responsible for implementing and maintaining quality assurance and quality control systems with written SOPs to ensure that trials are conducted and data are generated, documented (recorded), and reported in compliance with the protocol, GCP, and the applicable regulatory requirement(s) through written agreement from all involved parties to ensure direct access to sites, documents, and reports. Quality control should be applied to each stage of data handling to ensure that all data are reliable and have been processed correctly.
Contract Research Organization (CRO)	A sponsor may transfer any or all of the sponsor's trial-related duties and functions to a CRO in written, but the ultimate responsibility for the quality and integrity of the trial data always resides with the sponsor. The CRO should implement quality assurance and quality control. Any trial-related duties and functions not specifically transferred to and assumed by a CRO are retained by the sponsor.
Medical Expertise	The sponsor should designate appropriately qualified medical personnel who will be readily available to advise on trial-related medical questions or problems. If necessary, outside consultant(s) may be appointed for this purpose.
Trial Design	The sponsor should utilize qualified individuals (e.g., biostatisticians, clinical pharmacologists, and physicians) as appropriate, throughout all stages of the trial process, from designing the protocol and CRFs and planning the analyses to analysing and preparing interim and final clinical trial reports.
Trial Management, Data Handling, and Recordkeeping	The sponsor should utilize appropriately qualified individuals to supervise the overall conduct of the trial, to handle the data, to verify the data, to conduct the statistical analyses, and to prepare the trial reports. The sponsor may consider establishing an independent data monitoring committee (IDMC) to assess the progress of a clinical trial, including the safety data and the critical efficacy endpoints at intervals, and to recommend to the sponsor whether to continue, modify, or stop a trial. The IDMC should have written operating procedures and maintain written records of all its meetings.

Contd...

	Electronic trial data handling and/or remote electronic trial data systems, the sponsor should: Ensure and document that the electronic data processing system(s) conforms to the sponsor's established requirements for completeness, accuracy, reliability, and consistent intended performance (i.e., validation). System should be designed so that should provide unambiguous subject identification, no deletion of entered data, prevents unauthorized access, Maintain adequate backup, Safeguard the blinding, allow to compare the original data and observations with the processed data.
Investigator Selection	The sponsor is responsible for selecting the investigator(s)/institution(s) even for multicenter trials. Each investigator should be qualified by training and experience and should have adequate resources to properly conduct the trial for which the investigator is selected. The sponsor should obtain the investigator's/institution's agreement: • To conduct the trial in compliance with GCP, with the applicable regulatory requirement(s) and with the protocol agreed to by the sponsor and given approval/favourable opinion by the IRB/IEC. • To comply with procedures for data recording/reporting; • To permit monitoring, auditing, and inspection and • To retain the trial-related essential documents until the sponsor informs the investigator/institution these documents are no longer needed.
Allocation of Responsibilities	Prior to initiating a trial, the sponsor should define, establish, and allocate all trial-related duties and functions.
Compensation to Subjects and Investigators	If required by the applicable regulatory requirement(s), the sponsor should provide insurance or should indemnify (legal and financial coverage) the investigator/the institution against claims arising from the trial, except for claims that arise from malpractice and/or negligence. The sponsor's policies and procedures should address the costs of treatment of trial subjects in the event of trial-related injuries in accordance with the applicable regulatory requirement(s). When trial subjects receive compensation, the method and manner of compensation should comply with applicable regulatory requirement(s).
Financing	The financial aspects of the trial should be documented in an agreement between the sponsor and the investigator/institution.
Notification/Submission to Regulatory Authority	Before initiating the clinical trial, the sponsor (or the sponsor and the investigator, if required by the applicable regulatory requirement(s)) should submit any required application(s) to the appropriate authority for review, acceptance, and/or permission (as required by the applicable regulatory requirement to begin the trial. Any notification/submission should be dated and contain sufficient information to identify the protocol.
Confirmation of Review by IRB/IEC	The sponsor should obtain from the investigator/institution: (a) The name and address of the investigator's/institution's IRB/IEC with a statement that it is organized and operates according to GCP and the applicable laws and regulations. The sponsor should obtain from the investigator/institution IRB/IEC approved or re-approved protocol, written informed consent form(s) and any other written information to be provided to subjects, subject recruiting procedures,

Contd...

	and documents related to payments and compensation available to the subjects, and any other documents.
Information on Investigational Product(s)	When planning trials, the sponsor should ensure that sufficient safety and efficacy data from nonclinical studies and/or clinical trials are available to support human exposure by the route, at the dosages, for the duration, and in the trial population to be studied. The sponsor should update the Investigator's Brochure as significant new information becomes available.
Manufacturing, Packaging, Labelling, and Coding Investigational Product	The sponsor should ensure that the investigational product (including active comparator and placebo, if applicable) is manufactured in accordance with any applicable GMP, and is coded and labelled in a manner that protects the blinding, if applicable and regulatory requirement. The investigational product(s) should assure packaging to prevent contamination and unacceptable deterioration during transport and storage. The sponsor should determine, for the investigational product(s), acceptable storage temperatures, storage conditions (e.g., protection from light), storage times, reconstitution fluids and procedures, and devices for product infusion, if any. The sponsor should inform all involved parties (e.g., monitors, investigators, pharmacists, storage managers) of these determinations.
Supplying and Handling Investigational Product	The sponsor is responsible for supplying, timely delivery of sufficient the investigator(s)/institution(s) with the investigational product(s) only after getting all required documentation (e.g., approval/favourable opinion from IRB/IEC and regulatory authority. The sponsor should maintain essential records, written instructions for the handling and storage of investigational product(s) for the trial and documentation thereof. The sponsor should ensure stability of products over the period of use, maintain a system for retrieving (e.g., for deficient product recall, reclaim after trial completion, expired product reclaim) and disposition of unused investigational product(s) and for the documentation of same.
Record Access	The sponsor should ensure that it is specified in the protocol or other written agreement that the investigator(s)/institution(s) provide direct access to source data/documents for trial-related monitoring, audits, IRB/IEC review, and regulatory inspection. The sponsor should verify that each subject has consented, in writing, to direct access to his/her original medical records for trial-related monitoring, audit, IRB/IEC review, and regulatory inspection.
Safety Information	The sponsor is responsible for the ongoing safety evaluation of the investigational product(s). The sponsor should promptly notify all concerned investigator(s)/institution(s) and the regulatory authority of findings that could affect adversely the safety of subjects, impact the conduct of the trial, or alter the IRB/IEC's approval/favourable opinion to continue the trial.
Adverse Drug Reaction Reporting	The sponsor should expedite the reporting to all concerned investigator(s)/institutions(s), to the IRB(s)/IEC(s), where required, and to the regulatory authority of all adverse drug reactions (ADRs) that are both serious and unexpected. Such expedited reports should comply with the applicable regulatory requirement(s) and with the ICH Guideline for Clinical Safety Data Management: Definitions and Standards for Expedited Reporting.

Contd...

Monitoring	The purposes of trial monitoring are to verify that rights and well-being of human subjects are protected, reported trial data are accurate, complete, and verifiable from source documents and conduct of the trial is in compliance with the currently approved protocol/amendment(s), with GCP, and with the applicable regulatory requirement(s). Trained Monitors familiar with the investigational product(s) should be appointed by the sponsor. The sponsor should ensure that the trials are adequately monitored (In general before, during, and after the trial). **Monitors are** the main line of communication between the sponsor and the investigator.
Audit	The sponsor should appoint qualified and trained individuals, who are independent of the clinical trials/systems, to conduct audits to evaluate trial conduct and compliance with the protocol, SOPs, GCP, and the applicable regulatory requirements. Regulatory authority(ies) may seek access to an audit report on a case-by-case basis when evidence of serious GCP non-compliance exists, or in the course of legal proceedings. Potential noncompliance harmful to human subject protection or reliability of trial results is discovered, the sponsor should terminate the investigator's/institution's participation in the trial, notify promptly the regulatory authority and perform a root cause analysis and implement appropriate corrective and preventive actions.
Premature Termination or Suspension of a Trial	Sponsor should promptly inform authority about the premature termination or suspension with the reason(s).
Clinical Trial/Study Reports	Whether the trial is completed or prematurely terminated, the sponsor should ensure that the clinical trial reports are prepared and provided to the regulatory agency(ies) as required by the applicable regulatory requirement(s). The sponsor should also ensure that the clinical trial reports in marketing applications meet the standards of the ICH Guidance for Structure and Content of Clinical Study Reports.
Multicentre Trials	For multicentre trials, the sponsor should ensure that: documented responsibilities and communication of all participating investigator(s), conduct of trial by all investigators in strict compliance with the protocol and given approval/favourable opinion by the IRB/IEC and CRFs are designed to capture the required data at all multicentre trial sites.

Clinical Trial Protocol and Protocol Amendment

The contents of a trial protocol should generally include the following topics. However, site specific information may be provided on separate protocol page(s), or addressed in a separate agreement, and some of the information listed below may be contained in other protocol referenced documents, such as an Investigator's Brochure.

General Information	• Protocol title, protocol identifying number, and date. Any amendment should also bear the amendment number(s) and date. • Name and address of the sponsor and monitor (if other than the sponsor). • Name and title of the person(s) authorized to sign the protocol and the protocol amendment(s) for the sponsor. • Name, title, address, and telephone number(s) of the sponsor's medical expert (or dentist when appropriate) for the trial.

Contd...

	• Name and title of the investigator(s) who is (are) responsible for conducting the trial, and the address and telephone number(s) of the trial site(s). • Name, title, address, and telephone number(s) of the qualified physician (or dentist, if applicable), who is responsible for all trial-site related medical (or dental) decisions (if other than investigator). • Name(s) and address(es) of the clinical laboratory(ies) and other medical and/or technical department(s) and/or institutions involved in the trial.
Background Information	• Name and description of the investigational product(s). • A summary of nonclinical studies, potential risks and benefits, • route of administration, dosage, dosage regimen, and treatment period(s), Description of the population and References to literature relevant to the trial.
Trial Objectives and Purpose	A detailed description of the objectives and the purpose of the trial.
Trial Design	
Selection and Withdrawal of Subjects	• Subject inclusion criteria. • Subject exclusion criteria. • Subject withdrawal criteria (i.e., terminating investigational product treatment/trial treatment) and procedures specifying:
Treatment of Subjects	• The treatment(s) to be administered, including the name(s) of all the product(s), the dose(s), the dosing schedule(s), the route/mode(s) of administration, and the treatment period(s), including the follow-up period(s) for subjects for each investigational product treatment/trial treatment group/arm of the trial. • Medication(s)/treatment(s) permitted (including rescue medication) and not permitted before and/or during the trial.
Assessment of Efficacy	• Specification of the efficacy parameters. • Methods and timing for assessing, recording, and analysing efficacy parameters.
Assessment of Safety	• Specification of safety parameter. • The methods and timing for assessing, recording, and analysing safety parameters. • Procedures for eliciting reports of and for recording and reporting adverse event and intercurrent illnesses. • The type and duration of the follow-up of subjects after adverse events.
Statistics	• A description of the statistical methods to be employed, including timing of any planned interim analysis.
Direct Access to Source Data/Documents	The sponsor should ensure that it is specified in the protocol or other written agreement that the investigator(s)/institution(s) will permit trial-related monitoring, audits, IRB/IEC review, and regulatory inspection(s), providing direct access to source data/documents.

Contd...

Quality Control and Quality Assurance	
Ethics	• General ethical considerations related to the study • informed consent procedure • Possible reasons for not seeking informed consent
Data Handling and Recordkeeping	
Financing and Insurance -	Financing and insurance if not addressed in a separate agreement.
Publication Policy	Publication policy, if not addressed in a separate agreement.
Supplements	

Investigator's Brochure

Introduction

The Investigator's Brochure (IB) is a compilation of the clinical and nonclinical data on the investigational product(s) that are relevant to the study of the product(s) in human subjects. Its purpose is to provide the investigators and others involved in the trial with the information to facilitate their understanding of the rationale for, and their compliance with, many key features of the protocol, such as the dose, dose frequency/interval, methods of administration: and safety monitoring procedures.

The IB also provides insight to support the clinical management of the study subjects during the course of the clinical trial. The information should be presented in a concise, simple, objective, balanced, and non-promotional form that enables a clinician, or potential investigator, to understand it and make his/her own unbiased risk-benefit assessment of the appropriateness of the proposed trial. For this reason, a medically qualified person should generally participate in the editing of an IB, but the contents of the IB should be approved by the disciplines that generated the described data.

This guidance delineates the minimum information that should be included in an IB and provides suggestions for its layout. It is expected that the type and extent of information available will vary with the stage of development of the investigational product.

If the investigational product is marketed and its pharmacology is widely understood by medical practitioners, an extensive IB may not be necessary. Where permitted by regulatory authorities, a basic product information brochure, package leaflet, or labelling may be an appropriate alternative, provided that it includes current, comprehensive, and detailed information on all aspects of the investigational product that might be of importance to the investigator. If a marketed product is being studied for a new use (i.e., a new indication), an IB specific to that new use should be prepared.

The IB should be reviewed at least annually and revised as necessary in compliance with a sponsor's written procedures. More frequent revision may be appropriate depending on the stage of development and the generation of relevant new information. However, in accordance with GCP, relevant new information may be so important that it should be communicated to the investigators, and possibly to the Institutional Review Boards (IRBs)/Independent Ethics Committees (IECs) and/or regulatory authorities before it is included in a revised IB.

Generally, the sponsor is responsible for ensuring that an up-to-date IB is made available to the investigator(s) and the investigators are responsible for providing the up-to-date IB to the responsible IRBs/IECs.

In the case of an investigator sponsored trial, the sponsor-investigator should determine whether a brochure is available from the commercial manufacturer. If the investigational product is provided by the sponsor-investigator, then he or she should provide the necessary information to the trial personnel. In cases where preparation of a formal IB is impractical, the sponsor-investigator should provide, as a substitute, an expanded background information section in the trial protocol that contains the minimum current information described in this guidance.

Essential Documents for the Conduct of Clinical Trial

Essential Documents are those documents that individually and collectively permit evaluation of the conduct of a trial and the quality of the data produced. These documents serve to demonstrate the compliance of the investigator, sponsor, and monitor with the standards of GCP and with all applicable regulatory requirements.

Essential Documents also serve a number of other important purposes. Filing essential documents at the investigator/institution and sponsor sites in a timely manner can greatly assist in the successful management of a trial by the investigator, sponsor, and monitor. These documents are also the ones that are usually audited by the sponsor's independent audit function and inspected by the regulatory authority as part of the process to confirm the validity of the trial conduct and the integrity of data collected.

The minimum list of essential documents that has been developed follows. The various documents are grouped in three sections according to the stage of the trial during which they will normally be generated:

- before the clinical phase of the trial commences,
- during the clinical conduct of the trial, and
- after completion or termination of the trial. A description is given of the purpose of each document, and whether it should be filed in either the investigator/institution or sponsor files, or both. It is acceptable to combine some of the documents, provided the individual elements are readily identifiable.

Trial master files should be established at the beginning of the trial, both at the investigator/institution's site and at the sponsor's office. A final close-out of a trial can only be done when the monitor has reviewed both investigator/institution and sponsor files and confirmed that all necessary documents are in the appropriate files. Any or all of the documents addressed in this guidance may be subject to, and should be available for, audit by the sponsor's auditor and inspection by the regulatory authority.

Further Reading

1. European Medicines Agency. ICH Harmonised Tripartite Guideline E6: Note for Guidance on Good Clinical Practice (PMP/ICH/135/95) London: European Medicines Agency; 2002.
2. https://cdsco.gov.in/opencms/opencms/en/Clinical-Trial/clinical-trials/ Accessed in Dec 2020
3. https://database.ich.org/sites/default/files/E6_R2_Addendum.pdf Accessed in Dec 2020
4. Kumar M, Kher S. Regulatory Considerations for Conducting Clinical Trials in India. Regulatory Affairs Focus. 2007;12(3):26-31.
5. Kumar M, Tate K. Designing a Global Product Development strategy. Regulatory Affairs Focus. 2008;13(6):16-21.
6. Kumar M. Agencies Involved in Approving Clinical Trials in India. Regulatory Affairs Focus. 2007;12(8):34-9.
7. Office of Human Subjects Research. The Nuremberg Code [Web Page] 1949. Available at http://ohsr.od.nih.gov/guidelines/nuremberg.
8. Otte A, et al. Good Clinical Practice: Historical background and key aspects. 2005;26:563–74.
9. Schedule – Y, Amendment version 2005, Drugs and Cosmetics Rules, 1945 Available online https://rgcb.res.in/documents/Schedule-Y.pdf. Accessed Feb. 2021
10. The Doctors Trial (the Medical Case of the Subsequent Nuremberg Proceedings) [Web Page] Available at http://www.ushmm.org/research/doctors/Nuremberg_Code.htm.
11. The World Medical Association. Declaration of Helsinki [Web Page] 2004. Available at http://www.wma.net/e/policy/b3.htm.
12. Vadivale M. ICH-GCP Guidelines for Clinical Trials. Berita MMA. 1999;7(29)
13. Vijayananthan A, Nawawi O. The importance of Good Clinical Practice guidelines and its role in clinical trials. Biomed Imaging Interv J. 2008;4(1):e5. doi:10.2349/biij.4.1.e5
14. www.clinicaltrials.gov Accessed Feb. 2021
15. WHO 1995. Guidelines for Good Clinical Practice (GCP) for Trials on Pharmaceutical Products. World Health Organization, WHO Technical Series, No. 850, 1995, Annex 3

Scan QR code to view the website/guidelines

- ICH GCP Guidelines-
GUIDELINE FOR GOOD CLINICAL PRACTICE (ich.org)

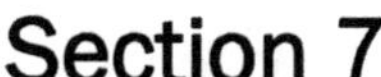

Section 7

Herbal Industry, IPR and Regulatory Affairs

CHAPTER 28

Herbal Industry: Infrastructure, Formulation, Production and Pilot Plant Scale-Up Management of Herbal Products

Introduction

Worldwide the herbal industry is picking up at a fast pace, due to the exponential growth in the field of herbal medicines. As the demand and commercial value of herbal medicines is increasing tremendously. The growth of herbal industry is increased. There is a growing demand for natural products including items of medicinal value/pharmaceuticals, food supplements and cosmetics in both domestic and international markets. India with its diversified biodiversity has a tremendous potential and advantage in this emerging area.

The increased demand of herbal medicines has led to a sudden increase in herbal manufacturing unit. There is a complex of large number of manufacturing units using herbal material for various purposes. Whereas the largest number of such manufacturing units are registered as 'pharmaceuticals', there are others that are engaged in making plant based cosmetics herbal and food supplements. . Another group of manufacturing units is engaged in making extracts and distilling oils for use by other industries and for exports. Raw materials for all these diverse industries are largely derived from botanical sources.

Several research works are going on the ASU drugs. Basic research to preclinical or clinical study, investigation on standardization and formulation on ISM are a hot area of research in current time. Central Council for Research in Ayurvedic Sciences, Central Council for Research in Unani Medicine, Central Council for Research in Siddha, Central Council for Research in Yoga & Naturopathy, CSIR, Central Drug Research Institute (CDRI), several private research centre, institution and universities are actively engaged in research, development and promotion of traditional herbal medicine.

Nearly, 9000 manufacturing units of Indian Traditional Medicine are present in the India as on April 2013. Though the majority of them (7744) are involved in manufacturing of Ayurveda drugs, whereas, 485, 344 and 323 manufacturing units were engaging in manufacturing of Unani, Siddha and Homoeopathy drugs respectively. Statistics also suggest that only 0.1% per annum growth was observed realized in total AYUSH drug manufacturing units during last two decade. A recent statistics showed that among the 10,000 Ayurvedic, Siddha and Unani medicine manufacturing unit about 54% is GMP complying units.

Herbal Industry in India uses about 8000 medicinal plants out of them some of the important plants are widely used in preparation of various herbal formulations. This plants are enlisted below.

Plants	Formulations
Terminalia chebula(Haritaki)	219
Emblica officinalis.(Amla)	141
Piper longum(Pipali)	135
Adhatoda vasaka.(Vasaka)	110
Withania somnifera(Ashwagandha)	109

Herbal preparations includes powdered substances, tinctures, extracts essential oils, expressed juices. Herbal Formulation can be divided as follows:

- Solid dosage form- herbal extracts, powders, tablets, capsules.

- Liquid dosage form-syrup, solution, suspension, medicated oils.
- Semi solid dosage form-ointments, paste, cream.

These herbal preparations are obtained by subjecting to treatments such as extractions, distillation, expression, fractionation, purification, and concentration or fermentation methods.

Herbal Industry Infrastructure

For manufacturing and processing of herbal medicine it is important to make proper infrastructure of industry. The requirements used for setting of herbal industry are as follows:

- Layout of herbal industry according to types of dosage form(solid, liquid, semi -solid)
- Raw Materials.
- Space Requirements
- Machinery and equipments
- Other resources
    - Building
    - Water supply
    - Storage
- Regulatory and Quality control Evaluation

The Layout **of herbal industry** should have adequate space for-receiving and storing raw material, manufacturing process areas, quality control section, finished goods store/drug store and office

Space Requirements for Manufacturing of Herbal Medicines

1200 sq ft covered area with separate cabins/partitions for each activity is required. Minimum space requirement for manufacturing individual category of medicine of Herbal as per GMP requirements has been further explained in Table below.

No.	Category of Medicine	Minimum space required
1.	Powder drugs	100 sq ft
2.	Tablets	200 sq ft
3.	Pills	100 sq ft
4.	Capsules	100 sq ft
5.	Liquid Dosage form(syrup)	150 sq ft
6.	Herbs extracts	100 sq ft
7.	Medicated oils	100 sq ft
8.	Ointment	100 sq ft

Buildings The factory building is an important aspect. The total building plan should have due consideration for dosage forms to be manufactured (product range), scale of operation, (small medium and large) and type of equipments (manufacturing of medicine should qualify following conditions along with conformity with the Factory act.

- Building should be designed constructed and maintained in such way to prevent entry of insects/rodents, flies and dust.
- Proper sanitary and drainage system in the unit is required.
- Adequate provision of light, electrical fixtures, proper ventilation/chimney and fire safety measures/exits.

Water Supply: Water used in manufacturing should be pure and of portable quality. Adequate provision for washing of premises should be made. Portable water should conform to prescribed standards (ICMR standards). Large quantities of water required for cooling, washing, and steam generation .Temperature, mineral content, cost of supply and purification treatment must also be considered while choosing a water supply.

Sterile Products requirement: There should be provision of separate enclosed area specifically designed for sterile products. **Manufacturing Area for sterile products should have a**ir locks for entry and should be free from dust and ventilated with an air supply.

Raw Material Stores: For the storage of raw materials appropriate containers as per material (physical and chemical properties) may be used to prevent from dampness, microbiological contamination, rodents and insect infestation, In ISM manufacturing unit raw material may be categorized as follows for their appropriate storage:

1. Fresh herbs
2. Dry herbs
3. Plant extracts and exudates/resins etc
4. Volatile oils/perfumes and flavours
5. Animal origin
6. Metallic origin
7. Mineral origin
8. Excipients

Packing Materials Stores: There should be separate space for storage of bottles, jars, capsules, etc. All the containers and closures lids should be adequately cleaned and dried before packing the products.

Finished Goods Stores: The finished products from the production area after proper packaging should be stored in the finished goods store. As per GMP(Good Manufacturing practice)packing, finished products are stored in hygeinic place (Quarantine) Area. After the quality control laboratory and the experts have checked the correctness of finished goods with reference to its packing/labeling as well as finished product quality as prescribed then it will be moved to “Approved Finished Goods Stock” area.

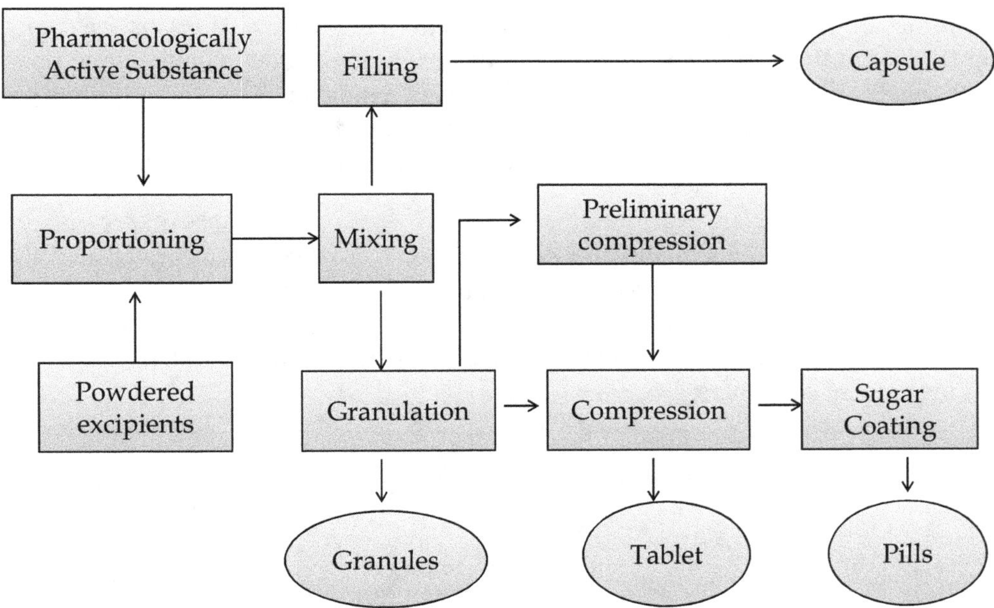

Figure 28.1 Pharmaceutical manufacturing of dosage-form products.

Manufacturing Steps in Herbal Industry

Extraction

Large volumes of natural materials, such as plant and animal matter, may be processed to extract substances which are pharmacologically active. In each step of the process, the volumes of materials are reduced by a series of batch processes, until the final drug product is obtained. Typically, processes are performed in campaigns lasting a few weeks, until the desired quantity of finished product is obtained. Solvents are used to remove insoluble fats and oils, thereby extracting the finished drug substance.

Manufacturing of dosage forms

Drug substances are converted into dosage-form [Figure 1] products before they are dispensed or administered to humans or animals. Active drug substances are mixed with pharmaceutical necessities, such as binders, fillers, flavouring and bulking agents, preservatives and antioxidants. These ingredients may be dried, milled, blended, compressed and granulated to achieve the desired properties before they are manufactured as a final formulation. Tablets and capsules are very common oral dosage forms; another common form is sterile liquids for injection or ophthalmic application.

Sterile manufacturing

Sterile products are manufactured in pharmaceutical manufacturing plants with modular design, clean workplace and equipment surfaces, and high efficiency particulate air (HEPA) filtered ventilation systems. The principles and practices of controlling contamination in sterile liquid manufacturing are similar to those in the microelectronics industry. Workers wear protective clothing to prevent them from contaminating products during sterile manufacturing operations. Sterile pharmaceutical technologies to control contamination involve freeze-drying products, using liquid germicides and sterilizing gases, installing laminar flow ventilation, isolating modules with differential air pressures and containing manufacturing and filling equipment.

Packaging

Pharmaceutical packaging operations are performed with a series of integrated machines and repetitive manual tasks. Finished dosage-form products may be packaged in many different types of containers (e.g., plastic or glass bottles, foil blister packs, pouches or sachets, tubes and sterile vials). The mechanical equipment fills, caps, labels, cartons and packs the finished products in shipping containers.

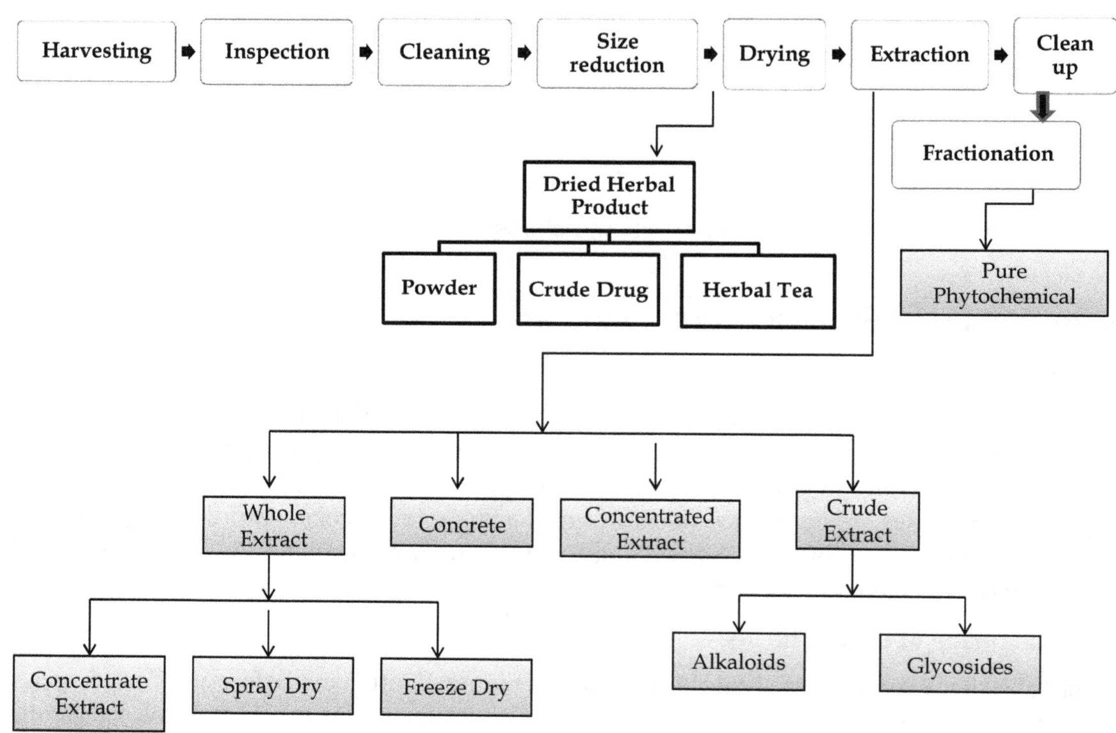

Figure 28.2 Steps involved in processing of herbs and value added products.

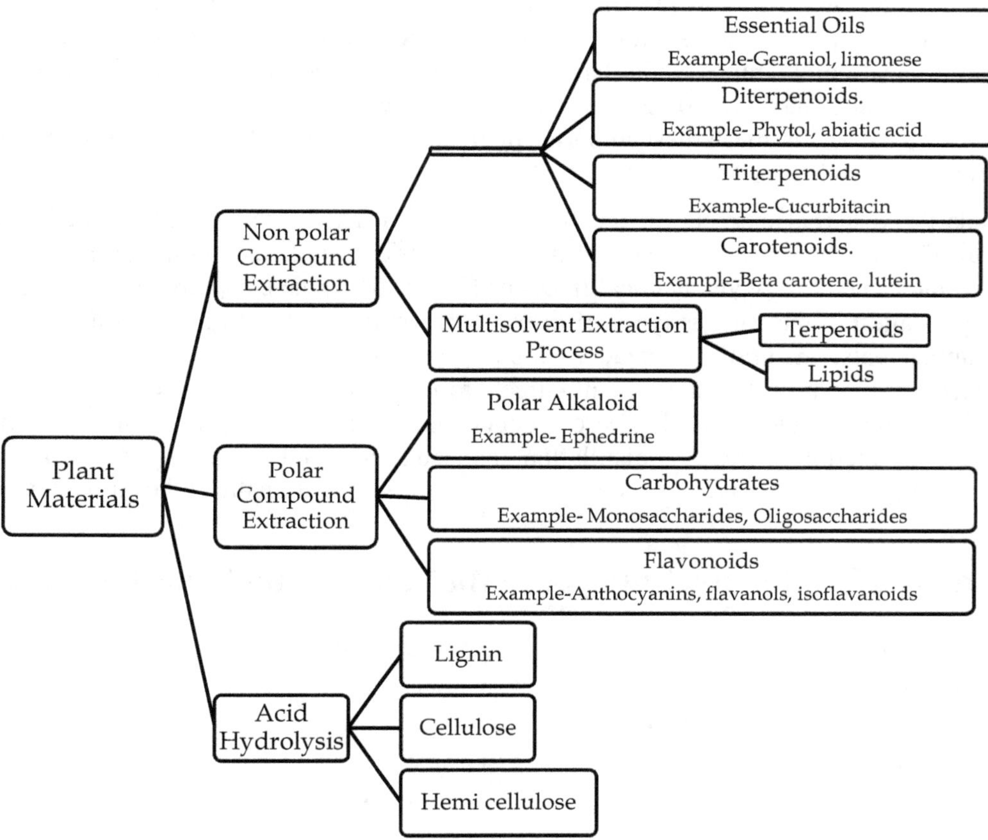

Figure 28.3 Phytochemical/s separation from plant material.

Formulation and Production Management of Herbal Products

Solid Dosage Form

Extracts

The medicinal plants sector has traditionally occupied an important position in the sociocultural, spiritual and medicinal background of rural and tribal lives of India. Besides meeting national demands, India caters to 12% of the global trade in herbal sector. In recent years, trade in herbal-based products has quantum leaped, particularly with respect to the volume of plant materials traded within and outside the country. Although India possesses one among the 12-mega biodiversity hotspots, the growing demand for medicinal plants is undoubtedly putting heavy strain on the existing resources, causing a number of species to become rare, threatened or endangered. Some rapid assessment of the threat status of medicinal plants using the IUCN-designed CAMP methodology has revealed that about 112 species in Southern India, 74 species in Northern and Central India and 42 species in the high altitudes of the Himalayas are threatened in the wild. Every year thousands of tonnes of these plant resources are being exploited from the natural habitat either legally or illegally, while very little of the benefits flow back to the local communities. India has large biodiversity and is endowed with 45,000 plant species out of which about 15,000-20,000 plants are known to have medicinal properties. With a share 46.4%, the US is the largest importer of medicinal herbs value added products [Figure 31.2] from India in 2013.

Standardized herbal extracts, in the form of dry powder, paste and liquid used as active additives in food, pharmaceutical, and cosmetics industries are planned in the project. Presently herbal extracts and pure phytochemical fractions [Figure 31.3] have captured a major consumer sector application in the various types of diseases preventing & health promotion zero calories food supplements, natural sweeteners, food supplement s, nutraceuticals, antioxidants, pharmaceutical, body fat reducer, anti-street formulations, harmless food colours, taste enhancer, perfumery additives, skin care products and even lifesaving anti-cancer & antiviral medicines. Extraction, filtration, distillation, concentration and or drying equipments may be batch, semi continuous and fully continuous, manual, semi automatic and or fully automatic

Equipments for Manufacturing of Herbal Extracts and Powder Drugs

Herbal extracts	**Powder Drugs**
Herbal pulverizer	Cutter mill
Extractors, Automatic grinder, cutter mill	Pulverizer
Rotary drum filter, flame and plate filter	Grinders
Spray drier, tray drier	Hammer mill
Distillation apparatus	Sieve sifter

Tablet: Tablets are solid preparations in which the herbal extract powder, plant powder or granule is blended with excipients and formed into a defined shape and size by compression.

Layout and of Tablet production section The tablet production department shall be divided in to three distinct and separate sections as follows:

1. Granulation section
2. Tablet compression section
3. Coating section.

- **Granulation Section:** 1) The numerous steps in granulating procedures increase the possibility of cross-contamination , in-correct product identification and or mix-up. To eliminate these possibilities, a separate room or booth is recommended for each step. A washing facility should be provided for cleaning of portable equipment such as granulators and mills. And to facilitate cleaning of non-portable equipments such as fluid-bed driers and mixers, each room should provided with floor drains.
- **Compression section:** separate room for tablet compression machines is necessary step to avoid cross contamination. Space should also be provided for in process testing of equipments such as balance and tablet hardness testers. Suitable physical, procedural and

labelling arrangements shall be made to prevent mix up of materials, granules and tablets on compression machinery. Tablets shall be de-dusted, preferably by automatic device and shall be monitored for the presence of foreign materials. Accurate and calibrated weighting equipment shall be readily available and used for in-process monitoring of tablet weight variation.

- **Coating Section:** Air supplied to coating pans for drying purposes shall be filtered air and of suitable quality. Coating solutions and suspensions shall be made afresh and used in a manner, which shall minimize the risk of microbial growth. Enclosing pans in groups have advantage to muffle the noise level to acceptable limits. The noise level can also be reduced in open pans by the use of insulating material around the outside of coating pans.

Other areas required for manufacturing of tablet are

- Raw material warehouse
  - Receiving quarantine
  - Approved raw material section
- Dispensary
- Quality control section
- Packaging Section.

Materials are weighed into batch quantities in dispensing and then moved into manufacturing area. After completion of manufacturing the finished tablets are place in **quarantine** and moved to bulk stock upon release. When packaging is done then are place in approved storage area.

- Temperature control and air control should be such that there should be comfortable working environment and no impact on characteristics of in process materials such as granulations, raw materials.
- Humidity should be lowered for specific products like moisture sensitive drugs. All areas should be properly ventilated with the use of roof fan.[6]

Equipments for Preparation of Tablets

Process	For preparation	For quality control
Size Reduction	Hammer mill, roller mill, edge runner mill	Tablet thickness tester
Mixing	V-blender, Ribbon blender.	Friability tester
Granulation	Fluidized granulator, Dry granulator, Roller compact granulator.	Weighing balance
Compression	Single punching machine	Disintegrator Apparatus
Coating	Coating pan, sugar coating pan	Dissolution apparatus
Drying	Spray drier, tray drier	

Capsule: Capsules are solid dosage forms in which the herbal substance is enclosed in either a hard or soft, soluble shell of gelatin or other suitable materials. Hard-shell capsules (also known as two-piece capsules) consist of two pieces (a body and a cap) in a range of standard sizes;

soft-shell capsules (also known as one-piece or gel capsules) comprise an outer case encapsulating a liquid or paste. The exact composition of the capsule varies with the nature of the content.

Preparation of capsules

Capsules are prepared by enclosing a plant powder, or homogeneous dry extract powder or granules with excipients in a suitable capsule base such as gelatin, of a particular shape and size. In the case of gel capsules, liquid extract or soft extract can also be encapsulated. The process is carried out using specialized equipment.

Layout of Capsules manufacturing area

- A separate enclosed areas
- Suitably air-conditioned
- Dehumidified
- An airlock arrangement is required.
- Empty capsules shall be stored under conditions which shall ensure their safety from the effects of excessive heat and moisture.
- Separate area for filling, drying, and storage.
- Packing area divided into two sections: blister packing area, strip packing area.
- Temperature and Humidity controls
- For Hard and Soft Gelatin Capsule Humidity-not more than 35%RH and Temperature-Not more than 25 %.[3]

Equipments for Preparation of Capsule

For preparation	For quality control
Capsule filling machine	Weighing balance
Automatic filling machine	Disintegrating tester
Capsule Polishing machine	Dissolution apparatus
Capsule Sealing machine	
Dehumidifier	

Liquid Dosage form

Syrup

Liquid herbal dosage forms may be prepared by dissolving the herbal preparation in an aqueous or non-aqueous solvent, by suspending it in an appropriate medium or by incorporating it into one of the two phases of an oil and water system. The layout required for preparation of liquid dosage and typical manufacturing facilities for liquid dosage form includes

- ❖ The premises and equipment shall be designed, constructed and maintained to suit the manufacturing of Oral liquids.

- Manufacturing personnel should wear non-fiber shedding clothing to prevent contamination of the product.
- Care shall be taken to maintain the homogeneity of emulsions by use of appropriate emulsifier and suspensions by use of appropriate stirrer during filling.
- Special care should be taken at the beginning of the filling process to ensure that the product is uniformly homogenous during filling.
- When the bulk product is not immediately packed, the maximum period of storage and storage conditions shall be specified.
- Manufacturing area shall have entry through double door airlock facility.
- There should be separate area for each section which included empty bottle storage area, washing area, raw material, liquid solvent storage area, labeling and packaging area. Temperature and Humidity should maintain.
- Drainage shall be of adequate size and have adequate traps, without open channels and design shall be such as to prevent back flow. Drains shall be shallow facilitate cleaning and disinfecting.
- The production area shall be cleaned and sanitized at the end of every
- production process.

Equipments required for preparation of Syrup

For preparation	For quality control
Stainless steel vessel	Hydrometer
Dry syrup powder filling machine	Cone and plate viscometer, Brookfield viscometer
Storage tank	Digital pH meter
Syrup filling machine	

Equipments for preparation of oils

For preparation	For quality control
Steam distillation	Hydrometer(density)
Hydrodistillation	Refractive index meter
Aroma oil distillator	
Soxlet Extraction	
Super critical fluid extraction	

Semi Solid Dosage Form

Ointment

Ointments and creams can be formulated with a herbal extract or powder and a variety of oils and emulsifying agents. Preparation usually involves heating, mixing and stirring the lipid and aqueous portions until the mixture has congealed. They usually require the addition of preservative unless they are intended to be used within a relatively short period of time.

Layout of semi solid dosage form (ointment)

The typical manufacturing facilities required for this forms includes:

- The entrance to the area where these products are manufactured should be through a suitable airlock.
- The area shall be fitted with an exhaust system of suitable capacity to effectively remove vapours, fumes, floating dust particles.
- The equipment used shall be designed and maintained to prevent the product from being accidentally contaminated with any foreign matter or lubricant.
- Water used in compounding should be Purified Water
- Powders where used, shall be suitably sieved before use.
- Heating vehicles and base like petroleum jelly should be done in separate mixing area in suitable stainless steel vessels.
- A separate packaging section may be provided for primary packaging of the products.[3]

Equipments used for preparation of semi solid dosage form (ointment)

For preparation	For quality control
Roller mill	Brookfield Viscometer
Planetary mixer	PH meter
Electric mortar and pestle	Spreadability testing
Ointment mill	
Colloidal mill	
Ointment filling machine	

As herbal medicines are in huge demand in both developed and developing countries, the growth of herbal industry is growing rapidly. It is important to have knowledge of all the legal and regulatory requirements for setting of herbal industry as per WHO, FDA and GMP norms. List of various basic machines and equipments for establishing manufacturing unit of solid, semisolid and liquid dosage form is also discussed in brief. In conclusion, this chapter will help in getting idea about infrastructure of herbal industries involved in production of herbal tablets, capsules, extracts, ointments and creams.

Pilot Plant Scale Up Techniques

Introduction

The Pilot plant is a hybrid development facility and manufacturing unit, which integrates development, early development activities, clinical supply manufacture, technology evaluation, scale up and transfer to production sites. A **pilot plant** is the part of the pharmaceutical industry where a lab scale formula is transformed into a viable product by development of liable and practical procedure of manufacture. **Scale-up** is the process of increasing the batch size or a procedure for applying the sameprocess to different output volumes. It is also defined as the art for designing of prototype using the data obtained from the pilot plant model. The Pilot plant studies must include;

- Current Good Manufacturing Practices (cGMP) environment,
- Highly trained and skilled staffs,
- Equipment support,
- Facility of through and close examination of the formula.

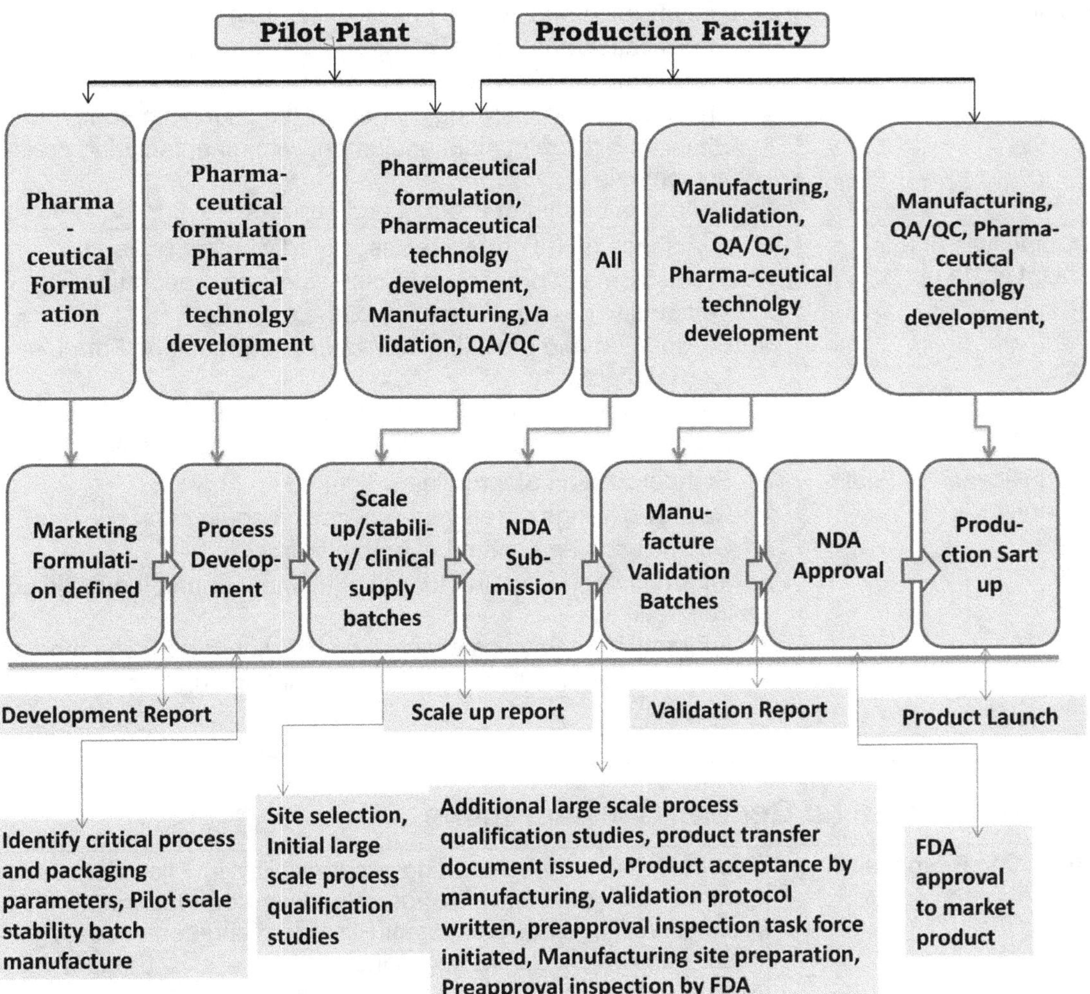

Figure 28.4 Pilot plant facility utilization.

The factors that must be determine for successful product scale up are- requirements, Training, reporting relationships and responsibility of personnel. The pilot plant, production and process control must be evaluated, validated and finalizedduring the scale up. The pilot plant plays an important role in the technology evaluation, scale up and transfer activities of new products.

Pilot plant scale up activities	➤ Technical aspects of process development and scale up ➤ Determination of responsibility of Organization and technology transfer team, ➤ Documentation of Technology transfer ➤ Preparation for FDA pre-approval inspection.
Major technical aspects:	➤ Identification and control of critical components ➤ Identification and control of formulation variables, ➤ Identification of critical process parameters. ➤ Identification of operating ranges for the pilot plant equipment ➤ Simulating the pilot plant equipment with manufacturing areas equipment. ➤ Collection of data of Product and process.
Objectives of Pilot plant scale up:	➤ Avoidance of the problems associated with the scale-up. ➤ Production and process controls guidelines preparation. ➤ To identify the critical features of the process ➤ Preparation and providing of Master Manufacturing Formula for manufacturing. ➤ Evaluation and Validation for process and equipment. ➤ Examination of the formula to assess the batch stability.
Significance of Pilot Plant:	➤ Standardization of formulae. ➤ Review of range of relevant processing equipment. ➤ Optimization and control of production rate. ➤ Information on infrastructure of equipment during the scale up batches. ➤ Information of batches physical space required for equipment. ➤ Identification of critical features to maintain quality of a product. ➤ Appropriate records and reports to support GMP.

Pilot Plant Scale up General Considerations

Reporting Responsibility:	The objective of the reporting responsibility in Pilot plant is to facilitate the transfer of a product from the laboratory into production. The effectiveness of Pilot plant is determined by the ease with which the new product or process is brought into routine production. This could be possible if a good relationship exists between the pilot plant group with other groups (Research & Development, Processing, Packaging, Quality Assurance, Quality Control, Regulatory and Packaging) of the company. The formulator who developed the product can take the product into the production. The formulator continues to provide the support to the other departments even after the transition into the production has been completed.

Contd...

Personnel requirements:	The individual responsibilities should be clearly understood and must be recorded. The qualification required for a person to work in pilot plant organization are: • Good theoretical knowledge of GMP Practices, physical, chemical, biochemical and medical attributes of dosage form and relevant experiences in production areas about formulation, process and equipment. • Good communication (Writing and speaking) and soft skills
Space requirements:	The space required in pilot plant is divided into 4 areas that are as follows; • *Administration and information area*: Adequate office and desk space should be provided for both scientists and technicians. The space should be adjacent to the working area. • *Physical testing area*: This area should provide permanent bench top space for routinely used physical- testing equipment. • *Standard equipment and floor space*: The sufficient specified space must be there for free installation, operation and easymaintenance of the equipment. • *Storage area:* Separate storage area for API, excipients, stability samples, in process materials, finished bulk products, retained samples, experimental production batches, packaging materials. Areas must be segregated into approved and unapproved areas according to GMP.
Training:	New employees, Employees assigned with a new job and Employees with poor performance of various departments: engineering, quality control, material handling, warehousing and distribution and purchasing should be trained on following activities as per the GMP and FDA guidelines that are: ➢ Manufacturing, Processing, packaging and holding of a drug product ➢ Technical environment, dealing with potent or dangerous chemicals ➢ Working with system of weights and measures ➢ Checking of manufacturing steps, containers, equipment and drying racks. ➢ Identification of packaging, proper stock rotation system. ➢ Raw material inspection, quality validation.
Review of the Formula	The objective of each ingredient and its contribution to the final product manufactured on small scale equipment must be thoroughly understood. The modification in formulation during the scale up is possible to be done in phase III trial, so that sufficient time could be available for generation of meaningful long term stability data in support of a proposed New Drug Application (NDA).

Contd...

<table>
<tr><td>Raw materials:</td><td>One major responsibility of a Pilot plant is the approval and validation of active and excipient raw materials used in the Pharmaceutical products. This is because the raw materials used during the small-scale formulation trials may not be representative of the large volume shipment of material due to change in raw materials properties like particle size, shape, morphology, bulk density, static charges, rate of solubility, flow property and color. An alternative supplier must be arranged as stand by basis which must validate the batches formanufactured products.</td></tr>
<tr><td>Relevant Processing Equipment:</td><td>The selection criteria for one equipment to produce effective product within the proposed specifications are equipment must be economic, simple (In installation, handling, cleaning and maintenance), efficient and most capable of consistently producing a product. The size of the equipment should be such that experimental trials can be run that are meaningful and relevant to the production sized batches.</td></tr>
<tr><td>Production Rate:</td><td>For determination of production rate, size and type of equipment required, the immediate and future market requirement must be considered. The selection of process and equipment to produce batches at a frequency need following considerations that are;<ul><li>The time required to clean the equipment between the batches.</li><li>The product loss in the equipment during the manufacture.</li><li>The number of batches that need to be tested before release of product.</li></ul></td></tr>
<tr><td>Process Evaluation:</td><td><ul><li>➢ Things that should be critically examined during the Process Evaluation are;<ul><li>Order of addition of the components including adjustment of their amount.</li><li>Mixing speed ant time.</li><li>Rate addition of granulating agent, solvents and drug solutions.</li><li>Heating and cooling rates.</li><li>Filter size for liquids.</li><li>Type and nature of filter media used for liquids.</li><li>Screening size for solids.</li><li>Drying temperature and time.</li><li>Fan speed.</li></ul></li><li>➢ The basis for process optimization and validation is the knowledge on effect of above mentioned parameters on the in process and finished product quality.</li></ul></td></tr>
</table>

Contd...

<table>
<tr><td></td><td>
➢ The objective of process validation to ensure the selected process could be able to produce quality products at various critical stages of production.
➢ This is possible by critically monitoring the within the batch variation of measurable parameters like content uniformity, moisture content and compressibility.
➢ Some measurable change in the materials may take place during the processes like milling, mixing, heating, cooling, drying, sterilizing, compacting and filling, should be evaluated.
➢ The process remains validated only if there is no change in the formula, quality of the ingredients and equipment configuration.
➢ The manufacturing process and quality control information should be reviewed on an annual basis and should be followed by re-validation to ensure that changes have not occurred.
</td></tr>
<tr><td>Preparation of Master Manufacturing Procedure</td><td>
The Master Manufacturing Procedure includes followings;
➢ The Process or Manufacturing Direction.
• Process direction should be precise and explicit.
• Must be written in a simple manner which should be easily understood by the operator.
➢ The Chemical Weight Sheet.
• Identification of chemical required.
• Quantities of chemical to be added.
• Order of chemicals to be added.
• The name and Identification number of the ingredient must be mentioned.
➢ The Sampling Direction.
• Time of sampling of finished product.
• Manner of sampling of finished products.
➢ The Batch record direction.
• The batch record directions should include specification for addition rates, mixing times, mixing speeds, heating and cooling rates and temperature.
➢ The In-Process Specification.
• Must mention a simple and easy access specification for easy understanding of operators.
➢ The Finished Product Specification.
• The drug in the dose specified.
• The self-life of the product.
</td></tr>
</table>

Contd...

	• The capability of the process. • The reliability of the test methods. • The stability kinetics of the product. The periodic revalidation, GMP and monitoring of finished product test results via control chartsare essential to maintaining consistent product quality.
GMP Consideration:	The check list of the GMP items that should be a part of the scale-up or new product or process introduction including following; • Equipment qualification. • Process Validation. • Regulatory schedule preventive maintenance. • Regular process review and revalidation. • Relevant writing standard operating procedures. • The use of competent, technically qualified personnel. • Adequate provision for training of personnel. • A well-defined technology transfer system. • Validated cleaning procedures. • Arrangement of material to avoid cross contamination.
Transfer of Analytical Methods to Quality Assurance	Analytical methods developed in research must be transferred to the QA department. • Transfer process includes the following aspects; • Review the process to make sure that the proper analytical instrument is available. • Personnel should be trained to perform the test. • Reliability of the test should be checked. • At last assay procedure should be reviewed before transfer.

Pilot Plant Scale up Considerations for Solids

The following points to be carefully consider during scaling up the solid dosage forms: batch size from intermediate to large scale production, each stage of operation, different types of equipment, use of sophisticated instruments with larger volume load and various sizes of equipment.

Material Handling:	Any material handling system must deliver the accurate amount of the ingredient to the destination. The cross contamination must be prevented if a system uses transfer of materials for more than one product step. This is accomplished by use of validated cleaning procedure for the equipment.

Contd...

Chemical Weighing:	The incorrect weighing can cause contamination and or misbranded product. Hence central weighing department in all the processing areas can avoid duplication, appropriate responsibility and reduced labor cost. A chemical weighing department should be designed to provide supervision, checkers, lightening, dust collection, adequate sanitation, proper weighing equipment, supply of sink and drain board, cabinets, vacuum supply system, printing scale facility and meters for liquids. For weighing of dye and high potent drugs, a separate room must be equipped.
Tablet blending and Granulation:	
Blending and Granulation:	Well blended material which is free of lumps and agglomerates results in good drug distribution and thus avoids content variation. In blending depends on particle size, shape, hardness and density.
Dry Blending and Direct Compression:	Different blenders used in blending are V- blender, double cone blender, Ribbon blender, Slant cone blender, Bin blender, Orbiting screw blenders, and vertical and horizontal high intensity mixers. The factors affect the optimization of blending operation of directly compressible materials are: order of addition of components, mixing speed, time and action and or blender loads.
Slugging (Dry Granulation):	The dry powder cannot be compressed directly due to poor flow and compression properties. The slugging is done by using the Tablet Press of 15 tones. After compression, slugs are broken down by Hammer Mill with suitable particle size distribution. The granulation by dry compaction can also be achieved by passing powders between two roller which put pressure of 10 Tones per linear inch.
Wet Granulation:	Granulation helps to give uniform dispersion of active ingredients, good flow properties, change the particle size distribution and increases the apparent density of the powders. Wet granulation has been carried out using Sigma blade mixer, heavy-duty planetary mixer, tumble blenders or by multifunctional "processors" The factors that affecting the Fluidized Bed Granulator are: inlet air temperature, atomization air pressure, air volume, liquid spray rate, nozzle position and number of spray heads, product and exhaust air temperature, filter porosity.
Drying	The important factors to consider as part of scale-up of a most common conventional method i.e. oven drying operation is airflow, air temperature, and the depth of the granulation on the trays. For too deep or too dense the drying process will be inefficient and can cause migration of soluble dyes to the surface of the granules. Drying times at specified temperatures and airflow rates must be established for each product, and for each particular oven load. For fluidized bed dryers, scales up factors are optimum loads, rate of airflow, inlet air temperature and humidity. For tray dryers, scale up factors are air flow, air temperature, depth of the granulation on the trays,

Contd...

Reduction of Particle size:	Compression factors that may be affected by the particle size distribution are flowability, compressibility, uniformity of weight, content, hardness, and color. Particle size reduction can be carried out using a series of "stacked" sieves of decreasing mesh openings or by passing all the material through an oscillating granulator, a hammer mill, a mechanical sieving device, or in some cases, a screening device. As part of the scale-up of a milling or sieving operation, the lubricants and glidants, which in the laboratory are usually added directly to the final blend, are usually added to the dried granulation during the sizing operation. This is done because some of these additives, especially magnesium stearate, tend to agglomerate when added in large quantities to the granulation in a blender.
Facilities:	To avoid cross contamination in scale up and to facilitate the cleaning of equipment effectively, following facilities must be available that are; • Multifunctional processing system • Separate room with availability of more space, • Granulation as unit operation, • Washing and drainage facilities, • Cold, hot water and steam supply system, • Stainless steel or non-dust material platforms should be with system, • Air condition system or screened windows
Granulation Handling and Feed System:	The handling of the finished granulation in the compression area is either by Hand scooping for small scale or by sophisticated automated handling system (long transfer tubes, valves, vacuum and pneumatic pumps) with vacuum or mechanical system for large scale. The properties of material like size, size distribution and flow property affect the tablet properties like drug content uniformity, tablet weight, thickness and hardness.
Tablet Compression:	The tablet press performs following functions during the compression are; • Filling of an empty die cavity with granulation. • Pre-compression of granulation. • Compression of granules. • Ejection of the tablet from the die cavity and take-off of the compressed tablet. The prolonged trial runs at press speeds is generally adopted to find out the potential compression problems like sticking, hardness, capping, and weight variation detected. High-speed press criteria depends on granulation feed rate, delivery system based particle size distribution, segregation of course and fine particles if any and induction of static charges. The smaller the tablet, the more difficult it is to get a uniform to fill high press

Contd...

	speeds. High levels of lubricant or over blending can result in a soft tablet, decrease in wettability of the powder and an extension of the dissolution time. Binding to die walls can also be overcome by designing the die to be 0.001 to 0.005 inch wider at the upper portion than at the center in order to relieve pressure during ejection.
Tablet Coating:	Many changes are happening in Sugar coating (Carried in conventional coating pans), due to new developments in coating technology (Conventional sugar-coating pan changed to perforated pans or fluidized-bed coating columns), changes in safety and environmental regulations. Lab level film coating solution may be totally unacceptable on a production scale. The tablets must be sufficiently hard to withstand the tumbling during coating. Film coating with an aqueous system for hydrophobic tablet core materials may require special formulation of the tablet core and/or the coating solution.
Encapsulation of Hard Gelatin Capsules:	
	The High-Speed equipment is used to prepare the capsule by using the processed powder blend with following particle characteristics like particle size distribution, bulk density, compressibility to promote good flow property. This facilitates the formation of compacts of the right size and of sufficient cohesiveness to be filled into capsule shells. Weight variation in capsules may come due to poor flow characteristics, improper lubrication and plug sticking to plunger surface. Overlay lubrication may create problems in weight variation, disintegration, dissolution and Bioavailability. The characteristics of granulation and the finished products are greatly influenced by the type and size of equipment used for blending, granulating, drying, sizing and lubrication. For better encapsulation, need of controlled environmental conditions that are Controlled humidity (RH 45 to 55 %) system in processing and encapsulation (RH 35 to 65 %) room and appropriate temperature condition of 15 to 25 °C.

Pilot Plant Scale up Considerations for Liquid Orals

The physical form of a drug product that can be incorporated demonstrates Newtonian or Pseudoplastic flow behavior. It conforms to its container at room temperature. Liquid dosage forms may be dispersed systems or solutions. In dispersed systems there are two or more phases, where one phase is distributed in another. A solution refers to two or more substances mixed homogeneously.

Steps of liquid manufacturing process	• Planning of material requirements. • Liquid preparation. • Filling and Packing. • Quality assurance.
Critical aspects of liquid manufacturing	• Physical Plant. • Heating, ventilation and air controlling system. ➢ The effect of long processing times at suboptimal temperatures should be considered in termsof consequences on the physical or chemical stability of ingredients as well as product.
Solution	➢ The parameters to be considered are for scale up of solutions are; • Impeller diameter. • Tank size (diameter). • Number of impellers. • Impeller type. • Mixing capability of impeller. • Rotational speed of the impeller. • Height of the filled volume in the tank. • Number of baffles. • Transfer system. • Clearance between Impeller Blades and wall of the mixing tank. • Filtration equipment (should remove desired materials but should not remove active oradjuvant ingredients). • Passivation of Stainless Steel (Pre-reacting the SS with acetic acid or nitric acid solutionto remove. the surface alkalinity of the Stainless Steel).
Suspension	➢ The parameters to be considered are for scale up of suspension are; • Variator (To avoid air entrapment). • Wetting of suspending agent. • Addition and dispersion of suspending agents. • Selection of the equipment according to batch size. • Time and temperature required for hydration of the suspending agent. • Mixing speeds (High speed should not be used as it leads to air entrapment). • Mesh size (Must be able to remove the foreign particulates and sieve selected based onproduction batch size trials).

Contd…

Emulsion	➢ The parameters to be considered are for scale up of emulsion are; • Homogenizing equipment. • Temperature. • Mixing equipment. • Phase densities. • In-process or final product filters. • Phase volumes. • Screens, pumps and filling equipment. • Phase viscosities.

Pilot Plant Scale up considerations for Semi Solids

Parameters are to be considered during the scale up of semisolid products	• Mixing speed. • Mixing equipment (Could be able to move semisolid mass from outside walls to thecenter and from bottom to top of the kettle). • Motors (Drive mixing system with appropriate handling system at its most viscous stage). • Heating and cooling process. • Component homogenization. • Product transfer. • Addition of active ingredients. • Working temperature range. • Shear during handling and transfer from manufacturing to holding tank to filling lines. • Transfer pumps (Easily must move viscous material without applying excessive shear andfree of entrapped air).
Parameters must be consider during choosing the size and type of pump	• Pumping rate. • Pumping pressure required should be considered. • Product compatibility with the pump surface. • Product viscosity.

SUPAC Guidelines

Any significant change in a process of making a pharmaceutical dosage form is a regulatory concern. The scale-up process and the changes made after approval in the composition, manufacturing process, manufacturing equipment, and change of site have become known as Scale-Up and Post approval Changes, or SUPAC. Scale-Up and Post approval Changes

(SUPAC) are of special interest to the FDA, as is evidenced by a growing number of regulatory documents released in the past several years by the Center for Drug Evaluation and Research (CDER), including Immediate Release Solid Oral Dosage Forms (SUPAC-IR), Modified Release Solid Oral Dosage Forms (SUPAC-MR), and Semisolid Dosage Forms (SUPAC-SS). Additional SUPAC guidance documents being developed include: Transdermal Delivery Systems (SUPAC-TDS), Bulk Actives (BACPAC), and Sterile Aqueous Solutions (PAC-SAS). Collaboration between the FDA, the pharmaceutical industry, and academia in this and other areas has recently been launched under the framework of the Product Quality Research Institute (PQRI).

The SUPAC Guidelines defines:

- The level of changes – Minor, Moderate and Major Changes.
- Test – Application test, *in vitro* dissolution and *in vivo*
- Filing – Annual report, changes being affected supplement and Prior Approval Supplement.
- The level of changes may impact on formulation and quality performance in following levels;
    - Level 1: unlikely to have detectable Impact.
    - Level 2: could have significant impact.
    - Level 3: likely to have significant impact.

SUPAC guidelines provide recommendations for post approval changes as follows:

1. The components or composition changes	➢ This section focuses on changes in excipients in the drug product. ➢ SUPAC-MR - Excipient critical or non-critical to the Modified drug release. • Changes in non-release and release controlling excipients. ➢ SUPAC-SS - Changes in preservative in semisolid formulations. ➢ SUPAC-IR Changes for immediate-release solid oral dosage forms.
2. The site changes of manufacture:	➢ Changes in location of the site of manufacture, packaging operations and/or analytical testinglaboratory. ➢ Do not include any scale-up changes, changes in manufacturing (including process and/orequipment), or changes in components or composition. ➢ Current Good Manufacturing Practice (CGMP) inspection.
Level I Changes -	*Classification*-Single facility where the same equipment, standard operating procedures (SOP's), environmental conditions (e.g., Temperature and humidity) and controls, and personnel common. *Test Documentation* - Application/ compendia requirements in chemistry, dissolution and *in vivo* Bioequivalence - None. ➢ *Filing Documentation*- Annual report.
Level II Changes -	*Classification*–Same continuous campus, Common personnel, No other changes. *Test Documentation*– o Application/ compendial requirements

Contd...

	○ Notification of Location of new site ○ Updated batch records ○ SUPAC – MR - Multi-point dissolution profiles (15, 30, 45, 60 and 120 min) USP buffer media at pH 4.5-7.5 for extended release). Three different Media (e.g., Water, 0.1N HCl, ands buffer media at pH 4.5 and 6.8for delayed release) until 80% of Drug Released. *Filing Documentation*- Annual report.
Level III Changes -	• *Classification*– Different campus, Different personnel. • *Test Documentation* – Application/compendial requirements, notification of location of new site, updated batch record. ○ SUPAC - IR: Multi-point dissolution profile in the application/compendia medium. ○ SUPAC - MR: Multi-point dissolution profiles (15, 30, 45, 60 and 120 min) USP buffer media at pH 4.5-7.5 for extended release). Three different Media (e.g., Water, 0.1N HCl, and USP buffer media at pH 4.5 and 6.8 for delayed release) until 80 % of Drug Released. • *Filing Documentation*- Annual report prior approval of supplement.
3. Changes in batch size (Scale-Up/Scale-Down):	Post-approval changes in the size of a batch from the pivotal/pilot scale bio batch material to larger or smaller production batches call for submission of additional information in the application. Scale-down below 100,000 dosage units is not covered by this guidance.
Level I Changes -	• *Classification*- Change in batch size, up to and including a factor of 10 times the size of thepilot/bio batch. • *Test Documentation* – Updated batch records application/compendial requirements stability. • *Filing Documentation*- Annual report (long term stability data).
Level II Changes -	• *Classification*- Changes in batch size beyond a factor of ten times the size of the pilot or bio batch,No other changes. • *Test Documentation –* Chemistry Documentation Application/ compendial release requirements. Notification of change and submission of updated batch records. Stability testing: One batch with three months accelerated stability data and one batch on long-term stability. ○ Dissolution Documentation-Case B testing. ○ In Vivo Bioequivalence - None. • *Filing Documentation*- Changes being affected supplement; annual report (long-term stabilitydata).
4. Manufacturing (process and equipment) Changes	Manufacturing changes may affect both equipment used in the manufacturing process and theprocess itself.
i) Equipment -	***Level I Changes:*** *Classification*- Alternate equipment of the same design and principles as automated equipment.

Contd...

	Test Documentation – Updated batch records, Application/compendial requirements and stability. *Filing Documentation*- Prior approval supplement with justification for change; annual report(long-term stability data). ***Level II Changes:*** *Classification*- Change to equipment of different design and principle. *Test Documentation* – Updated batch records, Application/compendial requirements and stability. o SUPAC – IR - Multi-point dissolution profiles in multiple media. o SUPAC – MR - Multi-point is solution profiles in multiple media. *Filing Documentation*- Annual report and changes being Affected Supplement.
ii) Process -	***Level I Changes:*** *Classification*- Alternate equipment of the same design and principles as automated equipment. *Test Documentation* – Updated batch records, Application/compendial requirements and stability. *Filing Documentation*- Annual report. ***Level II Changes:*** *Classification*- This category includes process changes including changes such as mixing times and operating speeds outside of application/ validation ranges. *Test Documentation* – Updated batch records, Application/compendial requirements and stability. o SUPAC - IR - Multi-point dissolution profile. o SUPAC- MR - Multi-point dissolution profiles in multiple media. o SUPAC – SS - *In vitro* release test Documentation. *Filing Documentation*- Changes being affected supplement; annual report (long term stabilitydata). ***Level III Changes*:** *Classification*- Changes in the type of process used (e.g. wet granulation to direct compression). *Test Documentation* – Updated batch records, Application/compendial requirements, stability,bio-study and IVIVC. o SUPAC - IR - Multi-point dissolution profile. o SUPAC- MR - Multi-point dissolution profiles in multiple media. *Filing Documentation*- Prior approval supplement with justification; annual report (long-termstability data).

Further Reading

1. Agalloco JP, Carleton FJ; Validation of Pharmaceutical Processes; 3rd edition, 2007: 417- 428.
2. Ahmed M.Faheem, Dalia H.Abdelkader.Novel drug delivery systems. Engineering Drug Delivery Systems. 2020, Pages 1-16
3. Amit J, Sunil C, Vimal K, Anupam P. The Pharma Review. New Delhi: Kongposh Publications Pvt. Ltd; 2008. Phytosomes: A revolution in herbal drugs; pp. 24–8.

4. Bhabani Shankar Nayak. Bp 702 t. Industrial pharmacy II (Theory) -Unit-I pilot plant scale up techniques. Institute of Pharmacy& Technology. Salipur, Cuttack,Odisha. Accessed-https://www.iptsalipur.org/wp-content/uploads/2020/08/BP702T_IP_I.pdf.
5. Block LH; Medicated Applications. In Gennaro AR editor; Remington: The Science and Practice of Pharmacy. 19th edition, Mack Publishing Company, Easton, Pennsylvania, 1995: 1590–1597.
6. Block LH; Medicated Applications. In Gennaro AR; Remington: The Science and Practice of Pharmacy. Mack Publishing Company, Easton, Pennsylvania, 1995:1577–1597.
7. Collett M, Aulton EA; Text Book of Pharmaceutical Practice. 2nd edition, 2002.
8. Dhobale AV, Mahale AM, Shirsat M, Pethkar S, Chakote V. Recent Advances in Pilot Plant Scale Up Techniques - A Review. Indo Am J Pharm Res 2018; 8(4): 1060-1068.
9. Durgesh Nandini Chauhan, Madhu Gupta, Nagendra Singh Chauhan, Vikas Sharma. Novel Drug Delivery Systems for Phytoconstituents.CRC Press, 2019.
10. FDA. Center for Drug Evaluation and Research,Guidance for Industry: Immediate Release Solid OralDosage Forms. Scale-up and Post-Approval Changes:Chemistry, Manufacturing and Controls, In VitroDissolution Testing, and In Vivo BioequivalenceDocumentation [SUPAC-IR]; 1995.
11. FDA; Guidance for Industry, Non-sterile Semisolid Dosage Forms, Scale-Up and Postapproval Changes: Chemistry, Manufacturing, and Controls, in vitro Release Testing and in vivo Bioequivalence Documentation, Rockville, MD, May 1997.
12. Gomez AL, Strathy WA. Engineering Aspects of Process Scale-Up and Pilot Plant Design. In: Michael Levin, editor. PharmaceuticalProcess Scale-Up. New York: Marcel Dekker Inc; 2002. p. 311-324.
13. Idson B, Lazarus J; Semisolids in the Theory and Practice of Industrial Pharmacy. In Lachman L, Lieberman HA, Kanig JL editors; Varghese Publishing House, Bombay, India, 1991: 534–563.
14. Idson B, Lazarus J; Semisolids. In The Theory and Practice of Industrial Pharmacy. In Lachman L, Lieberman HA, Kanig JL editors, Varghese Publishing House, Bombay, India, 1991: 534–563.
15. Lachman L, Lieberman HA, Kenig JL; The Theory & Practice of Industrial Pharmacy. 3rd edition, Varghese Publishing house, 1987.
16. Lieberman HA, Rieger MM, Banker GS; Pharmaceutical Dosage Forms: Disperse System, 2nd edition, Volume 3, 473-511
17. Mounica NVN, Sharmila RV, Anusha S, Evangeline L, Nagabhushanam MV, Nagarjunareddy D, et al. Scale up and Postapproval changes (SUPAC) Guidance for Industry: A Regulatory note. Int J Drug RegulAff 2017; 5(1): 13-19.
18. Mukherjee, S et al. "Solid lipid nanoparticles: a modern formulation approach in drug delivery system." Indian journal of pharmaceutical sciences vol. 71,4 (2009): 349-58.
19. Nash RA, Wachter AH; Pharmaceutical Process Validation; 3rd edition, 2003.
20. Rafiee TM, Mehramizi A; In vitro release studies of piroxicam from oil-in-water creams and hydroalcoholic gel topical formulations. Drug Dev Ind Pharm., 2000; 64: 409–414.
21. Roop K Khar, Farhan J Ahmad, A Vashishtha, S. Harder, GV Buskirk, JV Battista. Pilot Plant Scale-up and Production Management. In: Roop K Khar, SP Vyas, Farhan J Ahmad, Gaurav K Jain, Editors. Industrial Pharmacy. 4th edition. New Delhi: CBS Publishers & Distributors Pvt Ltd, 2013. pp. 947-1002.
22. Ryan F. Donnelly, Thakur Raghu Raj Singh. Novel Delivery Systems for Transdermal and Intradermal Drug Delivery. Willey, 2015.

23. Sahoo SK, Labhasetwar V. Nanotech approaches to drug delivery and imaging. Drug Discov Today. 2003;8:1112–20.
24. Shah VP, Skelly JP, Barr WH, Malinowski H, Amidon GL. Scale-up of Controlled ReleaseProducts - Preliminary Considerations. Pharm Technol1992; 16(5):35-40.
25. Sherman R. Technology & Product Architectures. In: Business Intelligence Guidebook. Science Direct; 2015.
26. Singhal P, Singhal R, Kumar V, Goel KK, Jangra AK, Yadav R. Transdermal Drug Delivery System: A Novel Technique To Enhance Therapeutic Efficacy And Safety Of Drugs. Am J Pharm tech Res. 2012; 2: 106-125.
27. Yie Chien. Novel Drug Delivery Systems. CRC Press LLC, 2019.
28. Zatz JL, Kushla P; Gels. In In: Lieberman HA, Rieger MM, Banker GS, editors; Pharmaceutical Dosage Forms: Disperse Systems. Voume 2, New York: Marcel Dekker, 1988:: 495-510.

Scan QR code to view the website/guidelines

- Herbal Sector in India-
Cover Design - Final.cdr (echarak.in)

CHAPTER 29

Herbal Entrepreneurship

Project

Introduction

The dictionary meaning of Project is that it is a scheme of something intended to be done; a Proposal for an Undertaking, design, speculative imagination etc. In simple words, a project is an idea or a plan that is intended to be carried out. The very foundation of an enterprise is the Project. Hence, the Success or Failure of an enterprise largely depends upon the Project. Few other definitions of "Project' are as follows:

- ***Definition 1***: The World Bank has defined Project as an approval for a capital investment to develop facilities to provide Goods & Services.
- ***Definition 2:*** A Project is an appraisal for Investment with the definite aim of producing a flow of Output over a specified period of time.
- ***Definition 3***: A Project is defined as the whole complex of activities involved in using resources to gain benefits.
- ***Definition 4***: A Project can be defined as a scientifically evolved work plan devised to achieve a specific objective within a specified period of time etc.

A Project is a combination of humanand non-human resources put together in a temporary organization to achieve a specified purpose. Project is a system involving co-coordination of a number of interrelated activities to achieve a specific objective. There are different types of projects as shown in figure 1.

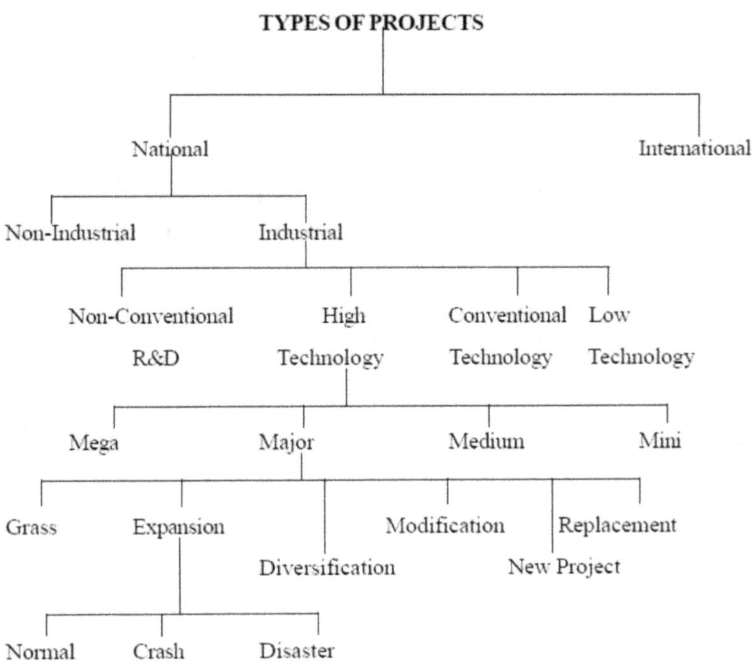

Figure 29.1 Types of projects.

Project Cycle

Project cycle has five stages-identification, formulation, appraisal, implementation and monitoring and evaluation.

(i) **Identification:** Identify feasible and promising business opportunities based on collection, compilation and analysis of economic data from sources like entrepreneurs, technical experts, local leaders, progressive farmers, bankers, mass media, extension agencies and national policies and plans.

(ii) **Fomlulation:** Advanced techniques of project planning like Programme Evaluation and Review of techniques (PERT) and Critical path Method (CPM) are used in capital intensive and complex project of long duration.

(iii) **Appraisal:** Project appraisal means analysis and scrutiny of several aspects like technical, financial, commercial, managerial, economic, distributive and environmental.

(iv) **Implementation**: The phases of Implementation from idea to establishment are:

  (a) Pre development phase: this involves getting registration, licenses and loan disbursement,

  (b) Development phase: construction of structures and starting up of production, and

  (c) Operational phase: starts with production and concludes when the economic life of the project comes to an end.

(v) **Monitoring and Evaluation:** Monitoring phase exercise indicators to check project performance according to the plan, identifying problem areas and finding possible solutions. There are two types of monitoring which banks undertake:

  (a) Desk monitoring based on collected data and

  (b) Field monitoring, based on actual field visit.

Evaluation is conducted for the purpose of learning lessons of success and failure from the project. There are several organizations (like NABARD or training establishments) which conduct such evaluations studies and publish them for wider circulation.

Project Identification/Selection or Ideation

Project identification is the first step of a new venture. A right direction may enable an entrepreneur to scale new height. Otherwise, he has to undergo a number of hurdles in his way. It is therefore, very crucial to entrepreneurs to identify project. Project identifications concerned with collection, compilation and analysis of economic data for the eventual purpose of locating possible opportunities for investment.

Design thinking is a non-linear, iterative process that teams use to understand users, challenge assumptions, redefine problems and create innovative solutions to prototype and test. Involving five phases—Empathize, Define, Ideate, Prototype and Test.

Ideation, or "Ideate", is the third step in the Design Thinking process – after "Empathize" (gaining user insights from research/observation) and "Define" (finding links/patterns within those insights to create a meaningful and workable problem statement or point of view).

STEP I: Generation of Ideas

It involves search for promising project idea or business opportunity though SWOT analysis, ideation individually or brainstorming with group of people. Performance of existing industries, inputs and outputs of various Industries, review imports and exports, Government initiatives and economic and social trends

Sample SWOT (acronym for Strength, Weaknesses, Opportunities and Threat) analysis		
Internal factors	**Strengths** • Political support • Funding available • Market experience • Strong leadership • Any foreign collaboration • Industrial contacts	**Weaknesses** • Project is very complex • Likely to be costly (huge inves1n1ent) • Lack of experience • Lack of trained personnel. • Inability to forecast market trends.
External factors	**Opportunities** • Project may improve local economy • Competitor weakness. • Project will boost company's public image • Government & other incentives. • New technology (create new market)	**Threats** • Environmental constraints • Time delays • New Technology (make the previous product outdated) • National and global economic conditions • Stiff competition in market.

Herbal business ideas:

- Aloe Vera Juice, Gel & Powder Production
- Cultivation and Processing of Medicinal Plants
- Production of Herbal Cosmetics
- Herbal Formulation
- Ayurvedic Medicine Formulations

STEP 2: Short Listing Ideas

After searching a number of business opportunities,best idea can be selected on following points:

1. **Compatibility with the Promoter:** According to Murphy, a real opportunity has three characteristics:
    - It fits the personality of the entrepreneur (abilities, training etc)
    - It is accessible to him

- It offers him the rapid growth and high returns

2. **Consistency with Governmental Priorities:**
    - Is the project consistent with national goals and priorities?
    - Is there any environmental effect contrary to governmental regulation?
    - Can the foreign requirements of the project be easily accommodated?
    - Will there be any difficulty in obtaining the Licenses for the project?
3. **Availability of Inputs:**
    - Are the capital requirements of the project within manageable Limits?
    - Can the technical know - how required for the project can be obtained?
    - Are the raw materials required for the project available domestically at reasonable cost?
    - Is the power supply for the project reasonably obtainable from external sources?
4. **Adequacy of the market**
    - Total present domestic market
    - Competitors and their market shares
    - Export market
    - Quality-price profile of the product vis-a-vis competitive product
    - Sales and distribution system
    - Projected increase in consumption
    - Patent protection
5. **Acceptability of Risk Level**
    - Vulnerability to business cycle.
    - Technological Changes
    - Competition from substitutes
    - Competition from imports
    - Governmental control over price
6. **Socio-Demographic Sector**
    - Population trends
    - Income distribution
    - Educational Framework
    - Attitude toward consumption and investment

STEP: 3 Assessment of Viability/Project Appraisal

1. **Feasibility Study:** Identified project must have technical, economic and financial viability, environmental compliance and social acceptability; as well as its conformity with the

national development objectives and priorities and the relevant policy, legal and regulatory frame work.

2. **Market Analysis:** Market analysis is concerned with aggregate demand, market share, past and present supply, imports and exports, competition, Cost structure, Consumer behavior, Distribution channels, Administrative, technical, and legal constraints
3. **Technical Analysis:** This examines aspects like availability of raw materials, power, and other inputs, optimal selected scale of operation, suitable' production process, appropriate equipment and machines, treatment of effluents, sound layout of the site, work schedules and social impact of proposed technology.
4. **Financial Analysis:** This helps to determine whether the project satisfies the investment criteria of generating acceptable level of profitability through aspects like: Investment outlay and cost of project, sources of financing, projected profitability, break-even point and level of risk
5. **Economic Analysis:** This implies social cost benefit analysis, for direct economic benefits in terms of shadow (efficiency) prices vs market prices, distribution of income in the society and social contribution
6. **Ecological Analysis:** Ecological analysis should be done particularly for major projects which have significant ecological implications/damage (like power plants and irrigation schemes) and environment-polluting industries (like bulk drugs, chemicals, and leather processing). It should satisfy restoration measures to keep damage within acceptable limit

Project Formulation

Project formulation is done to ensure the best utilization of minimum possible resource to yield the maximum possible results. Project formulation lays the foundation for the final selection of an investment proposal after a comparative analysis of all the investment proposal selected doe the purpose.

- Project involves step by step investigation and development of project idea.
- It provides a controlled mechanism for restricting expenditure on project development.
- Project formulation is a process involving the joint efforts of a team of experts. Each member of the team should be familiar with the broad strategy, objectives and other ingredients of the project.
- Project team should consist of experts in major substantive fields of the project.
- A well-formulated feasibility report provides a medium, for successful implementation of a project.

Project formulation is defined as "taking a first look carefully and critically at a project idea by an entrepreneur to build up an all-round beneficial to the project after carefully weighing its various components." In short Project Formulation is a process whereby the entrepreneur makes an objective and independent assessment of the various aspects of an investment proposition of a project idea for determining its total impact and also its liabilities.

Stages of Project Formulation

Feasibility Analysis:	First stage of screening to decide further for detailed project design or investment plan for internal and external constraints,
Project Design and Network Analysis	This helps to identify project inputs, finance requirement, cost-benefit, sequence and Time of events of the project
Input Analysis:	Its assesses the input requirements for materials, human resources
Financial Analysis:	Its assesses project costs, operating cost and fund requirements, discounted cash flow, cost-volume-profit relationship and ratio analysis, caution and foresight in developing financial forecasts
Cost- Benefit Analysis:	Its assesses overall worth of a project through costs that all entities have to bear and the benefit connected to
Pre-investment Analysis:	It helps sponsors, consultants or implementing bodies to accept/ reject the proposal

Project Financing/Capital Venture

Project finance can be a loan from a bank or it can be generated through sale of new shares through IPOs.

Capital Structure

The capital structure of a company refers as long-term finances used by the firm. The decision regarding the capital is based on the objective of achieving the maximization of shareholders wealth. Factors determining capital structure are: *Minimization of Risk*, *Control* over the firm, *Flexibility* for changing situations, *Profitability*, *Solvency* and satisfactory timely return.

Sources (Capital mix)	Amount	Cost	Percentage of total capital
Owners fund	25,000,000	12%	7.14
Equity share	75,000,000	15%	21.43
Preference share	50,00,000	16%	14.29
Borrowed fund:			
Debenture	40,00,000	14%	I 1.43
Term loans	J ,000,00,000	18%	28.58
Leasing finance	30,00,000	18%	8.57
Other advances	30,00,000	15%	8.57
	3,50,00,000		100

Owner Fund/ Owners Capital: Capital contributed by the owner or entrepreneur of a business, by means of savings or inheritance, is known as own capital or equity. Owner's capital refers to the sum of the business resources owned by the business owners. It is calculated through the subtraction of assets from liabilities. When a business pays all its debts, the amount remaining belongs to the business owner and it is the one that is referred to as owners Capital.

Equity Shares: A unit of ownership that represent equal proportion of company's capital. It entitles its holder (theshareholder) to an equal claim on the company's profits and losses.Two major types of shares are:

1. ***Ordinary shares (Common stock),*** share in the earnings of the company as and when they occur with voting rights
2. ***Preference shares (preferred stock)*** fixed periodic income (interest) to shareholder without voting rights.

Borrowed funds: Fund, in the form of debenture (certificate or a loan bond), term loan and financial lease, which are granted by another person or institution such as banks, financial institutions, public or by issuing bonds or debentures are called borrowed capital to be paid back with interest. The ratio between debt and equity is named leverage. Higher leverage higher the profit but create solvency risk. This can be in

Factors Determining Capital Structure

- Type and size of the enterprise.
- Future prospects of enterprise.
- Financial soundness of entrepreneur.
- Volume of capital required.
- Cost of capital and cost of its procurement.
- Pay-back period of the project.
- Availability of alternative sources.
- Rate of return on investment.
- Reputation of the entrepreneur.
- Risk involved in tJ1e project.
- Flexibility needed in the capital structure.

Cost of Capital

All capital has a cost but it varies from one sources of capital to another, from one company to another and from one period of time to another. Cost of capital can be equal to the average minimum rate of return that an investor in a company will expect for providing fund.

Importance of Cost of Capital

The cost of capital is a guideline for determining the optimum capital structure of a company, acceptance or rejection of project. Projects which earn higher than or equal to cost of capital are selected for investment.

Venture Capital

Harvard Business School professor Georges Doriot is generally considered the "Father of Venture Capital". He started the American Research and Development Corporation (ARD) in 1946 and raised a $3.5 million fund to invest in companies that commercialized technologies developed during WWII. ARDC's first investment was in a company that had ambitions to use x-ray technology for cancer treatment. The $200,000 that Doriot invested turned into $1.8 million when the company went public in 1955.

Venture Capital has emerged as a new financial method of financing during the 20th century. Venture capital is the capital provided by firms of professionals who invest alongside management in young, rapidly growing or changing companies that have the potential for high growth. Venture capital is a form of equity financing especially designed for funding high risk and high reward projects. There is a common perception that venture capital is a means of financing high technology projects. However, venture capital is investment of long term finance made in:

- Ventures promoted by technically or professionally qualified but unproven entrepreneurs, or
- Ventures seeking to harness commercially unproven technology, or
- High risk ventures.

The term 'venture capital' represents financial investment in a highly risky project with the objective of earning a high rate of return. In fact, the venture capitalist acts as a partner with the entrepreneur. Thus, a venture capitalist (VC) may provide the seed capital for unproven ideas, products, technology oriented or start up firms. The venture capitalists may also invest in a firm that is unable to raise finance through the conventional means.

Types of Venture Capitalists

Generally, there are three types of organized or institutional venture capital funds –

(i) angel investors- high network individual investors

(ii) subsidiaries of corporations- major corporations; commercial bank holding companies and other financial institutions

(iii) Private capital firms/funds- investing in an early stage company with little or no history for higher return through high-risk equity investments in the venture.

Modes of Finance by Venture Capitalists

Venture capitalists provide funds for long-term in any of the following modes- *Equity, Conditional loan or Convertible loans.*

Stages of Investment Financing

"Venture capital firms finance both early and later stage investments to maintain a balance between risk and profitability." Venture capital firms usually recognise the following two main stages when the investment could be made in a venture namely:

A. ***Early Stage Financing***: i. Seed Capital & Research and Development Projects. ii. Start Ups ii. Second Round Finance

B. *Later Stage Financing*: i. Development Capital ii. Expansion Finance iii. Replacement Capital iv. Turn Arounds

The venture capital funding procedure gets complete in six stages of financing corresponding to the periods of a company's development

- ***Seed money***: Low level financing for proving and fructifying a new idea
- ***Start-up:*** New firms needing funds for expenses related with marketing and product development
- ***First-Round***: Manufacturing and early sales funding
- ***Second-Round***: Operational capital given for early stage companies which are selling products, but not returning a profit
- ***Third-Round***: Also known as Mezzanine financing, this is the money for expanding a newly beneficial company
- ***Fourth-Round***: Also called bridge financing, 4th round is proposed for financing the "going public" process

Factors Affecting Investment Decisions

The venture capitalists usually take into account the following factors while making investments:

1. Strong Management Team
2. A Viable Idea
3. Business Plan
4. Project Cost and Returns
5. Future Market Prospects
6. Existing Technology
7. Miscellaneous Factors- availability of raw material and labor, pollution control measures undertaken, government policies, rules and regulations applicable to the business/industry, location of the industry etc

Procedure Followed by VCs

(a) *Receipt of proposal:* A proposal is a detailed and well-organised business plan.

(b) *Appraisal of plan:* It is based on credit worthiness, the nature of the product or service, the markets and or cost-benefit analysis.

(c) *Investment:* investment of funds from VCs.

(d) *Provide value added services:* Venture capitalists not only invest money but also provide managerial and marketing assistance and operational advice. They also make efforts to accomplish the set targets which consequently results in appreciation of their capital.

(e) *Exit*: After some years, when the assisted company has reached a certain stage of profitability the VC sells his shares in the stock market at high premium, thus earning profits as well as releasing locked up funds for redeployment in some other venture and this cycle continues.

Capitalization (Financial Structure, Capital Structure or Total Capitalization)

Definition According to Gestenberg, "Capitalizations means the total accounting value of all the capital regularly employed in the business". The entire amount of fund to be invested in an enterprise is known as capital. The capital requirement of an organization usually depends on the size of the unit, nature of project, volume of production, technology, nature of product etc. Capitalization implies the process of determining the plan of financing. In this sense capitalization includes:

- Estimation of total amount of capital to be raised.
- Determining the type of securities to be issued.
- Determining the composition of various securities

Types of capital

- **Fixed capital**: portion of capital utilized to create physical infrastructure i.e. creation or purchase or procurement of fixed assets
- **Blocked capital**: usually huge amount of money is blocked or along time
- **Working capital**: amount of capital utilized to run the enterprise on day to day basisi.e.in the payment of salaries rent, wages etc. is known as (working capital = current assets-current liabilities).

Both inadequate as well as surplus capitalis harmful for the financial health of an enterprise

Project Evaluation

Project evaluation refers to the systematic collection, analysis and use of information to answer questions about a project. It involves the analysis of costs, outcome or impact, implementation as well as the need for the project. In general terms it checks:

- Methods for controlling the cost, time, quality and performance
- Sound and effective initial to post completion assessment
- Prompt, adequate and accurate information Management
- Assets and interests are properly controlled and .safeguarded from all losses;
- Adequate safeguards against losses, fraud, error and impropriety
- Identification and recovery form of waste or inefficiency
- Sound basis for the funding of the project:
- Internal guidance and Standard SOPs for each operation

1. **Project Appraisal (Project Financial Evaluation):** To take a decision to a start a project, methods to determine the return of investment plays crucial role
   (a) Investment and Cash Flow Concept

(b) Return on Investment (ratio of profit to initial capital)

(c) Discounted Cash Flow Technique:

(d) Measures of Financial Viability

- Net Present value (NPV)
- Benefit Cost Ratio (BCR)
- Profitability Index
- Internal Rate of Return (IRR)

2. **Network Analysis (Project Time consumption evaluation):** Rough estimate of time taken by the project to complete is calculated with the help of:
   - CPM (Critical Path Method)
   - PERT (Program Evaluation Review Technique)

3. **Project Demand Analysis:** Methods of demand forecasting are as follows:

Opinion polling methods	Consumer Service method
	Collective opinion method
	Expert opinion Method (Delphi technique)
Statistical methods	Barometric Technique
	Simultaneous equation
	Regression Method
	Trend Projection Method Graphical Method ➢ Moving average Method ➢ Least Square Method

Global Marketing Management

Introduction

Global marketing management is of great importance to a company that is looking to offer its product in an international market.Global marketing requires a firm to understand the requirements associated with servicing customers locally with global standard solutions or products and localizes that product as required to maintain an optimal balance of cost, efficiency, customization and localization in a control-customization continuum to meet local, national and global requirements.

Global marketing and global branding are integrated. Branding involves a structured process of analyzing "soft" assets and "hard" assets of a firm's resources. The strategic analysis and development of a brand includes customer analysis (trends, motivation, unmet needs, segmentation), competitive analysis (brand image/brand identity, strengths, strategies, vulnerabilities), and self-analysis (existing brand image, brand heritage, strengths/capabilities, organizational values).

Global brand identity development is the process of establishing brands of products, the firm, and services locally and worldwide with consideration for scope, product attributes, quality, uses, users and country of origin; organizational attributes; personality attributes, and brand-customer relationship; and important symbols, trademarks metaphors, imagery, mood, photography and the company's brand heritage.

A global marketing and branding implementation system distributes marketing assets, affiliate programs and materials, internal communications, newsletters, investor materials, event promotions and trade shows to deliver integrated, comprehensive and focused communication, access and value to the customers.

Elements of Global Marketing

- **Product:** The product must deliver a minimum level of performance. A global company must be able to tweak elements of a product for different markets. For example, Coca-Cola uses two formulas (one with sugar, one with corn syrup) for all markets. The product packaging in every country incorporates the contour bottle design and the dynamic ribbon in some way, shape, or form. The bottle can also include the country's native language and is the same size as other beverage bottles or cans in that same country.
- **Price:** The price of a product varies based on factors such as costs of production, target segment, and supply-demand dynamics. There can be several types of pricing strategies, each tied in with an overall business plan. Pricing can also be used as a demarcation, to differentiate and enhance the image of a product. The price will always vary from market to market.
- **Place:** Refers to the point of sale. How the product is distributed is influenced by how the competition is being offered to the target market. With Coca-Cola, not all cultures use vending machines. In the United States, beverages are sold by the pallet via warehouse stores. In India, this is not an option. Placement decisions are also affected by the product's position in the market place. For example, a high-end product would not be distributed via a dollar store in the United States. Conversely, a product promoted as the low-cost option in France would find limited success in a pricey boutique.
- **Promotion:** Activities undertaken to make the product or service known to the user and trade including advertising, word of mouth, press reports, incentives, commissions and awards to the trade. It can also include consumer schemes, direct marketing, contests and prizes.
- **People:** A firms's arguably most valuable asset is its people. The personality forms the company's brand personality which engages with customers (customer experience), vendors, partners, shareholders and other "publics." The firm's core values, (integrity, honesty, leadership, social responsibility, drive for profit, drive for quality products and services) are reasons why customers choose to buy from one firm or another. And a reason why firms fail (e.g., dishonesty and fraud of Enron, Arthur Anderson, Worldcom).

- **Processes:** Processes for creative and delivering products and services have inherent value. It is an intangible asset that improves the quality of the product and service if well-designed.
- **Physical Evidence**: In today's digital economy, may firms provide non-physical services over the internet and companies' products are Software-as-a-Service (Saas). Historically, banks have many retail locations to signal the financial strength of their institution. Retail locations for consumer brands give evidence of the popularity and reach of their brands.
- Because there is a requirement for trust before a customer buys from a company, some companies without brick and mortar understand that they must provide some proof of existence that their software company is real, significant or legitimate.

Advantages

- Economies of scale in production and distribution
- Lower marketing costs
- Power and scope
- Consistency in brand image
- Ability to leverage ideas quickly and efficiently
- Uniformity of marketing practices
- Helps to establish relationships outside of the 'political arena'
- Helps to encourage ancillary industries to be set up to cater to the needs of the global player
- Benefits of eMarketing over traditional marketing

Project Report

Introduction

The Project Report is a Business Plan, this is an Outcome of an exercise meant to check the viability of an enterprise, analyzeand firm up its essential parameters. In other words, Project report or business plan is a written document of what an entrepreneur proposes to take up andhis course of action to establish his enterprise. The Project report serves like a road map to reach the destination determined by the entrepreneur. Thus, a Project Report can best be defined as a well evolved course of action devised to achieve the specified objectives within a specified period of time. A Project Report needs to be done / prepared with great care and consideration.

Purpose

- Its helps an entrepreneur judge the profitability of a given enterprise proposal. If it reveals a proposal to be unviable, the entrepreneur will avoid a grave error of investing in an unsound venture.
- It is the basis for a development bank to sanction long term financial assistance and a commercial bank to provide working capital assistance

- It aids the process of firming up technical arrangement, choosing a location, selecting plant & machinery, determining man powerandutility needs required for Project Implementation.
- It generates a knowledge base for the entrepreneur concerning such diverse facets as structure of enterprise – industry, market, raw material supply & technology etc.
- It educates the entrepreneur regarding the degree of risk underlying the enterprise proposal.
- It brings into sharp focus the key performance determinants in the chosen line of Business & thus makes the entrepreneur realize the need to pay special attention to such determinants.

Contents

- ***General Information:*** Information on product profile & product details
- ***Promoter(s):*** Educational qualification, work experience, project related experience, special achievements
- ***Location***: Exact proposed location of the project, lease or freehold, location advantages.
- ***Land &Building***: Land areas, built up area, type of construction, cost of construction, detailed plan & cost estimate along with Plant layout
- ***Plant &machinery***: Details of machinery required, capacity, suppliers, cost, various alternatives available, and cost of other miscellaneous assets
- ***Production process***: description of production process, process chart, technical knowhow, technology alternatives available, production programme etc
- ***Utilities***: Sources of utilities and cost estimates: water, power, steam, compressed air requirements, fuel etc
- ***Transport & Communication***: mode, costs
- ***Raw Material:*** list of raw materials required by quality & quantity, sources of procurement, cost of raw materials, tie up arrangements, if any, for procurement of raw materials, alternative raw materials, if any.
- ***Man Power***: the requirement such as skilled, semi skilled, & un-skilled (helpers), places of manpower availability, requirement of training & its cost.
- ***Products***: product mix, product standard, estimated production & sales figures, alternative product substitutes, if any.
- ***Market***: End users of products, distribution of market as local, national, international, trade practices, sales promotion devices etc.
- ***Requirement of Working Capital***: working capital required, sources of working capital, need for collateral security, nature & extent of credit facilities offered & available.
- ***Requirement of Funds***: break up of total project cost in terms of costs of land, building, plant & machinery, misc. fixed assets, preliminary & pre -operative expenses, contingencies & margin money for working capital, financial arrangements for meeting the cost of setting up of the project.
- ***Cost of Production & Profitability of first five years***: break even analysis, schedule of implementation

Project Report for Nishigandha Essential Oil Extraction

1. **Introduction of the Project**

   Nishigandha essential oil Extraction

   "Nishigandha" (*Polianthes tuberosa* L. Family-Amaryllidaceae) that is also known as "Tuberose" is globally famous plant because of its pleasant aroma. In aroma therapy, Nishigandha oil is mainly used to releive stress and brings calmness, joy and harmony in thoughts. It is also widely used in the manufacturing of the bath soaps, perfumes, hair oils and other cosmetic products. It has also wide applications in food industry as flavourant and fragrant for breverages. Tuberose flowers exude perfume for longer period even after detached from the parent plant. Tuberose essential oil can be extracted by Enfluerange method and solvent extraction with Petrolium ether or hydro distillation.

   150 kg of the flowers yeilds approximately 1 kg brown, semisolid absolute of enfleurage containing 11-15% steam volatile oil. For preparation of tuberose absolute, flowers generally picked up before they open to resume maximum quantity of essential oil. Extraction of tuberose flowers with petroleum ether yields 0.08 – 0.14 per cent of concrete, which gives 18 – 23% of absolute on treatment with alcohol and contains 3 – 5% steam volatile oil. Out of the approximate total yield of 30,000 kg of loose flowers from one hectare, in three years, 27.5 kg of 'concrete' could be obtained. This concrete in turn will yield about 5.50 kg of absolute. One hectare of tuberose plantation may yield up to 12 kg of concrete (Cost of 1 kg concrete is US $1350-1450 or Rs. 89805.68/- per Kg). Graded spikes are usually stored less than 24 hours before they are packed and shipped to the markets.Most tuberose flowers are shipped in refrigerated trucks. Spikes must be held in an upright position, during storage and transportation.

2. **Plant Capacity Per Annum** – ....

3. **Market and Demand Aspects**

   Today in 2021, the global essential oil market size is estimated of value of about 10.3 billion USD. It is also estimated that it will reach up to 16 billion USD by 2026. This clearly indicates the market potential of essential oils because of their continuosly increasing demand in aromatherapy, pharmaceuticals and cosmetics.

   One hectare of tuberose plantation may yield up to 12 kg of concrete (Cost of 1 kg concrete is US $1350-1450 or Rs. 89805.68/- per Kg).

4. **Basis and Presumption**

   (a) The scheme is based on two or three shifts of 8 hours per day and 300 working days per annum

   (b) The intrest rate on the borrowed capital has been taken as 12 % per annum

   (c) The cost in respect of Raw Materials, Packing Materials, and Machinery & Equipments has been taken at the time of preparation of project profile and may vary from place to place and time to time.

(d) The rental Value of production shed is taken as per the prevailing rates and may vary from place to place.

(e) The plant capacity utilization has been taken as 75 %, since plant used for oil extraction is continuous plant.

(f) Recovery of has been taken as .... % for the calculation purposes.

5. Implementation Schedule

The project implementation will take about nine months. The break-up of activities with relative time for each activity is as follows:

Sr. No	Activity	Estimated Time Period (Months)
1	Scheme preparation & approval	0 – 2
2	Registration under MSME Act 2006 and sanction of loan	2 - 5
3	Placement of Orders for Machines	4 - 5
4	PFA License	5 - 7
5	Power Connection	5 - 7
6	Installation of Machines	7 - 8
7	Recruitment of Staff & Trial run	8 – 9
8	Commercial Production	10th onwards

6. Legal Aspects:

The general requirements for obtaining License are as under:

(a) Land and Plant Layout.

(b) Proof of Ownership of Land of Consent letter of owner, if the land is taken on rent.

(c) Copy of Memorandum of articles of association or partnership dead, list of Directors etc. as the case may be.

(d) Photocopy of the packing material specimen. e. Clearance from State Pollution Control Board.

7. Technical Aspects

(a) PRODUCTION CAPACITY: ....Metric Ton (MT) P.A.

(b) QUALITY CONTROL & STANDARDS : As per Customer Specifications.

(c) MANUFACTURING PROCESS:

Generally the essential oil is extracted from the particular plant part by Solvent Extraction. However, this method is less advantageous on commercial scale due to the loss of essential oil during process, contamination with the extracting solvent, involvement of too many critical steps of purification and energy consumption. Hence today supercritical fluid chromatography is highly preffered method for isolation of essential oils in industry due to production of the pure oil without any contamination of the solvent and involves very few steps fo the purification if required and assurity of the best quality product. The principle, Method and instrumentation of supercritical fluid chromatography are as follows:

Principle: Supercritical fluid extraction (SFE) is the process of separating one component (the extractant) from another (the matrix) using supercritical fluids as the extracting solvent. Extraction is usually from a solid matrix, but can also be from liquids. SFE can be used as a sample preparation step for analytical purposes, or on a larger scale to either strip unwanted material from a product (e.g. decaffeination) or collect a desired product (e.g. essential oils). These essential oils can include limonene and other straight solvents. Carbon dioxide (CO2) is the most used supercritical fluid, sometimes modified by co-solvents such as ethanol or methanol. Extraction conditions for supercritical carbon dioxide are above the critical temperature of 31 °C and critical pressure of 74 bars. Addition of modifiers may slightly alter this. The discussion below will mainly refer to extraction with CO2, except where specified.

Procedure and Instrumentation

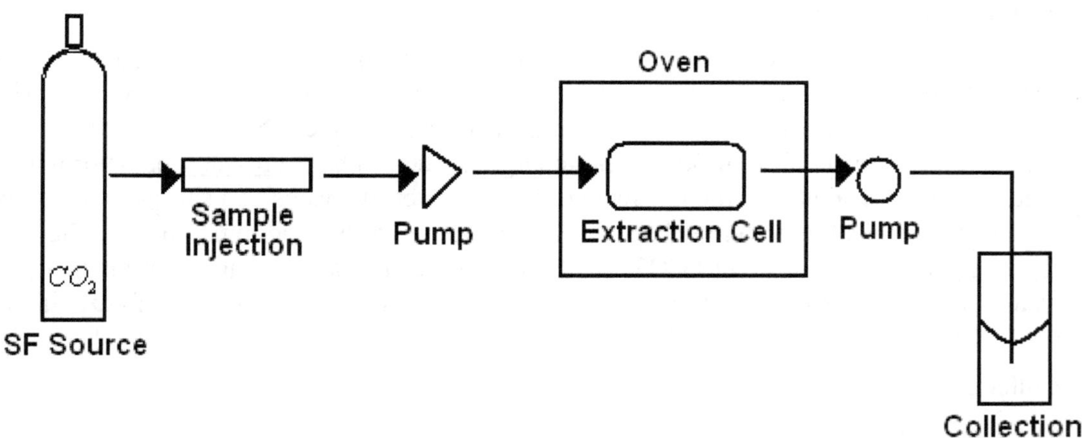

The system contains a pump for the CO2, a pressure cell to keep the sample, a means of maintaining pressure in the system and a collecting vessel. The liquid is pumped to a heating zone, where it is heated to supercritical conditions. It then passes into the extraction vessel, where it rapidly diffuses into the solid matrix and dissolves the material to be extracted. The dissolved material is swept from the extraction cell into a separator at lower pressure, and the extracted material settles out. The CO2 can then be cooled, re-compressed and recycled, or discharged to atmosphere.

Pumps

Carbon dioxide (CO_2) is usually pumped as a liquid, usually below 5 °C (41 °F) and a pressure of about 50 bars. The solvent is pumped as a liquid as it is then almost incompressible; if it were pumped as a supercritical fluid, much of the pump stroke would be "used up" in compressing the fluid, rather than pumping it. For small scale extractions (up to a few grams / minute), reciprocating CO_2 pumps or syringe pumps are often used. For larger scale extractions, diaphragm pumps are most common. The pump heads will usually require cooling, and the CO_2 will also be cooled before entering the pump.

Pressure vessels

Pressure vessels can range from simple tubing to more sophisticated purpose built vessels with quick release fittings. The pressure requirement is at least 74 bars, and most extractions are conducted at less than 350 bar. However, sometimes higher pressures will be needed, such as extraction of vegetable oils, where pressures of 800 bars are sometimes required for complete miscibility of the two phases.

The vessel must be equipped with a means of heating. It can be placed inside an oven for small vessels, or an oil or electrically heated jacket for larger vessels. Care must be taken if rubber seals are used on the vessel, as the supercritical carbon dioxide may dissolve in the rubber, causing swelling, and the rubber will rupture on depressurization.

Pressure maintenance

The pressure in the system must be maintained from the pump right through the pressure vessel. In smaller systems (up to about 10 mL / min) a simple restrictor can be used. This can be either a capillary tube cut to length, or a needle valve which can be adjusted to maintain pressure at different flow rates. In larger systems a back pressure regulator will be used, which maintains pressure upstream of the regulator by means of a spring, compressed air, or electronically driven valve. Whichever is used, heating must be supplied, as the adiabatic expansion of the CO2 results in significant cooling. This is problematic if water or other extracted material is present in the sample, as this may freeze in the restrictor or valve and cause blockages.

Collection

The supercritical solvent is passed into a vessel at lower pressure than the extraction vessel. The density, and hence dissolving power, of supercritical fluids varies sharply with pressure, and hence the solubility in the lower density CO2 is much lower, and the material precipitates for collection. It is possible to fractionate the dissolved material using a series of vessels at reducing pressure. The CO2 can be recycled or depressurized to atmospheric pressure and vented. For analytical SFE, the pressure is usually dropped to atmospheric, and the now gaseous carbon dioxide bubbled through a solvent to trap the precipitated components.

Heating and cooling

This is an important aspect. The fluid is cooled before pumping to maintain liquid conditions, and then heated after pressurization. As the fluid is expanded into the separator, heat must be provided to prevent excessive cooling. For small scale extractions, such as for analytical purposes, it is usually sufficient to pre-heat the fluid in a length of tubing inside the oven containing the extraction cell. The restrictor can be electrically heated, or even heated with a hairdryer. For larger systems, the energy required during each stage of the process can be calculated using the thermodynamic properties of the supercritical fluid.

On industrial scale, generally essential oil is obtained by CO2 extraction machine by using following steps:

1. Grinding of the raw material in to powder by using herbal grinder

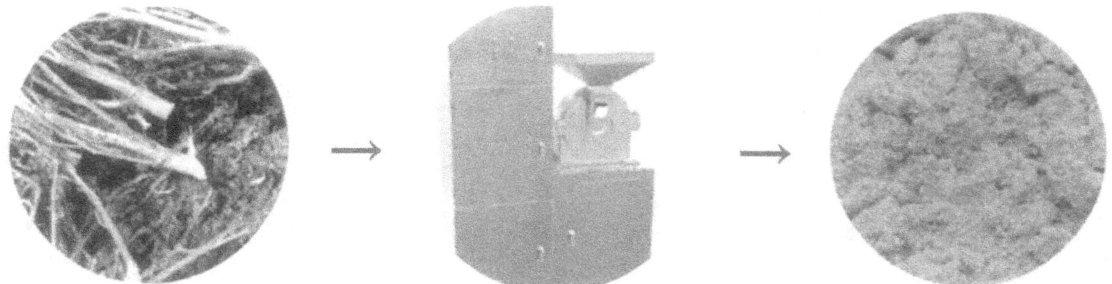

2. Extraction of the essential oil using CO2 extraction machine

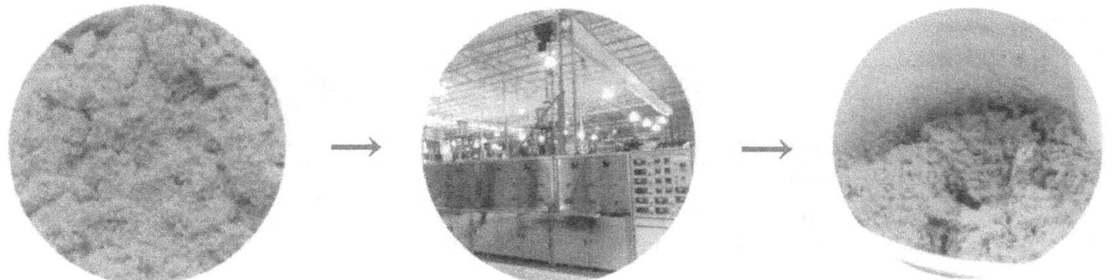

3. Preliminary filtering and removal of fatty material with Filter or Rotary evaporator

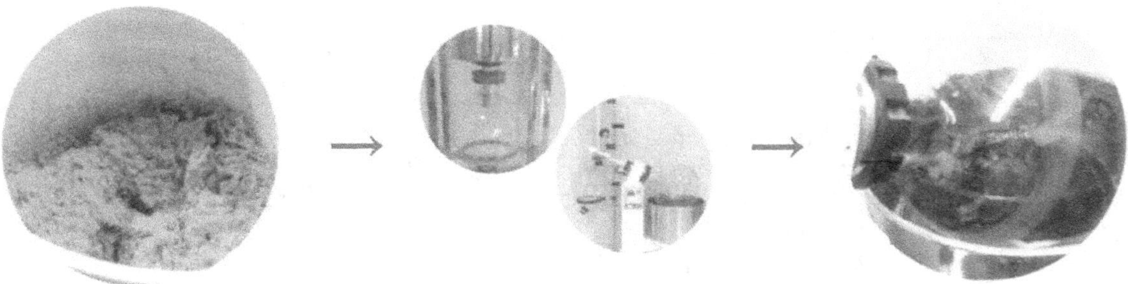

4. Full spectrum essential Oil through short path evaporators

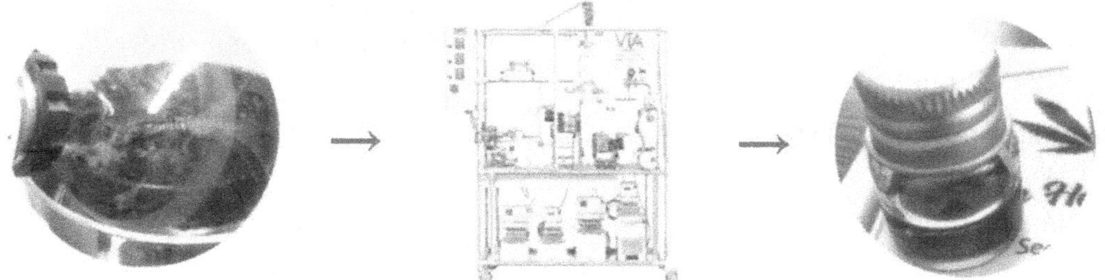

5. Analysis and purification of essential oil by HPLC

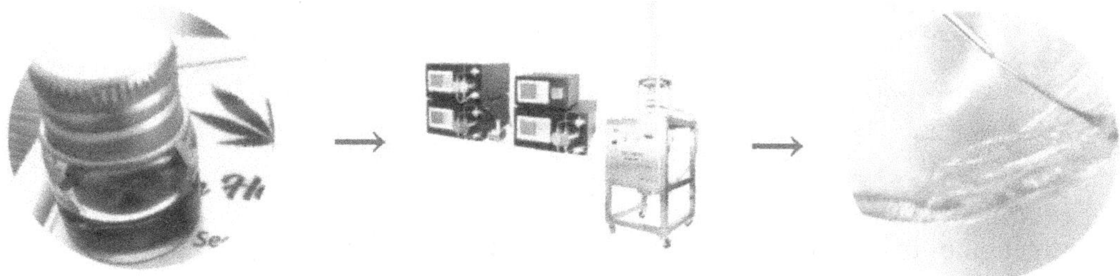

8. Financial Aspects:

Sr. No	Description	Quantity	Value (Rs.)
a.	Land & Building Covered area of ....Sq. Mtrs. on rent	L.S.	
b.	Machinery & Equipments		
1	Herbal Grinder of the required capacity, Supercritical extraction CO2 machine, CO2 Cylinders, collector for processed material, Rotary evaporators of specific capacity, short path distillation system, HPLC systems, filter dryer, Packaging machines, printers, conveyor	L.S	
2	Preoperative Expenses	L.S	
		Total	

(c) Raw & Packing Materials per Month

Sr. No.	Description	Quantity	Value (Rs.)
1	Tuberose flowers material		
2	Distilled water, CO2 gas		
3	Other chemicals		
4	Packaging materials		
		Total	

(d) Salary & Wages per Month

Sr. No.	Description	Quantity	Value (Rs.)
1	Manager		
2	Supervisor / Chemist		
3	Skilled labour		
4	Semi – skilled labour		
5	Unskilled labour		
		Total	

(e) Utilities per Month:

Sr. No.	Description	Quantity	Value (Rs.)
1	Power		
2	Water		
3	White Coal		
		Total	

(f) Other Expenses per Month:

Sr. No.	Description	Quantity	Value (Rs.)
1	Rent		
2	Postage & Stationery		
3	Telephone		
4	Repair & Maintenance		
5	Insurance @ 2% of Machinery & Equipment Cost		
6	Marketing & Travelling Expenses		
		Total	

(g) Working Capital for One Month (c+d+e+f):

(h) Working Capital for three Months:

(i) Total Capital Investment (b+h):

9. Financial Analysis

(a) Cost of production per Annum

Sr. No.	Description	Value (Rs.)
1	Raw & Packing Materials	
2	Salary & Wages	
3	Utilities	
4	Other Expenses	
5	Depreciation on Machinery & Equipments @ 10% p.a	
6	Interest on borrowed capital @ 12 % p.a.	
	Total	

(b) Turnover per Annum:

Sr. No.	Description	Value (Rs.)
1	Nishigandha essential oil @ ....Rs. MT	
2	Miscellaneous @ ....Rs. MT	
	Total	

(c) Net Profit per Year:

Net Profit = Total turnover – Total cost of production =

(d) Profit Ration on Sales:

$$\text{Profit Ratio on Sales} = \frac{\text{Net Profit}}{\text{Total Turnover}} \times 100$$

(e) Rate of Return (ROR) on Total Capital Investment:

$$\text{ROR} = \frac{\text{Net Profit per annum}}{\text{Total Capital Investment}} \times 100$$

(f) Break Even Analysis:

(i) Fixed Cost:

Sr. No.	Description	Value (Rs.)
1	Depreciation on Machinery & Equipments @ 10% p.a.	
2	Interest on Total Capital Investment @ 12 % p.a.	
3	40 % of Salary & Wages	
4	40 % of Other Expenses	
	Total	

(ii) Break Even Point (B.E.P.)

$$\text{B.E.P.} = \frac{\text{Fixed Cost}}{\text{Fixed Cost} + \text{Profit}} \times 100$$

Name and Addresses of Plant and Machinery Suppliers:

1. Hyperbaric Technologies Pvt. Ltd.Plot No 26, Shreenidhi, Kulashree Col. No. 1 Karvenagar, Pune, Maharashtra, India, 411052, response@hyperbarictechnologies.com, Tel No. 020 - 25463914 / 9923320599, +(91) - 94220 88839, 97666 36756
2. Manish Mahakalkar (Manager-Business Devt.), Ajit Burangey. Address: EL-47, Electronics Zone, T. T. C. Industrial Area, Mahape, Navi Mumbai - 400710, Maharashtra, India. 08046050982

Name and Addresses of Raw Material Suppliers:

Locally available

Plant Layout, Design and Construction

Plant layout

Plant layout refers to the arrangement of physical facilities such as machinery, equipment, furniture etc. within the factory building in such a manner so as to have quickest flow of material at the lowest cost and with the least amount of handling in processing the product from the receipt of material to the shipment of the finished product.

Definition

According to Riggs, "the overall objective of plant layout is to design a physical arrangement that most economically meets the required output – quantity and quality." According to J. L. Zundi, "Plant layout ideally involves allocation of space and arrangement of equipment in such a manner that overall operating costs are minimized.

Determinants of Plant Layout

1. Type of product (size, shape and quality)
2. Type of process (technology employed, sequencing etc)
3. Volume of productions- (increase or decrease)

Objectives

- It is long-term commitment with better inter department relationship which leads to increase in the output of the existing product
- Introduction of a new product and diversification is simplified due to well identified expansion possibilities.
- Unnoticed deficiencies can be identified at beginning and technological advancements in machinery, material, processes, product design, fuel etc can be easily introduced.
- It minimizes material handling, time and cost, and allows flexibility of operations
- It facilitates easy production flow, makes economic use of the building, promotes effective utilization of manpower, and provides for employee's convenience, safety, comfort at work, maximum exposure to natural light and ventilation.
- It allows efficient utilization of space, material, processes, labor efficiency, and supervision control.

Factors Influencing Plant Layout

- ***Factory building: -*** The nature and size of the building determines the floor space available for layout. While designing the special requirements, e.g. air conditioning, dust control, humidity control etc. must be kept in mind.

- ***Nature of product ort process:* -** Product layout is suitable for assembly line industries, uniform products whereas process layout is more appropriate for intermittent manufacturing, custom-made or batches of products.
- ***Type of machinery:*** General purpose machines are often arranged as per process layout while special purpose machines are arranged according to product layout.
- ***Repairs and maintenance:*** - Machines should be so arranged that adequate space is available between them for movement of equipment and people required for repairing the machines.
- ***Human needs:* -** Adequate arrangement should be made for clock room, washroom, lockers, drinking water, toilets and other employee facilities. Proper provision should be made for disposal of effluents, if any.
- ***Plant environment:* -** Heat, light, noise, ventilation and other aspects should be duly considered, e.g. paint shops and plating section should be located in another hall so that dangerous fumes can be removed through proper ventilation etc. Adequate safety arrangement should also be made.
- ***Management policies:* -** management policies regarding size, quality, employee facilities and delivery schedules should be considered while deciding plant layout.

Principles of Plant Layout

Principle of minimum movement	Minimum distance movement of materials and labour
Principle of flow	Permit sequence of operations with continuous flow of materials without congestion, interruption or delay.
Principle of space	Effectively use both vertically and horizontally.
Principle of safety	Provision for safety and convenience of workers.
Principle of flexibility	Allow rearrangement, expansion and or technological advancement in future .
Principle of interdependence	Interdependent operations should be in close proximity
Principle of overall integration	Facilities should be fully integrated to maximize efficiency and minimize costs of production.
Principle of minimum investment	Allow savings in fixed capital investment through optimum utilization of available facilities

Types of Layouts

1. Product or Line Layout	Machines and equipments are arranged as per sequence of operations required for the product. **Advantages**: 1. Optimum use of space and time 2. Economic, quick, smooth, uninterrupted continuous operations 3. Simple and effective production control as well as inspection **Disadvantages** 1. Breakdown of one machine affects complete production process 2. Large initial capital investment for special purpose machine 3. Less flexible to introduce new products

Contd...

2. Process Or Functional Layout	Similar type and or functions machines are arranged together at one place especially when many products in relatively small volumes or batches are to be produced. **Advantages** 1. Lower initial capital investment, maximum utilization, variety in products due to scope for expansion 2. Breakdown of one machine does not result in complete work stoppage **Disadvantages:** 1. Costly due to material handling, skilled labour and frequent inspection requirement 2. Large storage space required for progress inventory
3. Fixed Position or Location Layout	Major product, material, or components remain at fixed location and tools, machinery, equipment, labour and components are brought and arranged around it. **Advantages** 1. Relatively time and cost saving 2. Multi-order, multi-stage projects operations can be executed simultaneously 3. Flexible to change the sequence of operations to meet shortage of materials or labour **Disadvantages** 1. Long production period, high capital investment 2. Simultaneous multi-operations need different workgroups 3. Large space for storage of material and equipment near the product. 4. Not suitable for small scale entrepreneur
4. Combined Or Group Layout	It is combination of the product layout and process layout. **Advantages**: 1. Effective machine operation and productivity 2. Satisfactory component standardization, rationalization, reliability of estimates and customer service 3. Decrease overall production time. **Disadvantages:** This type of layout may not be feasible for all situations. If the product mix is completely dissimilar, then we may not have meaningful cell formation.

Recent Trends in Plant Layout

Plant layout is the art and science of bringing to gather men, materials, methods and supporting facilities in the form of a given arrangements that suits individuals industrial activity to have the benefits of profits maximizations through economy, efficiency, effectiveness and productivity. The recent trends in layout are as follows –

- **Use of computerized techniques**: The various techniques have been developed and used in layout engineering to save time and effort in large and complex layout problems such as ALDEP (Automated layout design program), CORELAP (Computerized relationship layout planning), CRAFT (computerized related allocation of facilities technique), CALP (computer Aided layout planning) etc.
- **Use of planning tools and techniques:**
    - ***Templates***: It is a pattern which consists of thin plate of wood or metal which serves as gauge or guide in mechanical work. A plant layout template is a scaled representation of physical object in a layout.

- ***Model equipment***: Model or three dimensional models represents machinery installed in a factory. It is a replica or a miniature prototype of machine and equipment. These show minor details and can be mounted on a thick plastic sheet.
- ***Layout drawing***: Layout drawings are the replica of a factory floor plan showing the space management. It is blue print which indicates the total square feet where all the equipment has to be arranged.
- ***Plot plan:*** Is a miniature of the entire factory building including the facilities of workers.
- ***Line balance***: is phase of assembly line study that equally divides then works to be done among workers so that the total number of employees required is minimum. OR concepts like linear programming, dynamic programming and optimal methods are used to study line balance problem.

Plant Design and Construction

A ideal plant design/building is the one which is built to house the most efficient layout that can be provided for the process involved, and artificially attractive and of such standard shape and design which is flexible its use and expansive units construction. The building ensures functional smoothness of the operation. It should be strong enough to withstand damages, vibrations and heavy machines.

Factors in Designing in Factory Building: Adaptability, expandability, product and equipment, facilities and services areas for employees, materials handling, lighting, ventilation and air-conditioning, fire protection, security, and maintenance.

Types of Buildings

The decision on choosing a suitable type for a particular firm depends among other things on the manufacturing process, the area of land, and the cost of construction. The industrial building can be grouped under four types –

1. ***Single storey building***
2. ***High bay and monitor types***
3. ***Multi-storey building***
4. ***Special building***

Utilities

Plant utilities refer to such services as lighting, ventilation, air-conditioning etc. All these deserve due consideration from operations management as they contribute to increased efficiency and greater output. The types of plant facilities and services are as follow:

- ***Plant lighting***: Adequate lighting (Day light or Artificial light)
- ***Ventilation*** – Ventilation (natural, mechanical or air conditioning)
- ***Industrial Sanitation*** – to maintain health of employees

- ***Noise Control*** – To control pollution
- **Health and Safety Considerations-** to avoid or control hazards

Herbal Product Project Management

The complex herbal product development process from lab to launch includes management of several steps raw material supply to regulatory strategy, clinical studies, and supply chain. Project management becomes more complex due to known as well as unknown risks. Lack of effective risk management can result in turbulence (chaos) in the project that can be incontrollable. The identification of risks at the right stage and an effective mitigation plan are key factors for success, both financially and technically. The use of available techniques, such as Program Evaluation and Review Technique (PERT) and Gantt charts, helps in identifying risks and developing a mitigation and contingency plan, which is beneficial in managing the known or foreseeable risks.

Elements Herbal Project Management	
Project definition and Objectives	This first element of a project management framework is used to define project scope and objectives. Objectives can be formulated as S.M.A.R.T. • Specific, • Measurable (or at least evaluable) achievement, • Achievable (recently Acceptable is used regularly as well), • Realistic and • Time terminated (bounded).
Project team and organization	Every member of project tram must have specific responsibility & proper authority to perform his/her job.
Project planning, scheduling and control	Methods for such planning are Work Breakdown Structure (WBS), Critical Path method, Project Evaluation and Review Technique (PERT). The Work Breakdown Structure (WBS) is a tree structure, which shows a subdivision of effort required achieving an objective; for example a program, project, and contract. • PERT method: critical path, worst case, and best case • Gantt chart: horizontal-bar schedule showing activity start, duration, and completion • Yellow sticky method: use of network diagram
Problem solving and Decision making using Prototypes	• Identify the problem (Raw material supply, Analysis, Regulatory permissions, • Transport facilities etc) • Find out the solutions (Contract farming, Govt. analytical laboratories, pre-clinical and clinical trials, experienced consultant services etc) • Choose the best solutions with the help of prototyping
Senior management review and control	Regular monitoring to get feedback on project performance, risk, errors, innovations, corrections required

Contd...

Proactive, real time change Management	Based on feedbacks from stakeholders, change management can minimize losses and related risks too.
Major queries/ questions should be answered in herbal product project report	1. What is the Project Feasibility, Market Opportunities? 2. What are the requirements of Working Capital, project cost, operating costs? 3. What raw material/s, machinery and equipment/s are required? 4. Who are the Suppliers of Raw materials, machinery and equipment/s? 5. What will be the income and expenditures for the plant? 6. What are the Projected Balance Sheets of the plant? 7. What is the requirement of utilities and overheads for setting up the plant? 8. What is the Built-up Area Requirement and cost for setting up the plant? 9. What is Manpower Requirements for setting up the plant? 10. What are Statistics of Import & Export for the Industry? 11. What is the time required to break-even? 12. What is the Break-Even Analysis of the plant? 13. What are the Project financials of the plant? 14. What are the Profitability Ratios of the plant? 15. What is the Sensitivity Analysis-Price/Volume of the plant? 16. What are the Projected Pay-Back Period and IRR of the plant? 17. What is the Plant Layout and Process Flow Sheet Diagram for setting up the plant?

Further Reading

1. Ahern, T. , Leavy, B. , & Byrne, P. J. (2014). Knowledge formation and learning in the management of projects: A problem solving perspective. International Journal of Project Management, 32(8), 1423–1431.
2. Cardinal, Laura B. "Technological Innovation in the Pharmaceutical Industry: The Use of Organizational Control in Managing Research and Development." Organization Science 12, no. 1 (2001): 19-36. Accessed May 2, 2021.
3. David I. Cleland, Roland Gareis (2006). Global Project Management Handbook. McGraw-Hill Professional, 2006
4. Dennis Lock (2007) Project Management (9th ed.) Gower Publishing, Ltd., 2007.
5. Hall, N.G. Project management: Recent developments and research opportunities. J. Syst. Sci. Syst. Eng. 21, 129–143 (2012).
6. House, C.; Price, R. The return map: tracking product teams. Harvard Bus. Rev. 1991, Jan/Feb.
7. Issacs, W. Dialogue, The Art of Thinking Together; Currency Doubleday, 1999.
8. James P. Lewis (2000). The project manager's desk reference: : a comprehensive guide to project planning, scheduling, evaluation, and systems. p.185

9. Jerome, J. G.; Cara, R. F.; Project management, Encyclopedia of Pharmaceutical Technology, pp. 3015-3026 (2006)
10. Jonas Söderlund. What project management really is about: alternative perspectives on the role and practice of project management? Int. J. Technology Management. 200;532 (3/4).
11. Katzenbach, J.R.; Smith, D.K. The Wisdom of Teams; Harper Business, 1994.
12. Meredith, J. R. ,& Mantel, S. J. (2006). Project management: A managerial approach. Hoboken, NJ: John Wiley.
13. Mikkola, J. H. (2001). Portfolio management of R&D projects: Implications for innovation management. Technovation, 21(7), 423–435.
14. Pattanaik, A.Complexity of project management in the pharmaceutical industry. Paper presented at PMI® Global Congress 2014—EMEA, Dubai, United Arab Emirates. Newtown Square, PA: Project Management Institute. - Available at: https://www.pmi.org/learning/library/project-management-complexity-pharmaceutical-industry-1487
15. Project management institute (PMI) standards committee. In Project Management Body of Knowledge; PMI, 1995.
16. Reinertsen, D.G. Managing the Design Factory; Free Press: New York, 1997.
17. Santos, Dusica. 2019. Evaluation of Project Management in EarlyDrug Discovery in Pharmaceutical Industry: Understanding the Cost and Benefit of Early Assignments of Project Managers. Master's thesis, Harvard Extension School.
18. Tanzeena Sara. Project Management in Pharmaceuticals. International Journal of Pharmaceutical and Life Sciences. 1(1), Serial 4: August 2012
19. The Harvard Gazette. The Talented Georges Doriot. 2015. Accessed Dec. 2020.
20. Tripathy, Swagat& Mohanty, Bishnu. (2018). Project management values driven in pharma industry. International Journal of Drug Regulatory Affairs. 4. 27-32. 10.22270/ijdra.v4i2.183.
21. Wheelwright, S.C.; Clark, KB. Revolutionizing Product Development; Free Press: New York, 1992.
22. Wheelwright, S.C.; Clark, KimB..Leading Product Development; Free Press: New York, 1994.
23. Niir Project Consultancy Services (NPCS). AN ISO 9001 : 2015 Certified Company. 106-E, KamlaNagar, Opposite Spark Mall, New Delhi-110007, India.

Scan QR code to view the website/guidelines

- Herbal Processing Charges-
  ICAR-Directorate of Medicinal and Aromatic Plants Research

- Herbal Business Development-
  Welcome to Central Institute of Medicinal and Aromatic Plants (CSIR-CIMAP)-Lucknow

CHAPTER 30

Herbal Raw Material Trade

Herbal Raw Material Trade in India

In 2000, Government of India's Report of the Task Force on Conservation & Sustainable Use of Medicinal Plants reported that 70% of medicinal plant collection activity is following destructive practices in India.

Good cultivation and collection practices of medicinal plants should be encouraged to limit collection and avoid overexploitation, price rise, non-availability of enough quantities and making few species endangered due to destruction of the resources by over-collection. Conservation strategies should also be implemented to tackle these issues.

Indiscriminate harvesting from wild sources of commercially important medicinal plants is leading to threat of extinction of such species.

The Foundation for Revitalisation of Local Health Traditions (FRLHT), Bangalore under the guidance of National Medicinal Plants Board (NMPB), department of AYUSH, Government of India, has assessed the demand and supply data of medicinal plants in India in 2007. This data is collected from literature, herbal manufacturing units and Mandis. Of the 960 (source of 1289 botanical raw drugs) traded medicinal plant species, following178 species with above 100 MT consumption per year fulfills the about 80% of the total industrial demand of all botanicals in the country. Analysis of these species based on their major sources of supply is as follows:

Table 30.1 Trade details of Important Medicinal plants.

Percentage	Source	Species
21 (12%)	**Temperate Forests**	Abiesspectabilis, Aconitum ferox, Aconitum heterophyllum, Berberisaristata, Bergeniaciliata, Cedrusdeodara, Cinnamomumtamala, Ephedra gerardiana, Juniperuscommunis, Jurineamacrocephala, Nardostachysgrandiflora, Onosmahispidum, Parmeliaperlata, Picrorhizakurroa, Pistaciaintegerrima, Rheum austral, Rhododendron anthopogon, Swertiachirayita, Taxuswallichiana, Valerianajatamansi, Viola pilosa
70 (40%)	**Tropical Forests**	*Commiphorawightii, Aquilariaagallocha, Acacia catechu, Acacia nilotica, Acacia sinuata, Aeglemarmelos, Albizziaamara, Alstoniascholaris, Anogeissuslatifolia, Asparagus racemosus, Baliospermummontanum, Bombaxceiba, Boswelliaserrata, Buchnanialanzan, Buteamonosperma, Careyaarborea, Cassia fistula, Celastruspaniculatus, Chlorophytumtuberosum, Cinnamomumsulphuratum, Clerodendrumphlomides, Cosciniumfenestratum, Cycleapeltata, Decalepishamiltonii, Desmodiumgangeticum, Embeliatsjerium-cottam, Emblicaofficinalis, Garciniaindica, Gardenia resinifera, Gmelinaarborea, Gymnemasylvestre, Helicteresisora,*

Contd...

Percentage	Source	Species
		Holarrhenapubescens, Holopteleaintegrifolia, Holostemmaada-kodien (Jeevanti), Ipomoea mauritiana (Palmudhukkankizhangu), Ixoracoccinea (Thechippoovu), Lanneacoromandelica (Jhinganjingini), Litseaglutinosa (Maida chhal), Lobelia nicotianaefolia (Lobelia leaves), Madhucaindica (Madhuka), Messuaferrea (Nagakesar), Mimusopselengi (Bakul), Morindapubescens (Manjanathi), Mucunapuriens (Kaunchbeej), Nilgirianthusciliatus (Kurinji), Operculinaturpethum (Nishoth), Oroxylumindicum (Tetuchhal), Premnaserratifolia (Arnimool), Pterocarpusmarsupium (Vijaysaar), Pterocarpussantalinus (Raktachandan), Rauvolfia serpentine (Sarpagandha), Rubiacordifolia (Manjishtha), Santalum album (Chandan), Sapindusmukorossi(Reetha), Saracaasoca (AshokaChhal), Schreberaswietenioides (Ghantiphool), Semecarpusanacardium (Balave), Shorearobusta (Raal), Smilax glabra (Chopchini), Soymidafebrifuga (Rohan), Sterculiaurens (Karaya), Stereospermumchelonoides (Patala), Strychnosnux-vomica (Kuchla), Strychnospotatorum (Nirmali), Symplocosracemosus (Lodhpathani), Terminaliaarjuna (Arjan), Terminaliabellirica (Behra), Terminaliachebula (Harda), Vateriaindica (Mandadhoopa), Wrightiatinctoria (Inderjau), Ziziphusxylocarpus (Ghontaphala)
36 (20%)	**Cultivation**	*Abelmoschusmoschatus (Muskdana), Acoruscalamus (Bach), Adhatodazeylanica (Adusa), Aloe barbedensis (Kumari), Alpiniacalcarata (Chittartha), Azadirachtaindica (Neem), Caesalpiniasappan(Pathimugam), Cassia angustifolia (Sonamukhi), Catharanthusroseus (Sadabahar), Cichoriumintybus (Kasani), Croton tiglium (Jamalghota), Curcuma angustifolia (Tikhur), Curcuma zerumbet(Kachur), Ficusbenghalensis (VadaChhal), Ficusreligiosa (Aralichakki), Gloriosasuperba (Kalihari), Indigoferatinctoria (Nil), Inularacemosa (Pushkarmool), Jatrophacurcas(Nepalam seed), Kaempferiagalanga (Kacholum), Lawsoniainermis (Henna), Lepidiumsativum (Halim), Ocimumbasilicum (Sweet basil), Ocimumtenuiflorum (Tulasi), Piper longum(Pippali), Plantagoovata (Isabgol), Plectranthusbarbatus (Gandhira), Pongamiapinnata (Karanj), Prunusarmeniaca (Chuli), Saussureacostus (Kuth), Silybummarianum (Milk thistle), Simmondsiachinensis (Jojoba), Trachyspermumammi (Ajwain), Vitexnegundo (Neergundi), Withaniasomnifera (Ashvagandha), Ziziphusjujuba (Ber)*

Contd...

Percentage	Source	Species
5 (5%)	Imports	*Aquilariaagallocha, Commiphorawightii, Glycyrrhizaglabra, Piper chaba and Quercusinfectoria*
46 (25%)	Wastelands	*Abrusprecatorius, Achyranthesaspera, Aervalanata, Andrographispaniculata, Bacopamonnieri (Brahmi), Boerhaviadiffusa (Punarnava), Cardiospermumhalicacabum (Mudakkatham), Cassia absus (Chaksoo), Cassia tora (Chakodabeeja), Centellaasiatica (Brahmibooti), Centratherumanthelminticum (Kali zeeri), Citrulluscolocynthis (Indrayan), Convolvulus microphyllus (Shankhapushpi), Curculigoorchioides (Kali musli), Cynodondactylon(Durva), Cyperusesculentus(Musta), Cyperusrotundus (Nagar motha), Daturametel (Dhatura), Ecliptaprostrata (Bhringraj), Fumariaindica (Shatara), Hedyotiscorymbosa (Pitpapra), Hemidesmusindicus (Anatmool), Hygrophyllaschulli (Tal makhana), Ipomoea nil (Kaladana), Merremiatri dentate (Prasarani), Ocimumamericanum (Ban tulsi), Peganumharmala (Harmal), Phyllanthusamarus(Bhumiamla), Pluchealanceolata (Rasna), Plambagozeylanica (Chitrak), Pseudarthia viscid (Moovila), Psoraleacorylifolia (Bawachi), Sidarhombifolia (Bala), Sisymbriumirio (Khubkalan), Solanumanguivi (Kathelibadi), Solanumnigrum (Makoi), Solanumvirginianum (Kateli), Sphaeranthusindicus (Gorakh mundi), Tephrosiapurpurea (Sarpankha), Tinosporacordifolia (Giloy), Tragiainvolucrata (Kodithoova), Tribulusterrestris (Gokshura), Trichosanthescucumerina (Patolpanchang), Vetiveriazizanioides (Lavancha), Withaniacoagulens (Panirdodi), Woodfordiafruticosa(Dhatki)*

Import and Export of Herbal Material

International Trade of Herbal **material** is subject to compliance with the International treaties like Convention on International Trade in Endangered Species of Wild Fauna and Flora (CITES). CITES, who regulate the international trade of certain species, which are threatened with extinction or which would be reaching the status of being endangered, if their overexploitation is not checked.

The trade data of medicinal and aromatic plants can be obtained from COMTRADE database, (https://comtrade.un.org/ -UN Statistics Division, New York) and Export Import Data Bank (DGCI&S Kolkata, India). Both the databases furnish data according to Harmonized Commodity Description and Coding System (HS) classification, adopted by the Customs Co-operation Council (World Customs Organization) since June 1983 which came into force on 1 January 1988 (Brussels, 1989).

According to HS convention, merchandise products are classified to names and unique eight digit numbers: up to 2 digit (01-96) called chapters reflecting major classification; headings, broad commodity groupings within the chapters are denoted by next two digits; subheadings, the next two digits give account of more specific classification of any commodity within headings; last two digits are left to more specification of particular goods under subheading, and left to the nation states to assign as per need. COMTRADE database keep records up to universal 6 digit HS numbers while Export Import Data Bank of India compiles data up to 8 digit level classification.

India is the second largest exporter of MAPs based commodities after China with more than 30 unique HS numbers allotted to them. Under other MAPs (HS121190: Plants & parts, pharmacy, perfume, insecticide use n.e.s.) category, total international trade is increasing with annual growth rate of 6.1%, from US$ 1.8b in 1996 to US$ 5.1b in 2013. The total trade of Medicinal plants (HS1211) have increased from US$ 2.4bn (billion) in 1996 to US$ 6.2bn in 2013 with annual growth rate of 5.4% in past 18 years, and growth rate of 10.7% is registered in recent years.

According to the Export and Import Policy, 2002-07, export of wild harvested serpentine roots are prohibited, but cultivated varieties are allowed for export subject to production of Certificate of Cultivation from competent authority as well as CITES permit. Since 2006, its import is subject to provisions of CITES. As per Schedule II of Export and Import Policy, 2002-07, export of plants, plant portions and derivatives and extracts obtained from wild Red sandal (Pterocarpus santalinus) is prohibited. Agarwood has been placed under restricted category since 2006 and import is subject to the provisions of Convention of International Trade in Endangered Species of Wild Flora and Fauna (CITES) and Wildlife (Protection) Act 1972.

Examples of Export and Import of few medicinal plants

Medicinal Plants	HS Code	Export value (2013-14)
Rauwolfia roots	HS12119044	26.5t valued at 5L
Senna leaves and pods	HS12119022	11214.6t valued at 7769.6L
Mint, incl. leaves (all species)	HS12119070	09.2t valued at 303.7L
Garcinia	HS1211 9096	03.1t valued at ` 577.3L
Sandal wood chips and dust	HS12119050	78.3t valued at `1504.5L
Agarwood (including chips and dust)	HS12119080	62.6t valued at 139.1L
Gal an gal rhizomes and roots incl. Greater galangal	HS12119042	1874.8t valued at` 1801.3L
Cubeb	HS12112002	505.2t at 444L
Ginseng roots	HS12112000	3.1t valued at ` 33.1L
Pyrethrum	HS12119026	96t valued at 150.8L
Ipecac dried rhizome and roots	HS12119043	9.5t valued at 214.3L

Nearly 30% of the global trade is made up by top two countries of the import and export. China and India from Asia; Egypt and Morocco from Africa; Poland, Bulgaria and Albania from Europe; Chile and Peru from South America are important supply sources. The USA, Japan and Europe are the major consumers of the world.

For India, Exporting Company has to apply for Free Sale Certificate for exporting Ayurvedic medicines. "Form of Free Sale Certificate and Non-Conviction Certificate. – The State Drug Controller or Licensing Authority shall, on request by the Ayurveda, Siddha and Unani Drugs manufacturer, issue, within 15 days; from the date of application, Free Sale Certificate in Form 26 E2-I for original License holder or in Form 26 E2-II for loan license and Non Conviction Certificate for both original and loan license holder in Form 26 E3 or in the format as specified by the importing country or tenderer respectively, after fulfillment of all requisite formalities as required in the respective formats.

Further Reading

1. Ved, D.K. & G.S. Goraya, 2007. Demand and Supply of Medicinal Plants in India. NMPB, New Delhi & FRLHT, Bangalore, India.
2. Mrozek-Szetela A, Rejda P, Wińska K. A Review of Hygienization Methods of Herbal Raw Materials. Applied Sciences. 2020; 10(22):8268
3. Berginc, K.; Kreft, S. Dietary Supplements. Safety, Efficacy and Quality; Woodhead Publishing: Sawston/Cambridge, UK, 2014.
4. Cheng, W.-C.; Ng, C.-S.; Poon, N.-L. Herbal Medicines and Phytopharmaceuticals–Contaminations. In Encyclopedia of Forensic Sciences; Academic Press: Cambridge, MA, USA, 2013; pp. 280–288.
5. Herbal Medicine Market Research Report—Global Forecast Till 2023; Market Research Future, Maharashtra MRFR/Pharma: Pune, India, 2019.
6. WHO Global Report on Traditional and Complementary Medicine 2019; World Health Organization: Geneva, Switzerland, 2020.
7. Phillipson, J.D. Quality assurance of medicinal plants. Acta Hort. 1993, 333, 117–122.
8. Hossain, M.B.; Brunton, N.P.; Rai, D.K. (Eds.) Herbs, Spices and Medicinal Plants: Processing, Health Benefits and Safety; Wiley: West Sussex, UK, 2020.
9. GS Kumar. KN Jayaveera. A Textbook of Pharmacognosy and Phytochemistry. S Chand & Company Limited. India. 2014.
10. Simone BadalMccreath. RupikaDelgoda. Pharmacognosy-Fundamentals, Applications and Strategies. Elsevier Science. 2017
11. Biren Shah, Avinash Seth. Textbook of Pharmacognosy and Phytochemistry. Elsevier Health Sciences. 2014

12. AshutoshKar. PharmacognosyandPharmacobiotechnology. New Age International (P) Limited. 2003
13. Michael Heinrich, Elizabeth M. Williamson, Joanne Barnes, Simon Gibbons, Jose Prieto-Garcia Fundamentals of Pharmacognosy and Phytotherapy E-Book. Elsevier Health Sciences. 2017
14. W.C.Evans, Trease and Evans Pharmacognosy, 16th edition, W.B. Sounders & Co., London, 2009.
15. Jean Bruneton. Pharmacognosy, Phytochemistry, Medicinal Plants. Technique & Documentation. 1999
16. Luqi Huang. Molecular Pharmacognosy. Springer Netherlands. 2012
17. Gunnar Samuelsson. Drugs of Natural Origin-A Textbook of Pharmacognosy. Apotekarsocieteten. 1999
18. A.N.M. Alamgir. Therapeutic Use of Medicinal Plants and Their Extracts: Volume 1
19. Pharmacognosy- Volume 1. Springer International Publishing. 2017
20. Michael Heinrich, Joanne Barnes, Simon Gibbons. Fundamentals of Pharmacognosy and Phytotherapy. Churchill Livingstone/Elsevier. 2012
21. K. Mangathayaru. Pharmacognosy: An Indian perspective. Pearson Education India. 2013
22. Mohammad Ali. Pharmacognosy and Phytochemistry, CBS Publishers & Distribution, New Delhi.
23. C.K. Kokate, Purohit, Gokhlae. Text book of Pharmacognosy, 37th Edition, NiraliPrakashan, Pune. 2007
24. Kaliya.A. Text Book of Industrial Pharmacognosy. CBS Publishers & Distributors, Delhi. 2009
25. Rangari VD. Pharmacognosy& Phytochemistry. Career Publication, Nashik. 2008
26. James Bobbers, Marilyn KS, VE Tylor. Pharmacognosy&Pharmacobiotechnology. Williams & Wilkins. 1996.
27. H. Ansari. Essentials of Pharmacognosy. Second edition, Birla publications, New Delhi, 2007
28. S. S. Handa. Pharmacognosy. VallabhPrakashan, New Delhi. 1989
29. N P S Sengar, Ashwini Singh, RiteshAgrawal. A Textbook of Pharmacognosy. PharmaMed Press. 2018
30. Kendall Jefferson. Pharmacognosy and Phytotherapy. Foster Academics.2019
31. C. S. Shah, J. S. Qadry. A Textbook of Pharmacognosy. Messrs B.S. Shah 1971
32. Alice Kurian, M. AshaSankar Medicinal Plants. New India Publishing Agency. 2007
33. T. C. Denston. A Textbook of Pharmacognosy. Read Books. 2012
34. S. S. Agarwal, M. Paridhavi. Herbal Drug Technology. Universities Press. 2012
35. SaikatSen, Raja Chakraborty Herbal Medicine in India-Indigenous Knowledge, Practice, Innovation and Its Value. Springer Singapore. 2019

36. Hamrell MR. 2. Vol. 14. California: On Clinical Research and Regulatory Affairs; 1997. An Update on the Generic Drug Approval Process; pp. 139–54. Available from: http://www.informahealthcare.com/doi/abs/10.3109/10601339709019635?journalCode=crr . [Last accessed on Dec 2020].
37. K. Dubey, Rajesh Kumar and Pramila Tripathi , Global promotion of herbal medicine: India's opportunity - Current Science, 2004, 86(1).
38. Kumar, M. & Janagam, D.. (2011). Export and import pattern of medicinal plants in India. 4. 245-248. 10.17485/ijst/2011/v4i3/29975.
39. Leon S, Kanfer I. Generic drug product development Solid Oral Dosage forms. New York: Marcel Dekker Inc; 2005. Introduction to Generic drug product development; p. 8.
40. Perera PK (2017) Traditional Medicine Based Drug Development. Biochem Anal Biochem 6: 311. doi: 10.4172/2161-1009.1000311
41. Praveen K, Ramesh T, Saravanan D. ON Pharma Times. Goa: Sanofi-Synthelabo (India) Limited; 2011. Regulatory perspective for entering global pharma markets; p. 43.
42. Ramawat, Kishan & Goyal, Shaily. (2008). The Indian Herbal Drugs Scenario in Global Perspectives. 10.1007/978-3-540-74603-4_18.
43. Ravi Kiran and Sunita Mishra, Research and Development, Exports and Patenting in the Indian Pharmaceutical Industry: a Post TRIPS Analysis, Eurasian Journal of Business and Economics 2011, 4 (7): 53-67.
44. Redmond K. The US and European Regulatory Systems: A Comparison: ON JAmbul Care Manage.;2004 27:105
45. S.B. Kayne. Traditional Medicine: a Global Perspective. Pharmaceutical Press, London (2010)
46. Sahoo N, Manchikanti P. Herbal drug regulation and commercialization: an Indian industry perspective. Journal of Alternative and Complementary Medicine (New York, N.Y.). 2013 Dec;19(12):957-963. DOI: 10.1089/acm.2012.0275.
47. Sahoo, N., Manchikanti, P., Dey, S. Herbal drugs: Standards and regulation (Review). Fitoterapia. 2010;81(6):462-471.
48. Senthil V, Priyadharshini RB, Ramachandran A, Ganesh GNK and Shrivastava A: Regulatory Process for Import and Export of Drugs in India. Int J Pharm Sci Res 2015; 6(12): 4989-99.doi: 10.13040/IJPSR.0975-8232.6(12).4989-99.
49. Shraddha Thakkar, Elke Anklam, Alex Xu, Franz Ulberth, Jing Li, Bo Li, Marta Hugas, Nandakumara Sarma, Scott Crerar, Sibyl Swift, Takashi Hakamatsuka, Valeriu Curtui, William Yan, Xingchao Geng, William Slikker, Weida Tong. Regulatory landscape of dietary supplements and herbal medicines from a global perspective. Regulatory Toxicology and Pharmacology. 2020;114.104647.ISSN 0273-2300.

50. Tripathi, Himanshu & Suresh, Ram & Kumar, Sanjay & Khan, Feroz. (2017). International trade in medicinal and aromatics plants: A case study of past 18 years. Journal of Medicinal and Aromatic Plant Sciences. 39. 1-17.
51. Uma Vasireddy, G. Krishna Mohan, M. Lakshmi Narasu and P. V. Appaji, Impact of India's formulation and bulk drug registrations with U.S. FDA on it exports: A stochastic analysis - Scholars Research Library, Der Pharmacia Lettre, 2011,3 (4):84-100
52. Vasisht K, Sharma N, Karan M. Current Perspective in the International Trade of Medicinal Plants Material: An Update. Curr Pharm Des. 2016;22(27):4288-336. doi: 10.2174/1381612822666160607070736. PMID: 27281331.

Scan QR code to view the website/guidelines

- Import and export of cosmetics-
Guidance-Document-on-Registration-and-Import-of-cosmetics-into-India-converted.pdf (cdsco.gov.in)

-

- Marketing of Herbal Drugs-
e.Charak (echarak.in)

- Foreign Trade (Export and Import) of Herbal Raw Drugs-
Cover Design - Final.cdr (echarak.in)

- Trade of Medicinal plants-
Medicinal plant HS Codes | HS Code of Medicinal plant Import | Medicinal plant HS Code for Export (seair.co.in)

CHAPTER 31

GMP, GLP, TQM and ISO for Herbal Medicines

Good Manufacturing Practices (GMP)

Introduction

Unlike conventional pharmaceutical products, which are usually produced from synthetic materials by means of reproducible manufacturing techniques and procedures, herbal medicines are prepared from materials of herbal origin, which are often obtained from varied geographical and/or commercial sources. As a result it may not always be possible to ascertain the conditions to which they may have been subjected. In addition, they may vary in composition and properties. Furthermore, the procedures and techniques used in the manufacture and quality control of herbal medicines are often substantially different from those employed for conventional pharmaceutical products. Because of the inherent complexity of naturally grown medicinal plants and the often variable nature of cultivated ones, the instances of contamination with toxic medicinal plants and/or plant parts and the large numbers of active ingredients, few of which have been defined, the production and primary processing has a direct influence on the quality of herbal medicines. For this reason, application of GMPs in the manufacture of herbal medicines is an essential tool to assure their quality.

These new *Good manufacturing practices (GMP) for the manufacture of herbal medicines* guidelines are intended to complement those provided in Good *manufacturing practices for pharmaceutical products* and should be read in conjunction with the parent guide. The additional standards addressed by the present guidelines should therefore be considered supplementary to the general requirements. They relate specifically to the production and control of herbal medicines, in so far as they mainly focus on identifying the critical steps needed to ensure good quality. The supplementary guidelines are intended to provide WHO Member States with general and minimum technical requirements for quality assurance and control in the manufacture of herbal medicines. Each Member State should develop its own national GMP for manufacturing herbal medicines that are appropriate to its particular situation. These guidelines deal exclusively with herbal medicines. They do not cover combination of herbal materials with animal materials, mineral materials, chemicals and other substances.

1. **Quality assurance in the manufacture of herbal medicines:** In addition to the use of modern analytical techniques (chromatography, spectrometry etc.) to characterize herbal medicines, quality assurance requires the control of starting materials as well as of storage and processing.
2. **Good manufacturing practice for herbal medicines:** Parent guidelines are a reference general principle for herbal medicines. GACP Guidelines are applicable for starting materials for herbal medicines, as well as processing of herbal medicines are covered by other guidelines. This is of particular importance for those products that consist solely of comminuted or powdered herbal materials.
3. **Sanitation and hygiene:** Maintain a high standard of hygiene in the manufacturing area to avoid alterations and to reduce contamination due to microbiological contaminants during harvesting, processing and storage.

4. **Qualification and validation:** Qualification of critical equipment, process validation and change control are required for ensuring consistency of quality, efficacy and safety between batches.
5. **Complaints:** product quality complaints and complaints about adverse reactions or events should be handled by trained and experienced person. Records of action taken should be maintained.
6. **Product recalls:** The product recall should be processed in accordance with national regulations through well-defined standard operating procedure.
7. **Contract production and analysis:** The contract partner should have adequate and separate premises and equipments if required for the production, quality control of herbal medicines according to GMP.
8. **Self-inspection:** At least one member of the self-inspection team should possess a thorough knowledge of herbal medicines.
9. **Personnel:** Personnel dealing with the production and quality control of herbal medicines should have adequate experience and qualification on the specific issues relevant to herbal medicines.
10. **Training:** Personnel dealing with the production and quality control of herbal medicines should have adequate training on the specific issues relevant to herbal medicines.
11. **Personal hygiene:** Personnel dealing with the production and quality control of herbal medicines should have adequate training on high degree of personal hygiene, dealing with infectious diseases or skin diseases and protective clothing for toxic irritants and potentially allergenic plant materials.
12. **Premises:** Premises should be designed, located, constructed, adapted and maintained to suit the operations, to avoid degradation and infestation with certain pests, moisture and temperature. **Storage area** set-up should be well organized, tidy, allow separate material storage, minimize the risk of cross- contamination of other materials, have special conditions of humidity and temperature or protection from light. Storage area should work on principal "first in, first out" (FIFO), monitoring and record keeping. **Production areas** should feasible for various process of production like sampling, weighing, mixing, powdering, heating, boiling etc., facilitate cleaning and avoid cross-contamination.
13. **Equipment:** Effective cleaning of the equipment is important. Equipment should not come into direct contact with chemicals or contaminated material. If the use of wooden equipment is unavoidable, special consideration must be given to its cleaning as wooden materials may retain odours, be easily discoloured and are easily contaminated.
14. **Materials:** All incoming herbal materials should be quarantined and stored under appropriate conditions that take into account the degradability of herbal materials and herbal preparations. The reference standard (sample of herbal material, preparation-extract

or a chemically defined substance a marker substance or a known impurity) should be stored under appropriate conditions to prevent degradation and of appropriate quality of known expiry and/or revalidation date

15. **Documentation:** The documentation for herbal materials should as far as possible include, as a minimum, the following information:

    Herbal materials: The family and botanical name of the plant used according to the binomial system (genus, species, variety and the authority, i.e. the reference to the originator of the classification, for example, Linnaeus). It may also be appropriate to add the vernacular name and the therapeutic use in the country or region of origin of the plant. Details of the geographical source, processing, identification tests, active constituents or markers, , Tests for pesticide contamination, toxic metals, microbiological contamination, fumigant residues (if applicable), mycotoxins, pest infestations, radioactivity and and Qualitative and quantitative information on the active ingredients or constituents with known therapeutic activity.

    Herbal preparations and finished herbal products

    - Tests for microbiological contamination and tests for other toxicants.
    - Uniformity of weight (for example, for tablets, single-dose powders, suppositories, capsules and herbal tea in sachets), disintegration time (for tablets, capsules, suppositories and pills), hardness and friability (for example, for uncoated tablets), viscosity (for internal and external fluids), consistency (semisolid preparations), and dissolution (for tablets or capsules), if applicable.
    - Physical appearance such as colour, odour, form, shape, size and texture.
    - Loss on drying, or water content.
    - Identity tests, qualitative determination of relevant constitutents of the plants (for example, fingerprint chromatograms).
    - Quantification of relevant active ingredients, if they have been identified, and the analytical methods that are available.
    - Limit tests for residual solvents.

16. **Good practices in production:** To ensure not only the quality, but also the safety and efficacy of herbal medicines, it is essential that the steps in their production be as per well-defined SOPs.

17. **Good practices in quality control:** The quality control of the herbal material, herbal preparations and finished herbal products should establish their quality but this does not imply the control of every single constituent. Stability data are always required to support the shelf life proposed for the finished herbal products. Packaging materials and labelling should be in accordance to maintain quality, safety and efficacy of herbal medicines.

Good Laboratory Practice (GLP)

Good Laboratory Practice (GLP) Principles set out the requirements for the appropriate management of nonclinical safety studies. This helps the researcher to perform his/her work in compliance with his/her own pre-established scientific design. GLP Principles help to define and standardise the planning, performance, recording, reporting, monitoring and archiving processes within research institutions. The regulations are not concerned with the scientific or technical content of the studies per se. The regulations do not aim to evaluate the scientific value of the studies: this task is reserved first for senior scientists working on the research programme, then for the Registration Authorities, and eventually for the international scientific community as a whole. The GLP requirements for proper planning, for controlled performance of techniques, for faithful recording of all observations, for appropriate monitoring of activities and for complete archiving of all raw data obtained, serve to eliminate many sources of error. Whatever the industry targeted, GLP stresses the importance of the following main points:

1. Resources	
Organisation and Personnel	GLP regulations require clear definitions of the structure of the research organisation and the responsibilities of the research personnel. GLP also stresses that the number of personnel sufficient to perform the tasks with defined and recorded in job descriptions and their qualifications and competence defined in education and training records.
Facilities and equipment	The GLP Principles emphasise that facilities and equipment must be sufficient, spacious and adequate to avoid overcrowding, cross contamination or confusion between projects. Utilities (water, electricity etc.) must be adequate and stable. All equipment must be in working order; a programme of validation/ qualification, calibration and maintenance attains this. Keeping records of use and maintenance is essential in order to know, at any point in time, the precise status of the equipment and its history.
2.Characterisation	
Test items and test systems	In order to perform a study correctly, it is essential to know non-clinical studies to evaluate the safety, Characteristics such as identity, potency, composition, stability, impurity profile, etc. should be known.
3. Rules	
Protocol or study plan	The approved study plan or protocol outlines the design and conduct of the study and provides evidence that the study has been properly thought through and planned.
Written Procedures	The details of all routine procedures should be described in Standard Operating Procedures (SOPs) which must be reviewed regularly, and modified if required.

Contd...

4. Results	
Raw data	The results and their interpretations provided by the scientist in the study report must be a true and accurate reflection of the raw data.
Study Report	The GLP Principles list the essential elements to be included in a final study report.
Archives	The storage of records must enable their restricted safekeeping for long periods of time without loss or deterioration and, preferably, in a way which allows quick retrieval.
5. Quality Assurance	Quality Assurance (QA) – sometimes also known as the Quality Assurance Unit (QAU) - as defined by GLP is a team of persons charged with assuring management that GLP compliance has been attained in the test facility as a whole and in each individual study. QA must be independent of the operational conduct of the studies, and functions as a "witness" to the whole preclinical research process

Total Quality Management (TQM)

Total quality management (TQM) has been defined as an integrated organizational effort designed to improve quality at every level. The process to produce a perfect product by a series of measures requires an organized effort by the entire company to prevent or eliminate errors at every stage in production is called total quality management. According to international organization for standards defined TQM as, "TQM is a management approach for an organization, centered on quality, based on the participation of all its members and aiming at long-term success through customer satisfaction and benefits to all members of the organization and to the society. Imprints of TQM concepts can be found in modern approaches to quality management, such as the Malcolm Baldrige National Quality Award (MBNQA) criteria, ISO 9001, Six Sigma and lean manufacturing,

Characteristics of TQM

- Committed management
- Adopting and communicating about total quality management
- Closer customer relations
- Closer provider relations
- Benchmarking
- Increased training
- Open organization
- Employee empowerment

- Flexible production
- Process improvements
- Process measuring

Traditional Approach and TQM

With traditional quality management, the company defines its quality standards and determines whether a particular product is acceptable. In total quality management, customers determine a product's quality. A company can change its standards, train employees or revise its processes, but if customers aren't satisfied, then the organization isn't producing a quality product.

Principles of TQM

1. Produce quality work the first time and every time.
2. Focus on the customer.
3. Have a strategic approach to improvement.
4. Improve continuously.
5. Encourage mutual respect and teamwork

Key Elements of TQM

These elements are considered so essential to TQM that many organizations define them, in some format, as a set of core values and principles on which the organization is to operate. The methods for implementing this approach come from the teachings of such quality leaders as Philip B. Crosby, W. Edwards Deming, Armand V. Feigenbaum, Kaoru Ishikawa, and Joseph M. Juran.

Customer-focused	It is important to identify the organization's customers. External customers consume the organization's product or service. Internal customers are employees who receive the output of other employees.
Total employee involvement	Front line employees are likely to have the closest contact with external customers and thus can make the most valuable contribution to quality. All employees participate in working toward common goals. Total employee commitment can only be obtained after fear has been driven from the workplace, when empowerment has occurred, and when management has provided the proper environment. High-performance work systems integrate continuous improvement efforts with normal business operations. Self-managed work teams are one form of empowerment.
Process-centered	A fundamental part of TQM is a focus on process thinking. A process is a series of steps that take inputs from suppliers (internal or external) and transforms them into outputs that are delivered to customers (internal or external). The steps required to carry out the process are defined, and performance measures are continuously monitored in order to detect unexpected variation.

Contd...

Integrated system:	Although an organization may consist of many different functional specialties often organized into vertically structured departments, it is the horizontal processes interconnecting these functions that are the focus of TQM. Micro-processes add up to larger processes, and all processes aggregate into the business processes required for defining and implementing strategy. Everyone must understand the vision, mission, and guiding principles as well as the quality policies, objectives, and critical processes of the organization. Business performance must be monitored and communicated continuously. Every organization has a unique work culture, and it is virtually impossible to achieve excellence in its products and services unless a good quality culture has been fostered. Thus, an integrated system connects business improvement elements in an attempt to continually improve and exceed the expectations of customers, employees, and other stakeholders.
Strategic and systematic approach:	A critical part of the management of quality is the strategic and systematic approach to achieving an organization's vision, mission, and goals. This process, called strategic planning or strategic management, includes the formulation of a strategic plan that integrates quality as a core component.
Continual improvement:	A large aspect of TQM is continual process improvement. Continual improvement drives an organization to be both analytical and creative in finding ways to become more competitive and more effective at meeting stakeholder expectations.
Fact-based decision making:	In order to know how well an organization is performing, data on performance measures are necessary. TQM requires that an organization continually collect and analyze data in order to improve decision making accuracy, achieve consensus, and allow prediction based on past history
Communications:	During times of organizational change, as well as part of day-to-day operation, effective communications plays a large part in maintaining morale and in motivating employees at all levels. Communications involve strategies, method, and timeliness.

Benefits of TQM:

Total quality management benefits and advantages:

- Strengthened competitive position
- Adaptability to changing or emerging market conditions and to environmental and other government regulations
- Higher productivity
- Enhanced market image

- Elimination of defects and waste
- Reduced costs and better cost management
- Higher profitability
- Improved customer focus and satisfaction
- Increased customer loyalty and retention
- Increased job security
- Improved employee morale
- Enhanced shareholder and stakeholder value
- Improved and innovative processes

Importance of TQM in Pharma Industry

- ***Handling***: Containers should be opened carefully and subsequently resealed in an approved manner. Highly sensitising material should be handled in separate production areas. Highly active or toxic API should be manufactured in a dedicated area and using dedicated equipment. Pure and final API should be handled in an environment giving adequate protection against contamination.
- ***Storage***: Secure storage facilities should be designated for use to prevent damage or deterioration of materials. These should be kept clean and tidy and subject to appropriate pest control measures. Environmental conditions should be recorded. The condition of stored material should be assessed at appropriate intervals. Storage conditions for API should be based upon stability studies taking into account time, temperature, humidity, light etc
- ***Packaging***: Labelling and packaging processes should be defined and controlled to ensure that correct packaging materials are used correctly and other specified requirements are met. Printed labels should be securely stored to avoid mix-ups arising. Marking and labelling should be legible and durable, provide sufficient information, for accurate identification and indicate, if appropriate, required storage conditions, retest and/or expiry date.
- ***Facilities and equipment***: The location, design, and construction of buildings should be suitable for the type and stage of manufacture involved, protecting the product from contamination (including cross-contamination) and protecting operators and the environment from the product. Equipment surfaces in contact with materials used in API manufacture should be non-reactive.
- ***Sterile area***: Personnel suffering from an infectious disease or having open lesions on the exposed surface of the body should avoid activities which could compromise the quality of API. Smoking, eating, drinking, chewing and storage of food should be restricted to designated areas separated from production or control areas.

- ***Labelling***: Each container should be identified by an appropriate label, showing at least the product identification and the assigned batch code, or any other easily understandable combination of both. Containers for external distribution may require additional labels.
- **Computerised systems**: Computer systems should be designed and operated to prevent unauthorised entries or changes to the programme. In the case of manual entry of quality critical data there should be a second independent check to verify accuracy of the initial entry. A back-up system should be provided of all quality critical data.

Disadvantages of TQM

- Initial introduction cost.
- Benefits may not be seen for several years.
- Workers may be resistant to change.

TQM encourages participation amongst employees, managers and organization as whole. Using Quality management reduces rework nearly to zero in an achievable goal. The responsibilities either its professional, social, legal one that rest with the pharmaceutical manufacturer for the assurance of quality of product are tremendous and it can only be achieved by well organised. Work culture and complete engagement of the employees at the work place. It should be realised that national & international regulations must be implemented systematically and process. Control should be practiced rigorously. Thus quality is critically important ingredient to organisational success today which can be achieved by TQM, an organisational approach that focusses on quality as an over achieving goals, aimed at aimed at the prevention of defects rather than detection of defects..

International Organization for Standardization (ISO)

ISO is an independent, non-governmental international organization with a membership of 163 national standards bodies. ISO is derived from the Greek "isos" meaning equal. Whatever the country, whatever the language, we are always ISO.

Through its members, it brings together experts to share knowledge and develop voluntary, consensus-based, market relevant International Standards that support innovation and provide solutions to global challenges.

ISO International Standards ensure that products and services are safe, reliable and of good quality. For business, they are strategic tools that reduce costs by minimizing waste and errors and increasing productivity. They help companies to access new markets, level the playing field for developing countries and facilitate free and fair global trade.

ISO 9000 - Quality management: The ISO 9000 family addresses various aspects of quality management and contains some of ISO's best known standards. The standards provide guidance and tools for companies and organizations who want to ensure that their products and services consistently meet customer's requirements, and that quality is consistently improved. There are many other standards in the ISO 9000 series that can help you reap the full benefits of a quality management system and put customer satisfaction at the heart of your business. ISO 9000 contains detailed explanations of the seven quality management principles with tips on how to ensure these are reflected in the way you work. It also contains many of the terms and definitions used in ISO 9001.

ISO 9001:2015 sets out the criteria for a quality management system and is the only standard in the family that can be certified to (although this is not a requirement). It can be used by any organization, large or small, regardless of its field of activity. In fact, there are over one million companies and organizations in over 170 countries certified to ISO 9001. This standard is based on a number of quality management principles including a strong customer focus, the motivation and implication of top management, the process approach and continual improvement. Using ISO 9001:2015 helps ensure that customers get consistent, good quality products and services, which in turn brings many business benefits. ISO 9004 provides guidance on how to achieve sustained success with your quality management system. ISO 19011 gives guidance for performing both internal and external audits to ISO 9001. This will help ensure your quality management system delivers on promise and will prepare you for an external audit, should you decide to seek third-party certification.

Seven quality management principles (QMPs):

ISO 9000, ISO 9001 and related ISO quality management standards are based on these seven QMPs.

Customer focus	***Statement***: The primary focus of quality management is to meet customer requirements and to strive to exceed customer expectations. ***Rationale***: Sustained success is achieved when an organization attracts and retains the confidence of customers and other interested parties. Every aspect of customer interaction provides an opportunity to create more value for the customer. Understanding current and future needs of customers and other interested parties contributes to sustained success of the organization. **Key benefits** ➢ Increased customer value ➢ Increased customer satisfaction ➢ Improved customer loyalty ➢ Enhanced repeat business ➢ Enhanced reputation of the organization ➢ Expanded customer base ➢ Increased revenue and market share **Actions you can take** ➢ Recognize direct and indirect customers as those who receive value from the organization. ➢ Understand customers' current and future needs and expectations.

Contd...

	➢ Link the organization's objectives to customer needs and expectations. ➢ Communicate customer needs and expectations throughout the organization. ➢ Plan, design, develop, produce, deliver and support goods and services to meet customer needs and expectations. ➢ Measure and monitor customer satisfaction and take appropriate actions. ➢ Determine and take actions on interested parties' needs and expectations that can affect customer satisfaction. ➢ Actively manage relationships with customers to achieve sustained success.
Leadership	***Statement***: Leaders at all levels establish unity of purpose and direction and create conditions in which people are engaged in achieving the organization's quality objectives. ***Rationale***: Creation of unity of purpose and direction and engagement of people enable an organization to align its strategies, policies, processes and resources to achieve its objectives. **Key benefits** ➢ Increased effectiveness and efficiency in meeting the organization's quality objectives ➢ Better coordination of the organization's processes ➢ Improved communication between levels and functions of the organization ➢ Development and improvement of the capability of the organization and its people to deliver desired results **Actions you can take** ➢ Communicate the organization's mission, vision, strategy, policies and processes throughout the organization. ➢ Create and sustain shared values, fairness and ethical models for behaviour at all levels of the organization. ➢ Establish a culture of trust and integrity. ➢ Encourage an organization-wide commitment to quality. ➢ Ensure that leaders at all levels are positive examples to people in the organization. ➢ Provide people with the required resources, training and authority to act with accountability. ➢ Inspire, encourage and recognize people's contribution.
Engagement of people	***Statement***: Competent, empowered and engaged people at all levels throughout the organization are essential to enhance its capability to create and deliver value. ***Rationale***: To manage an organization effectively and efficiently, it is important to involve all people at all levels and to respect them as individuals. Recognition, empowerment and enhancement of competence facilitate the engagement of people in achieving the organization's quality objectives.

Contd...

	Key benefits ➢ Improved understanding of the organization's quality objectives by people in the organization and increased motivation to achieve them ➢ Enhanced involvement of people in improvement activities ➢ Enhanced personal development, initiatives and creativity ➢ Enhanced people satisfaction ➢ Enhanced trust and collaboration throughout the organization ➢ Increased attention to shared values and culture throughout the organization ***Actions you can take*** ➢ Communicate with people to promote understanding of the importance of their individual contribution. ➢ Promote collaboration throughout the organization. ➢ Facilitate open discussion and sharing of knowledge and experience. ➢ Empower people to determine constraints to performance and to take initiatives without fear. ➢ Recognize and acknowledge people's contribution, learning and improvement. ➢ Enable self-evaluation of performance against personal objectives. ➢ Conduct surveys to assess people's satisfaction, communicate the results, and take appropriate actions.
Process approach	***Statement***: Consistent and predictable results are achieved more effectively and efficiently when activities are understood and managed as interrelated processes that function as a coherent system. ***Rationale***: The quality management system consists of interrelated processes. Understanding how results are produced by this system enables an organization to optimize the system and its performance. ***Key benefits*** ➢ Enhanced ability to focus effort on key processes and opportunities for improvement ➢ Consistent and predictable outcomes through a system of aligned processes ➢ Optimized performance through effective process management, efficient use of resources, and reduced cross-functional barriers ➢ Enabling the organization to provide confidence to interested parties as to its consistency, effectiveness and efficiency ***Actions you can take*** ➢ Define objectives of the system and processes necessary to achieve them. ➢ Establish authority, responsibility and accountability for managing processes. ➢ Understand the organization's capabilities and determine resource constraints prior to action. ➢ Determine process interdependencies and analyse the effect of modifications to individual processes on the system as a whole.

Contd...

	➢ Manage processes and their interrelations as a system to achieve the organization's quality objectives effectively and efficiently. ➢ Ensure the necessary information is available to operate and improve the processes and to monitor, analyse and evaluate the performance of the overall system. ➢ Manage risks that can affect outputs of the processes and overall outcomes of the quality management system.
Improvement	***Statement***: Successful organizations have an ongoing focus on improvement. ***Rationale***: Improvement is essential for an organization to maintain current levels of performance, to react to changes in its internal and external conditions and to create new opportunities. **Key benefits** ➢ Improved process performance, organizational capabilities and customer satisfaction ➢ Enhanced focus on root-cause investigation and determination, followed by prevention and corrective actions ➢ Enhanced ability to anticipate and react to internal and external risks and opportunities ➢ Enhanced consideration of both incremental and breakthrough improvement ➢ Improved use of learning for improvement ➢ Enhanced drive for innovation **Actions you can take** ➢ Promote establishment of improvement objectives at all levels of the organization. ➢ Educate and train people at all levels on how to apply basic tools and methodologies to achieve improvement objectives. ➢ Ensure people are competent to successfully promote and complete improvement projects. ➢ Develop and deploy processes to implement improvement projects throughout the organization. ➢ Track, review and audit the planning, implementation, completion and results of improvement projects. ➢ Integrate improvement considerations into the development of new or modified goods, services and processes. ➢ Recognize and acknowledge improvement.
Evidence-based decision making	***Statement***: Decisions based on the analysis and evaluation of data and information are more likely to produce desired results. ***Rationale***: Decision making can be a complex process, and it always involves some uncertainty. It often involves multiple types and sources of inputs, as well as their interpretation, which can be subjective. It is important to understand cause-and-effect relationships and potential unintended consequences. Facts, evidence and data analysis lead to greater objectivity and confidence in decision making.

Contd...

	Key benefits ➢ Improved decision-making processes ➢ Improved assessment of process performance and ability to achieve objectives ➢ Improved operational effectiveness and efficiency ➢ Increased ability to review, challenge and change opinions and decisions ➢ Increased ability to demonstrate the effectiveness of past decisions **Actions you can take** ➢ Determine, measure and monitor key indicators to demonstrate the organization's performance. ➢ Make all data needed available to the relevant people. ➢ Ensure that data and information are sufficiently accurate, reliable and secure. ➢ Analyse and evaluate data and information using suitable methods. ➢ Ensure people are competent to analyse and evaluate data as needed. ➢ Make decisions and take actions based on evidence, balanced with experience and intuition.
Relationship management	***Statement***: For sustained success, an organization manages its relationships with interested parties, such as suppliers. ***Rationale***: Interested parties influence the performance of an organization. Sustained success is more likely to be achieved when the organization manages relationships with all of its interested parties to optimize their impact on its performance. Relationship management with its supplier and partner networks is of particular importance. **Key benefits** ➢ Enhanced performance of the organization and its interested parties through responding to the opportunities and constraints related to each interested party ➢ Common understanding of goals and values among interested parties ➢ Increased capability to create value for interested parties by sharing resources and competence and managing quality-related risks ➢ A well-managed supply chain that provides a stable flow of goods and services **Actions you can take** ➢ Determine relevant interested parties (such as suppliers, partners, customers, investors, employees, and society as a whole) and their relationship with the organization. ➢ Determine and prioritize interested party relationships that need to be managed. ➢ Establish relationships that balance short-term gains with long-term considerations.

Contd...

	➢ Pool and share information, expertise and resources with relevant interested parties. ➢ Measure performance and provide performance feedback to interested parties, as appropriate, to enhance improvement initiatives. ➢ Establish collaborative development and improvement activities with suppliers, partners and other interested parties. ➢ Encourage and recognize improvements and achievements by suppliers and partners.

Further Reading

1. Ameh SJ, Tarfa F, Ayuba S, Gamaniel KS: Herbal Product Realization in accordance with WHO and ISO Guidelines. Int J Pharm Sci Res. 3(10); 4019-4035.
2. Anderson J.C., Rungtusanatham M., & Schroeder R.G. (1994). A theory of quality management underlying the deming management method. Academy of Management Review, 19(3), 472-509.
3. Andrea Burton, Michael Smith, Torkel Falkenberg. Building WHO's global Strategy for Traditional Medicine. European Journal of Integrative Medicine. 2015; 7 (1):13-15.
4. Bergman., Master's thesis, Department of Economics, School of Economics and Management, 2006
5. General guidelines for methodologies on research and evaluation of traditional medicine. Geneva: World Health Organization; 2000.
6. Good laboratory practice (GLP) for safety tests on chemicals. Medicines and Healthcare products Regulatory Agency. 20 January 2017.
7. Good manufacturing practices for pharmaceutical products: main principles. In: WHO Expert Committee on Specifications for Pharmaceutical Preparations: thirty-seventh report. Geneva: World Health Organization; 2003: Annex 4 (WHO Technical Report Series, No. 908).
8. Good manufacturing practices: supplementary guidelines for the manufacture of herbal medicinal products. In: WHO Expert Committee on Specifications for Pharmaceutical Preparations: thirty- fourth report. Geneva: World Health Organization; 1996: Annex 8 (WHO Technical Report Series, No. 863).
9. Guidelines for the assessment of herbal medicines. In: WHO Expert Committee on Specifications for Pharmaceutical Preparations: thirty-fourth report. Geneva: World Health Organization; 1996: Annex 11 (WHO Technical Report Series, No. 863). These guidelines were reproduced in Quality assurance of pharmaceuticals. A compendium of guidelines and related materials. Volume 1. Geneva: World Health Organization; 1997.
10. Hasan M. & Kerr R.M. (2003). The relationship between total quality management practices and organizational performance in service organizations. The TQM Magazine, 15(4), 286-291.
11. https://asq.org/quality-resources/total-quality-management Accessed on 2 May 2021.
12. https://www.iso.org/files/live/sites/isoorg/files/store/en/PUB100080.pdf Accessed on 2 May 2021.

13. https://www.who.int/tdr/publications/documents/glp-handbook.pdf Accessed on 2 May 2021.
14. Jacqueline Wiesner, Werner Knöss. Future visions for traditional and herbal medicinal Products—A global practice for evaluation and regulation? Journal of Ethnopharmacology. 2014;158, Part B:516-518.
15. J-K. Chen and I-S. Chen., TQM measurement model for the biotechnology industry in Taiwan. Expert Systems with Applications, 2009, 36, 8789–8798.9. J.M. Juran., Quality Control Handbook/McGraw-Hill, New York, 195110. R. Buzzell and B. Gale., The PIMS Principles: Linking Strategy to Performance, New York: Free Press. 1987
16. M. Gabriel Antony Raj., M.S. Thesis, Quality Management, BITS, Pilani. 2007.
17. Quality assurance of pharmaceuticals. A compendium of guidelines and related materials. Volume 2. Geneva: World Health Organization; 1999 (Volume 2, Updated edition, 2004).
18. Tian-Tian He, Carolina Oi Lam Ung, Hao Hu, Yi-Tao Wang. Good manufacturing practice (GMP) regulation of herbal medicine in comparative research: China GMP, cGMP, WHO-GMP, PIC/S and EU-GMP. European Journal of Integrative Medicine. 2015;7 (1): 55-66.

Scan QR code to view the website/guidelines

- WHO GMP Guidelines of herbal Medicines-
trs1010-annex2-who-gmp-manufacture-herbal-medicines.pdf

- WHO guidelines on good manufacturing practices (GMP) for herbal medicines-
WHO guidelines on good manufacturing practices (GMP) for herbal medicines

- GLP Practices Guidelines-
OECD Principles of Good Laboratory Practice (GLP) and GLP Compliance Monitoring - OECD

- What is ISO?-
ISO - About us

CHAPTER 32

Intellectual Property Rights and Herbal Products

Introduction

IPR Organisations

- WTO
- WIPO
- TRIPS
- Paris Convention for the Protection of Industrial Property (1883)

TRIPS Patentable and Non-Patentable (Exclusion) Inventions

Patent Search and Literature

TRIPS Patentable and Non-patentable (exclusion) Inventions

Patent Filing Procedures

PCT, Comparison of Paris and PCT Route, Overview of Indian Patent Filing

Indian Patent's Act 1970

Patent Rules

Indian Patent Filing, Processing and Grant of Patents

Indian and International IPR laws Applicable to Herbal Drugs and Natural Products

Patent, Copyright, Trade Secret, Trademarks, Geographical Indication

Legislative Provisions for Protecting Traditional Medical Knowledge

Convention on Biological Diversity (CBD) Law 1993

Sui Generis Laws 2002

Protection of Plant Variety and Farmers Right Act, 2001 (PPVFR Act)

Plant Beeders' Rights (PBR) or Plant Variety Rights (PVR)

Traditional Knowledge Digital Library (TKDL) and Traditional Knowledge Resource Classification (TKRC)

Further Reading

Introduction

IPR are legal rights to intellectual creations of the mind like inventions, artistic works, symbols, names, images, and designs used in commerce. Thus, IPR matters to everyone which has the following main types:

Patent: A patent is a set of exclusive rights granted by a state to a person for a fixed period of time in exchange for the regulated, public disclosure of certain details of a device, method, process or composition of matter (substance) known as an invention which is new, inventive and useful. It is mainly used for protection to one's invention (novel, non-obviousness and utility) for technological, economical advances as well as promotion to creativity with award of sole benefits.

Copyright: This is legal right granted to a work of authorship/creator. Example: music, writing, dance, software and web sites etc.

Industrial design: These are eye appealing designs of useful articles (ornamental or aesthetic) of distinctive or functional necessity. Example: novel designs of teapot, chair etc.

Trademark: This is a distinctive and deceptive sign to distinguish goods and services, Example: Star of Mercedes, logo of university, brand names etc.

Geographical indication: The indication and appellation of origin of goods and service is called as geographical indication. Example: Made in India, Champagne, Darjeeling Tea (word and logo) etc.

IPR Organizations

WTO

The World Trade Organization (WTO) is the only global international organization dealing with the rules of trade between nations. At its heart are the WTO agreements, negotiated and signed by the bulk of the world's trading nations and ratified in their parliaments. The goal is to ensure that trade flows as smoothly, predictably and freely as possible. The WTO officially commenced on 1 January 1995 under the Marrakesh Agreement, signed by 123 nations on 15 April 1994, replacing the General Agreement on Tariffs and Trade (GATT), which commenced in 1948. It was established after World War II in the wake of other new multilateral institutions dedicated to international economic cooperation – notably the Bretton Woods institutions known as the World Bank and the International Monetary Fund. The headquarters of the World Trade Organization is in Geneva, Switzerland.

Principles of the trading system

The WTO establishes a framework for trade policies; it does not define or specify outcomes. That is, it is concerned with setting the rules of the trade policy games. Five principles are of particular importance in understanding both the pre-1994 GATT and the WTO:

1. Non-discrimination

2. Reciprocity
3. Binding and enforceable commitments
4. Transparency
5. Safety values

WTO Agreements

The WTO oversees about 60 different agreements which have the status of international legal texts. Member countries must sign and ratify all WTO agreements on accession. A discussion of some of the most important agreements follows.

- The Agreement on Agriculture came into effect with the establishment of the WTO at the beginning of 1995. The AoA has three central concepts, or "pillars": domestic support, market access and export subsidies.
- The General Agreement on Trade in Services was created to extend the multilateral trading system to service sector, in the same way as the General Agreement on Tariffs and Trade (GATT) provided such a system for merchandise trade. The agreement entered into force in January 1995.
- The Agreement on Trade-Related Aspects of Intellectual Property Rights sets down minimum standards for many forms of intellectual property (IP) regulation. It was negotiated at the end of the Uruguay Round of the General Agreement on Tariffs and Trade (GATT) in 1994.
- The Agreement on the Application of Sanitary and Phytosanitary Measures—also known as the SPS Agreement—was negotiated during the Uruguay Round of GATT, and entered into force with the establishment of the WTO at the beginning of 1995. Under the SPS agreement, the WTO sets constraints on members' policies relating to food safety (bacterial contaminants, pesticides, inspection and labelling) as well as animal and plant health (imported pests and diseases).
- The Agreement on Technical Barriers to Trade is an international treaty of the World Trade Organization. It was negotiated during the Uruguay Round of the General Agreement on Tariffs and Trade, and entered into force with the establishment of the WTO at the end of 1994. The object ensures that technical negotiations and standards, as well as testing and certification procedures, do not create unnecessary obstacles to trade".
- The Agreement on Customs Valuation, formally known as the Agreement on Implementation of Article VII of GATT, prescribes methods of customs valuation that Members are to follow. Chiefly, it adopts the "transaction value" approach.
- In December 2013, the biggest agreement within the WTO was signed and known as the Bali Package.

WIPO

- The World Intellectual Property Organization (WIPO) is one of the 15 specialized agencies of the United Nations (UN). Pursuant to the 1967 Convention Establishing the World

Intellectual Property Organization, WIPO was created to promote and protect intellectual property (IP) across the world by cooperating with countries as well as international organizations. It began operations on 26 April 1970 when the convention entered into force. That date is commemorated annually as World Intellectual Property Day, which raises awareness of the importance of IP. Under Article 3 of this Convention, WIPO seeks to "promote the protection of intellectual property throughout the world". WIPO became a specialized agency of the UN in 1974.

- WIPO's activities including hosting forums to discuss and shape international IP rules and policies, providing global services that register and protect IP in different countries, resolving transboundary IP disputes, helping connect IP systems through uniform standards and infrastructure, and serving as a general reference database on all IP matters; this includes providing reports and statistics on the state of IP protection or innovation both globally and in specific countries. WIPO also works with governments, nongovernmental organizations (NGOs), and individuals to utilize IP for socioeconomic development.
- WIPO administers 26 international treaties that concern a wide variety of IP issues, ranging from the protection of broadcasts to establishing international patent classification.
- Headquartered in Geneva, Switzerland, WIPO has "external offices" around the world, including in Algiers, Algeria; Rio de Jainero, Brazil; Beijing, China, Tokyo, Japan; Moscow, Russia; and Singapore. Unlike most UN organizations, WIPO does not rely heavily on assessed or voluntary contributions from member states; 95 percent of its budget comes from fees related to its global services.
- WIPO currently has 193 member states, including 190 UN member states and the Cook Islands, Holy See and Niue; Palestine has permanent observer status. The only nonmembers are the Federated States of Micronesia, Palau and South Sudan.
- The predecessor to WIPO was the United International Bureaux for the Protection of Intellectual Property (Bureaux Internationaux Réunis pour la Protection de la Propriété Intellectuelle, with the French acronym for "BIRPI"), which had been established in 1893 to administer the Berne Convention for the Protection of Literary and Artistic Works and the Paris Convention for the Protection of Industrial Property.

TRIPS

The Agreement on Trade-Related Aspects of Intellectual Property Rights (TRIPS) is an international legal agreement between all the member nations of the World Trade Organization (WTO). It sets down minimum standards for the regulation by national governments of many forms of intellectual property (IP) as applied to nationals of other WTO member nations. TRIPS was negotiated at the end of the Uruguay Round of the General Agreement on Tariffs and Trade (GATT) between 1989 and 1990 and is administered by the WTO.

The TRIPS agreement introduced intellectual property law into the multilateral trading system for the first time and remains the most comprehensive multilateral agreement on intellectual property to date. In 2001, developing countries, concerned that developed countries were insisting on an overly narrow reading of TRIPS, initiated a round of talks that resulted in the Doha Declaration. The Doha declaration is a WTO statement that clarifies the scope of TRIPS, stating for example that TRIPS can and should be interpreted in light of the goal "to promote access to medicines for all."

Specifically, TRIPS requires WTO members to provide copyright rights, covering authors and other copyright holders, as well as holders of related rights, namely performers, sound recording producers and broadcasting organisations; geographical indications; industrial designs; integrated circuit layout-designs; patents; new plant varieties; trademarks; trade names and undisclosed or confidential information. TRIPS also specifies enforcement procedures, remedies, and dispute resolution procedures. Protection and enforcement of all intellectual property rights shall meet the objectives to contribute to the promotion of technological innovation and to the transfer and dissemination of technology, to the mutual advantage of producers and users of technological knowledge and in a manner conducive to social and economic welfare, and to a balance of rights and obligations.

TRIPS require member states to provide strong protection for intellectual property rights. For example, under TRIPS:

- Copyright terms must extend at least 50 years, unless based on the life of the author. [Article (Art.) 12 and 14]
- Copyright must be granted automatically, and not based upon any "formality", such as registrations, as specified in the Berne Convention. (Art. 9)
- Computer programs must be regarded as "literary works" under copyright law and receive the same terms of protection.
- National exceptions to copyright (such as "fair use" in the United States) are constrained by the Berne three-step test
- Patents must be granted for "inventions" in all "fields of technology" provided they meet all other patentability requirements (although exceptions for certain public interests are allowed (Art. 27.2 and 27.3) and must be enforceable for at least 20 years (Art 33).
- Exceptions to exclusive rights must be limited, provided that a normal exploitation of the work (Art. 13) and normal exploitation of the patent (Art 30) is not in conflict.
- No unreasonable prejudice to the legitimate interests of the right holders of computer programs and patents is allowed.
- Legitimate interests of third parties have to be taken into account by patent rights (Art 30).
- In each state, intellectual property laws may not offer any benefits to local citizens which are not available to citizens of other TRIPS signatories under the principle of national treatment (with certain limited exceptions, Art. 3 and 5). TRIPS also has a most favored nation clause.
- The TRIPS Agreement incorporates by reference the provisions on copyright from the Berne Convention for the Protection of Literary and Artistic Works (Art 9), with the exception of moral rights. It also incorporated by reference the substantive provisions of

the Paris Convention for the Protection of Industrial Property (Art 2.1). The TRIPS Agreement specifically mentions that software and databases are protected by copyright, subject to originality requirement (Art 10).

- Article 10 of the Agreement stipulates: "1. Computer programs, whether in source or object code, shall be protected as literary works under the Berne Convention (1971). 2. Compilations of data or other material, whether in machine readable or other form, which by reason of the selection or arrangement of their contents constitute intellectual creations shall be protected as such. Such protection, which shall not extend to the data or material itself, shall be without prejudice to any copyright subsisting in the data or material itself."

Paris Convention for the Protection of Industrial Property (1883)

The Paris Convention applies to industrial property in the widest sense, including patents, trademarks, industrial designs, utility models (a kind of "small-scale patent" provided for by the laws of some countries), service marks, trade names (designations under which an industrial or commercial activity is carried out), geographical indications (indications of source and appellations of origin) and the repression of unfair competition. The substantive provisions of the Convention fall into three main categories: national treatment, right of priority, common rules.

1. Under the provisions on national treatment, the Convention provides that, as regards the protection of industrial property, each Contracting State must grant the same protection to nationals of other Contracting States that it grants to its own nationals. Nationals of non-Contracting States are also entitled to national treatment under the Convention if they are domiciled or have a real and effective industrial or commercial establishment in a Contracting State.

2. The Convention provides for the right of priority in the case of patents (and utility models where they exist), marks and industrial designs. This right means that, on the basis of a regular first application filed in one of the Contracting States, the applicant may, within a certain period of time (12 months for patents and utility models; 6 months for industrial designs and marks), apply for protection in any of the other Contracting States. These subsequent applications will be regarded as if they had been filed on the same day as the first application. In other words, they will have priority (hence the expression "right of priority") over applications filed by others during the said period of time for the same invention, utility model, mark or industrial design. Moreover, these subsequent applications, being based on the first application, will not be affected by any event that takes place in the interval, such as the publication of an invention or the sale of articles bearing a mark or incorporating an industrial design. One of the great practical advantages of this provision is that applicants seeking protection in several countries are not required to present all of their applications at the same time but have 6 or 12 months to decide in which countries they wish to seek protection, and to organize with due care the steps necessary for securing protection.

3. The Convention lays down a few common rules that all Contracting States must follow. The most important are:
   - **(a)** ***Patents***. Patents granted in different Contracting States for the same invention are independent of each other: the granting of a patent in one Contracting State does not oblige other Contracting States to grant a patent; a patent cannot be refused, annulled or terminated in any Contracting State on the ground that it has been refused or annulled or has terminated in any other Contracting State. The inventor has the right to be named as such in the patent. The grant of a patent may not be refused, and a patent may not be invalidated, on the ground that the sale of the patented product, or of a product obtained by means of the patented process, is subject to restrictions or limitations resulting from the domestic law.

     Each Contracting State that takes legislative measures providing for the grant of compulsory licenses to prevent the abuses which might result from the exclusive rights conferred by a patent may do so only under certain conditions. A compulsory license (a license not granted by the owner of the patent but by a public authority of the State concerned), based on failure to work or insufficient working of the patented invention, may only be granted pursuant to a request filed after three years from the grant of the patent or four years from the filing date of the patent application, and it must be refused if the patentee gives legitimate reasons to justify this inaction. Furthermore, forfeiture of a patent may not be provided for, except in cases where the grant of a compulsory license would not have been sufficient to prevent the abuse. In the latter case, proceedings for forfeiture of a patent may be instituted, but only after the expiration of two years from the grant of the first compulsory license.
   - **(b)** ***Trade Marks***. The Paris Convention does not regulate the conditions for the filing and registration of marks which are determined in each Contracting State by domestic law. Consequently, no application for the registration of a mark filed by a national of a Contracting State may be refused, nor may a registration be invalidated, on the ground that filing, registration or renewal has not been effected in the country of origin. The registration of a mark obtained in one Contracting State is independent of its possible registration in any other country, including the country of origin; consequently, the lapse or annulment of the registration of a mark in one Contracting State will not affect the validity of the registration in other Contracting States.

     Where a mark has been duly registered in the country of origin, it must, on request, be accepted for filing and protected in its original form in the other Contracting States. Nevertheless, registration may be refused in well-defined cases, such as where the mark would infringe the acquired rights of third parties; where it is devoid of distinctive character; where it is contrary to morality or public order; or where it is of such a nature as to be liable to deceive the public. If, in any Contracting State, the use of a registered mark is compulsory, the registration cannot be canceled for non-use until after a reasonable period, and then only if the owner cannot justify this inaction.

Each Contracting State must refuse registration and prohibit the use of marks that constitute a reproduction, imitation or translation, liable to create confusion, of a mark used for identical and similar goods and considered by the competent authority of that State to be well known in that State and to already belong to a person entitled to the benefits of the Convention. Each Contracting State must likewise refuse registration and prohibit the use of marks that consist of or contain, without authorization, armorial bearings, State emblems and official signs and hallmarks of Contracting States, provided they have been communicated through the International Bureau of WIPO. The same provisions apply to armorial bearings, flags, other emblems, abbreviations and names of certain intergovernmental organizations.

Collective marks must be granted protection.

(c) **Industrial Designs**. Industrial designs must be protected in each Contracting State, and protection may not be forfeited on the ground that articles incorporating the design are not manufactured in that State.

(d) **Trade Names**. Protection must be granted to trade names in each Contracting State without there being an obligation to file or register the names.

(e) **Indications of Source**. Measures must be taken by each Contracting State against direct or indirect use of a false indication of the source of goods or the identity of their producer, manufacturer or trader.

(f) **Unfair competition**. Each Contracting State must provide for effective protection against unfair competition.

The Paris Union, established by the Convention, has an Assembly and an Executive Committee. Every State that is a member of the Union and has adhered to at least the administrative and final provisions of the Stockholm Act (1967) is a member of the Assembly. The members of the Executive Committee are elected from among the members of the Union, except for Switzerland, which is a member ex officio. The establishment of the biennial program and budget of the WIPO Secretariat – as far as the Paris Union is concerned – is the task of its Assembly. The Paris Convention, concluded in 1883, was revised at Brussels in 1900, at Washington in 1911, at The Hague in 1925, at London in 1934, at Lisbon in 1958 and at Stockholm in 1967, and was amended in 1979. The Convention is open to all States. Instruments of ratification or accession must be deposited with the Director General of WIPO.

Patent Search and Literature

Categories of Patent Searches

- Landscape Search
- Patentability or Novelty Search
- Prior Art Search
- Validity Search

- FTO or Clearance Search
- Infringement Search
- Miscellaneous

Landscape Search: To identify business opportunities for products and services, general state-of-the-art, comprehensive patent landscape. Data sources include patent literature and non-patent literature databases. Information for the search is derived from business development and scientific leadership. Results are used to support development of business plan and are not intended for an opinion on patentability

Patentability or Novelty Search: Search to determine whether or not an inventive concept is known (Novelty and Obviousness). Data sources include patent and non-patent literature including expired and unexpired anywhere in the world. Information for search is derived from inventors and from invention disclosures Results are used to decide whether a patent application should be filed and to help draft claims that avoid the prior art

Prior Art Search: Search to determine whether any prior art patents or other publications exist that would bar issuance of a valid patent. Data sources include patent and non-patent literature. Information for search is derived from proposed draft patent application. Results are used to draft claims that avoid the prior art and to focus the application on the novel and non-obvious features of the invention

Validity Search: Search to find invalidating references for a patent.Data sources include patent and non-patent literature published before the earliest priority date of the patent in question. Ideally a year or more before the priority date. Information for the search is derived from the claims in the patent in question. Experts in the art are consulted to identify potential references, research groups, or inventors. Results are used To invalidate patents in infringement cases, to prepare for patent enforcement, prior to licensing, to draft an FTO opinion

FTO Search: Search to provide reassurance that you will not infringe the valid IP rights of another. Data sources include non-expired patents that potentially read on your product or service only in countries of interest. Information for your search is derived from an analysis of your product or service. Results are used to draft an opinion. Often an invalidity search is performed on some of the identified patents

Infringement Search: Search to determine whether an enforceable patent claims the same subject matter as your concept or unpatented invention. Data sources include unexpired patents only in countries of interest. Information for the search is derived from a draft or actual claim set. Results are used for an opinion prior to making, using, or selling a product or service

Other Patent-Related Searches: To search legal status and expiry dates, to identify the members and status of a patent family, to identify proper ownership (assignments), to calculate when a patent will expire, maintenance fees, file histories, to identify limitations on the claims, to identify conditions of terminal disclaimer, court records and identify any previous or current litigation

Database Selection: Determine which databases should be searched-US, WIPO, Other Countries. Perform non-patent literature too. Access databases like patent office sites, free providers and or paid services. Search published applications, issued patents, or both.

Patent Databases

- Patent Databases – US- USPTO http://patft.uspto.gov/
- Free Patents On-Line http://www.freepatentsonline.com/
- Patent Lens http://www.patentlens.net http://www.lens.org
- Thomson Innovation http://www.thomsoninnovation.com
- PatBase* http://www.patbase.com

Patent Databases - International

- Delphion is a patent information service platform developed by omson Reuters in the United States
- WIPO PatentScope http://patentscope.wipo.int
- EPO http://worldwide.espacenet.com/advancedSearch?locale=en_EP
- Directories of International Offices
- http://members.pcug.org.au/~arhen/ } http://www.wipo.int/directory/en/urls.jsp }
- Sequence Searching (BLAST)
- http://blast.ncbi.nlm.nih.gov/

Fee Based Commercial Patent Databases & Added Value Service

- Anacubis
- BizInt
- Chemical Abstract Service
- Dialog
- FIZ Karlsruhe
- GetIPDL Patent Downloader from IP Digital Libraries
- IFI Claims
- Lexis-Nexis Patent and Trademark Solutions
- Micropatent
- Minesoft
- Paterra
- Patolis and (Patolis-e)
- Questel-Orbit
- STN
- VantagePoint

TRIPS Patentable and Non-patentable (exclusion) Inventions

Patentable Inventions

Patent will be granted to all inventions, whether products or processes, in all fields of technology, if the invention (Art. 27.1):

- New or Novel – the invention should be new and not disclosed to the public anywhere in the world.
- Non-obvious – the invention should not be obvious to a person skilled in the art in the relevant area of technology and should involve an inventive feature over previous inventions made in the same field.
- Industrial utility – the new product or process should be capable of being made or used in an industry and it should have economic significance.

And Disclosure under Article 29.1: Details of the invention have to be described in the application and therefore have to be made public. Member governments have to require the patent applicant to disclose details of the invention and they may also require the applicant to reveal the best method for carrying it out.

An invention is new when:

- it is not in the prior art (technical status);
- it has inventive level that is not obvious, or obviously derived from prior art, to a person skilled in the relevant technical field; and
- it is considered to have industrial application where its subject matter may be produced or used in any productive activity, including services.

Non-Patentable (Exclusion) Inventions

Those fields of technology in which patents may be denied by members are listed in Art. 27.216 and 27.3 17. Art. 27.3 specific provisions also deal with biotechnological technologies (including the human medical field), allowing Members to exclude patents in the assigned areas:

(a) the one "necessary to protect or dre public or morality", including when intended to protect human, animal or plant life or health or to avoid serious prejudice to the environment, provided that necessity is at stake, and not just convenience; and

(b) a second group including: (i) diagnostic, therapeutic and surgical methods for the treatment of humans or animals, as well as (ii) plants and animals other than microorganisms , and (iii) plant or animal production essentially biological processes other than non-biological and microbiological processes

Patent Filing Procedures

"Patent filing" can be defined as a process of submitting an application in a patent office requesting grant of patent rights to invention. There are following patent filing options:

- Filing a provisional or complete patent application in own country
- Filing a patent application in a foreign country
    - Paris Convention filing
    - Filing a Patent Cooperation Treaty (PCT) application

A provisional application is a temporary application which is filed when the invention is not finalized and is still under experimentation. An application for patent filed in the Patent Office without claiming any priority of application made in a convention country or without any reference to any other application under process in the office is called an ordinary application. An ordinary application must be accompanied with a complete specification and claims. When an applicant feels that he has come across an invention which is a slight modification of the invention for which he has already applied for or has obtained patent, the applicant can go for patent of addition if the invention does not involve a substantial inventive step. There is no need to pay separate renewal fee for the patent of addition during the term of the main patent and it expires along with the main patent. When an application made by applicant claims more than one invention, the applicant on his own or to meet the official objection may divide the application and file two or more applications, as applicable for each of the inventions. This type of application, divided out of the parent one, is called a Divisional Application. The priority date for all the divisional applications will be same as that claimed by the Parent Application (Ante-dating).

Paris Convention Filing

The Paris Convention for the Protection of Industrial Property, signed in Paris, France, on 20 March 1883, was one of the first intellectual property treaties. It established a Union for the protection of industrial property. The Convention is currently still in force. The substantive provisions of the Convention fall into three main categories: national treatment, priority right and common rules. As of January 2019, the Convention has 177 contracting member countries, which makes it one of the most widely adopted treaties worldwide. The Paris Convention is administered by the World Intellectual Property Organization (WIPO), based in Geneva, Switzerland.

The Paris Convention applies to industrial property in the widest sense, including patents, trademarks, industrial designs, utility models (a kind of "small-scale patent" provided for by the laws of some countries), service marks, trade names (designations under which an industrial or commercial activity is carried out), geographical indications (indications of source and appellations of origin) and the repression of unfair competition.

Paris Convention patent filing (convention application) is also known as direct filing. The International treaty of the Paris Convention enables the candidates to document the application in their nation of origin first as the domestic patent application. It very well may be considered as an option in contrast to the PCT patent application. The application for the patent is known as the "priority document" and the date on which the equivalent is documented is known as the "priority date". Paris Convention is truly appropriate for the patent applicants who have a limited spending plan and need the patent protection promptly.

PCT Patent Filing Procedure

The PCT is an international treaty with more than 150 Contracting States. The PCT makes it possible to seek patent protection for an invention simultaneously in a large number of countries by filing a single "international" patent application instead of filing several separate national or regional patent applications. The granting of patents remains under the control of the national or regional patent Offices in what is called the "national phase".

The PCT procedure includes:

- **Filing**: file an international application with a national or regional patent Office or WIPO, complying with the PCT formality requirements, in one language, and pay one set of fees.
- **International Search**: an "International Searching Authority" (ISA) (one of the world's major patent Offices) identifies the published patent documents and technical literature ("prior art") which may have an influence on whether your invention is patentable, and establishes a written opinion on your invention's potential patentability.
- **International Publication**: as soon as possible after the expiration of 18 months from the earliest filing date, the content of international application is disclosed to the world.
- **Supplementary International Search (optional):** a second ISA identifies, at request, published documents which may not have been found by the first ISA which carried out the main search because of the diversity of prior art in different languages and different technical fields.
- **International Preliminary Examination (optional):** one of the ISAs at request carries out an additional patentability analysis, usually on a version of your application which you have amended in light of content of the written opinion.

National Phase: after the end of the PCT procedure, usually at 30 months from the earliest filing date of your initial application, from which claim priority, start to pursue the grant of patents directly before the national (or regional) patent Offices of the countries in which applicant want to obtain them.

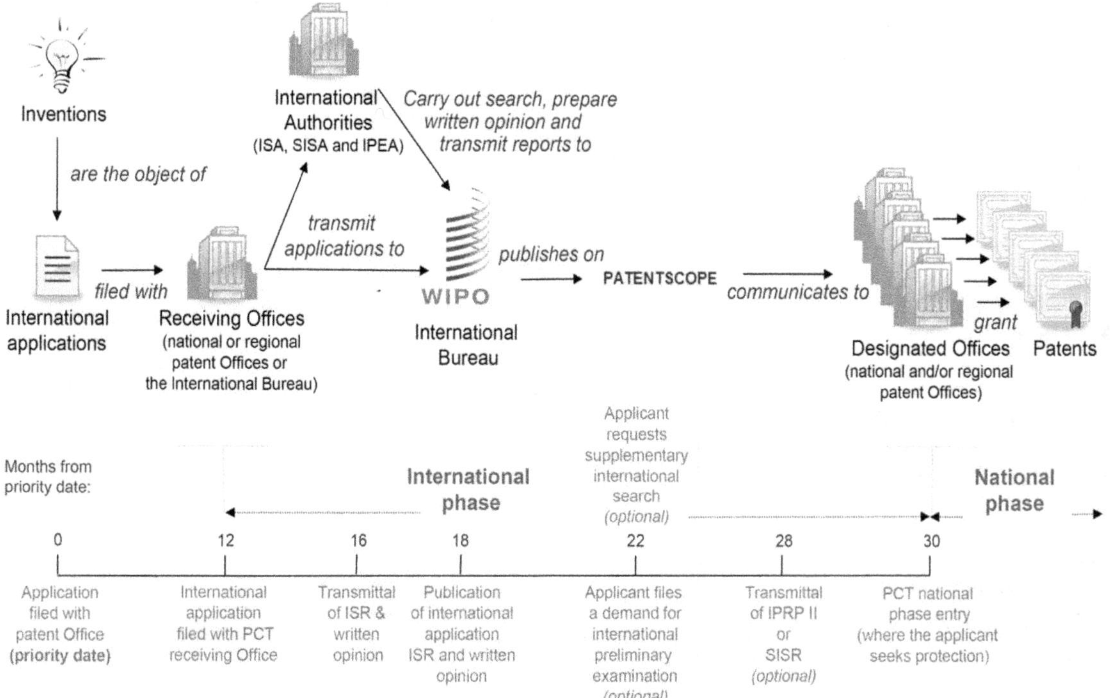

Figure 32.1 Overview of PCT patent filing [Courtesy-WIPO].

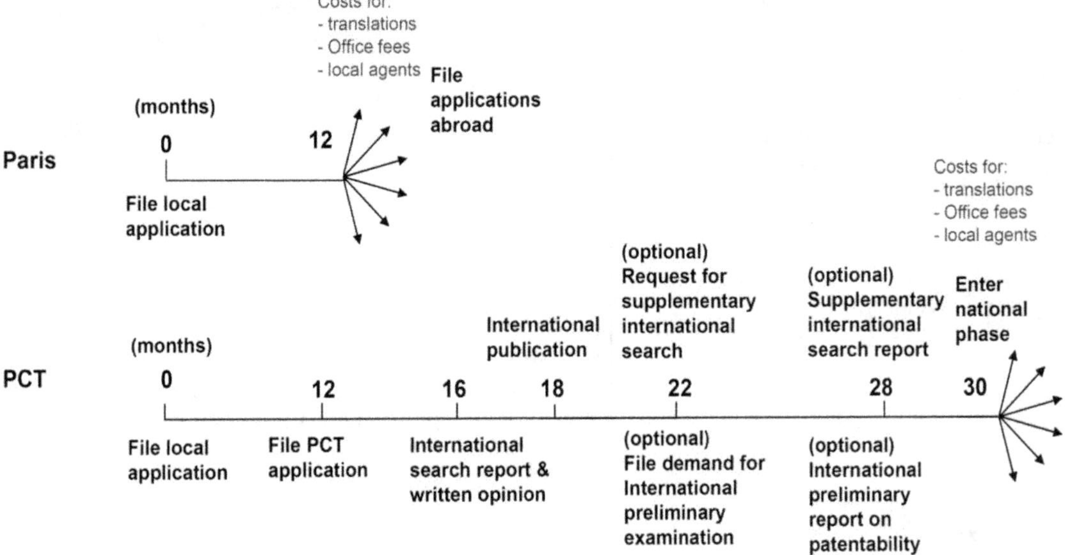

Figure 32.2 Comparison of Paris and PCT Route [Courtesy-WIPO].

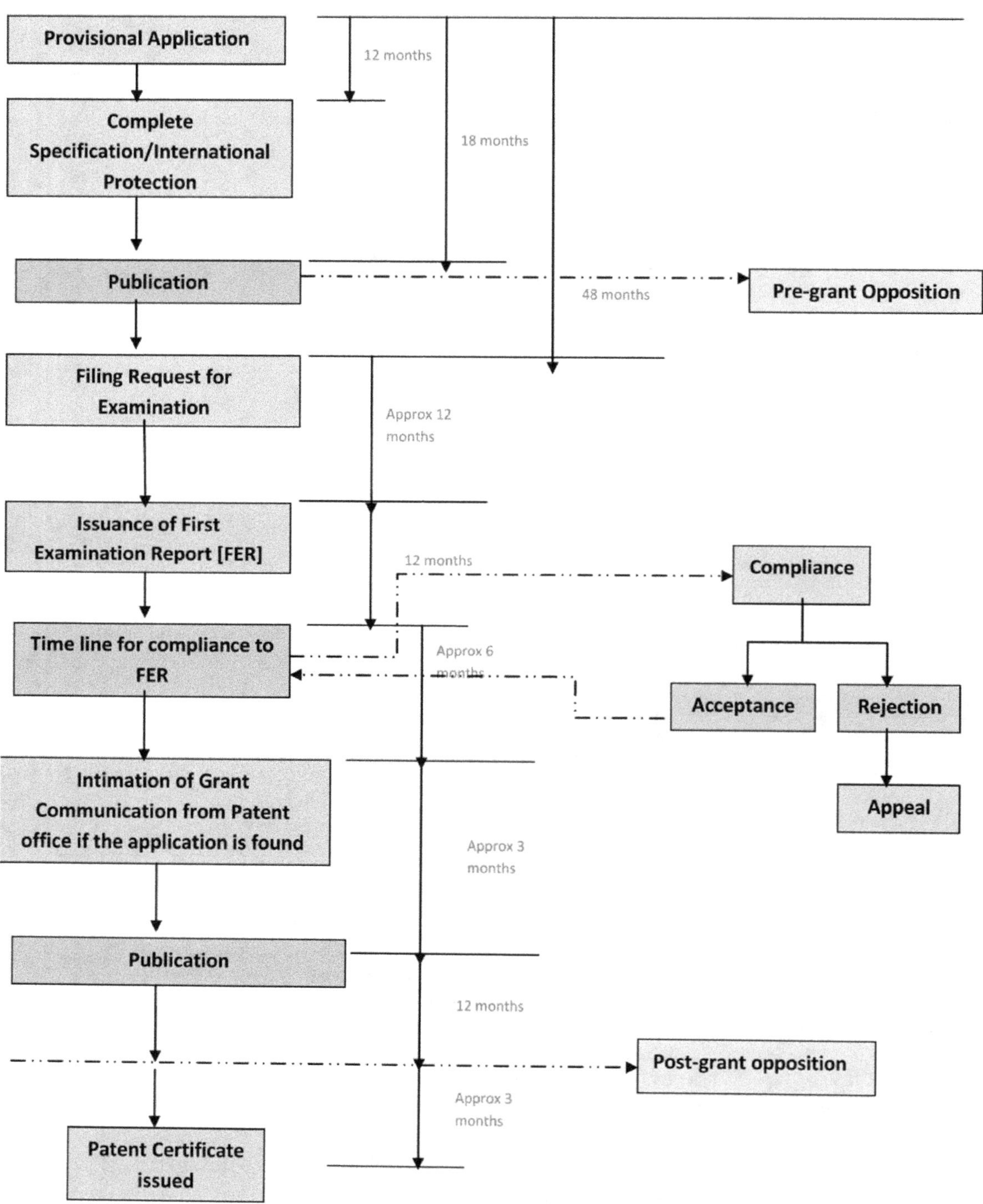

Figure 32.3 Overview of Indian patent filing.

Indian Patent's Act 1970

- The first legislation in India relating to patents was the Act VI of 1856. The objective of this legislation was to encourage inventions of new and useful manufactures and to induce inventors to disclose secret of their inventions. The Act was subsequently repealed by Act IX of 1857 since it had been enacted without the approval of the British Crown . Fresh legislation for granting 'exclusive privileges' was introduced in 1 859 as Act XV of 1859. This legislation contained certain modifications of the earlier legislation, namely, grant of exclusive privileges to useful inventions only and extension of priority period from 6 months to 12 months. This Act excluded importers from the definition of inventor. This Act was based on the United Kingdom Act of 1852 with certain departures which include allowing assignees to make application in India and also taking prior public use or publication in India or United Kingdom for the purpose of ascertaining novelty.
- In 1872, the Act of 1859 was consolidated to provide protection relating to designs. It was renamed as "The Patterns and Designs Protection Act" under Act XIII of 1872. The Act of 1872 was further amended in 1883 (XVI of 1883) to introduce a provision to protect novelty of the invention, which prior to making application for their protection were disclosed in the Exhibition of India. A grace period of 6 months was provided for filing such applications after the date of the opening of such Exhibition.
- This Act remained in force for about 30 years without any change but in the year 1883, certain modifications in the patent law were made in United Kingdom and it was considered that those modifications should also be incorporated in the Indian law. In 1888, an Act was introduced to consolidate and amend the law relating to invention and designs in conformity with the amendments made in the U.K. law.
- The Indian Patents and Designs Act, 1911, (Act II of 1911) replaced all the previous Acts. This Act brought patent administration under the management of Controller of Patents for the first time. This Act was further amended in 1920 to enter into reciprocal arrangements with UK and other countries for securing priority. In 1930, further amendments were made to incorporate, inter-alia, provisions relating to grant of secret patents, patent of addition, use of invention by Government, powers of the Controller to rectify register of patent and increase of term of the patent from 14 years to 16 years. In 1945, an amendment was made to provide for filing of provisional specification and submission of complete specification within nine months.
- After Independence, it was felt that the Indian Patents & Designs Act, 1911 was not fulfilling its objective. It was found desirable to enact comprehensive patent law owing to substantial changes in political and economic conditions in the country. Accordingly, the Government of India constituted a committee under the Chairmanship of Justice (Dr.) Bakshi Tek Chand, a retired Judge of Lahore High Court, in 1949 t o review the patent law

in India in order to ensure that the patent system is conducive to the national interest. The terms of reference included —

- o To survey and report on the working of the patent system in India;
- o To examine the existing patent legislation in India and to make recommendations for improving it, particularly with reference to the provisions concerned with the prevention of abuse of patent rights;
- o To consider whether any special restrictions should be imposed on patent regarding food and medicine;
- o To suggest steps for ensuring effective publicity to the patent system and to patent literature, particularly as regards patents obtained by Indian inventors;
- o To consider the necessity and feasibility of setting up a National Patents Trust;
- o To consider the desirability or otherwise of regulating the profession of patent agents
- o To examine the working of the Patent Office and the services rendered by it to the public and make suitable recommendations for improvement; and
- o To report generally on any improvement that the Committee thinks fit to recommend for enabling the Indian Patent System to be more conducive to national interest by encouraging invention and the commercial development and use of inventions.

- The committee submitted its interim report on 4th August, 1949 with recommendations for prevention of misuse or abuse of patent right in India and suggested amendments to sections 22, 23 & 23A of the Patents & Designs Act, 1911 on the lines of the United Kingdom Acts 1919 and 1949. The committee also observed that the Patents Act should contain clear indication to ensure that food and medicine and surgical and curative devices are made available to the public at the cheapest price commensurate with giving reasonable compensation to the patentee.
- Based on the above recommendation of the Committee, the 1911 Act was amended in 1950(Act XXXII of 1950) in relation to working of inventions and compulsory licence/revocation. Other provisions were related to endorsement of the patent with the words 'licence of right' on an application by the Government so that the Controller could grant licences. In 1952 (Act LXX of 1952) an amendment was made to provide compulsory licence in relation to patents in respect of food and medicines, insecticide, germicide or fungicide and a process for producing substance or any invention relating to surgical or curative devices. The compulsory licence was also available on notification by the Central Government. Based on the recommendations of the Committee, a bill was introduced in the Parliament in 1953 (Bill No.59 of 1953). However, the Government did not press for the consideration of the bill and it was allowed to lapse.
- In 1957, the Government of India appointed Justice N. Rajagopala Ayyangar Committee to examine the question of revision of the Patent Law and advise government accordingly. The report of the Committee, which comprised of two parts, was submitted in September,

1959. The first part dealt with general aspects of the Patent Law and the second part gave detailed note on the several clauses of the lapsed bills 1953. The first part also dealt with evils of the patent system and solution with recommendations in regards to the law. The committee recommended retention of the Patent System, despite its shortcomings. This report recommended major changes in the law which formed the basis of the introduction of the Patents Bill, 1965. This bill was introduced in the Lok Sabha on 21st September, 1965, which however lapsed. In 1967, again an amended bill was introduced which was referred to a Joint Parliamentary Committee and on the final recommendation of the Committee, the Patents Act, 1970 was passed. This Act repealed and replaced the 1911 Act so far as the patents law was concerned. However, the 1911 Act continued to be applicable to designs. Most of the provisions of the 1970 Act were brought into force on 20 th April 1972 with publication of the Patent Rules, 1972.

- This Act remained in force for about 24 years without any change till December 1994. An ordinance effecting certain changes in the Act was issued on 31 st December 1994, which ceased to operate after six months. Subsequently, another ordinance was issued in 1999. This ordinance was subsequently replaced by t he Patents (Amendment) Act, 1999 that was brought into force retrospectively from 1 st January, 1995. The amended Act provided for filing of applications for product patents in the areas of drugs, pharmaceuticals and agro chemicals though such patents were not allowed. However, such applications were to be examined only after 31-12-2004. Meanwhile, the applicants could be allowed Exclusive Marketing Rights (EMR) to sell or distribute these products in India, subject to fulfilment of certain conditions.
- The second amendment to the 1970 Act was made through the Patents (Amendment) Act, 2002 (Act 38 0f 2002). This Act came into force on 20 th May 2003 with the introduction of the new Patent Rules, 2003 by replacing the earlier Patents Rules, 1972
- The third amendment to the Patents Act 1970 was introduced through the Patents (Amendment) Ordinance, 2004 w.e.f. 1 st January, 2005. This Ordinance was later replaced by the Patents (Amendment) Act 2005 (Act 15 of 2005) on 4th April, 2005 which was brought into force from 1-1-2005.

Patents Rules

Under the provisions of section 159 of the Patents Act, 1970 the Central Government is empowered to make rules for implementing the Act and regulating patent administration. Accordingly, the Patents Rules, 1972 were notified and brought into force w.e.f. 20.4.1972. These Rules were amended from time to time till 20 May 2003 when new Patents Rules, 2003 were brought into force by replacing the 1972 rules. These rules were further amended by the Patents (Amendment) Rules, 2005 and the Patents (Amendment) Rules, 2006. The last amendments are made effective from 5th May 2006.

Indian Patent's Act 1970 Chapters and Sections

Chapter I - Preliminary	
1	Short title, extent and commencement
2	Definitions and interpretation
Chapter II - Inventions Not Patentable	
3	What are not inventions
4	Inventions relating to atomic energy not patentable
5	[Omitted]
Chapter III - Applications for Patents	
6	Persons entitled to apply for patents
7	Form of application
8	Information and undertaking regarding foreign applications
9	Provisional and complete specifications
10	Contents of specifications
11	Priority dates of claims of a complete specification
Chapter IV - Publication and Examination of Applications	
11A 11B	Publication of applications Request for examination
12	Examination of application
13	Search for anticipation by previous publication and by prior claim
14	Consideration of the report of examiner by Controller
15	Power of Controller to refuse or require amended applications, etc., in certain case
16	Power of Controller to make orders respecting division of application
17	Power of Controller to make orders respecting dating of application
18	Powers of Controller in cases of anticipation
19	Powers of Controller in case of potential infringement
20	Powers of Controller to make orders regarding substitution of applicants, etc.
21	Time for putting application in order for grant
22	22-24. [Omitted]
Chapter IVA [Omitted]	
Chapter V - Opposition Proceedings to Grant of Patents	
23-24	Section 24A-24F. [Omitted]
25	Opposition to the patent
26	In cases of "obtaining" Controller may treat the patent as the patent of opponent
27	[Omitted]
28	Mention of inventor as such in patent

Contd...

Chapter VI -Anticipation	
29	Anticipation by previous publication
30	Anticipation by previous communication to Government
31	Anticipation by public display, etc
32	Anticipation by public working
33	Anticipation by use and publication after provisional specification
34	No anticipation if circumstances are only as described in sections 29,30,31 and 32
Chapter VII - Provisions for Secrecy of Certain Invention	
35	Secrecy directions relating to inventions relevant for defense purposes
36	Secrecy directions to be periodically reviewed
37	Consequences of secrecy directions
38	Revocation of secrecy directions and extension of time
39	Residents not to apply for patents outside India without prior permission
40	Liability for contravention of section 35 or section 39
41	Finality of orders of Controller and Central Government
42	Savings respecting disclosure to Government
Chapter VIII - Grant of Patents and Rights Conferred Thereby	
43	Grant of patents
44	Amendment of patent granted to deceased applicant
45	Date of patent
46	Form, extent and effect of patent
47	Grant of patents to be subject to certain conditions
48	Rights of patentees
49	Patent rights not infringed when used on foreign vessels etc., temporarily or accidentally in India
50	Rights of co-owners of patents
51	Power of Controller to give directions to co-owners
52	Grant of patent to true and first inventor where it has been obtained by another in fraud of him
53	Term of patent
Chapter IX Patents of Addition	
54	Patents of addition
55	Term of patents of addition
56	Validity of patents of addition
Chapter X - Amendment of Applications and Specifications	
57	Amendment of application and specification or any document related thereto before Controller

Contd...

58	Amendment of specification before Appellate Board or High Court
59	Supplementary provisions as to amendment of application or specification
Chapter XI – Restoration of Lapsed Patents	
60	Applications for restoration of lapsed patents
61	Procedure for disposal of applications for restoration of lapsed patents
62	Rights of patentees of lapsed patents which have been restored
Chapter XII – Surrender and Revocation of Patents	
63	Surrender of patents
64	Revocation of patents
65	Revocation of patent or amendment of complete specification on directions from Government in cases relating to atomic energy
66	Revocation of patent in public interest
Chapter XIII - Register Of Patents	
67	Register of patents and particulars to be entered therein
68	Assignments, etc., not to be valid unless in writing and duly executed
69	Registration of assignments, transmissions, etc
70	Power of registered grantee or proprietor to deal with patent
71	Rectification of register by Appellate Board
72	Register to be open for inspection
Chapter XIV - Patent Office and Its Establishment	
73	Controller and other officers
74	Patent office and its branches
75	Restriction on employees of patent office as to right or interest in patents
76	Officers and employees not to furnish information, etc
Chapter XV - Powers of Controller Generally	
77	Controller to have certain powers of a civil court
78	Power of Controller to correct clerical errors, etc
79	Evidence how to be given and powers of Controller in respect thereof
80	Exercise of discretionary powers by Controller
81	Disposal by Controller of applications for extension of time
Chapter XVI - Working of Patents, Compulsory Licenses And Revocation	
82	Definition of "patented articles" and "patentee"
83	General principles applicable to working of patented inventions
84	Compulsory licensess
85	Revocation of patents by the Controller for non-working
86	Power of Controller to adjourn applications for compulsory licences, etc., in certain cases

Contd...

87	Procedure for dealing with applications under sections 84 and 85
88	Powers of Controller in granting compulsory licenses
89	General purposes for granting compulsory licenses
90	Licensing of related patents
91	Special provision for compulsory licenses on notifications by Central Government
92 (A)	Compulsory license for export of patented pharmaceutical products in certain exceptional circumstances
93	Order for license to operate as a deed between parties concerned
94	Termination of compulsory license
95-98	[Omitted]
Chapter XVII - Use of Inventions for Purposes of Government and Acquisition of Inventions by Central Government	
99	Meaning of use of invention for purposes of Government
100	Power of Central Government to use inventions for purposes of Government
101	Rights of third parties in respect of use of invention for purposes of Government
102	Acquisition of inventions and patents by the Central Government
103	Reference to High Court of disputes as to use for purposes of Government
Chapter XVIII- Suits Concerning Infringement of Patents	
104	Jurisdiction
104 (A)	Burden of proof in case of suits concerning infringement
105	Power of court to make declaration as to non-infringement
106	Power of court to grant relief in cases of groundless threats of infringement proceedings
107	Defenses, etc., in suits for infringement
107(A)	Certain acts not to be considered as infringement
108	Reliefs in suit for infringement
109	Right of exclusive licensee to take proceedings against infringement
110	Right of licensee under section 84 to take proceedings against infringement
111	Restriction on power of court to grant damages or account of profits for infringement
112	[Omitted]
113	Certificate of validity of specification and costs of subsequent suits for infringement thereof
114	Relief for infringement of partially valid specification
115	Scientific advisers

Contd...

Chapter XIX- Appeals to the Appellate Board	
116	Appellate Board
117(A)	Staff of Appellate Board
117(B)	Appeals to Appellate Board
117(C)	Bar of jurisdiction of courts, etc.
117(D)	Procedure for application for rectification, etc., before Appellate Board
117(E)	Appearance of Controller in legal proceedings
117 (F)	Costs of Controller in proceedings before Appellate Board
117 (G)	Transfer of pending proceedings to Appellate Board
117 (H)	Power of Appellate Board to make rules
Chapter XX- Penalties	
118	Contravention of secrecy provisions relating to certain inventions
119	Falsification of entries in register, etc
120	Unauthorized claim of patent rights
121	Wrongful use of words "patent office"
122	Refusal or failure to supply information
123	Practice by non-registered patent agents
124	Offences by companies
Chapter XXI - Patent Agents	
125	Register of patent agents
126	Qualifications for registration as patent agents
127	Rights of patent agents
128	Subscription and verification of certain documents by patent agents.
129	Restrictions on practice as patent agents
130	Removal from register of patent agents and restoration
131	Power of Controller to refuse to deal with certain agents
132	Savings in respect of other persons authorised to act as agents
Chapter XXII- International Arrangements	
133	Convention countries
134	Notification as to countries not providing for reciprocity
135	Convention applications
136	Special provisions relating to convention application
137	Multiple priorities
138	Supplementary provisions as to convention applications
139	Other provisions of Act to apply to convention applications

Contd...

Chapter XXIII- Miscellaneous	
140	Avoidance of certain restrictive conditions
141	Determination of certain contracts
142	Fees
143	Restrictions upon publication of specification
144	Reports of examiners to be confidential
145	Publication of official journal
146	Power of Controller to call for information from patentees
147	Evidence of entries, documents, etc.
148	Declaration by infant, lunatic etc
149	Service of notices, etc., by post
150	Security for costs
151	Transmission of orders of courts to Controller
152	[Omitted]
153	Information relating to patents
154	Loss or destruction of patents
155	Reports of Controller to be placed before Parliament
156	Patent to bind Government
157	Right of Government to sell or use forfeited articles
157(A)	Protection of security of India
158	Power of High Courts to make rules
159	Power of Central Government to make rules
160	Rules to be placed before Parliament
161	[Omitted]
162	Repeal of Act 2 of 1911 in so far as it relates to patents and savings
163	[Omitted]

Indian Patent Filing, Processing and Grant of Patents

The first step in securing a patent is the filing of a patent application. Many patent offices provide a specific form to fill in. In some patent offices, you can file a patent application on line. In the patent application, in general, you must describe the title of the invention, as well as provide an indication of its technical field. You must also include the background to and a description of the invention, in clear language and enough detail that a person with an average understanding of the field could use or reproduce the invention. Such descriptions are usually accompanied by visual materials such as drawings, plans, or diagrams to better describe the invention and an abstract, which contains a brief summary of the invention. You must also clearly and concisely define the matter for which patent protection is sought in the "claims" part of the patent application.

In addition, depending on the applicable patent law, you may need to submit various kinds of statements, declarations or supporting documents to a patent office. In view of the complexity it is recommended that you consult a patent attorney or a patent agent to prepare a patent application.

- **Filing:** applicants choose a submission category – i.e., national, regional or international – and file an application. The initial filing is considered the "priority filing" from which further successive national, regional or international filings may be made within the 'priority period' of one year, in accordance with the Paris Convention for the Protection of Industrial Property.
- **Formal examination:** the patent office ensures that all administrative formalities have been met, that the relevant documentation has been included in the application, and that all associated fees have been paid.
- **Prior art search:** in many countries the patent office carries out a search of the prior art – all relevant technological information publicly known at the time of filing the application. Using extensive databases and expert examiners in the specific technical field of the application, a 'search report' is drafted that compares the technical merits of the claimed invention with that of the known prior art.
- **Publication:** in most countries, the patent application is published 18 months after the priority date; i.e., after the date of first filing.
- **Substantive examination:** if a prior art search report is available, the examiner checks that the application satisfies the requirements of patentability – that the invention is novel, inventive and susceptible to industrial application, compared to the prior art as listed in the search report.
- **Grant/refusal:** the examiner may either grant the patent application without amendments, change the scope of the claims to reflect the known prior art, or reject the application.
- **Opposition:** many patent offices allow third parties to oppose the granted patent within a specified period on the grounds that it does not satisfy patentability requirements.
- **Appeal:** many offices provide the opportunity for an appeal after the substantive examination or after the opposition procedure.

A patent owner has the right to decide who may – or may not – use the patented invention for the period in which the invention is protected. In other words, patent protection means that the invention cannot be commercially made, used, distributed, imported, or sold by others without the patent owner's consent.

Indian and International IPR Laws Applicable to Herbal Drugs and Natural Products

Medicinal plants are an important part of human health care history, culture and tradition. They are widely used in traditional cultures all over the world and are becoming increasingly popular in modern society as natural alternatives to synthetic chemicals on the understanding that these are soundly based on empirical observation over many generations. Natural products and their derivatives represent more than 50 % of all drugs in clinical use in the world. Rauwolfia for hypertension, vinca for cancer, gymnema for diabetis, digitalis for heart failure, opium for pain, colchicine for gout, artemisinin for malaria are just a few examples of medicines derived from plant sources.

With the tremendous advancement in the *Information Technology* and market value of herbal products, the safety, efficacy and quality of herbal traditional medicines have become the subject of research. The patentability of traditional medicines and associated knowledge is the major reason of increasing international attention in recent years. However, issues relating to the protection of herbal knowledge, biodiversity, inventions and practices of traditional and indigenous medicine must be solved with some modifications in present Intellectual Property Rights and implementing some new amendments.

A majority of the herbal patents applications and grants in India are with individual inventors. Claim analysis indicates that these patents include novel multi-herb compositions with synergistic action. Indian research organizations are more active than companies in filing for patents. CSIR has maximum numbers of applications not only in India but also in the US and EU. Patents by research organizations and herbal companies are on development of new processes for active compound isolation and standardization of such components in addition to new compositions for therapeutic use. Pharmaceutical companies such as Ranbaxy, Lupin and Panacea Biotech are increasingly patenting on herbal drugs. There is increased patenting activity related to diabetes, cancer, cardiovascular diseases, asthma and arthritis in India and abroad.

Patents

Holders of traditional medical knowledge can nevertheless face significant obstacles in satisfying the conditions required to obtain a patent, especially the requirements of novelty and inventiveness. Because many traditional medicines have been used for generations, disseminated in local communities and documented in publicly available sources, these medicines may fail to qualify for patent protection for lack of novelty.

Moreover, because herbal medicines typically comprise natural products in their raw form, it can be difficult to claim that a remedy involves an inventive step. Identifying how the claimed invention differs from prior art can also be problematic. That said, pharmaceutical drugs derived from natural products usually involve some form of alteration or purification, which may be considered a novel and inventive step making the drugs eligible for patent protection.

Several common ways that inventors can obtain patents for herbal medicines are if they can:

1. find new uses for an existing herb;
2. isolate a new active ingredient or
3. improve the method for extraction of the active ingredient(s).

There are several ways to patent natural or herbal medicines such as by claiming new uses for old compounds. The basic recipe or composition for most traditional herbal medicine has been known for years and, therefore, is not patentable. Researchers who can find something new about herbal medicines, e.g. a new use for old compounds, may be able to apply for patent protection.

One problem with patenting natural or herbal medicines, particularly traditional herbal medicines, is that most of the herbs have been described previously; therefore, they are what we call "publicly known". Many of them may have also been publicly used, i.e. people at different levels have used the herbs for different purposes. An herbal medicine composition, the process of making the composition, and the uses of the composition may not be novel since they are either publicly known or have been publicly used.

In medicinal and aromatic plant research: patents are not granted for - Non-obvious inventions means those which are known already – documented, traditional knowledge; occurring in nature itself like phytochemicals Reserpine, taxol, baccosides, cultivars, etc; new use of a known substance and Frivolous inventions.

But Patents are grantable for – "Processes" like better extraction processes, better dosage forms, stable formulations, better tastes/aroma, producing higher yields; involving biotechnological interventions, improving bioavailability, providing synergy/antagonistic activity and Processes for standardization, fractionation, isolation, etc.

Patents are grantable for "products" like novel formulations, novel combinations of specific ingredients; specific proportions; novel combinations that show synergy/antagonisms - resulting in better activity or lesser adverse effects; better stability, better absorption/bioavailability; Novel combinations with formulation aids that show inventive steps - can be even addition of - stabilizers or penetration enhancers to provide unique benefit to users etc; Uniquely standardized to provide specific quality responsible for therapeutic activity, Unique drug delivery tubings etc.

In China, patent law protects new traditional medicine-based products, methods of process and new uses of traditional medicine, including herbal preparations, extracts from herbal medicines, foods containing herbal medicines and methods for preparing herbal formulas.

Indian law has adequate provisions for the protection of TK and Biological Resources. Traditional knowledge, by its very definition, is in the public domain and hence, any application for patent relating to TK does not qualify as an invention under section 2 (1) (j) of the Patents Act, 1970, which defines that "invention means a new product or process involving an inventive step and capable of industrial application". Further, under section 3(e) of the Patents Act "a substance obtained by a mere admixture resulting only in the aggregation of the properties of the components thereof or process for producing such substances" is not an invention and hence, not patentable. The Indian Patents Act also has a unique provision under Section 3 (p), wherein "an invention which, in effect, is traditional knowledge or which is an aggregation or duplication of known properties of traditionally known component or components" is not an invention and hence, not patentable, within the meaning of the Patents Act. Additionally, sections 3 (b), (c), (d), (f), (h), (i) and (j) are of relevance with respect to the patent applications related to TK and/or biological material.

Indian applications for patents based on TK and/or biological material contravening the provisions of law can be refused under section 15 or in pre-grant opposition under clauses (d), (f) and (k) of Section 25 (1) and granted patents can be revoked in post-grant opposition under clauses (d), (f) and (k) of Section 25 (2) of the Patents Act, 1970. Nondisclosure or wrong mention of the source or geographical origin of biological material used for an invention in the complete specification also forms a ground for pre- and post- grant opposition under clause (j) of Sections 25 (1) and 25 (2) respectively of the Patents Act, 1970.

In India, patent screening accords appropriate IPC classification for such TK applications so that these applications can be properly routed for examination to the respective groups such as Chemistry, Pharmaceuticals, Agrochemicals, Biotechnology, Microbiology, Biochemistry, Food, Mechanical, etc. e.g., C07D, C07G5/00 (for Chemical), A61K, A61L (for Pharmaceuticals), A01N (for Agrochemcials), C12S, C12N, C07K4/00; 14/00 (for Biotechnology), C12N, C12P, C12Q (for Microbiology), C12F, C12G (for Biochemistry), A23C, A23L (for Food), B25F (for Mechanical), etc. The screening of an application as "Traditional Knowledge" is an administrative process for facilitating the examination and to indicate that the subject-matter of the application is important and has relevance in the context of traditionally known substances, articles or processes for preparing them or their use

Copyright: This is legal right can be granted to herbal drugs medicines related work of authorship/creator, e.g. music, writing, software and web sites etc RELATED TO

Trade Secret

A trade secret is information not generally known or reasonably discoverable, through which an IP holder can obtain some economic advantage. Once trade secrets become known, they generally cease to provide protection. Traditional medical knowledge holders may choose not to disclose their knowledge and keep it secret. In some communities, traditional medical knowledge is known and transmitted only to individual healers and not to the community at large.

Trademarks

Trademarks protect distinctive signs, such as words, phrases, symbols and designs that identify the source of a product. This helps consumers identify products with preferred characteristics, such as a specific brand of herbal medicine. Trademark rights are established through either registration or use in commerce. Trademarks have been used to market products based on traditional medical knowledge, such as Truong Son Balsam, a traditional balm of medical plants from Viet Nam. However, while trademarks can help distinguish authentic goods, they do not prohibit third parties from using traditional knowledge without the trademark or under a different mark. Trademarks cannot be used to protect traditional medical knowledge itself. Ayurvedic firms such as Dabur, Zandu, etc use trademarks. Medicinal plant cultivars and traders can use the route of trademarks. India Organic'' is a certification trademark granted by the Spices Board on the basis of compliance with the National Standards for Organic Production. The present AGMARK standards cover quality guidelines for 224 different commodities spanning a variety of pulses, cereals, essential oils, vegetable oils, Fruits and Vegetables and semi-processed products like vermicelli.

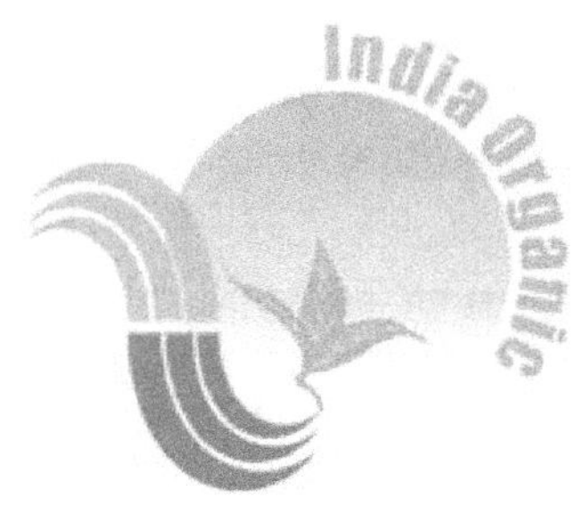

The 'India Organic' certification mark by Agricultural and Processed Food Products Export Development Authority (APEDA)

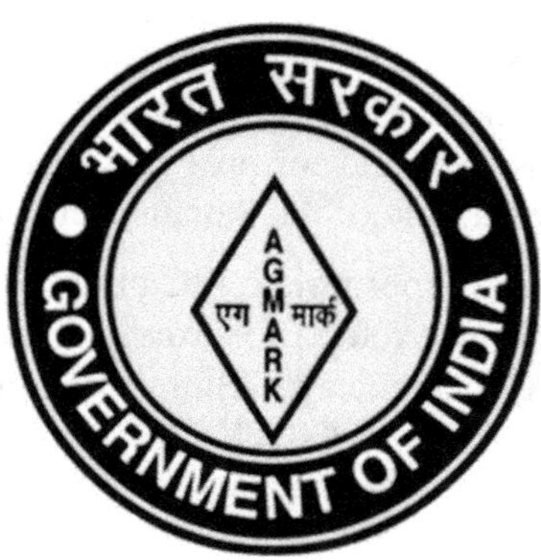

Agmark (Agriculture marketing) by Directorate of Marketing and Inspection, Government of India

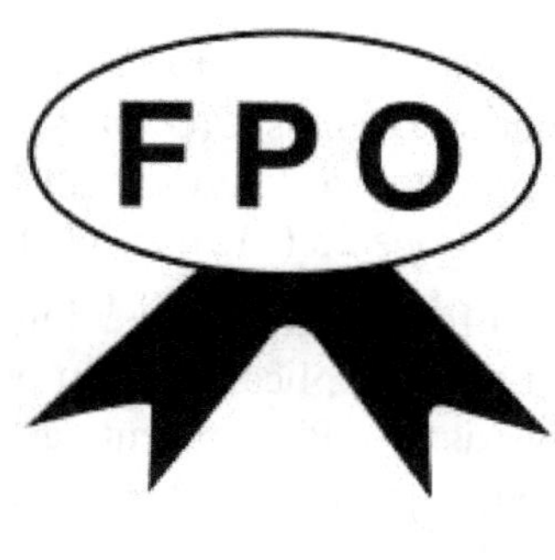

Fruit products order by Ministry of Food Processing Industries (India)

Geographical Indication

A geographical indication is another sort of IP right that can help to identify the source of goods. Geographical indications identify products as having characteristics associated with their place of origin. However, although geographical indications can be used to distinguish products based on traditional medical knowledge specific to a location, they cannot protect against the same use of traditional medical knowledge that is not associated with a place. The way in which geographical indications are protected varies by country, and may require registration or use in commerce. As with trademarks, geographical indications can be used only for the protection of products based on traditional medical knowledge, not the knowledge itself.

Legislative Provisions for Protecting Traditional Medical Knowledge

Convention on Biological Diversity (CBD) Law 1993:

The Convention on Biological Diversity (CBD), known informally as the Biodiversity Convention, is a multilateral treaty. The Convention has three main goals including: the conservation of biological diversity (or biodiversity); the sustainable use of its components; and the fair and equitable sharing of benefits arising from genetic resources. In other words, its objective is to develop national strategies for the conservation and sustainable use of biological diversity. CBD law of Costa Rica in 1993 gives sovereign rights over biological resources and communities rights over their knowledge also providing sharing of benefits arising from the utilization of the genetic resources. On the issue of Biological resources, section 6 (1) of the Biological Diversity Act, 2002 provides very clearly that "no person shall apply for any intellectual property right, by whatever name called, in or outside India for any invention based on any research or information on a biological resource obtained from India without obtaining the previous approval of National Biodiversity Authority before making such application; provided that, if a person applies for a patent, permission of the National Biodiversity Authority may be obtained after the acceptance of the patent but before the sealing of the patent1 by the patent authority concerned; provided further that the National Biodiversity Authority shall dispose of the application for permission made to it within a period of ninety days from the date of receipt thereof. The Indian Patent Law complements this provision of the Biological Diversity Act, 2002 by making it mandatory for the applicant of a patent to submit a declaration under Form-1 (Application for Grant of Patent) of the Patent Rules 2003 to the effect that "the invention as disclosed in the specification uses the biological material from India and the necessary permission from the Competent Authority shall be submitted by me/us before the grant of patent to me/us." The Biological Diversity Act, 2002 has a penal provision in this regard under section 55 (1) which provides that "whoever contravenes or attempts to contravene or abets the contravention of the provisions of the section 3 or section 4 or section 6 shall be punishable with imprisonment for a term which may extend to five years, or with fine which may extend to ten lakh rupees and where the damage caused exceeds ten lakh rupees such fine may commensurate with the damage caused, or with both."

Sui Generis Laws 2002

The sui generis regime of Peru was established by Law No. 27, 811 of 2002, whose objectives are to protect TK, to promote fair and equitable distribution of benefits, to ensure that the use of the knowledge takes place with the prior informed consent of the indigenous peoples, and to prevent misappropriation. It also protects the collective knowledge of indigenous peoples associated to biological resources. The law also foresees the payment of equitable compensation for the use of certain types of TK into a national Fund for Indigenous Development or directly to the TK holders.

Protection of Plant Variety and Farmers Right Act, 2001 (PPVFR Act)

The Protection of Plant Variety and Farmers Right Act, 2001 (PPVFR Act) is an Act of the Parliament of India that was enacted to provide to grant intellectual property rights as effective system for protection of plant varieties, the rights of farmers and plant breeders, and to encourage the development and cultivation of new varieties of plants. The period of protection for field crops is 15 years and for trees and vines is 18 years and for notified varieties it is 15 years from the date of notification under section 5 of Seeds Act, 1966.

The International Union for the Protection of New Varieties of Plants or UPOV is an intergovernmental organization with headquarters in Geneva, Switzerland. The UPOV Convention was adopted in 1961 as a result of the Diplomatic Conferences held in Paris in 1957 and 1961. The UPOV Convention entered into force in 1968 with the ratification of Germany, the Netherlands and the United Kingdom. The UPOV Convention was amended in 1972, 1978 and 1991. UPOV, which continues to be the only internationally harmonized, effective sui generis system of plant variety protection, is continuing to expand. In UPOV, rights are granted only to the breeder, which in today's context means the seed companies. There is no concept of Farmers' Rights in the UPOV (International Union for the Protection of New Varieties of Plants) system, particularly under 1991 Act. The PPVFR Act provides a balance between breeder's right and farmer's right, the provisions for compulsory licensing, researcher's rights, and exclusion of certain varieties from registration.

Plant Breeders' Rights (PBR) or Plant Variety Rights (PVR)

Plant breeders' rights (PBR), also known as plant variety rights (PVR), are a form of intellectual property rights granted to the breeder of a new variety of plant that give the breeder exclusive control over the propagating material (including seed, cuttings, divisions, tissue culture) and harvested material (cut flowers, fruit, foliage) of a new variety for a number of years.

Plant breeders' rights are now being granted by a large number of states throughout the world to protect breeders and encourage plant breeding. Most states that have plant breeders' rights are members of UPOV- the International Union for the Protection of New Varieties of Plants. UPOV acts as international spokesman on plant breeders' rights and as a co-ordinating body for member states. But there is conflict between UPOV (1991) and GATT 1994. UPOV (1991) provides for the grant of an exclusive exportation right over plant and other material and for the revival of this right after exhaustion. The exclusive exportation right constitutes an export restriction inconsistent with Article XI:1 of GATT 1994 that lacks a justification in Article XX(d) or any other GATT exception. Many WTO Members join UPOV (1991) as a means of implementing a TRIPS obligation but TRIPS neither requires nor authorizes the grant of exclusive exportation rights inconsistent with GATT 1994. Certain free trade agreements do require ratification of UPOV (1991) but paradoxically reiterate the obligation in Article XI:1 of GATT 1994 as well. Thus laws providing for exclusive exportation rights for plant breeders are vulnerable to challenge in the WTO dispute settlement mechanism.

Plant breeders' right (PBR) certificates provide legal rights for breeders over the varieties they produce which fulfill the criteria of novelty (not been commercialized for more than one year in the country of protection), distinctness (such as height, maturity, color, etc), uniformity (consistent characteristics from plant to plant), and stability (remain genetically fixed and same from generation to generation). With these rights, the breeder can choose to become the exclusive marketer of the variety, or to license the variety to others. Virtually all national PBR systems are based to a greater or lesser degree on the UPOV Convention.

The breeder must also give the variety an acceptable "denomination", which becomes its generic name and must be used by anyone who markets the variety. Typically, plant variety rights are granted by national offices, after examination. Seed is submitted to the plant variety office, who grow it for one or more seasons, to check that it is distinct, stable, and uniform. If these tests are passed, exclusive rights are granted for a specified period (typically 20/25 years (or 25/30 years, for trees and vines). Annual renewal fees are required to maintain the rights.

Traditional Knowledge Digital Library (TKDL) and Traditional Knowledge Resource Classification (TKRC)

Traditional Knowledge Digital Library (TKDL) is a pioneer initiative of India to prevent misappropriation of country's traditional medicinal knowledge at International Patent Offices on which healthcare needs of more than 70% population and livelihood of millions of people in India is dependent. Its genesis dates back to the Indian effort on revocation of patent on wound healing properties of turmeric at the USPTO. Besides, in 2005, the TKDL expert group estimated that about 2000 wrong patents concerning Indian systems of medicine were being granted every year at international level, mainly due to the fact that India's traditional medicinal knowledge which exists in local languages such as Sanskrit, Hindi, Arabic, Urdu, Tamil etc. is neither accessible nor comprehensible for patent examiners at the international patent offices.

Traditional Knowledge Digital Library* has overcome the language and format barrier by scientifically converting and structuring the available contents (till date 0.29 million medicinal formulations) of the ancient texts on Indian Systems of Medicines i.e. Ayurveda, Siddha, Unani and Yoga, into five international languages, namely, English, Japanese, French, German and Spanish, with the help of information technology tools and an innovative classification system - Traditional Knowledge Resource Classification (TKRC).

At present, as per the approval of Cabinet Committee on Economic Affairs, access of TKDL is available to nine International Patent Offices (European Patent Office, United State Patent & Trademark Office, Japan Patent Office, United Kingdom Patent Office, Canadian Intellectual Property Office, German Patent Office, Intellectual Property Australia, Indian Patent Office and Chile Patent Office), under TKDL Access (Non-disclosure) Agreement.

TKDL is proving to be an effective deterrent against bio-piracy and is being recognized as a global leader in the area of traditional knowledge protection.

Further Reading

1. A series of briefs, www.wipo.int/tk/en/briefs.html. • Consultation draft of the WIPO Traditional Knowledge Documentation Toolkit, www.wipo.int/tk/en/tk/TKToolkit.html.
2. Darrell Addison Posey, Graham Dutfield. Beyond Intellectual Property-Toward Traditional Resource Rights for Indigenous Peoples and Local Communities. International Development Research Centre (Canada). 1996.
3. Database of legislative texts on the protection of traditional knowledge and traditional cultural expressions and legislative texts relevant to genetic resources, www.wipo.int/tk/en/legal_texts/.

4. DB Anantha Narayana. Intellectual property rights for herbal products. PharmaBiz. May 22, 2013.
5. Deepa Goel, Shomini Parashar. IPR, Biosafety and Bioethics. Pearson Education India. 2013
6. Graham Dutfield, Uma Suthersanen. Global Intellectual Property Law. Edward Elgar Publishing, Incorporated. 2008
7. http://www.ipindia.nic.in/index.htm Accessed on May 2021
8. https://www.wipo.int/portal/en/index.html Accessed on May 2021
9. **https://www.wto.org/** Accessed on May 2021
10. Intellectual Property and Genetic Resources, Traditional Knowledge and Traditional Cultural Expressions: An Overview (WIPO Publication No. 933), www.wipo.int/export/sites/www/tk/en/publications/933e_booklet_1.pdf.
11. Neeraj Pandey, Khushdeep Dharni. Intellectual Property Rights. PHI Learning. 2014
12. Parintek Innovations. Unfolding Intellectual PRoperty Rights-A Practical Patent Guide for Researchers, Academicians and start-ups. Notion Press. 2019
13. Peter Ulvskov. Patenting in Biotechnology-A Laboratory Manual. Polyteknisk Boghandel og Forlag. 2019.
14. Prabuddha Ganguli. Gearing Up for Patents-The Indian Scenario. Universities Press. 1998
15. Promoting Access to Medical Technologies and Innovation: Intersections between Public Health, Intellectual Property and Trade (WIPO Publication No. 628), www.wipo.int/export/sites/www/freepublications/en/global_challenges/628/wipo_pub_628.pdf
16. Sahoo N, Manchikanti P, Dey SH. Herbal drug patenting in India: IP potential. J Ethnopharmacol. 2011 Sep 1;137(1):289-97. doi: 10.1016/j.jep.2011.05.022. Epub 2011 May 27. PMID: 21640810.
17. The WIPO Intergovernmental Committee on Intellectual Property and Genetic Resources, Traditional Knowledge and Folklore (IGC), www.wipo.int/tk/en/igc/index.html
18. Uma J. Lele, William Lesser, Gesa Horstkotte-Wesseler. Intellectual Property Rights in Agriculture-The World Bank's Role in Assisting Borrower and Member Countries. World Bank. 2000

Scan QR code to view the website/guidelines

- IPR-
About Us | Intellectual Property India | Government of India (ipindia.gov.in)

- IPR and Traditional Medicinal Knowledge-
Intellectual Property and Traditional Medical Knowledge (wipo.int)

CHAPTER 33

Geogrpahical Indications of Goods (Registration and Protection) Act, 1999

Introduction

Geographical Indications have been defined under Article 22(1) of the WTO Agreement on Trade-Related Aspects of Intellectual Property Rights (TRIPS) Agreement as: "Indications which identify a good as originating in the territory of a member, or a region or a locality in that territory, where a given quality, reputation or characteristic of the good is essentially attributable to its geographic origin."

The Geographical Indications of Goods (Registration and Protection) Act, 1999 No.48 of 1999 provides registration and better protection of geographical indications relating to goods. It is enacted by Parliament in the Fiftieth Year **(30th December, 1999)** of the Republic of India. It has total 9 chapters and 87 section.

Chapters	Sections	
Chapter I: Preliminary	1-2	1. Short Title, Extent and Commencement 2. Definitions and Interpretation
Chapter II: The Register and Conditions for Registration	3-10	3. Registrar of Geographical Indications 4. Power of Registrar to Withdraw or Transfer Cases etc. 5. Geographical Indications Registry and Offices Thereof 6. Register of Geographical Indications 7. Part A and Part B of the Register 8. Registration to be in Respect of Particular Goods and Area 9. Prohibition of Registration of Certain Geographical Indications 10. Registration of Homonymous Geographical Indications
Chapter III: Procedure for and Duration of Registration	11-19	11. Application for Registration 12. Withdrawal of Acceptance 13. Advertisement of Application 14. Opposition to Registration 15. Correction and Amendment 16. Registration 17. Application for Registration as Authorised User 18. Duration, Renewal, Removal and Restoration of Registration 19. 19. Effect of Removal from Register for Failure to Pay Fee for Renewal
Chapter IV: Effect of Registration	20-24	20. No Action for Infringement of Unregistered Geographical Indication 21. Rights Conferred by Registration 22. Infringement or Registered Geographical Indications 23. Registration to be Prima Facie Evidence of Validity 24. Prohibition of Assignment or Transmission, etc.

Contd...

Chapters	Sections	
Chapter V: Special Provisions Relating to Trade Marks and Prior Users	25-26	25. Prohibition of Registration of Geographical Indication as Trade Mark 26. Protection to Certain Trade Marks
Chapter VI: Rectification and Correction of the Register	27-30	27. Power to Cancel or Vary Registration and to Rectify the Register 28. Correction of Register 29. Alteration of Registered Geographical Indications 30. Adaptation of Entries in Register to Amend or Substitute Classification of Goods
Chapter VII: Appeals to the Appellate Board	31-36	31. Appeals to the Appellate Board 32. Bar of Jurisdiction of Courts, etc. 33. Procedure of the Appellate Board 34. Procedure for Application for Rectification etc., Before Appellate Board 35. Appearance of Registrar in Legal Proceedings 36. Costs of Registrar in Proceedings before Appellate Board
Chapter VIII: Offences, Penalties and Procedure	37-54	37. Meaning of Applying Geographical Indications 38. Falsifying and Falsely Applying Geographical Indications 39. Penalty for Applying False Geographical Indications 40. Penalty for Selling Goods to which False Geographical Indication is applied 41. Enhanced Penalty on Second or Subsequent Conviction 42. Penalty for Falsely Representing a Geographical Indication as Registered 43. Penalty for Improperly Describing a Place of Business as Connected with the Geographical Indications Registry 44. Penalty for Falsification of Entries in the Register 45. No Offence in Certain Cases 46. Forfeiture of Goods 47. Exemption of Certain Persons Employed in Ordinary Course of Business 48. Procedure where Invalidity of Registration is pleaded by the Accused 49. Offences by Companies 50. Cognizance of Certain Offences and the Powers of Police Officer for Search and Seizure

Contd...

		51. Costs of defense of Prosecution 52. Limitation of Prosecution 53. Information as to Commission of Offence 54. 54. Punishment for Abetment in India of Acts Done Out of India
Chapter IX: Miscellaneous	55-87	55. Protection of Action Taken in Good Faith 56. Certain Persons to be Public Servants 57. Stay of Proceedings where the Validity of Registration of the Geographical Indication is Questioned, etc. 58. Application for Rectification of Register be made to Appellate Board in Certain Cases 59. Implied Warranty on Sale of Indicated Goods 60. Power of Registrar 61. Exercise of Discretionary Power by Registrar 62. Evidence before Registrar 63. Death of Party to a Proceeding 64. Extension of Time 65. Abandonment 66. Suit for Infringement etc., to be instituted before District Court 67. Relief in Suit for Infringement or for Passing Off 68. Authorized User to be impleaded in Certain Proceedings 69. Evidence of Entries in Register, etc., and Things Done by the Registrar 70. Registrar and Other Officers not Compellable to Produce Register, etc. 71. Power to Require Goods to Show Indication of Origin 72. Certificate of Validity 73. Groundless Threats of Legal Proceedings 74. Address for Service 75. Trade Usages, etc., to be taken into Consideration 76. Agents 77. Index 78. Documents Open to Public Inspection 79. Reports of Registrar to be Placed Before Parliament 80. Fees and Surcharge 81. Savings in Respect of Certain Matters in Chapter VIII 82. Declarations as to Title of Geographical Indication not Registrable under the Registration Act, 1908 83. Government to be bound

Contd...

		84. Special Provisions Relating to Applications for Registration from Citizens of Convention Countries 85. Provisions as to Reciprocity 86. Powers of Central Government to Remove Difficulties 87. Power to Make Rules

Benefits of Registration of Geographical Indications

Registering Geographical Indication is always beneficial as the owner can prevent others from unauthorized usage or from commercializing of the registered product. However, the registration of GI is not mandatory in India, unregistered GI are protected under passing off cases, but it's always advisable to register the geographical origin as no further proof is required.

- It confers legal protection to Geographical Indications in India,
- It prevents unauthorized use of a registered Geographical Indication by others.
- It boosts exports of Indian Geographical indications by providing legal Protection.
- It enables seeking legal protection in other WTO member countries.
- It promotes economic Prosperity of Producers.
- It is widely believed that effective protection of a GI product, by way of preventing loss of value through copying or free riding, could go a long way in increasing the flow of cash income to the community involved in its production.
- Hence, GI is often cited as a tool that has the potential to contribute to rural development though indirectly through a reduction in income poverty.

Application and Registration of Geographical Indications

Any association of persons, producers, organization or authority established by under the law can apply. The applicant must represent the interest of the producers. Registration process is as shown in Figure :

9. *Prohibition of Registration of Certain Geographical Indications*

A geographical indication:

(a) the use of which would be likely to deceive or cause confusion; or

(b) the use of which would be contrary to any law for the time being in force; or

(c) which comprises or contains scandalous or obscene matter; or

(d) which comprise or contains any matter likely to hurt the religious susceptibilities of any class or section of the citizens of India; or

(e) which would otherwise be disentitled to protection in a court; or

(f) which are determined to be generic names or indications of goods and are, therefore, not or ceased to be protected in their country of origin, or which have fallen into disuse in that country; or

(g) which although literally true as to the territory, region or locality in which the goods originate, but falsely represent to the persons that the goods originate in another territory, region or locality, as the case may be, shall not be registered as a geographical indication.

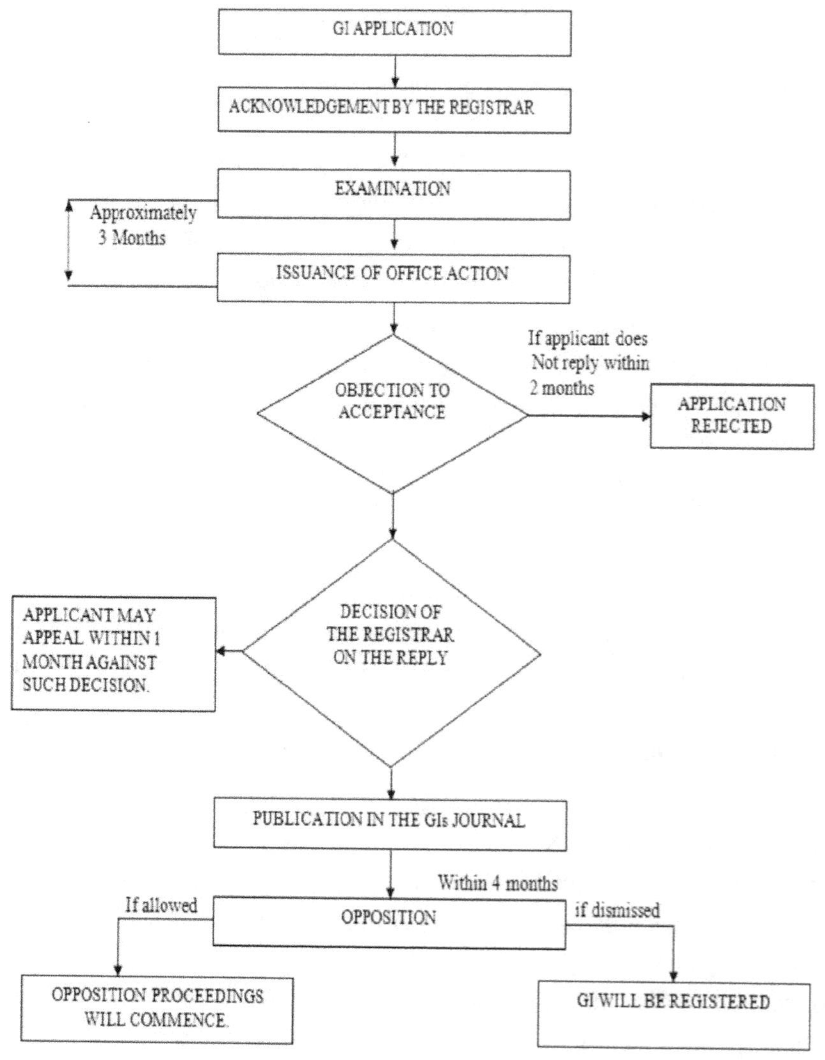

Geographical indication registration process

Explanation 1: For the purposes of this section, "generic names or indications", in relation to goods, means the name of a goods which, although relates to the place or the region where the goods was originally produced or manufactured, has lost its original meaning and has become the common name of such goods and serves as a designation for or indication of the kind, nature, type or other property or characteristic of the goods.

Explanation 2: In determining whether the name has become generic, account shall be taken of all factors including the existing situation in the region or place in which the name originates and the area of consumption of the goods.

39. Penalty for Applying False Geographical Indications, Selling Goods to which False Geographical Indication is Applied

punishable with imprisonment for a term which shall not be less than six months but which may extend to three years and with fine which shall not be less than fifty thousand rupees but which may extend to two lakhs rupees:

Provided that the court may, for adequate and special reasons to be mentioned in the judgement, impose a sentence of imprisonment for a term of less than six months or a fine of less than fifty thousand rupees.

punishable for the second and for every subsequent offence, with imprisonment for a term which shall not be less than one year but which may extend to three years and with fine which shall not be less than one lakh rupees but which may extend to two lakh rupees:

Provided that the court may, for adequate and special reason to be mentioned in the judgement, impose a sentence of imprisonment for a term of less than one year or a fine of less than one lakh rupees:

Provided further that for the purposes of this section, no cognizance shall be taken of any conviction made before the commencement of this Act.

Registered Geographical Indications of Medicinal/Aromatic Plants and Allied Products

Germany had the largest number of GIs in force (9,499), followed by China (7,566), the EU (4,914), the Republic of Moldova (3,442) and Bosnia and Herzegovina (3,147). Till now in India, around 365 products have been added to the GI list. Recently Kashmir saffron and black rice of Manipur got the GI tag.

Product	State	Reg.No.
Mysore Agarbathi	Karnataka	11
Mysore Sandalwood oil	Karnataka	23
Mysore Sandal soap	Karnataka	24
Mysore Betel leaf	Karnataka	28
Nanjanagud Banana	Karnataka	29

Contd...

Product	State	Reg.No.
Mysore Jasmine	Karnataka	37
Uduppi Jasmine	Karnataka	38
Hadagalli Jasmine	Karnataka	39
Navara rice	Karnataka	40
Coorg Green Cardamom	Karnataka	57
Kamalapur Red Banana	Karnataka	115
Devanahalli Pomelo (Chakkota)	Karnataka	113
Byadagi Chilli	Karnataka	147
Bangalore Rose Onion	Karnataka	217
Pokkali Rice	Kerala	86
Wayanad Jeerakasala Rice	Kerala	137
Wayanad Gandhakasala rice	Kerala	138
Kaipad Rice	Kerala	199
Khirsapati (Himsagar) Mango	West Bengal	95
Naga Mirchi	Nagaland	99
Ganjam Kewda Rooh	Odisha	171
Ganjam Kewda Flower	Odisha	172
Kalanamak Rice	Uttar Pradesh	194
Kannauj Perfume	Uttar Pradesh	203
Naga Tree Tomato	Nagaland	220
Sikkim Large Cardamom (Amomum subulatum)	Sikkim	222
Assam Karbi Anglong Ginger	Assam	226
Khasi Mandarin	Meghalaya	231

Further Reading

1. Brinckmann JA. Emerging importance of geographical indications and designations of origin - authenticating geo-authentic botanicals and implications for phytotherapy. Phytother Res. 2013 Nov;27(11):1581-7
2. Darrell Addison Posey, Graham Dutfield. Beyond Intellectual Property-Toward Traditional Resource Rights for Indigenous Peoples and Local Communities. International Development Research Centre (Canada). 1996.
3. Deepa Goel, Shomini Parashar. IPR, Biosafety and Bioethics. Pearson Education India. 2013
4. Graham Dutfield, Uma Suthersanen. Global Intellectual Property Law. Edward Elgar Publishing, Incorporated. 2008
5. http://www.ipindia.nic.in/index.htm Accessed on May 2021
6. https://www.wipo.int/portal/en/index.html Accessed on May 2021
7. https://www.wto.org/ accessed Accessed on May. 2021

8. Larson J. Relevance of geographical indications and designations of origin for the sustainable use of genetic resources. Rome, Italy: Global Facilitation Unit for Underutilized Species 2007.
9. National Institute for the Defense of Competition and for Protection of Intellectual Property Rights (INDECOPI). Geneva: International Bureau of the World Intellectual Property Organization (WIPO) 2013, 41: 19–21.
10. Neeraj Pandey, Khushdeep Dharni. Intellectual Property Rights. PHI Learning. 2014
11. Parintek Innovations. Unfolding Intellectual PRoperty Rights-A Practical Patent Guide for Researchers, Academicians and start-ups. Notion Press. 2019
12. Peter Ulvskov. Patenting in Biotechnology-A Laboratory Manual. Polyteknisk Boghandel og Forlag. 2019.
13. Prabuddha Ganguli. Gearing Up for Patents-The Indian Scenario. Universities Press. 1998
14. Uma J. Lele, William Lesser, Gesa Horstkotte-Wesseler. Intellectual Property Rights in Agriculture-The World Bank's Role in Assisting Borrower and Member Countries. World Bank. 2000

Scan QR code to view the website/guidelines

- Geographical Indication Act-
The Geographical Indications of Goods (Registration and Protection) Act, 1999 No.48 of 1999 (ipindia.gov.in)

CHAPTER 34

New Drug Application: NDA, INDA, ANDA, BLA, OTC

Introduction

There are two broad application categories for drugs and biologics regulated by Food and Drug Administration (FDA):

- Requests for authorization for clinical investigations
- Requests for marketing approval

The Investigational New Drug (IND) application falls into the first category, while the New Drug Application (NDA), Abbreviated New Drug Application (ANDA), and Biologics License Application (BLA) fall into the second category. Over-the-Counter (OTC) drugs are regulated slightly differently, either by conformance with an established OTC drug monograph or via the NDA process.

FDA Botanical Drug Development Guidance describes appropriate development plans for botanical drugs to be submitted in new drug applications (NDAs) and specific recommendations on submitting investigational new drug applications (INDs). The term botanical means products that include plant materials, algae, macroscopic fungi, and combinations thereof. FDA guidance recommends that IND must contain sufficient information to demonstrate that the drug is safe for testing in humans and that the clinical protocol is properly designed for its intended objectives. In addition to general regulatory requirements for an NDA - nonclinical pharmacology/toxicology studies, clinical evidence of efficacy and safety - for botanical drugs there are special requirements to ensure safety and quality of botanicals.

In India, ASU drugs have been under the purview of Department of AYUSH. In contrast, 2015 regulatory requirements for phytopharmaceuticals are under the purview of the Central Drugs Standards Control Organization (CDSCO). This gazette notification defines regulatory provisions for phytopharmaceuticals and regulatory submission requirements for scientific data on quality, safety, and efficacy to evaluate and permit marketing for an herbal drug on similar lines to synthetic, chemical moieties. The new phytopharmaceuticals regulation permits the development of the drug development using advanced techniques of solvent extraction, fractionation, potentiating steps, modern formulation development, etc. After NDA approval from CDSCO, the marketing status of the new phytopharmaceutical drug would be like that of a new chemical entity-based drug. The new regulation for phytopharmaceutical is in line with regulations in USA, China, and other countries involving scientific evaluation and data generation. The detail drug development process is explained in flowchart figure 34.1.

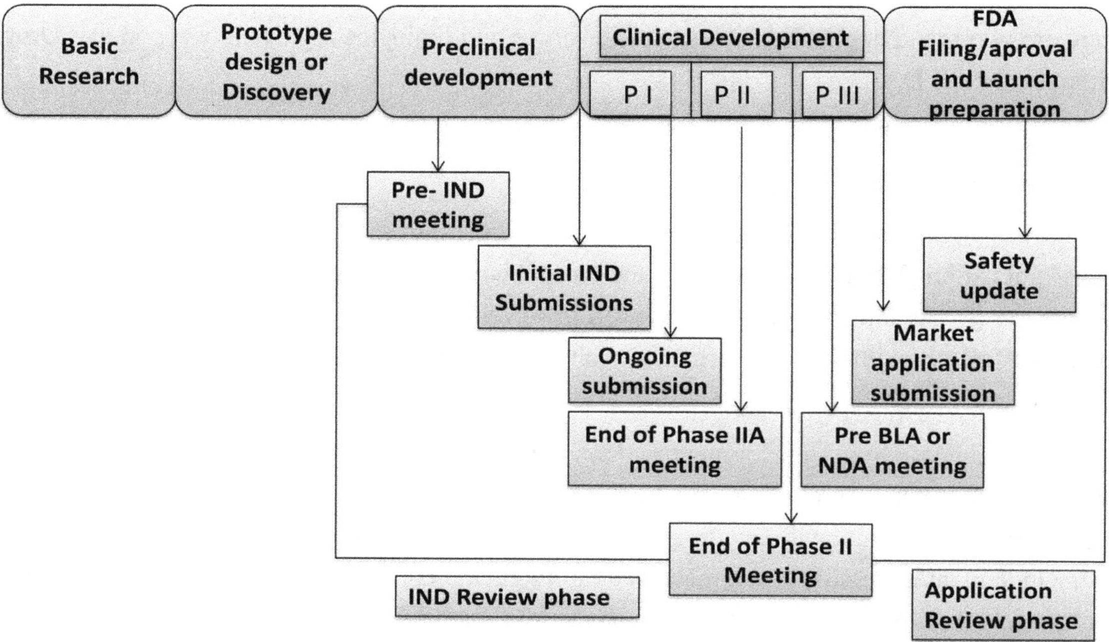

Figure 34.1 Drug Development process.

Investigational New Drug (IND)

There are two IND categories:

***Commercial INDs*•** These are applications that are submitted primarily by the companies to obtain marketing approval for a new product.

Noncommercial (Research)INDs • These INDs are filed for noncommercial research.

1. Investigator's IND- It is submitted by a physician who both initiates and conducts an investigation and who also administers and dispenses the IP. A physician might submit a research IND to propose studying an unapproved drug or an approved drug for new indications or in new patient population.
2. Emergency Use IND-This IND allows the use of an experimental drug in an emergency situation that does not allow submission of an IND in accordance with 21 CFR Sec312.23 or Sec 312.34. It can also be used for patients who do not meet the criteria of an existing study protocol or if an approved study protocol does not exist.
3. Treatment IND or Expanded Access IND- This IND may be submitted for experimental drugs showing promise in clinical testing of serious and immediately life threatening conditions while the final clinical work is conducted and the FDA review takes place (21 CFR 312.34).

The IND application must contain information in three broad areas:

- Animal Pharmacology and Toxicology Studies
- Manufacturing Information
- Clinical Protocols and Investigator Information

Once the IND is submitted, the sponsor must wait 30 calendar days before initiating any clinical trials. During this time, FDA has an opportunity to review the IND for safety to assure that research subjects will not be subjected to unreasonable risk. The detail IND Application review process is explained in flowchart figure 34.2.

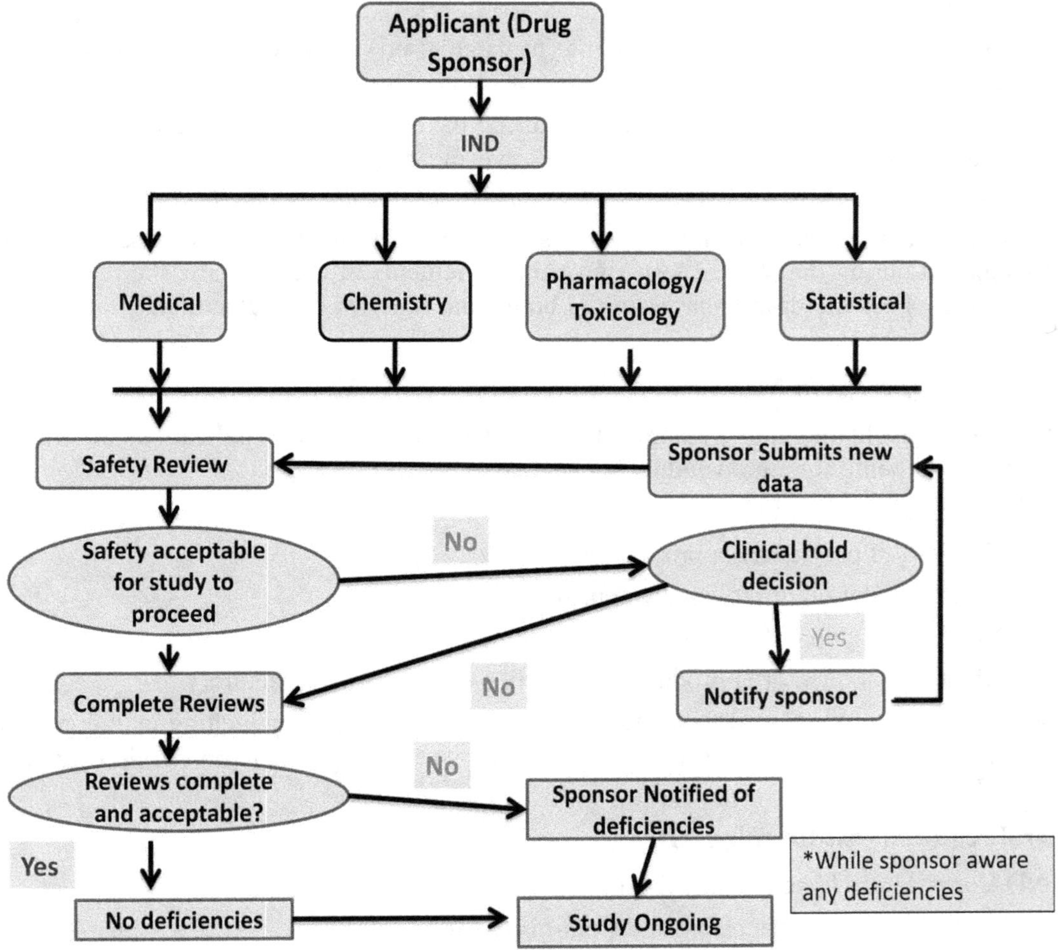

Figure 34.2 IND Application Review Process.

New Drug Application (NDA)

When the sponsor of a new drug believes that enough evidence on the drug's safety and effectiveness has been obtained to meet FDA's requirements for marketing approval, the sponsor submits to FDA a new drug application (NDA). The application must contain data from specific technical viewpoints for review, including chemistry, pharmacology, medical, biopharmaceutics, and statistics. If the NDA is approved, the product may be marketed in the United States. For internal tracking purposes, all NDA's are assigned an NDA number.

The goals of the NDA are to provide enough information to permit FDA reviewer to reach the following key decisions:

- Whether the drug is safe and effective in its proposed use(s), and whether the benefits of the drug outweigh the risks.
- Whether the drug's proposed labeling (package insert) is appropriate, and what it should contain.
- Whether the methods used in manufacturing the drug and the controls used to maintain the drug's quality are adequate to preserve the drug's identity, strength, quality, and purity.

The documentation required in an NDA is supposed to tell the drug's whole story, including what happened during the clinical tests, what the ingredients of the drug are, the results of the animal studies, how the drug behaves in the body, and how it is manufactured, processed and packaged.

Classification of drugs in NDA

Center of drug evaluation and Research (CDER) classifies new drug applications according to the type of drug being submitted and its intended use:

- New molecular entity
- New salt of previously approved drug
- New formulation of previously approved drug
- New combination of two or more drugs
- Already marketed drug product- Duplication (i.e., new manufacturer)
- New indication (claim) for already marketed drug (includes switching marketing status from prescription to OTC) g. Already marketed drug product (no previous approved NDA)

General requirements for filing NDA

The NDA application to be submitted following section wise information

(i) Chemistry, Manufacturing and Controls (CMC)

(ii) Nonclinical Pharmacology and Toxicology

(iii) Human Pharmacokinetics and Bioavailability

(iv) Microbiology (if required)
(v) Clinical data
(vi) Statistical data

The detail NDA Application review process is explained in flowchart figure 34.3.

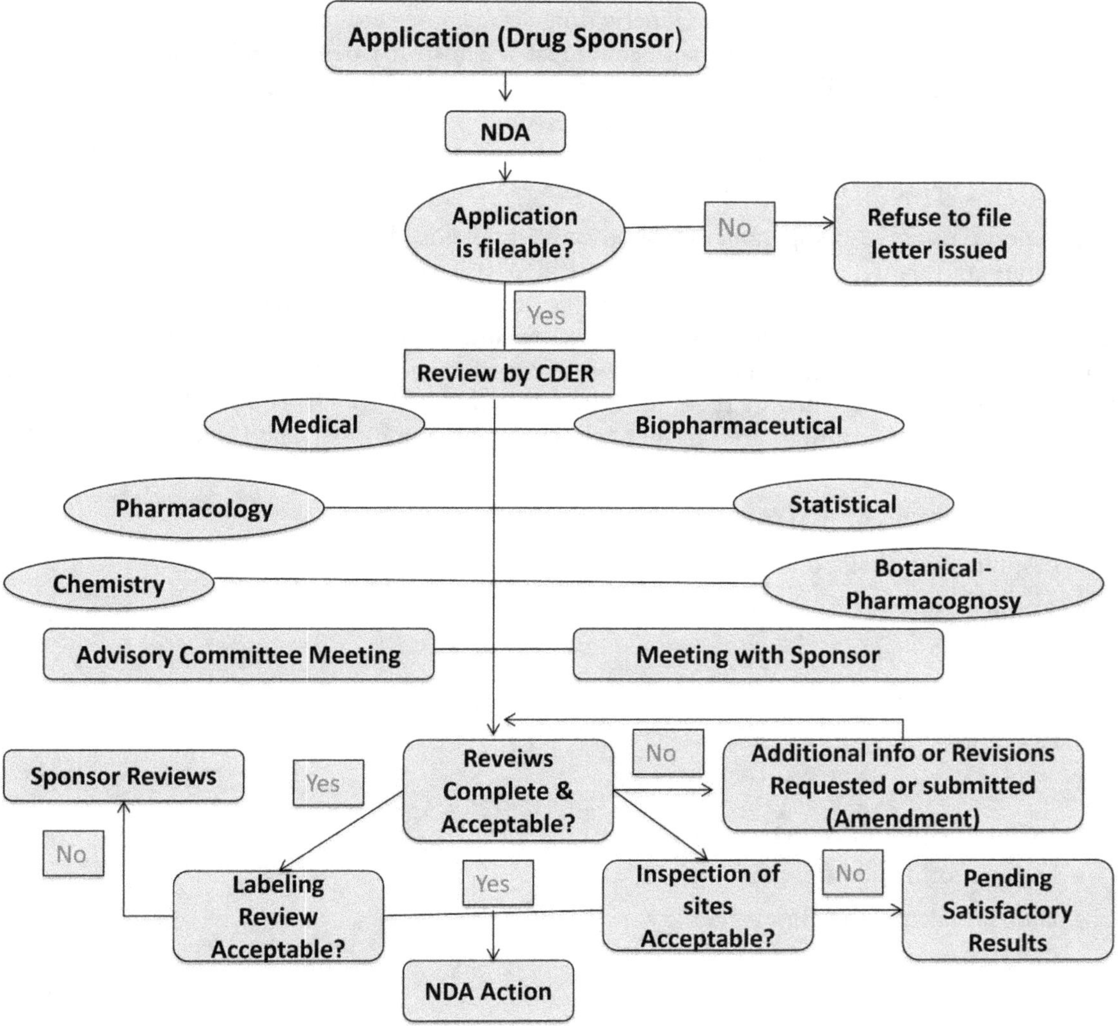

Figure 34.3 NDA Application Review Process.

Abbreviated New Drug Application (ANDA)

An Abbreviated New Drug Application (ANDA) contains data that, when submitted to FDA's Center for Drug Evaluation and Research, Office of Generic Drugs, provides for the review and ultimate approval of a generic drug product. Generic drug applications are called "abbreviated" because they are generally not required to include preclinical (animal) and clinical (human) data to establish safety and effectiveness. Generic drug applications are referred to Abbreviated New Drug Application. Instead, a generic applicant must scientifically demonstrate that its product is bioequivalent means performs in the same manner as the innovator drug. Once approved, an applicant may manufacture and market the generic drug product to provide a safe, effective, low cost alternative to the American public. Pharmaceutical companies must admit ANDAs and receive FDA's approval before marketing new generic drugs.

A generic drug is comparable to Innovator drug for dosage form, strength, route of administration, quality, performance and intended use. One of the ways to demonstrate bioequivalence is to measure the time taken by generic drug to reach bloodstream in 24-36 healthy volunteers. The time and amount of active ingredients in the bloodstream should be comparable to those of Innovator drug. Use of bioequivalence as base for approving generic drug products was established in 1984, also known as WAXMAN-HATCH ACT. It is because of this act that generic drugs are cheaper without conducting costly and duplicative clinical trials.

Format and Content of ANDA

ANDA Application shall contain the following:

- Application form
- Table of Contents
- Basis for ANDA submission
- Conditions of use
- Active Ingredients
- Route of Administration
- Dosage form and Strength
- Bioequivalence and Bioavailability
- Labeling
- Chemistry, Manufacturing and Controls
- Samples
- Patent Certification
- Financial Certification or disclosure statement.
- Other Information.

The detail ANDA Application review process is explained in flowchart figure 34.4.

Difference between submission of NDA and ANDA

ANDA requires submission of :	NDA requires submission of:
1. Detailed description of components. 2. Details of Manufacturing, Packaging and Labelling 3. Bioequivalence, bioavailability data	1. Preclinical and clinical safety and efficacy data 2. Details of Manufacturing and Packaging. 3. Proposed annotated Labelling

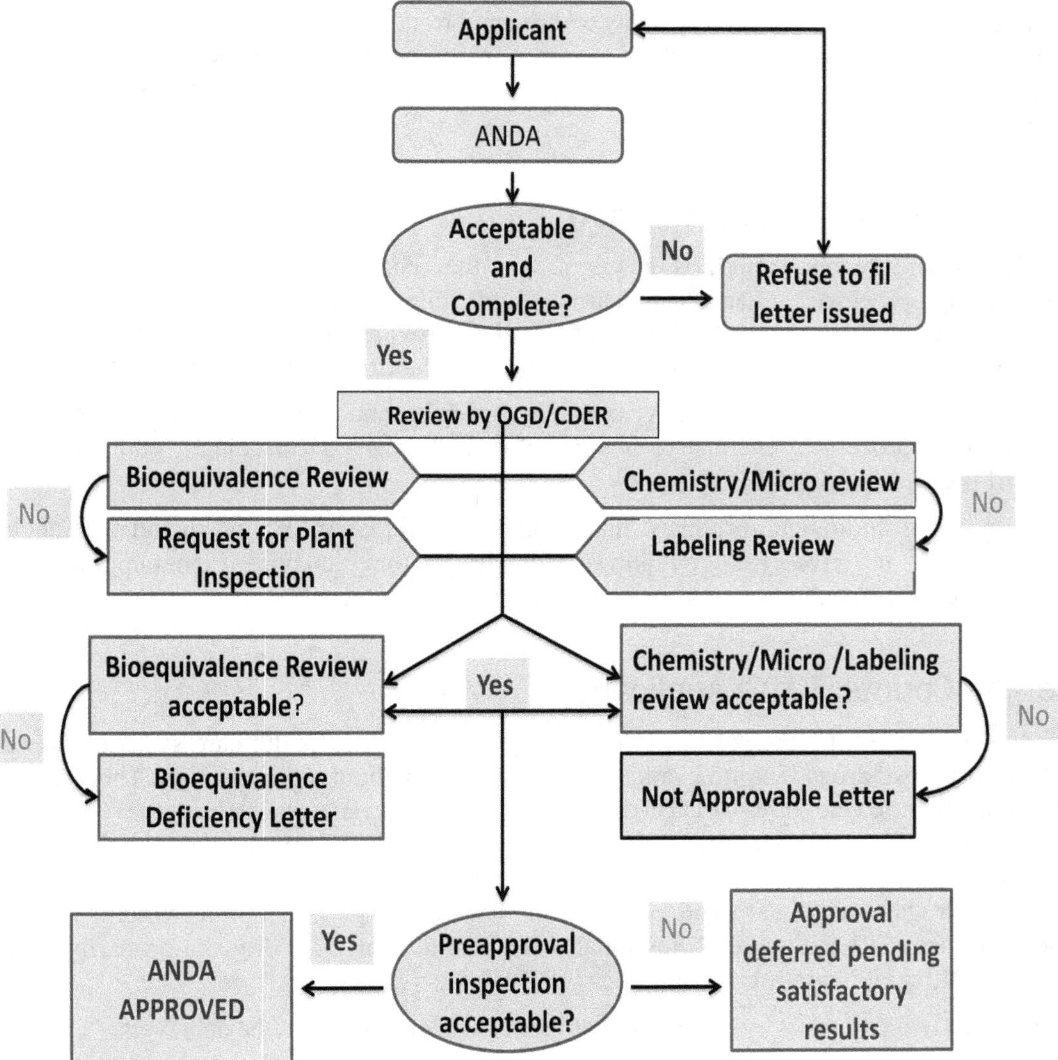

Figure 34.4 ANDA Application Review Process.

Before ***Hatch Waxman Amendment***, generic manufacturer could file ANDA only after innovator's patent expiry or cancellation. But under Sec 505(j)(5)(B) of Hatch Waxman amendment it permits preparation and filing of ANDA before patent expiration, so that the effective approval date of generic drug would be on expiration date of the patent of Innovator Original drug. The Act also establishes another procedure in which the generic company can challenge patent of the Innovator. For generic companies, the amendment provides an inventive 180-day exclusivity period in which no other ANDA for that drug can be approved. This 180-day period is to encourage generic companies to challenge validity of Orange book listed patents or to design around these patents to bring more quickly a generic drug to market. For Innovator Company, filing of an ANDA is an act of patent infringement. So, if Innovator Company brings suit within 45 days, the approval of generic company's ANDA is delayed for upto 30 months.

Biologic License Application (BLA)

A biologics license application is a submission that contains specific information on the manufacturing processes, chemistry, pharmacology, clinical pharmacology and the medical affects of the biologic product. If the information provided meets FDA requirements, the application is approved and a license is issued allowing the firm to market the product.

Similar to an NDA, the BLA contains specific and detailed information on the manufacturing processes, chemistry, pharmacology, clinical pharmacology, and the medical effects of the biological product.

Examples of biological products that would be subject to BLAs include monoclonal antibodies for in vivo use, cytokines, growth factors, enzymes, immunomodulators, thrombolytics, therapeutic proteins, and non-vaccine immunotherapies.

Over-the-Counter (OTC) Application

Over-the-counter (OTC) drugs play an increasingly vital role in health care system. OTC drug products are those drugs that are available to consumers without a prescription. There are more than 80 therapeutic categories of OTC drugs, ranging from acne drug products to weight control drug products. As with prescription drugs, FDA oversees OTC drugs to ensure that they are properly labeled and that their benefits outweigh their risks. Over-the-counter (OTC) drugs are defined as drugs that are safe and effective for use by the general public without needing a prescription from a health care professional. FDA's review of OTC drugs is primarily handled by FDA's Office of Nonprescription Drugs (ONPD).

There are two pathways by which marketing of OTC products may be achieved:

- Compliance with an OTC drug monograph
- Approval under an NDA or ANDA

An OTC monograph is a set of regulatory standards for different therapeutic drug classes that includes acceptable ingredients, doses, formulations, and labeling requirements. If the standards of an applicable OTC monograph are met, marketing pre-clearance is not required by the FDA. If the OTC drug deviates from the final monograph, however, a formal marketing application (e.g., NDA) or citizen petition may be used to request approval.

In India, most traditional medicinal products are available as over the counter (OTC) drugs. It may be noted that, in the year 2008, the Government of India took an initiative in establishing the National Pharmacovigilance Programme for Ayurveda, Siddha and Unani drugs in a structured way. Eight regional centers, 30 peripheral centers and 55 centers in various Ayurveda colleges along with a National Resource Centre at Jamnagar were established in between 2008 and 2011. Many awareness programmes were conducted by the centre itself and also in collaboration with WHO country office, New Delhi where more than 2000 teachers and medical officers were oriented towards the concept of pharmacovigilance. The centre received more than 300 suspected reports of adverse drug reactions and out of them 200 were scrutinized and analyzed by the National Pharmacovigilance Technical Advisory Committee. However, due to lack of continued support, this initiative has not been able to further its activities.

In 2016, a public notice was issued by the Department of Ministry of AYUSH. This notice advised the public to purchase and consume Ayurveda, Unani & Siddha drugs only on the prescription of the institutionally qualified and registered practitioner of the respective system. The notice also warned the public to avoid purchasing these drugs online, over the counter (OTC) and to avoid their use without medical consultation.

Frequently Asked Questions (FAQS) on Approval of New Phytopharmaceutical Drugs by CDSCO, India

1. What is a phytopharmaceutical drug?	"Phytopharmaceutical drug" includes purified and standard fraction with defined minimum four bio-active or phytochemical compound (qualitatively and quantitatively assessed) of an extract of a medicinal plant or its part, for internal or external use of human beings or animals for diagnosis, treatment, mitigation or prevention of any disease or disorder but does not include administration by parenteral route as specified in Rule 2 (eb) of the Drugs & Cosmetics (D&C) Rules, 1945.
2. When a phytopharmaceutical drug is considered as new drug?	As defined in the Rule 122E of D&C Rules, a phytopharmaceutical drug which has not been used in the country to any significant extent under the conditions prescribed, recommended or suggested in the labeling thereof and has not been recognised as effective and safe by the licensing authority mentioned under Rule 21 of D&C Rules for the proposed claims is considered as a new drug.

Contd...

3. How does phyto-pharmaceutical drug differ from ayurvedic, siddha or unani (ASU) under Section 3 (a) & (h) of Drugs & Cosmetic Act 1940?	Ayurvedic, Siddha or Unani drugs include all medicines intended for internal or external use for or in the diagnosis, treatment, mitigation or prevention of (disease or disorder in human beings or animals, and manufactured) exclusively in accordance with the formulae described in, the authoritative books of ayurvedic, siddha and unani tibb systems of medicine specified in the first Schedule. However, phytopharmaceutical drugs are fraction of crude extract and are distinctly differentiated by being purified and standardized.
4. The definition demands "with defined minimum four bio-active / phytochemical compounds (qualitatively & quantitatively assessed)". Should four bio-active / phytochemical compounds need to be assessed qualitatively & quantitatively?	Minimum four compounds shall be identified as bio-active / phyto chemical compounds. It is ideally if all of them are bio active, hence the condition of identification of minimum four compounds from fraction is non-negotiable. The number of compounds with bio activity may be considered on case to case basis, based on the justification submitted by the applicant. However the applicant should specify the limits of the bio-active / phyto chemical compounds for maintaining batch to batch consistency.
5. Does a new phytopharmaceutical drug undergo clinical trial in India?	The data requirements have been specified in the Appendix IB of Schedule Y of D&C Rules. (i) Clinical trials for phytopharmaceutical drugs to be conducted as per applicable rules and guidelines for new drugs. (ii) For all phytopharmaceutical drugs data from phase I (to determine maximum tolerated dose and associated toxicities) and the protocols shall be submitted prior to performing the studies. (iii) Data of results of dose finding studies performed and the protocols shall be submitted prior to performing the studies. Provided that in the case of phytopharmaceutical drug already marketed for more than five years or where there is adequate published evidence regarding the safety of the phytopharmaceutical drug, the studies may be abbreviated, modified or relaxed.
6. How and where to apply for grant of permission to import or manufacture new phytopharmaceutical drug (as new drug) in the country for sale or to undertake clinical trial?	Applications for grant of permission to import or manufacture new phytopharmaceutical drug are to be made in Form 44 prescribed in D&C Rule to Drugs Controller General (India), Central Drugs Standard Control Organization, Directorate General of Health Services, Ministry of Health and Family Welfare, Government of India, FDA Bhawan, ITO, Kotla Road, New Delhi -110002. Applicant shall submit all the documents specified under Appendix IB of Schedule Y of D&C Rules. (Checklist for submission is available on CDSCO website). Applications as per checklist can be mailed by Post to Drugs Controller General (India).
7. New drug applications are currently required to be filed online to DCG(I) Office. Whether online submission of applications for phytopharmaceutical drugs is available?	Work on providing access and necessary data entry for filing phytopharmaceutical application online is ongoing and will be made possible in due course of time. In the meantime interested stakeholders may file hard copy applications along with suitable covering letter to CDSCO. Such applications would be received and acknowledged by CDSCO after pre- screening as per the checklist.

Contd...

8. What are the fees to be paid along with the application for grant of permission to import / manufacture of new phyto-pharmaceutical drug?	(i) Application for grant of permission to import new phytopharmaceutical drug (Form 44) - Rs 50,000/-. (ii) Application for grant of permission to manufacture new phytopharmaceutical drug (Form 44) - Rs 50,000/- .
9. What are the fees to be paid along with the application for grant of permission to conduct clinical trial for new phyto-pharmaceutical drug?	(i) Clinical trial Phase-I application (Form 44) - Rs 50,000/- (ii) Clinical trial Phase-II application (Form 44) - Rs 25,000/- (iii) Clinical trial Phase-III application (Form 44) - Rs 25,000/- However, as specified under Rule 122DA (2) (c), no fees shall be required to be paid along with the application by Central Government or State Government Institutes involved in clinical research for conducing trials for academic or research purpose (iv) Application for import of new phytopharmaceutical drug for purpose of examination, test or analysis (Form 12) - Rs 100/- for single drug and additional fee of Rs 50/- for each additional drug.
10. Where and how to deposit the specified fees for the application?	The fees shall be paid through a Challan in the Bank of Baroda, Kasturba Gandhi Marg, New Delhi-110001 or any other branch or branches of Bank of Baroda, or any other bank, as notified, from time to time by the Central Government, to be credited under the Head of Account "0210-Medical and Public Health, 04-Public Health, 104-Fees and Fines". Following are the additional banks notified by the Govt. where fees can be deposited. 1. Bank of Baroda, Law Garden Branch, Bank of Baroda Towers, Ellis Bridge, Ahmedabad-380006. 2. Bank of Baroda, Plot No 8/3/2014/17, Annapurna Nilayam, B.K. Guda, S.R Nagar, Hyderabad Nagar 500038. 3. Bank of Baroda, Raj Nagar Branch, Raj Nagar, Ghaziabad-201002, Uttar Pradesh. 4. Bank of Baroda Tardeo Branch, Everest Building, D.J Dadaji Road, Tardeo, Mumbai 400034. 5. Bank of Baroda, India Exchange Branch, 4, India Exchange Place, Kolkata700001. 6. Bank of Baroda, Chennai Main Branch, 70, Rajaji Salai, Chennai-600001. 7. Bank of Baroda. SCO-212, Sector-40-D, Chandigarh-160036. 8. Bank of Baroda, Gandhinagar Branch, Fole Market, Gandhinagar, Jammu, Jammu Tawi. 9. Bank of Baroda, Vasco-Da-Gama Branch, P.O.-144, Swatantra Path, VascoDa-Gama, Goa-403802. 10. Bank of Baroda, Malleswaram Branch, 74, Seventh Cross, Malleswaram, Bangalore.

Contd...

11. What are the conventional preclinical study & safety document required to be submitted alongwith application for phytopharmaceutical drug?	Based on disease, nature of phytopharmaceutical drug and duration of treatment the applicant may submit as much as available documents to establish safety and efficacy of the phytopharmaceutical drug as specified under Appendix IB of Schedule Y of D&C Rules.
12. Whether parenteral formulation of phytopharmaceutical drugs can be considered for market authorization in India?	No. As per the definition specified under Rule 2 (eb) of the D & C Rules the parenteral dosage form of phytopharmaceutical drugs cannot be considered for market authorization.
13. Can phytopharmaceutical drug be sold as without prescription or is it prescription drug?	CDSCO would specify this aspect, whether any phytopharmaceutical drug for which marketing authorization is issued need to be sold only against prescription of a R.M.P. / specialist / or it can be sold without prescription.
14. What are the current GMP requirements to manufacture phytopharmaceutical drugs?	GMP requirements for manufacture of drugs are prescribed in the Schedule M of the D & C Rules. However, presently, there is no specific GMP guidelines finalised for Phytopharmaceutical drugs. The GMP requirements would depend on the ingredients and the stage of processing. It may be recognized that a common GMP requirements across the chain - raw herb (cultivation / collection / drying / minimal processing / storage and transport): processing of botanical (grinding / extraction / fractionation steps / other unit operations like spry drying, tray drying etc / packing and storage in bulk): formulation (compatibility with excipients / dosage form selected for product formulation / various steps involved in the production etc) should be implemented. It is expected that this area will be further developed in the future and currently applicants would need to adopt such procedures and documentation that would prevent contamination, degradation and protect the quality and integrity of the final phytopharmaceutical product.
15. What shall be the Pharmacopoeial standard of Phytopharmaceuticals?	Currently no phytopharmaceutical drug has been approved by the CDSCO as a new drug meeting the definition of phytopharmaceutical drug. As and when CDSCO will approve a phytopharmaceutical drug the aspect of including a monograph in IP would be considered keeping in mind various other factors.
16. What shall be the quality standard of raw material used for Phytopharmaceuticals, IP or USP etc.?	The applicant will need to provide adequate information including specifications and test methods for raw botanical, processed botanical forming the phytopharmaceutical and the formulation of the phytopharmaceutical as prescribed in Appendix IB of Schedule Y of the D&C Rules. The applicant should adopt monograph for any of these parameters as per the general standards prescribed in IP. If not prescribed in IP but included in the official Pharmacopoeia of any other country, same may be followed.

Contd...

17. Samples of new drugs normally go through a step of checking the specification and test method for the new drug in one of the central drugtesting laboratories. Would a similar step is involved for a phytopharmaceutical drug for quality?	Yes. In fact the applicant is required to send adequate quantity of phytopharmaceutical, phytopharmaceutical formulation / product along with adequate quantities of all the identified bio-active / phyto chemical compounds to the laboratories when demanded by the CDSCO for testing.

Further Reading

1. Ali A, Ali J, Sahni JK, Qureshi J. United States of America. In: International Licensing. New Delhi: Hamdard University, Excel Books Pvt Ltd 2007; pp. 51-110.
2. Anjan K. Mahapatra, N.H. Sameeraja and P.N. Murthy, "Drug Approval Process – In United States of America, European Union and India: A Review", Applied Clinical Research, Clinical Trials and Regulatory Affairs (2014) 1: 13. https://doi.org/10.2174/2213476X01666140123234357
3. Baboota S, Ahuja A, Ali A, Sultana Y, Aqil M. Study of Major Acts Enforced by the Indian FDA. In: Drug Regulatory Affairs in India. New Delhi: Jamia Hamdard University, Excel Books Pvt Ltd 2005; pp. 65-75.
4. Bhatt A. Phytopharmaceuticals: A new drug class regulated in India. Perspect Clin Res. 2016;7(2):59-61. doi:10.4103/2229-3485.179435
5. Bolar H, Bhatt A. India. In: Chambers AA, International Pharmaceutical Registration. Florida: CRC Press LLC 2000; pp. 193-203.
6. Chandra S. Ayurvedic research, wellness and consumer rights. Journal of Ayurveda and Integrative Medicine. 2016 Mar;7(1):6-10. DOI: 10.1016/j.jaim.2016.05.002.
7. Charles JM, Jayaraman C, Joseph WO, Jack DH, Benjamin BW. Strategies and tactics for optimizing the Hit-to-Lead process and beyond – A computational chemistry perspective. Drug Discov Today 2008; 13(3-4): 99-109.
8. Dec. 2020]
9. Food and Drug Administration Botanical Drug Development Guidance for Industry. 2015. Aug, [Accessed on Dec. 2020]
10. Food and Drug Administration. Investigational New Drug Application. Available from: http://www.fda.gov/drugs/developmentapprovalprocess/howdrugsaredevelopedandapproved/approvalapplications/investigationalnewdrugindapplication/ [Accessed on
11. Guidance for Industry – Requirements for permission of new drug approval; CDSCO, Document No. MA/71108; Version 1.1; Ministry of Health; Government of India. Available from: http://cdsco.nic.in/CDSCO-GuidanceForIndustry.pdf.
12. Guidance for Industry on submission of clinical trial application for evaluating safety and efficacy; Document No. CT/71108; Version 1.1; CDSCO, Ministry of Health; Government of India. Available from: http://cdsco.nic.in/CDSCO-GuidanceForIndustry.pdf. Accessed on Dec. 2020.

13. Handoo S, Arora V, Khera D, Nandi PK, Sahu SK. A comprehensive study on regulatory requirements for development and filing of generic drugs globally. International Journal of Pharmaceutical Investigation. 2012 Jul;2(3):99-105.
14. https://cdsco.gov.in/opencms/opencms/en/Home/Accessed on April 2021-05-05
15. https://cdsco.gov.in/opencms/opencms/system/modules/CDSCO.WEB/elements/download_file_division.jsp?num_id=MzI0MA==Accessed on April 2021-05-05
16. https://www.fda.gov/drugs/how-drugs-are-developed-and-approved/types-applicationsAccessed on April 2021-05-05
17. IRA RB, Robert PM. The Pharmaceutical Regulatory Process. 2nd ed. Informa healthcare. 2008.
18. Kishor Patwardhan, Jigyasa Pathak, Rabinarayan Acharya. Ayurveda formulations: A roadmap to address the safety concerns. Journal of Ayurveda and Integrative Medicine. 2017; 8(4):279-282.
19. Mulaje SS, Birajdar S, Patil BR, Bhusnure OG. Procedure for drug approval in different countries: a review. J Drug Deliv Ther 2013; 3(2): 233-8.
20. Peck GE, Poust R. Food and Drug Laws that affect Drug Product Design, Manufacture and Distribution. In: Gilbert SB, Christopher
21. Pisano DJ, David M. Overview of Drug Development and the FDA. In: Pisano DJ, FDA Regulatory Affairs: A Guide for Prescription Drugs, Medical Devices, and Biologics. Florida: CRC Press LLC 2004; pp. 2-20.
22. Pritchard JF, Jurima RM, Reimer ML, Mortimer E, Rolfe B, Cayen MN. Making better drugs: decision gates in non-clinical drug development. Nat Rev Drug Discov 2003; 2: 542-53.
23. Rick NG. Drugs from discovery to approval. 2nd ed. John Wiley & Sons, Inc.; 2008.
24. Sahoo N, Manchikanti P. Herbal drug regulation and commercialization: an Indian industry perspective. J Altern Complement Med. 2013;19(12):957-963. doi:10.1089/acm.2012.0275
25. Schedule Y. Amendment Version 2005, Drugs and Cosmetics Rules, 1945; pp. 503-47.
26. Sharma S. Current status of herbal product: Regulatory overview. J Pharm Bioallied Sci. 2015;7(4):293-296. doi:10.4103/0975-7406.168030
27. The Drugs and Cosmetics Act and Rules; Ministry of Health and Family Welfare; Government of India; corrected upto 30 April 2003; pp.1.
28. TR, Modern Pharmaceutics. 4th ed, New York: Marcel Dekker Inc 2002; pp. 930-46.
29. Troetel WM. Investigational New Drug Application and the Investigator's Brochure. In: Richard AG, New Drug Approval Process: Accelerating Global Registrations; 4th ed. New York: Marcel Dekker Inc 2004; pp. 54-86.
30. William RP, Raymond DM. Drug Regulatory Affairs. In: Lachman L, Lieberman HA, The theory and practice of Industrial Pharmacy. India: CBS Publishers and Distributors 2009; pp. 856-882.

Scan QR code to view the website/guidelines

- Types of Drug applications-
Types of Applications | FDA

CHAPTER 35

Master Formula SMF-Site Master File, DMF-Drug Master File, Dossier and CTD, Chemistry Manufacturing and Controls (CMC) Dossier

Master Formula (MF)

A document or set of documents specifying the starting materials with their quantities and the packaging materials, together with a description of the procedures and precautions required to produce a specified quantity of a finished product as well as the processing instructions, including the in-process controls. WHO identifies manufacturing instructions as "Master Formula. Other terms used in GMP guidelines and regulations are "Manufacturing Formula", "Master Production and Control Record", but all mean the same thing – an approved master document that describes the full process of manufacturing for the batch of product with at least cross reference to the support operations for a batch of a specific product. Individual companies may give internal names to these documents (manufacturing instructions, monographs, etc). In this guidance document the WHO term Master Formula (or MF) will be used.

A formally authorized master formula should exist for each product and batch size to be manufactured. The master formula should include:

- the name of the product, with a product reference code relating to its specification;
- a description of the dosage form, strength of the product and batch size;
- a list of all starting materials to be used (if applicable, with the INNs), with the amount of each, described using the designated name and a reference that is unique to that material (mention should be made of any substance that may disappear in the course of processing);
- a statement of the expected final yield with the acceptable limits, and of relevant intermediate yields, where applicable;
- a statement of the processing location and the principal equipment to be used;
- the methods, or reference to the methods, to be used for preparing and operating the critical equipment, e.g. cleaning (especially after a change in product), assembling, calibrating, sterilizing, use;
- detailed step-wise processing instructions (e.g. checks on materials, pretreatments, sequence for adding materials, mixing times, temperatures);
- the instructions for any in-process controls with their limits;
- where necessary, the requirements for storage of the products, including the container, the labelling, and any special storage conditions;
- any special precautions to be observed.

MF and Corresponding Batch Records

Master Formula give the complete production instructions for a specific batch and batch size of cell banks, virus seed lots, intermediates, final bulks, final formulated bulks or final container product that are made in one production run with definite start to finish steps. Blank spaces are provided for the entry of data as the production run progresses. Identification or cross-reference to required supporting data is included in the step-bystep instructions.

Formats for MF

The generally recommended MF format is to prepare a single continuous document that provides step-by-step production instructions, raw materials, equipment used, locations of production, dates, operators, etc for the product, with blank spaces to record the data and sign and date all entries, and at least cross-references to all supporting SOPs and operations. Many other formats are possible for a MF and will depend on the production process and supporting activities, as well as on the documentation system in place at the manufacturing company. Master formulae, once approved and signed, should remain under the control of QA.

Site Master File (SMF)

What is a site master file?

A Site Master File (SMF) is a document prepared by the manufacturer containing specific and factual Good Manufacturing Practice (GMP) information about the production and/or control of pharmaceutical manufacturing operations carried out at the named site. If only part of a manufacturing operation is carried out on the site, a SMF need only describe those activities, Example: analysis, packaging etc.

How Should A Site Master File Be Submitted?

A Site Master File should be concisely written in English and, as far as possible, not exceed 25-30 A4 sheets. The Site Master File should have an edition number and an effective date, and preferably be submitted on loose individually numbered A4 sheets. The sheets should be ring-bound to ensure the integrity of the document. Wherever possible, simple plans, outline drawings or schematic layouts should be used instead of narrative. These plans etc., should fit on A4 sheets of paper. The format and heading of the site master file should be set out as follows:-

Chapter 1 General Information Requirement

- Brief information on the site (including name and address), relation to other sites and, particularly, any information relevant to understand the manufacturing operations. Any other manufacturing activities carried out on the site.
- Name and exact address of the site, including telephone, fax and 24-hour telephone numbers. Type of actual products manufactured on the site and information about specifically toxic or hazardous substances handled, mentioning the way they are manufactured (in dedicated facilities or on a campaign basis).
- Number of employees engaged in quality assurance, production, quality control, storage and distribution. Use of outside scientific, analytical or other technical assistance in relation to manufacture and analysis. Short description of the quality management system of the company responsible for manufacture.

Chapter 2 Personnel

- Organization chart showing the arrangements for quality assurance, including production and quality control.
- Qualifications, experience and responsibilities of key personnel.
- Outline of arrangements for basic and in-service training and how records are maintained.
- Health requirements for personnel engaged in production.
- Personnel hygiene requirements, including clothing.

Chapter 3 Premises and Equipment

Premises

- Simple layout plan and description of manufacturing areas with indication of scale (architectural or engineering drawings not required).
- Nature of construction and finishes.
- Brief description of ventilation systems. More details should be given for critical areas with potential risks of airborne contamination (including schematic drawings of the systems). Classification of the rooms used for the manufacture of sterile products should be mentioned.
- Special areas for the handling of highly toxic, hazardous and sensitizing materials.
- Brief description of water systems (schematic drawings of the systems are desirable) including sanitation.
- Maintenance (description of planned preventive maintenance programmes and recording system).

Equipment

- Brief description of major production and quality control laboratories equipment (a list of the equipment is NOT required).
- Maintenance (description of planned preventive maintenance programmes and recording system).
- Qualification and calibration, including the recording system. Arrangements for computerized systems validation.

Sanitation

- Availability of written specifications and procedures for cleaning manufacturing areas and equipment.

Chapter 4 Documentation

- Arrangements for the preparation, revision and distribution of necessary documentation for manufacture, including storage of master documents.

- Any other documents related to product quality which is not mentioned elsewhere (e.g. microbiological controls on air and water).

Chapter 5 Production

- Brief description of production operations using, wherever possible, flow sheets and charts specifying important parameters (see at Appendix the list of products manufactured)
- Arrangements for the handling of starting materials, packaging materials, bulk and finished products, including sampling, quarantine, release and storage.
- Arrangements for reprocessing or rework.
- Arrangements for the handling of rejected materials and products.
- Brief description of general policy for process validation.

Chapter 6 Quality Control

- Description of the Quality Control system and of the activities of the Quality Control Department. Procedures for the release of finished products.

Chapter 7 Contract Manufacture and Analysis

- Description of the way in which the GMP compliance of the contract acceptor is assessed.

Chapter 8 Distribution, Complaints and Product Recalls

- Arrangements and recording system for distribution.
- Arrangements for the handling of complaints and product recalls.

Chapter 9 Self Inspection

- Short description of the self-inspection system

Appendix

Type of Products Manufactured

A. Sterile products

A.1 Liquid dosage forms (large volume solutions, including LVP and rinsing solutions)

A.1.1 Aseptically prepared

A.1.2 Terminally sterilized

A.2 Liquid dosage forms (small volume solutions, including SVP and eye drops)

A.2.1 Aseptically prepared

A.2.2 Terminally sterilized

A.3 Semi-solid dosage forms

A.4 Solid dosage forms

A.4.1 Solid fill

A.4.2 Freeze-dried

B. Non-sterile products

B.1 Liquid dosage forms

B.2 Semi-solid dosage forms

B.3 Solid dosage forms

B.3.1 Unit dose form (eg tablets, capsules, suppositories, pessaries)

B.3.2 Multi dose form (eg powders, granules)

C. Biological products

C.1 Vaccines

C.2 Sera

C.3 Blood products

C.4 Others (describe)

D. Specifically toxic and hazardous substances

D.1 Penicillins

D.2 Cephalosporins

D.3 Hormones

D.4 Cytostatics

D.5 Others (describe)

E. Packaging only

E.1 Liquid dosage forms

E.2 Semi-solid dosage forms

E.3 Solid dosage forms

F. Contract manufacturing (kind of products)

Company reported upon is:

F.1 Acceptor

F.2 Giver

G. Drugs for clinical trials

H. Others

Including products not subjected to registration/licensing by the Competent Authorities (e.g. veterinary products, cosmetics, health/dietary supplements, etc)

Drug Master File (DMF)

I. Introduction

A Drug master File (DMF) is a submission to the Food and Drug Administration (FDA) that may be used to provide confidential detailed information about facilities, processes, or articles used in the manufacturing, processing, packaging, and storing of one or more human drugs. The submission of a DMF is not required by law or FDA regulation. A DMF is submitted solely at the discretion of the holder. The information contained in the DMF may be used to support an Investigational New Drug Application (IND), a New Drug Application (NDA), an Abbreviated New Drug Application (ANDA), another DMF, an Export Application, or amendments and supplements to any of these.

A DMF is not a substitute for an IND, NDA, ANDA, or Export Application. It is not approved or disapproved. Technical contents of a DMF are reviewed only in connection with the review of an IND, NDA, ANDA, or an Export Application

This guideline does not impose mandatory requirements (21 CFR 10.90(b)). It does, however, offer guidance on acceptable approaches to meeting regulatory requirements. Different approaches may be followed, but the applicant is encouraged to discuss significant variations in advance with FDA reviewers to preclude spending time and effort in preparing a submission that FDA may later determine to be unacceptable.

Master Files are provided for in 21 CFR 314.420. This guideline is intended to provide DMF holders with procedures acceptable to the agency for preparing and submitting a DMF. The guideline discusses types of DMF's, the information needed in each type, the format of submissions to a DMF,, the administrative procedures governing review of DMF's, and the obligations of the DMF holder.

DMF's are generally created to allow a party other than the holder of the DMF to reference material without disclosing to those party contents of the file. When an applicant references its own material, the applicant should reference the information contained in its own IND, NDA, or ANDA directly rather than establishing a new DMF.

II. Definitions

For the purposes of this, guideline, the following definitions apply:

- Agency means the Food and Drug Administration.
- Agent or representative means any person who is appointed by a DMF holder to serve as the contact for the holder.
- Applicant means any person who submits an application or abbreviated application or an amendment or supplement to them to obtain FDA approval of a new drug or an antibiotic drug and any other person who owns an approved application (21 CFR 314.3 (b)).

- Drug product means a finished dosage form, for example, tablet, capsule, or solution, that contains a drug substance, generally, but not necessarily, in association with one or more other ingredients (21 CFR 314.3 (b)).
- Drug substance means an active ingredient that is intended to furnish pharmacological activity or other direct effect in the diagnosis, cure, mitigation, treatment, or prevention of disease or to affect the structure or any function of the human body, but does not include intermediates used in the synthesis of such ingredient (21 CFR 314.3 (b)).
- Export application means an application submitted under section 802 of the Federal Food, Drug, and Cosmetic Act to export a drug that is not approved for marketing in the United States.
- Holder means a person who owns a DMF.
- Letter of authorization means a written statement by the holder or designated agent or representative permitting FDA to refer to information in the DMF in support of another person's submission.
- Person includes individual, partnership, corporation, and association. (Section 201(e) of the Federal Food, Drug, and Cosmetic Act.)
- Sponsor means a person who takes responsibility for and initiates a clinical investigation. The sponsor may be an individual or pharmaceutical company, governmental agency, academic institution, private organization, or other organization (21 CFR 312.3 (b)).

Types of Drug Master Files

There are five types of DMF's:

- Type I Manufacturing Site, Facilities, Operating Procedures, and Personnel
- Type II Drug Substance, Drug Substance Intermediate, and Material Used in Their Preparation, or Drug Product
- Type III Packaging Material
- Type IV Excipient, Colorant, Flavor, Essence, or Material Used in Their Preparation
- Type V FDA-Accepted Reference Information

Each DMF should contain only one type of information and all supporting data.

Submissions to Drug Master Files

Each DMF submission should contain a transmittal letter, administrative information about the submission, and the specific information to be included in the DMF as described in this section. The DMF must be in the English language. Whenever a submission contains information in another language, an accurate certified English translation must also be included. Each page of each copy of the DMF should be dated and consecutively numbered. An updated table of contents should be included with each submission.

Drug Master File Contents

Type I: Manufacturing Site, Facilities, Operating Procedures, and Personnel	A Type I DMF is recommended for a person outside of the United States to assist FDA in conducting onsite inspections of their manufacturing facilities. The DMF should describe the manufacturing site, equipment capabilities, and operational layout. A Type I DMF is normally not needed to describe domestic facilities, except in special cases, such as when a person is not registered and not routinely inspected. The description of the site should include acreage, actual site address, and a map showing its location with respect to the nearest city. An aerial photograph and a diagram of the site may be helpful. A diagram of major production and processing areas in helpful for understanding the operational layout. Major equipment should be described in terms of capabilities, application, and location. Make and model would not normally be needed unless equipment is new or unique. A diagram of major corporate organizational elements, with key manufacturing, quality control, and quality assurance positions highlighted, at both the manufacturing site and corporate headquarters, is also helpful.
Type II Drug Substance. Drug Substance Intermediate, and Material Used in Their Preparation Or Drug Product	A Type II DMF should, in general, be limited to a single drug intermediate, drug substance, drug product, or type of material used in their preparation. Detailed guidance on what should be included in a Type II DMF for drug substances and intermediates may be found in the following guidelines: ➢ Guideline for Submitting Supporting Documentation in Drug Applications for the Manufacture of Drug Substances. ➢ Guideline for the Format and Content of the Chemistry, Manufacturing, and Controls Section of an Application. ➢ Guideline for the Format and Content of the chemistry, Manufacturing, and Controls Section of an Application. ➢ Guideline for Submitting Samples and Analytical Data for Methods Validation
Type III: Packaging Material	Each packaging material should be identified by the intended use, components, composition, and controls for its release. The names of the suppliers or fabricators of the components used in preparing the packaging material and the acceptance specifications should also be given. Data supporting the acceptability of the packaging material for its intended use should also be submitted as outlined in the "Guideline for Submitting Documentation for Packaging for Human Drugs and B Biologics." Toxicological data on these materials would be included under this type of DMF, if not otherwise available by cross-reference to another document.

Contd...

Type IV: Excipient, Colorant, Flavor,. Essence, or Material Used in Their Preparation	Each additive should be identified and characterized by its method of manufacture, release specifications, and testing methods. Toxicological data on these materials would be included under this type of DMF, if not otherwise available by cross-reference to another document. Usually, the official compendia and FDA regulations for color additives (21 CFR Parts 70 through 82), direct food additives (21 CFR Parts 170 through 173), indirect food additives (21 CFR Parts 174 through 178), and food substances (21 CFR Parts 181 through 186) may be used as sources for release tests, specifications, and safety. Guidelines suggested for a Type II DMF may be helpful for preparing a Type IV DMF. The DMF should include any other supporting information and data that are not available by cross-reference to another document
Type V: FDA-Accepted Reference Information	FDA discourages the use of Type V DMF's for miscellaneous information, duplicate information, or information that should be included in one of the other types of DMF's. If any holder wishes to submit information and supporting data in a DMF that is not covered by Types I through IV, a holder must first submit a letter of intent to the Drug Master File Staff (for address, see D.5.a. of this section). FDA will then contact the holder to discuss the proposed submission.

Processing and Reviewing Policies

A. Policies Related to Processing Drug Master Files

1. Public availability of the information and data in a DMF is determined under 21 CFR Part 20, 21 CFR 314.420(e), and 21 CFR 314.430.
2. An original DMF submission will be examined on receipt to determine whether it meets minimum requirements for format and content. If the submission is administratively acceptable, FDA will acknowledge its receipt and assign it a DMF number. If the submission is administratively incomplete or inadequate, it will be returned to the submitter with a letter of explanation from the Drug Master File Staff, and it will not be assigned a DMF number.

B. Drug Master File Review

A DMF is never approved or disapproved. The agency will review information in a DMF only when an IND sponsor, an applicant for an NDA, ANDA, or Export Application, or another DMF holder incorporates material in the DMF by reference. As noted, the incorporation by reference must be accompanied by a copy of the DMF holder's letter of authorization. If FDA reviewers find deficiencies in the information provided in a DMF, a letter describing the deficiencies is sent to the DMF holder. At the same time, FDA will notify the person who relies on the information in the deficient DMF that additional information is needed in the supporting DMF. The general subject of the deficiency is identified, but details of the deficiency are disclosed only to the DMF holder. When the holder submits the requested information to the DMF in response to the agency's deficiency letter, the holder should also send a copy of the accompanying transmittal letter to the affected persons relying on the DMF and to the FDA reviewing division that identified the deficiencies. The transmittal letter will provide notice that the deficiencies have been addressed.

Holder Obligations

Any change or addition, including a change in authorization related to specific customers, should be submitted in duplicate and adequately cross-referenced to previous submission(s). The reference should include the date(s), volume(s), section(s), and/or page number(s) affected.

Major Reorganization of a Drug Master File

A holder who plans a major reorganization of a DMF is encouraged to submit a detailed plan of the proposed changes and request its review by the Drug Master File Staff. The staff should be given sufficient time to comment and provide suggestions before a major reorganization is undertaken.

Closure of a Drug Master File

A holder who wishes to close a DMF should submit a request to the Drug Master File Staff stating the reason for the closure. See Section IV.D.5.a for the address.

Dossier and Common Technical Document (CTD)

The word 'Dossier' has the English meaning as a collection or file of documents on the particular subject, especially a file containing detailed information about a person or a topic. Any formulation is prepared for human use i.e. designated to modify or explore physiological systems or pathological states for the benefit of the recipient is called as "Pharmaceutical product for human use". Process of critiquing and assessing the dossier of pharmaceutical product containing its detailed about administrative, chemistry, preclinical & clinical information and the permission granted by the regulatory agencies of a country with a view to support its marketing or approval in a country is called as "Marketing approval or Registration", "Marketing Authorization or "Product Licensing".

"Registration Dossier" of the pharmaceutical product is a document that contains all technical data (administrative, quality, nonclinical, and clinical) of a pharmaceutical product to be approved / registered / marketed in a country. It is more commonly called as New Drug Application (NDA) in the USA or Marketing Authorization Application (MAA) in European Union (EU) and other countries as simply Registration Dossier. Thus, pharmaceutical Regulatory dossiers are of 2 types

- ***Clinical applications:***
  - IND- Investigational New Drug Applications (in USA)or
  - CTA- Clinical trial application (Ex USA)

➢ ***Market applications:***
- NDA- New Drug applications (FDA- for small molecules)
- BLA- Biologic license Application (FDA- for Large molecules)
- MAA- Market authorization application (Ex USA for both small and large molecules)

The Common Technical Document (CTD) is a set of specifications for an application dossier for the registration of Medicines and designed to be used across Europe, Japan and the United States. It is an internationally agreed format for the preparation of applications regarding new drugs intended to be submitted to regional regulatory authorities in participating countries. It was developed by the European Medicines Agency (EMA, Europe), the Food and Drug Administration (FDA, US) and the Ministry of Health, Labour and Welfare (Japan). The CTD is maintained by the International Conference on Harmonisation of Technical Requirements for Registration of Pharmaceuticals for Human Use (ICH).

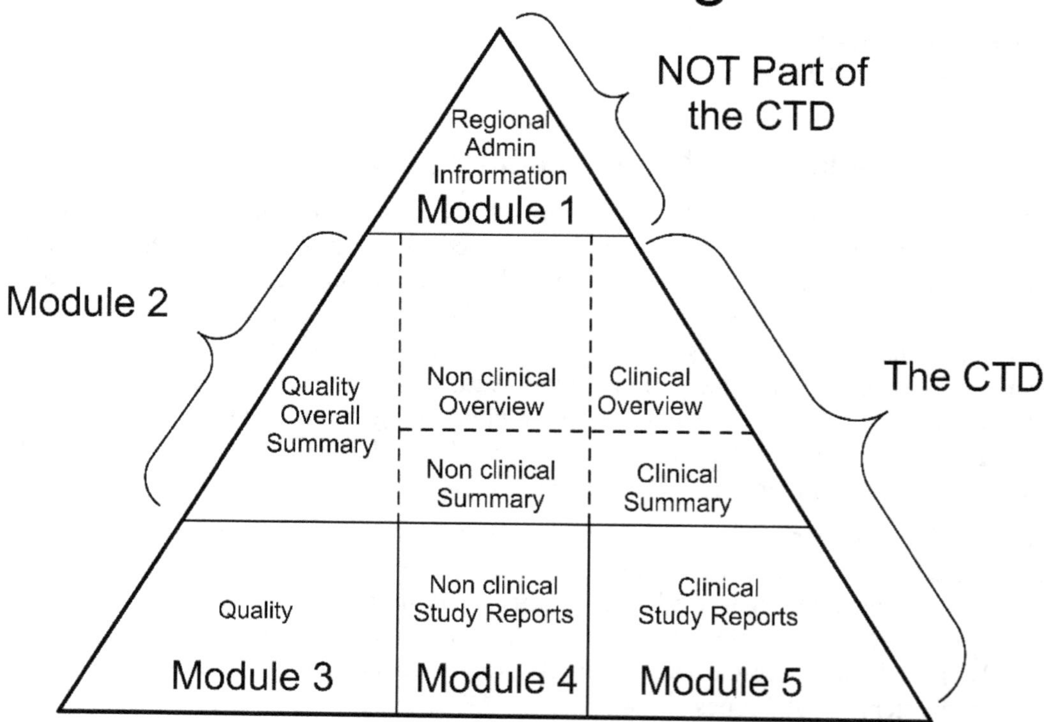

Pharmaceutical Dossier is an Important & Critical part of Product Registration process, which is needed to submit in Food & Drug Administration of the concerned Ministry of Health, of Regulatory Authority. Different Regulatory Authority published their Standard format according to country Guidelines. ICH-CTD is followed by ICH countries where as ACTD is usually adopted by ASEAN countries. The ICH-CTD has five modules. The ACTD has parts instead of module. They are four in number. These include summary of quality, nonclinical and clinical in part II, III, IV, respectively. The administrative data of Part I is part of ACTD whereas Module 1 of ICH-CTD is purely country specific. The summaries of the quality (Part II), nonclinical (Part III) and clinical (Part IV) are located at the beginning of each part of the ACTD. The ICH-CTD dedicates these summaries in a separate Module 2. As the ACTD does not have such summary part, it consists of only 4 Parts. Common Pharmaceutical Dossier which is widely used in the Pharmaceutical Industry are:

CTD Format Dossiers	This Format of Dossier is an Important & widely used Dossier format in most of the country, This format of any registration application for Marketing Authorization Dossier is submitted to Food and Drug Authority or Ministry of health or any other equivalent authority along with other required documents. Common Technical Document Consists of the following Modules with the number of the required Documents. Module 1 – Administrative Information & Prescribing Information Module 2 - Common Technical Documents Summaries Module 3 –Quality Module 4 – Non Clinical Study Report Module 5 – Clinical Study Report CTD Format Dossier is widely used in semi regulated & regulated market like CIS Countries, Middle East countries, European Union, USA , Australia, African Countries, Canada, Japan, etc
ACTD Format Dossiers	The Association of Southeast Asian Nations (ASEAN) comprises Brunei Darussalam, Cambodia, Indonesia, Laos, Malaysia, Myanmar, Philippines, Singapore, Thailand, and Vietnam. ACTD Format Dossier is also Described as ASEAN CTD Dossier, ASEAN Common Technical Dossier (ACTD) provides a common format for the preparation of well-structured Common Technical Dossier applications for submission in ASEAN regulatory authorities for the registration of pharmaceuticals for human use. ACTD format significantly reduce the time and resources needed to compile applications for registration. Regulatory reviews and communication with the applicant is facilitated by a standard document of common elements. This guideline merely demonstrates an appropriate write-up format for acquired data. However, applicants can modify, if needed, to provide the best possible presentation of the technical information, in order to facilitate the understanding and evaluation of the results upon pharmaceutical registration. Dossier writing and compilation as per ACTD Format. Asian Common Technical Documents consists of following parts: ➢ Part I – Administrative Data and Product Information ➢ Part II – Quality Documents ➢ Part III – Non Clinical Documents [Bibliographic review of Safety for Herbal CTD]

Contd...

	➢ Part IV – Clinical Documents. [Traditional use evidence for Herbal CTD] ACTD Format is Asian harmonization for Common technical Documents used in Asian Countries like Vietnam, Thailand, Singapore, and Malaysia, Philippines & in Member States. CTD-Herbal(Module 1-5) Module 1-Administrative data Module 2-CTD Summaries Module 3 Quality Module 4- Module 5-Traditional use evidence
eCTD Format Dossier	This format of Registration Dossier is an electronic format for CTD Dossier, Submission in eCTD format should be in accordance with the current ICH M2 EWG eCTD specification, Electronic files should be in accordance with the Guidance for Industry on Providing Regulatory Information in Electronic Format. The eCTD is an interface for the pharmaceutical industry to transfer regulatory information with various regulatory agencies. The content is based on the Common Technical Document (CTD) format. It was developed by the International Conference on Harmonisation (ICH) Multidisciplinary Group 2 Expert Working Group (ICH M2 EWG). NeeS format Dossier Requirements for the submission of Non-eCTD electronic Submissions (NeeS). A separate EU guidance document covering eCTD submissions, which is regarded as the principal electronic submission format in EU. Once the switch to this electronic format is made it is expected that further applications and responses relating to the particular medicinal product are submitted in NeeS format. Applicants can switch from NeeS to eCTD at the start of any new regulatory activity. Applicants should however not change from eCTD back to NeeS. There is no requirement to reformat the whole dossier into NeeS format when switching from paper to NeeS, but this could be done at the applicant's discretion.
Country Specific Format	This format of Registration Dossier is in accordance with the Specific Country Regulatory Guidelines.

The CTD is divided into five modules

Module 1	**Administrative Information and Prescribing Information:** This module should contain documents specific to each region; for example, application forms or the proposed label for use in the region. The content and format of this module can be specified by the relevant regulatory authorities. For information about this module see the guidance for industry, General Considerations for Submitting Marketing Applications According to the ICH/CTD Format.
Module 2	**Common Technical Document Summaries:** Module 2 should begin with a general introduction to the pharmaceutical, including its pharmacologic class, mode of action, and proposed clinical use. In general, the introduction should not exceed one page. Module 2 should contain 7 sections in the following order: 1. CTD Table of Contents

Contd...

	2. CTD Introduction 3. Quality Overall Summary 4. Nonclinical Overview 5. Clinical Overview 6. Nonclinical Written and Tabulated Summaries 7. Clinical Summary. The individual organization of the Module 2 summaries is described in three separate documents: ➢ M4Q: The CTD — Quality ➢ M4S: The CTD — Safety ➢ M4E: The CTD — Efficacy.
Module 3	**Quality:** Information on Quality should be presented in the structured format described in the guidance M4Q.
Module 4	**Nonclinical Study Reports:** The Nonclinical Study Reports should be presented in the order described in the guidance M4S.
Module 5	**Clinical Study Reports:** The human study reports and related information should be presented in the order described in the guidance M4E .

Chemistry Manufacturing and Control (CMC)

The Basics of CMC

Chemistry, Manufacturing and Controls (CMC) ensures that pharmaceutical and biopharmaceutical drug products are consistently effective, safe and high quality for consumers. It sustains a connection between the drug that is used in clinical studies and the commercial drug that is marketed and available to consumers. CMC isn't a one-size-fits-all checklist or list of tests to be performed on every product, but is instead tailored to the platform and delivery system (e.g. injectable, controlled release, inhalant, topical, solid dose, oral, etc.).

Chemistry, Manufacturing and Controls applies to both the drug product and the facility in which the product is being manufactured:

Drug Product

- The manufacturing process
- Quality control release testing
- Specifications and stability of the product

Manufacturing Facility

- Design
- Qualification
- Operation
- Maintenance

CMC is an integral part of any pharmaceutical product application to FDA. CMC is critical to attaining a successful registration filing. CMC is applicable to the entire product lifecycle – it starts during the drug candidate selection phase, and continues through post-approval and beyond. CMC information in dossier is detailed and an important section which support clinical trial as well as marketing applications.

- ***Chemistry***: Structure, synthesis of drug substance, the composition of drug product, the materials involved in it
- ***Manufacturing***: Description of manufacture of the product, equipment used, Facility information
- ***Controls***: Ensure the quality of the product

ICH guidelines gives general idea about CMC but there lack of exact content of guidance documents. Content depends upon the type of product like if it pharmaceutical, biological, Biosimilars, generics or vaccines. Details of the sections depend upon the type of the product and countries specific requirements. If it is Pharma product than it contains least content and it is well described/ characterized. In ICH all guidance documents are described in detail about CMC. The required format, data and content are also given in ICH.

Importance of CMC Section in CTD Dossier:

For any marketing application or clinical trials CMC (chemistry, manufacturing and controls) section is a very important and detailed section. If the manufacturing process cannot be shown to its highest quality standard and do not satisfied the regulators need as well as product have not their quality standard as mentioned in Pharmacopoeia than it might be chance to drug may lost the marketing approval. So it is important to show the standard quality process and parameter of drug manufacturing details and other parameter cover in module 3 Quality contain Chemistry, manufacturing and Control. The chemistry, manufacturing and controls (CMC) section is a very important part of any clinical trial or marketing application. Drugs can be denied marketing approval if the quality of the product and the manufacturing process cannot be shown to be of a sufficiently high standard to satisfy regulators. The ICH guideline Q1A(R2) (Stability Testing of New Drug Substances and Products) defines the stability data package required for new drug substances and products submitted for approval in each of the major regions that accept the ICH guidelines (i.e., US, Japan and EU).

Dossier Technical Section Compilation

One has to save time during product approval; process during filing an application & to get rid from unnecessary queries that may lengthen the approval process Therefore one has to focus on the probable queries that may arise after submission of marketing application. Once approved, the applicant may manufacture and market the generic drug product to provide safe, effective and stable & quality product with low cost to the public. The queries of CMC section compiled in CTD format as per ICH guideline: "The Common Technical Document for the Registration of Pharmaceuticals for Human Use [M4Q (R1)] which gives good understanding of critical aspects of marketing application in ICH harmonized countries like US, Europe and Japan and their market requirements.

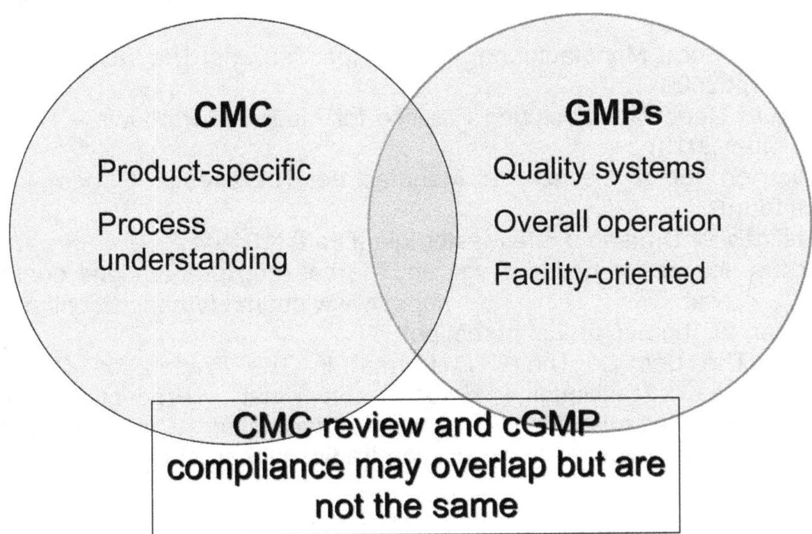

Further Reading

1. Guan, H.-F & Zhang, Y.-W. (2018). Establishment of CTD format content for CMC section of natural medicinal products application data. Chinese Journal of New Drugs. 27. 2137-2142.
2. Wang ZM, Liu JY, Liu XQ, Wang DQ, Yan LH, Zhu JJ, Gao HM, Li C, Wang JY, Li CY, Ni QC, Huang JS, Lin J. [Consideration about chemistry, manufacture and control (CMC) key problems in simplified registration of classical traditional Chinese medicine excellent prescriptions]. Zhongguo Zhong Yao Za Zhi. 2017 May;42(10):1819-1824.
3. https://www.fda.gov/media/71581/download Accessed on April 2021-05-05
4. Patel, Dhruvi & Badjatya, Jitendra & Patel, Amit. (2017). Preparation and review of chemistry, manufacturing and control (CMC) sections of CTD dossier for marketing authorization. International Journal of Drug Regulatory Affairs. 5. 1-12. 10.22270/ijdra.v5i2.196.
5. https://www.who.int/medicines/publications/qas_herbalmed/en/
6. https://cdsco.gov.in/opencms/opencms/en/Home/Accessed on April 2021-05-05
7. EU Good Manufacturing Practice Vol 4. Explanatory Notes for Pharmaceutical Manufacturers on the Preparation of a Site Master File (2010)
8. EU Good Manufacturing Practice Vol 4. Medicinal Products for Human and Veterinary Use – Chapter 4: Documentation (2010)
9. ICH Q10 Pharmaceutical Quality System (2008)
10. ISO 9001:2008 Quality Management Systems
11. ISO 13485:1996 Quality Systems – Medical Devices – Particular requirements for the application of ISO 9001.

12. PIC/S Explanatory Notes for Pharmaceutical Manufacturers on the Preparation of a Site Master File (2011)
13. PIC/S Guide to Good Manufacturing Practice for Medicinal Products – Part I Version 8 PE009-8 (15 Jan 2009)
14. PIC/S Guide to Good Manufacturing Practice for Medicinal Products – Part I Version 9 PE009-9 (1 Sept 2009)
15. PIC/S Guide to Good Manufacturing Practice for Medicinal Products – Part I Version 10 PE009-10 (1 Jan 2013)
16. TGA Application for a Licence to Manufacture Therapeutic Goods – 1413 (0406) (application form)
17. WHO Guidelines for Drafting a Site Master File (Draft) (2010)
18. Content of the dossier for herbal drugs and Herbal drug preparations quality evaluation. Available at - https://www.edqm.eu/medias/fichiers/cep_content_of_the_dossier_for_herbal_drugs_herbal.pdf
19. Guideline on The Use Of The CTD Format In The Preparation Of A Registration Application For Traditional Herbal Medicinal Products. Available at https://www.ema.europa.eu/en/documents/regulatory-procedural-guideline/guideline-use-ctd-format-preparation-registration-application-traditional-herbal-medicinal-products_en-0.pdf
20. PA/PH/CEP (02) 6 1R.https://www.gmp-compliance.org/files/guidemgr/cep_content_of_the_dossier_for_herbal_drugs_herbal.pdf

Scan QR code to view the website/guidelines

- CTC-
  ICH Official web site : ICH

- SMF-
  untitled (who.int)

- DMF-
  Drug Master Files (DMFs) | FDA

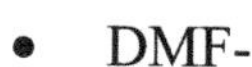

- CMC-
  Chemistry Manufacturing and Controls (CMC) Guidances for Industry (GFIs) and Questions and Answers (Q&As) | FDA

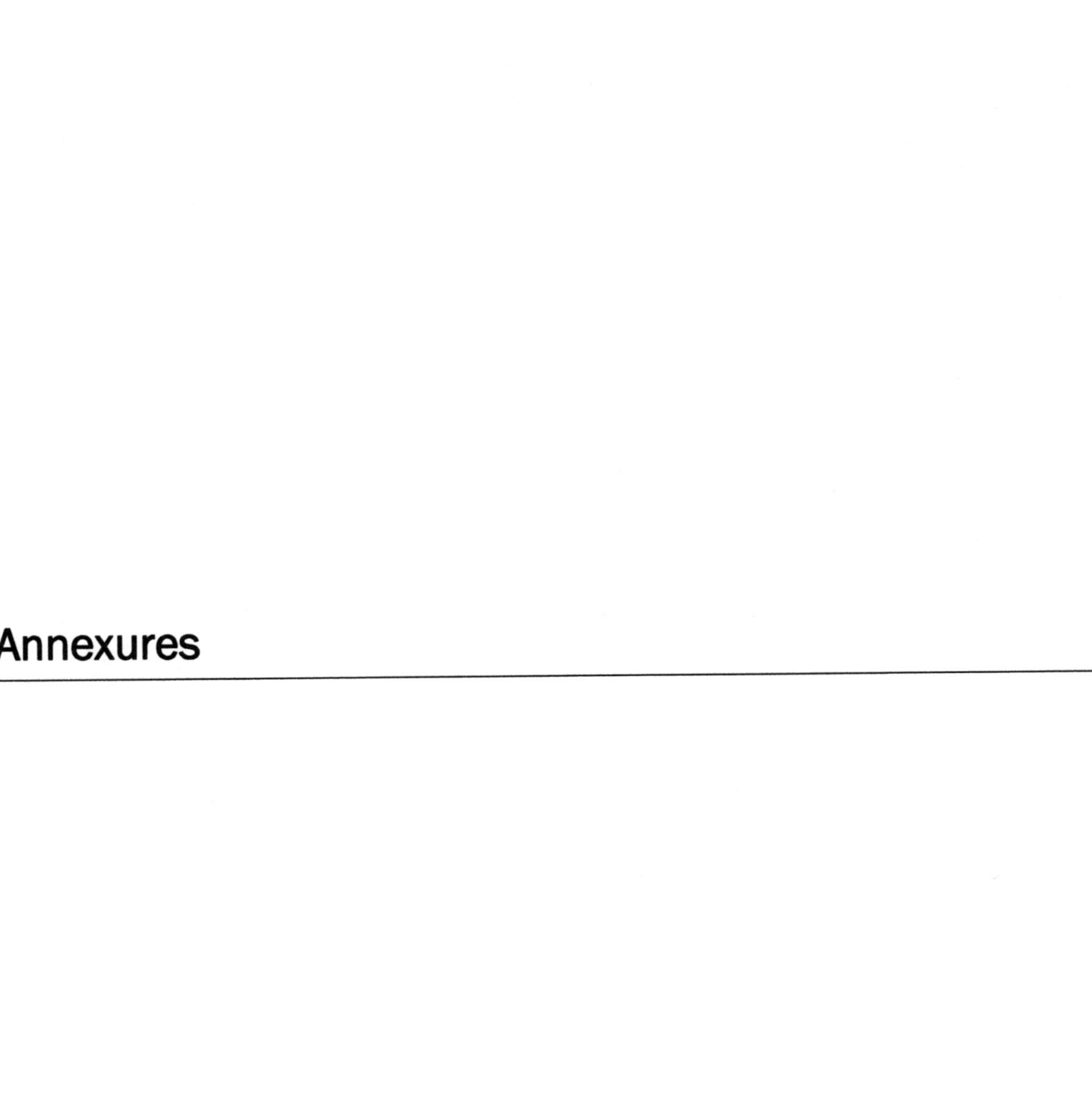

Annexures

ANNEXURE

1 Analytical Profiles of Herbal Drugs

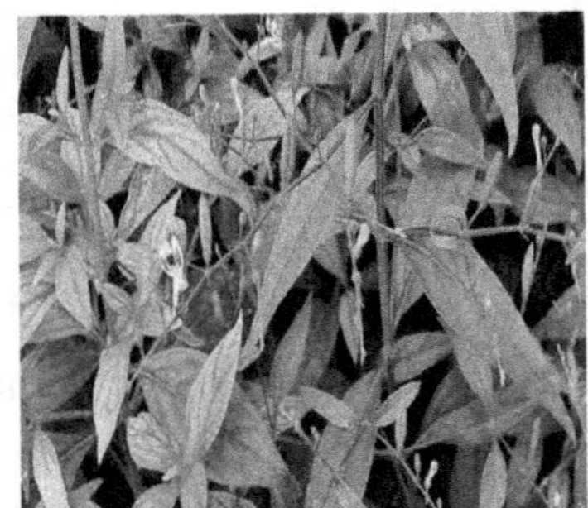

Kalmegh (*Andrographis Paniculata*):

Kalmegh consists of the dried aerial parts, mainly stems and leaves, of *Andrographis paniculata* Nees. (*Fam, Acanthaceae*). Kalmegh contains not less than 1.0 per cent w/w of andrographolide, calculated on the dried basis.

Description - Taste, intensely bitter.

Identification:

A. Macroscopic - Mixture of crisp, dark green - coloured broken leaves and quadrangular stems; leaves brittle. Stem fracture short, fibrous.

B. Microscopic - Stems quadrangular with collenchymas strands at angles and on side; small acicular crystals of calcium oxalate present in pith and cortex. Trichomes 1-3 celled, glandular hair disc-shaped and multicellular.

C. Determine by thin-layer chromatography, coating the plate with silica gel GF254.

Mobile phase: A mixture of 7 volumes of chloroform and 1 volume of methanol.

Test solution: Reflux 1 g of coarsely powdered substance under examination with 50 ml methanol for 15 minutes, cool and filter. Reflux the residue further with 2 × 50 ml of methanol.

Cool and filter: Combine all the filtrates and concentrate to 10 ml.

Reference solution: Reflux 0.5 g of kalmegh RS with 50 ml methanol for 15 minutes, cool and filter. Reflux the residue further with 2 × 50 ml of methanol, cool and filter. Combine all the filtrates and concentrate to 5 ml.

Apply to the plate 10 III of each solution as bands 10 mm by 2 mm. Allow the mobile phase to rise 8 cm. Dry the plate in air and examine in ultraviolet light at 254 Dill and 365 Dill, spray with methanolic sulphuric acid (20 per cent, v/v). Heat the plate at 1200 for 5-10 minutes and examine in day light. The chromatographic profile of the test solution is similar to that of the reference solution.

Tests:

- **Foreign organic matter** - Not more than 2.0 per cent.

- **Ethanol-soluble extractive** - Not less than 3.0 per cent.
- **Water-soluble extractive** - Not less than 12.0 per cent
- **Total ash** - Not more than 15 per cent.
- **Acid-insoluble ash** - Not more than 3.0 per cent.
- **Heavy metals** - 1.0 g complies with the limit test for heavy metals, Method B (20 ppm).
- **Loss on drying** - Not more than 12.0 per cent, determined on 5 g by drying in an oven at 105°.
- **Microbial contamination** - Complies with the microbial contamination tests.

Assay: Determine by liquid chromatography

Test solution: Reflux about 2.5 g of the coarsely powdered substance under examination with 50 ml of methanol on a water bath for 15 minutes, cool and filter. Reflux the residue further with methanol till the last extract turns colorless, cool and filter. Combine all the filtrates and concentrate to 50.0 ml.

Reference solution: A 0.1 per cent w/v solution of andrographolide RS in methanol.

Chromatographic system

- A stainless steel column 25 cm × 4.6 mm packed with octadecylsilane bonded to porous silica (5 um),
- Mobile phase: 65 volumes of methanol and 35 volumes of water,
- Flow rate. 1ml per minute,
- Spectrophotometer set at 223 nm,
- Injection volume 20 ul.

Inject the reference solution. The test is not valid unless the relative standard deviation for the replicate injections is not more than 2.0 per cent.

Inject the test solution and reference solution.

Calculate the content of andrographolide.

Storage: Store protected from heat, moisture and against attack by insects and rodents.

Kunduru (*Sallaki Gum*; Gum of *Boswellia Serrata*):

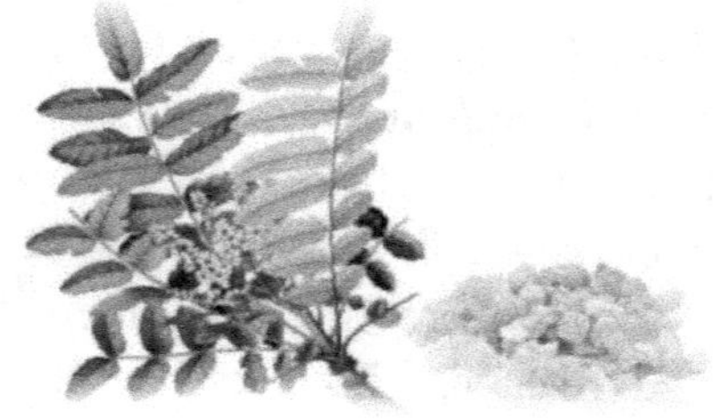

Kunduru is the gum-resin from *Boswellia serrata Roxb.* (*Fam. Burseraceae*).

Kunduru contains not less than 1.0 per cent w/w of total 11- keto-beta-boswellic acid and acetyl-ll-keto-beta-boswellic acid, calculated on the dried basis.

Description: Translucent, brittle, whitish yellow substance, in roundish, club-shaped, pear-shaped, or irregular tears.

Identification

A. Macroscopic: Fracture dull, slightly sticky to touch; odour, balsamic; taste slightly mucilaginous, bitter and aromatic.

B. Determine by thin-layer chromatography: coating the plate with silica gel GF254.

Mobile phase: A mixture of 7 volumes of hexane and 3 volumes of ethyl acetate.

Test solution: Reflux I g of coarsely powdered substance under examination with 50 ml methanol on a boiling water-bath for 30 minutes, cool and filter. Evaporate the filtrate to dryness and dissolve the residue in 10 ml of methanol.

Reference solution: Reflux 1 g of coarsely powdered kunduru RS with 50 ml methanol on a boiling water-bath for 30 minutes, cool and filter. Evaporate the filtrate to dryness and dissolve the residue in 10 ml of methanol.

Apply to the plate 10 ul of each solution as bands 10 mm by 2 mm. Allow the mobile phase to rise 8 cm. Dry the plate in air and examine in ultraviolet light 254 urn and 365 urn, spray with methanolic sulphuric acid (1 0 per cent, v/v). Heat the plate at 110° for 5-10 minutes and examine in day light. The chromatographic profile of the test solution is similar to that of the reference solution.

Tests:

Foreign organic matter: Not more than 2.0 per cent.

Ethanol-soluble extractive: Not less than 35 per cent.

Total ash: Not more than 10.0 per cent.

Acid-insoluble ash: Not more than 2.0 per cent.

Heavy metals: 1.0 g complies with the limit test for heavy metals, Method B (20 ppm).

Water: Not more than 12.0 per cent, determined on 0.2g.

Microbial contamination: Complies with the microbial contamination tests.

Assay: Determine by liquid chromatography

Test solution: Reflux about 2 g of the coarsely powdered substance under examination with 50 ml of methanol on a water bath for 15 minutes, cool and filter. Reflux the residue further with methanol till the last extract tums colorless, cool and filter. Combine all the filtrates and concentrate to 100.0 ml.

Reference solution (a): A 0.01 per cent w/v solution of ll-keto-b-boswellic acid RS in methanol.

Reference solution (b): A 0.05 per cent w/v solution of acetyl-ll-keto-b-boswellic acid RS in methanol.

Chromatographic system:

- A stainless steel column 25 cm × 4.6 rom packed with octadecylsilane bonded to porous silica (5 lum),
- Mobile phase: 90 volumes of methanol and 10 volumes o a mixture containing 5 ml of acetonitrile and 95 ml of water, adjusting the pH to 2.8 with dilute orthophosphoric acid,
- Flow rate. 1.5 ml per minute,
- Spectrophotometer set at 247 nm,
- Injection volume. 20 ul

Inject the reference solution (a) and (b). The test is not valid unless the relative retention times are about 0.65 for ll-keto-beta-boswellic acid and 0.1 for acetyl-11-keto-b-boswellic acid and the relative standard deviation for the replication injection is not more than 2.0 per cent.

Inject the test solution.

Calculate the sum of the contents of ll-keto-b-boswellic acid and acetyl-ll-keto-b-boswellic acid.

Storage: Store protected from heat, moisture and against attack by insects and rodents.

Coleus (*Coleus forskohlii*):

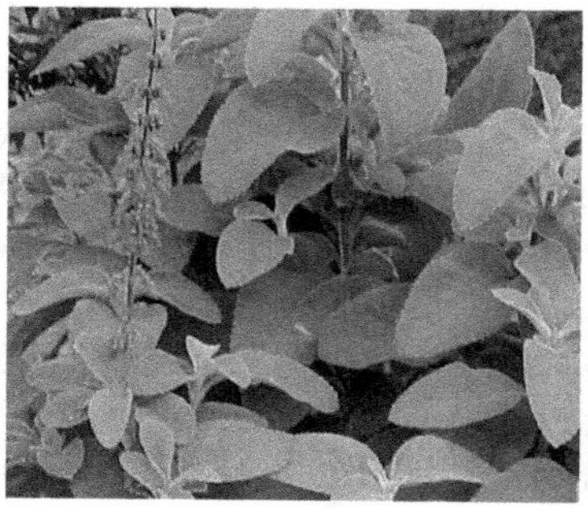

Coleus consists of the whole or cut dried roots of *Coleus forskohlii Briq.* (*Fam. Lamiaceae*).

Coleus contains not less than 0.4 per cent w/w of forskolin, calculated on the dried basis.

Description: The roots are light brown in color, generally long and radially spread. They have an aromatic characteristic odor and the taste is slightly pungent.

Identification:

A. Macroscopic: Roots are brown, longitudinally wrinlded, fracture short, cut surface yellowish white.

B. Microscopic: The outermost layer consists of rectangular cork cells, cork cambium, rectangular parenchymatous region containing sclereids and calcium oxalate crystals. Vascular cambium is present in the form of a continuous ring. The tracheids and tracheidal fibres have bordered pits.

C. Determine by thin-layer chromatography, coating the plate with silica gel GF254.

Mobile phase. A mixture of 75 volumes of benzene, and 25 volumes of ethyl acetate.

Test solution: To 5 g of the coarsely powdered substance under examination, add 50 ml of acetonitrile and reflux for 15 minutes, cool and filter. Reflux the residue further for two times with 50 ml of acetonitrile, cool and filter. Combine all the filtrates and concentrate under vacuum to 100 ml.

Reference solution: To 1 g of coleus RS add 50 ml of acetonitrile and reflux for 15 minutes cool and filter. Reflux the residue further for two times with 50 ml of acetonitrile, cool and filter. Combine all the filtrates and concentrate under vacuum to 20 ml.

Apply to the plate 20 ul of each solution as bands 10 mm by 2 rom. Allow the mobile phase to rise 8 cm. Dry the plate in air and examine in ultraviolet light at 254 nm and 365 nm, spray with vanillin glacial acetic acid reagent. Heat the plate at 100° for 5-10 minutes and examine in day light. The chromatographic profile of the test solution is similar to that of the reference solution.

Tests:

Foreign organic matter: Not more than 2.0 per cent.

Ethanol-soluble extractive: Not less than 15.0 per cent.

Water-soluble extractive: Not less than 18.0 per cent by method I.

Total ash: Not more than 15.0 percent.

Acid-insoluble ash: Not more than 5.0 per cent.

Heavy metals: 1.0 g complies with the limit test for heavy metals, Method B (20 ppm).

Loss on drying: Not more than 12.0 per cent, determined on 5 g by drying in an oven at 105°.

Microbial contamination: Complies with the microbial contamination tests.

Assay: Determine by liquid chromatography

Test solution: Weigh 3 g of coarsely powdered substance under examination, add 50 ml of acetonitrile and reflux on a water bath for 15 minutes cool and filter. Reflux the residue two times with 75 ml of acetonitrile, cool and filter, Concentrate the filterate to 100.0 ml.

Reference solution: A 0.1 per cent w/v solution off orskolin RS in acetonitrile.

Chromatographic system:

- A stainless steel column 25 cm x 4.6 rom packed with octadecylsilane bonded to porous silica (5 /lm),
- Mobile phase: filtered and degassed mixture of 45 volumes of acetonitrile and 55 volumes of water,
- Flow rate- 1.8 ml per minute,
- Spectrophotometer set at 220 nm,
- Injection volume. 20 ul

Inject the reference solution. The relative standard deviation for the replicate injections is not more than 2.0 per cent.

Inject the test solution and reference solution.

Calculate the content of forskolin.

Storage: Store protected from moisture and against attack by insects and rodents.

Haridra (*Haldi; Turmeric; Curcuma longa*):

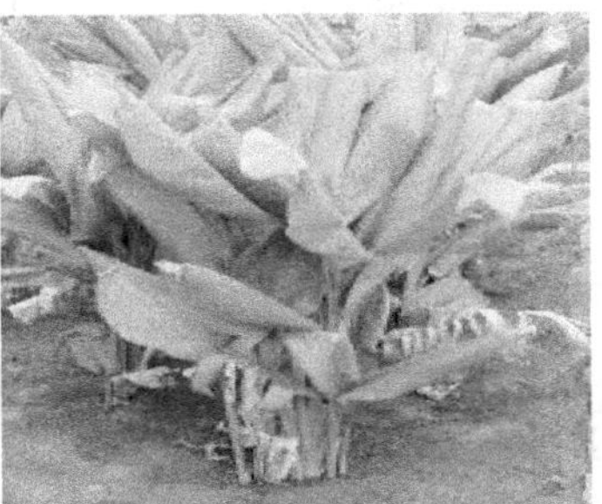

Haridra consists of the dried rhizomes of *Curcuma longa Linn.* (*Fam. Zingiberaceae*). Haridra contains not less than 1.5 per cent w/w of curcumin, calculated on the dried basis.

Description: Externally yellowish to yellowish brown with root scars and annulations. Odour, aromatic; taste, warmly aromatic and bitter.

Identification:

A. Macroscopic: Rhizome oblong, conical or cylindrical to elongate, finger-like; internally orange yellow. Texture hard and heavy; fracture short.

B. Microscopic: Ground tissue of parenchyma cells; cells filled with gelatinized starch grains and yellow pigment. Fibrovascular bundles and oil cells scattered throughout ground tissue. C. Determine by thin-layer chromatography, coating the plate with silica gel GF254. Mobile phase- A mixture of 94 volumes of chloroform, 5 volumes of ethanol and 1 volume glacial acetic acid.

Test solution: Extract 1 g of the coarsely powdered substance under examination with 5 ml methanol for 10 minutes with slight warming. Filter and use the filtrate.

Reference solution- Reflux 1 g of coarsely powdered haridra RS with 5 ml methanol for 15 minutes, cool and filter.

Apply to the plate 10 ul of each solution as bands 10 mm by 2 mm. Allow the mobile phase to rise 8 cm. Dry the plate in air and examine in ultraviolet light 254 run, 365 run and also under day light. The chromatographic profile of the test solution is similar to that of the reference solution.

Tests:

Foreign organic matter: Not more than 2.0 per cent.

Ethanol-soluble extractive: Not less than 6.0 per cent.

Water-soluble extractive: Not less than 12.0 per cent by Method 1.

Total ash: Not more than 10.0 per cent.

Acid-insoluble ash: Not more than 2.0 per cent.

Heavy metals: 1.0 g complies with the limit test for heavy metals, Method B (20 ppm).

Water: Not more than 12.0 per cent, determined on 0.2g.

Microbial contamination: Complies with the microbial contamination tests.

Assay: Determine by liquid chromatography.

Test solution: Reflux about 1 g of the coarsely powdered substance under examination with 50 ml of methanol on a water bath for 15 minutes cool and filter. Reflux the residue further with 5 × 25 ml of methanol, cool and filter. Combine all the filtrates and concentrate to 100ml

Reference solution: A 0.01 per cent w/v solution of curcumin RS in methanol.

Chromatographic system:

- A stainless steel column 25 cm x 4.6 mm packed with silicagel consisting of porous spherical particles with chemically bonded nitrile group,
- Mobile phase: a mixture of 35 volumes of tetrahydrofuran 65 volumes of a buffer solution prepared by dissolving 109 of citric acid in 1000 ml of water, adjusting the pH to 3.0 with dilute ammonia solution,
- Flow rate. 1.2 ml per minute,
- Spectrophotometer set at 430 nm,
- Injection volume. 20 ul

Inject the reference solution: The test is not valid unless the relative standard deviation for the replicate injections is not more than 2.0 per cent.

Inject the reference solution and the test solution.

Calculate the content of curcumin.

Storage: Store protected from moisture.

Amalaki (*Emblic Myrobalan; Indian Gooseberry*):

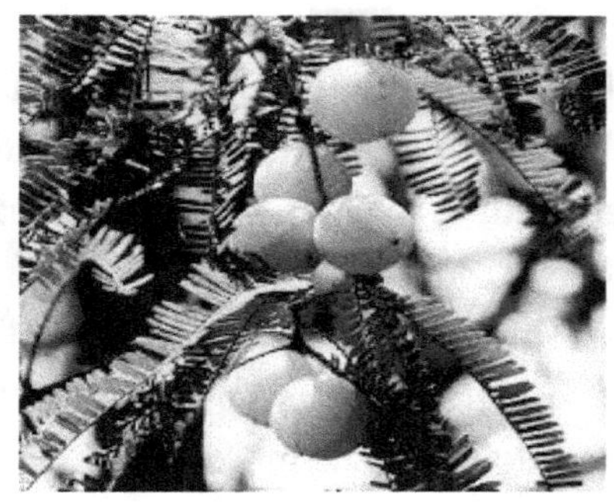

Amalaki consists of the dried fruit pericarp of Emblica officinalis Gaertn. (*Phyllanthus emblica Linn.*) (*Fam. Euphorbiaceae*). Amalaki contains not less than 1.0 per cent w/w gallic acid calculated on the dried basis.

Description: The dried fruit has a highly shriveled and wrinkled external surface. The taste is sour and astringent followed by delicately sweet tinge.

Identification:

A. Macroscopic: The dried fruit shows a broad, highly shriveled and wrinkled external convex surface, lateral surface transversely wrinlded, external surface exhibits few whitish specks, occasionally some pieces show a portion of stony testa.

B. Microscopic: The epicarpic cells are rectangular in shape and their walls are highly cuticularized. Anomocytic type of stomata is found rarely. Collateral fibrovascular bundles are scattered throughout the inner mesocarp. Pitted and helical tracheids with tapering ends are seen. At places in the phloem, large cavities filled with crystal mass are present.

C. Determine by thin-layer chromatography, coating the plate with silica gel GF254. Mobile phase - A mixture of 20 volumes oftoluene, 45 volumes of ethyl acetate, 20 volumes of glacial acetic acid and 5 volumes off ormic acid.

Test solution: Reflux 2 g of the coarsely powdered substance under examination with 50-75 ml of methanol for 15 minutes, cool and filter. Reflux the residue further for two times with 75 ml of methanol, cool and filter. Combine all the filtrates and concentrate under vacuum to 50 ml.

Reference solution: Reflux 0.4 g of the coarsely powdered amalaki RS with 50-75 ml of methanol for 15 minutes, cool and filter. Reflux the residue further for two times with 75 ml of methanol, cool and filter. Combine all the filtrates and concentrate under vacuum to 10 ml.

Apply to the plate 10 ul of each solution as bands 10 mm by 2 mm. Allow the mobile phase to rise 8 cm. Dry the plate in air and examine in ultraviolet light at 254 nm and 365 nm, spray with anisaldehyde sulphuric acid reagent. Heat the place at 100° for 5-10 minutes and examine in day light. The chromatographic profile of the test solution is similar to that of the reference solution.

Tests:

Foreign organic matter: Not more than 3 per cent.

Ethanol-soluble extractive: Not less than 30 per cent.

Water-soluble extractive: Not less than 40 per cent by Method I.

Total Ash: Not more than 5.0 per cent.

Acid-insoluble ash: Not more than 2.0 per cent.

Heavy metals: 1.0 g complies with the limit test for heavy metals, Method B(20 ppm).

Loss on drying: Not more than 12.0 per cent, determined on 5 g by drying in an oven at 105°.

Microbial contamination: Complies with the microbial contamination tests.

Assay: Determine by liquid chromatography

Test solution: Weigh accurately about 0.5 g of coarsely powdered substance under examination, add 50 ml of water, sonicate for 3 minutes and heat on a boiling water-bath for 15 minutes, cool and dilute to 100.0 ml with water and filter.

Reference solution: A 0.01 per cent w/v solution of gallic acid RS in water.

Chromatographic system:

- A stainless steel column 25 cm × 4.6 mm packed with octadecylsilane bonded to porous silica (5 /lm),
- Mobile phase: A. a solution prepared by dissolving 0.136 g of potassium di-hydrogen orthophosphate in 500 ml of water, add 0.5 ml of ortho phosphoric acid and dilute to 1000 ml with water, B. acetonitrile
- A linear gradient programme using the conditions given below,
- Flow rate. 1.5 ml per minute,
- Spectrophotometer set at 270 nm,
- Injection volume. 20 ul.

Inject the reference solution: The test is not valid unless the relative standard deviation for replicate injections is not more than 20 per cent.

Inject the test solution and the reference solution.

Calculate the content of gallic acid.

Storage: Store protected from light, heat, moisture and against attack by insects and rodents.

ANNEXURE

2 List of GMP Certified Herbal Raw Material and Phytochemical Suppliers in India

Sr. No	Name of Company	Address/contact Details	Key Role/Product
1	Yucca Enterprises	-246, Antop Hill Warehousing Co., Barkat Ali Naka, Wadala (E), Mumbai, Maharashtra, India	Manufacturer and supplier of Raw herbs, standardized extracts
2	Natural Remedies Pvt Ltd	5 B Veerasandra Industrial area, 19th K. M. Stone, House Road, Electronic City (Post), Bangaluru Tel – 080 – 40209999 www.naturalremedy.com Email – info@naturalremedy.com	Manufacturer of standardized herbal extracts, marker compounds
3	Indus Extracts, C/0 Impex	7, Devkaran Mansion, 24 Vithaldas Road, Princess street, Mumbai – 400002 Tel – 022 22014864 www.Indusextracts.com Email – info@indusextracts.com	Manufacturer of standardized Botanical Therapeutic Extracts, Phytochemicals, Spice Extracts (Oleoresins & Oils), Plant Enzymes, and Plant and Mineral based Nutrients.
4	Hill Green Herbals Pvt Ltd	No 17, 13th Cross, Vasanthnagar East, bengaluru – 560052 080 – 41235313 www.hillgreen.com	Manufacturer of standardized herbal extracts, herbal formulations, high purity herb cultivation, collection and packaging
5	Bio-syn Herbs Pvt Ltd	601 – Akash Kalyan Complex, Varsova, Andheri (W), Mumbai – 400061 Tel – 022 – 56210271 www.Biosynherb.com Email – info@biosynherb.com	Manufacturer of standardized herbal extracts, herbal formulations, high purity herb

Contd...

Sr. No	Name of Company	Address/contact Details	Key Role/Product
6	Bayir Group	No. 92/1/1, PVR Towers, Kathirguppa Main Road, BSK 3rd Stage, Bengaluru – 560085 Tel – 080 -26798464 www.bayirextracts.com Email – bayir@satyam.net.in, info@bayirextracts.com	Manufacturer of standardized herbal extracts
7	Coimbatore Flavones and Fragrances	5/82, P.G. Pudur, K. Vadamaduri Post, Coimbatore – 641017 Tel – 0422 2642076 www.cffindia.com Email – cffindia@vsnl.com	Producers and Exporters of Perfumery raw materials & Herbal Extracts
8	Herbotech Pharmaceuticals	PO Pandori Waraich, Majitha Road, Amritsar – 143008 Tel – 0183 – 3299196, 3250230	Leading supplier of Herbal Drug Intermediates ,Herbal Extracts
9	Bioprex Labs	389, J.M. Road, Sahil Arcade, Pune 411 005 020 25672347, 020 24265368 www.bioprex.com info@bioprex.com, bioprex@yahoo.com	Manufacturer of standardized herbal extracts and nutraceuticals
10	Arjuna Natural Extracts Ltd	P. B. No: 126, Bank Road, Aluva, Dist. Kochi Tel – 0484 2622644, 2622655 www.arjunnatural.com Email – mail@arjunnatural.com	Manufacturer of standardized herbal extracts and nutraceuticals
11	Amsar Pvt Ltd	2, Hormuz Mansion, 72, B Desai Road, Mumbai – 400026 Tel – 022 23673009 www.amsar.com amsar@amsar.com	Manufacturer of standardized herbal extracts
12	Anju Phytochemicals Pvt Ltd	104/1, Unit No. 3, 13th Km, Singasandra, Bengaluru 560006 Tel – 080 - 25731527	Manufacturer and exporters of pure herbs, herbal extracts, cosmoceuticals
13	Alkaloids Corporation	8, Bentinck Street, Kolkta – 700001 Tel – 033 22435841, 22485464 www.alkaloidscorp.com Email – alkacorp@vsnl.com	Dedicated to identification, development, production & distribution of potent Phytochemicals and Botanical extracts.

Contd...

Sr. No	Name of Company	Address/contact Details	Key Role/Product
14	Alchemy Chemicals	31/04 & 31/06, Industrial area, Maksi Road, Ujjain – 456010 Tel – 0734 2525870 www.alchemychemicals.net alchemychemicals@rediffmail.com	Manufacturer of Herbal Extracts, Phytochemicals & Oleoresins.
15	Indophytochem Pharmaceuticals	Near Moginand, Kala – Amb Nahan Road, Kala – Amb Distt. Sirmour, Himachal Pradesh Tel – 01702 – 238347 www.indophytochem.net Email – info@indophytochem.com, products@indophytochem.com	Manufactures and exports selective most potent Phytochemicals & Herbal Extracts in the field of Phytoceuticals for Pharmaceuticals, Nutraceuticals, Cosmoceuticals, Dietary Supplements and Medical Nutrition industry.
16	Kancor Flavours and Extracts Ltd	Kancor Road, Angamally South – 683573, Dist Kochi Tel – 0484 – 2452236, 2452237 https://manekancor.com/ mail@kancor.in	Manufactures Oleoresins, Essential oils, Natural anti-oxidants, Natural Colours, Culinary platforms, Delivery platforms and Organic Ingredients
17	KP Patel Phyto Extractions Pvt Ltd	A-101 'Alaknanda' Annasaheb Vartak Marg, Borivili, Mumbai Tel – 022 – 28994142 www.phytoextractskp.com Email – info@phytoextractskp.com	Manufacturer of standardized herbal extracts and herbal products
18	Min Chem India	117, Loha Bhawan, P.D'Mello Road, Curnac Bunder, Masjid (East), Mumbai 022 32908187, 23485439 www.minchm.in Email – minchem-USA@minchem.in	Manufacturer of Standardized Herbal Extracts
19	Mother Herbs Pvt Ltd	C-39, II & IV Floor, 13 Street, Madhu Vihar, Pratapganj, Gurgaon – 110 092 Tel – 0120 2424943 www.motherherbs.com info@motherherbs.com	Manufacturer of Herbal extracts and nutraceuticals

Contd...

Sr. No	Name of Company	Address/contact Details	Key Role/Product
20	Neutra India	Glen Angels, Bypass, Solan – 173212 www.neutra.in info@neutra.in	Manufacturer of nutritional supplements prepared from the best natural resources as a preventive therapy for people who are health conscious under the brand name of "NutraLeaf".
21	Phyto life sciences pvt. ltd	1145, Block No, Near Santej petrol pump., Santej Ta;Kalol, Gandhinagar, Gujarat 382721 079 4900 0066 https://plpl.in/	Manufacturer of Standardized Herbal Extracts and products
22	Pioneer Herbals	101, Raudat Tahera Street, Mumbai – 40003 Tel – 022 – 23472534 www.pioneerherbal.com Email – pioneerherbal@yahoo.com	Manufacturer of Standardized Herbal Extracts, essential oil, phytochemicals, medicinal herbs
23	Sami Labs	19/1 & 19/2, I Main, II phase, Peenya Industrial Area, Bengaluru – 560 058 Tel – 080 28397973 www.samilabs.com mail@samilabs.com	Manufacturer of Standardized Herbal Extracts, essential oil, phytochemicals, medicinal herbs
24	Verdure Herbals	485/2, Katra Ishwar Bhawan, Khari Baoli, New Delhi – 110 006 www.herbsnherbalextracts.com info@herbsnherbalextracts.com	Manufacturer and supplier of medicinal herbs, plant extracts, spices and vegetable seeds
25	Vidya Herbs	No: 30, 33rd Main, 16th Cross, J.P Nagar, 6th phase, Bengaluru Tel – 080 – 26534942, 26545385	Manufacturer of Standardized Herbal Extracts and essential oil
26	Himalaya Herbal Healthcare	The Himalaya Drug Company Makali, Bangalore - 562123 91 - 08 - 23714444/5/6/7/8 PHONE 0091 132 2661695	Manufacturer of Standardized Herbal Extracts, essential oil, phytochemicals, medicinal herbs
27	Ayush Herbs Pvt Ltd	25, Phase 1, Industrial Area, Nagrota Bagwan, District Kangra, Himachal Pradesh, India. 176047 Tel: +91 1892 252109, 252099 Mobile : 9816109919 , 9418028919, 8894959190 pharma@ayushherbs.com	Manufacturer of Standardized Herbal Extracts, essential oil, phytochemicals, medicinal herbs

Contd...

Sr. No	Name of Company	Address/contact Details	Key Role/Product
28	Aryavaidyasala	Vaidyaratnam P. S. Varier's Arya Vaidya Sala, Head office Kottakkal (P.O.), Malappuram (Dist.), Kerala - 676 503, India. Tel: +91 483 280 8000 E-mail : mail@aryavaidyasala.com	Arya Vaidya Sala Manufactures More Than 530 Classical Formulations Which Fall In The Nine Categories: Arishta / Asava (Fermented Formulation) / Bhasma (Calicinated Drug) / Churna (Powdered Herb) / Ghrita (Ghee Based) / Gulika (Pill) / Kashaya (Decoction) / Leha (Electuary) / Rasakriya (Collerium) / Kuzhampu (Oil Based).
29	Trividha Ayurveda	C-88, Sector-65, Noida 201301 0120-4265100 info@trividhaayurveda.com	supplier of raw herbs, quality patent products
30	Cultivator Natural Products Pvt. Ltd	Plot No. 24 to 31 & 25 to 30, Khasra No. 135/1, Sonamukhi Nagar, Sangaria Fanta, Jodhpur-342 005 (Rajasthan) India +91 291 2980406 Email: info@cultivator.in	Quality supplier of certified organic herbs and botanicals
31	Yashco Industries Private Ltd	Parag Jhaveri MD 31/h, Laxmi Industrial Estate, New Link Road Andheri West, Mumbai - 53 Maharashtra 912266929152/3	Herbal extracts, healthcare products, Organic extracts and powders manufacturer & Supplier
32	Sowparnika Herbal Extracts & Pharmaceuticals Pvt. Ltd.	No. 31-A /2A, North Phase, Sidco Industrial Estate, Chennai - 600 098 PH : 26252590 Fax : 26521607	Manufacturer of herbal extracts, healthcare products
33	Dave Pharmaceuticals	2, Aditya Apts, Plot no 107, MCCH Society Panvel - New Mumbai, Maharashtra	Manufacturers of Ayurvedic Product & Ayurvedic Herbal Medicines like Supplements, Cosmetic, Tisane, Crude Herbs, Fresh Herbs, Plant Extracts, Herbal Teas, Herbal products, Oils, etc.

Contd...

Sr. No	Name of Company	Address/contact Details	Key Role/Product
34	Harshal Ayur Pharma	Bambagher, Ram Nagar, Nanital, Uttaranchal Phone(S): 91 - 5947 - 251720/255055 Mobile : 09837057416 Fax(S) :	Manufacturers of Herbal products, Herbal Medicines, Herbal Syrup And Cough Syrup.
	Shiva International	Moka Road, Gandhinagar, Bellary, Karnataka Phone(S): 91 - 8392 - 256504 Mobile : 98451 50672 Reliance : 9342206361 Fax (S) : 91 - 8392 - 256926	Manufacturers of Herbal Product Like Herbal Beauty Products, Health Products like Oils, Spices, Herbs.
35	Ayrumed Biotec (p) Ltd	31, New Silver Home, 15, New Kantwadi Road, Bandra(West), Mumbai, Maharashtra Phone(S): 91 - 22 - 26421551 Mobile : +919869711527	Manufacturers of Medicinal Herbs, Aromatic Herbs, Ayurvedic Herbs, Western Herbs, Culinary Herbs, Herbal Products, Spices, Stevia products, Herbal Extracts, Seeds, Planting Material, Plant Material.
36	S M Heena Industries	H - 1 - 37 - 38, Phase - 3, Industrial Area, Sojat, Rajasthan Phone(S): 91 - 2960 - 223263 Mobile : +91 - 9829098255 Fax (S) : 91 - 2960 - 222817	Manufacturers of Herbal Products & Herbal Extracts Like Natural Heena Powder, Black Henna Powder, Green Henna powder, Brown Henna Powder, Henna Related Products etc.
37	Garlico Herbal Concentrate	187, Abhinandan Colony Mandsaur, Madhya Pradesh Phone(S): 91 - 7422 - 505804 Mobile : 098260 37205 Fax (S) : 91 - 7422 - 245421	Manufacturers of Herbal Extracts, Beauty & Health Products Like Garlic Oil, Kalongi Oil, Garlic Oleoresins, Dehydrated Vegetables, Ashwagadha Extract, Boswellia Extract, Gynema Extract, Onion Oleoresins, Shilajit, Safed Musli, Babchi Oil, Neem Oil etc.
38	Varun Biocel (p) Ltd	Gangotri - II, B 27/35-8, Ravindrapuri Ext, Varanasi, Uttar Pradesh. Phone(S): 91 - 542 - 2311721 Mobile : 91 - 9451221966 Fax (S) : 91 - 542 - 2314903	Manufacturers Of Herbal Ayurvedic Medicines for Diabetes, Enzymes ification of Oils, Enzymes, Bio Bleaching Systems, Enzymes Converting Vegetable Oils to Bio Diesel, Bio Surfactants.

Contd...

Sr. No	Name of Company	Address/contact Details	Key Role/Product
39	Urmi Herbals	3A, Samadhan Society, Senapati Bapat Road, Dadar (West), Mumbai - 400028, Maharashtra	Manufacturers Of Ayurvedic Products, Herbal Products, Hair Oil, Massage Oil, Face Massage Oil, Body MassageOil, Brain Tonic, Tooth Powder, Diabetic Powder, Herbal Heena Powder, Mehandi Powder and all Ayurvedic Single Ingredient Powder Like Neem Powder, Tulsi Powder, Shatavari Powder, Ashwagandha Powder, Jethimadh Powder etc
40	Indichem	7, Shamroz Ind. Estate, Ram Mandir Road, Goregaon West, Mumbai, Maharashtra	Manufacturers Of Aloe Vera Juice, Aloe Vera Water White Liquid Aloe Vera Thick Gel For Skin Products, Aloe Vera Shampoo, Aloe Vera Capsules, Aloe Vera Soap, Aloe Vera Cream, Sunscreen, Moisturiser, Aloe Vera Based Food Supplements For Diabetes, Joint Pain Acidity, Menopause, Cancer.
41	Ind Swift limited	781 Industrial Area Phase 2, Chandigarh	Manufacturers Of Ayurvedic Herbs Product & Herbal Products Like Vigorvit, Liver Nuture, Cardio Nurture, Vigorlife, Slimfit, Urilife, Respilife, Ashwagandha, Garlee, Natural Extracts, Ayurveda, Herbs, Herbal Products, Sexual Health, Shilajit, Arjuna, Tulasi, Amla, Shallaki, Guggul, Triphala, Neem, etc.
42	Admark Herbals Limited	4th Floor, Binori Corner, Jivrajpark, Ahmedabad, Gujrat	Manufacturers Of Diabetes Herbal Cure, Diabetes Herbal Medicine, Diabetes Mellitus, Medicine For Diabetes, Pure Herbs, Diabetes Cure India, Diabetes Medicine Herbs, Herbal Medicine.

www.ingramcontent.com/pod-product-compliance
Lightning Source LLC
LaVergne TN
LVHW082007150826
845684LV00005B/48

* 9 7 8 9 3 9 0 2 1 1 9 4 4 *